# Lecture Notes in Computer Science 1230

Edited by G. Goos, J. Hartmanis and J. van Leeuwen

Advisory Board: W. Brauer   D. Gries   J. Stoer

**Springer**
*Berlin*
*Heidelberg*
*New York*
*Barcelona*
*Budapest*
*Hong Kong*
*London*
*Milan*
*Paris*
*Santa Clara*
*Singapore*
*Tokyo*

James Duncan   Gene Gindi  (Eds.)

# Information Processing in Medical Imaging

15th International Conference, IPMI'97
Poultney, Vermont, USA, June 9-13, 1997
Proceedings

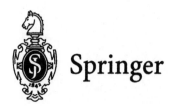

Springer

Series Editors

Gerhard Goos, Karlsruhe University, Germany

Juris Hartmanis, Cornell University, NY, USA

Jan van Leeuwen, Utrecht University, The Netherlands

Volume Editors

James Duncan
Department of Diagnostic Radiology, Yale University School of Medicine
333 Cedar Street, New Haven, CT 06520-8042, USA
E-mail: duncan.james@yale.edu

Gene Gindi
Department of Radiology, State University of New York
Stony Brook, NY 11794-8460, USA
E-mail: gindi@clio.rad.sunysb.edu

Cataloging-in-Publication data applied for


Die Deutsche Bibliothek - CIP-Einheitsaufnahme


**Information processing in medical imaging** : 15th international
conference ; proceedings / IPMI '97, Poultney, Vermont, USA, June
9 - 13, 1997. James Duncan ; Gene Gindi (ed.). - Berlin ; Heidelberg
; New York ; Barcelona ; Budapest ; Hong Kong ; London ; Milan ;
Paris ; Santa Clara ; Singapore ; Tokyo : Springer, 1997
  (Lecture notes in computer science ; Vol. 1230)
  ISBN 3-540-63046-5




CR Subject Classification (1991): I.4, I.2.5-6, J.3

ISSN 0302-9743
ISBN 3-540-63046-5 Springer-Verlag Berlin Heidelberg New York

© Springer-Verlag Berlin Heidelberg 1997
Printed in Germany

Typesetting: Camera-ready by author
SPIN 10548733    06/3142 – 5 4 3 2 1 0    Printed on acid-free paper

# Preface

The fifteenth international conference on Information Processing in Medical Imaging (IPMI) was held June 9-13, 1997 on the campus of Green Mountain College in Poultney, Vermont, USA. Following the very successful 1995 IPMI meeting held in Brest, France, this conference was the latest in a series of biennial meetings where new contributions to the processing and analysis of medical images were critically discussed and extended.

We received 96 full paper submissions to this meeting; of these, only 27 were accepted as oral presentations. The three or four papers in each section of the proceedings correspond to the actual oral sessions at the meeting, and each session comprises three or four representative works at the leading edge of an important area. ( However, this quantization led to a few cases of strange categorical bedfellows.) The papers were presented in a single track, received the bulk of the discussion time during the course of the meeting, and were each given 14 pages in the proceedings. This year, 31 submissions were accepted as poster presentations. For the first time at IPMI, the posters were each given 6 pages in the proceedings in order to better document some of the excellent submissions that could not be presented orally.

It was our intent that IPMI97 recapture some of the flavor of previous IPMIs, where the applied mathematics common to the separate areas of image analysis, image reconstruction, and image quality assessment would unify the meeting, and would encourage equal numbers of submissions from each of these areas. While the breadth of topics was considerable, the representation was not equal; as in recent IPMIs, image analysis continued as the dominant topic.

The first session concerns, in a general sense, the construction of shape models from examples, and matching procedures useful in these endeavors. The construction of abstract shape models, the topic of the first two papers, often depends ultimately on the operations of identifying, and then matching, homologous landmarks across sets of images. The third paper presents the formulation of an algorithm to carry out these procedures, and proposes a novel means of sidestepping the laborious task of identifying homologies.

While the three papers in session 1 deal mostly with analyses and models independent of specific medical applications, the topic of the related fifth session is concerned more with registration and mapping problems that arise in specific modalities. Of note here is the introduction of physical models of tissue deformation into the registration problem. The fourth paper in this session is not concerned with registration *per se*, but with efficient means of transforming images once suitable mappings have been computed.

Traditionally, IPMI has included a session on novel imaging methods and modalities, since these carry concomitant challenges in information processing. The papers in the second session concern the novel modalities of elastic imaging, electrical impedance tomography (the topic of the previous IPMI Erbsmann Award paper), and optical tomography. Image reconstruction is the problem that arises in the latter two modalities. The fourth paper, whose subject is actually a novel image representation rather than a modality, falls neatly into the spirit, if not the content, of this session.

Segmentation continues as a formidable challenge for medical image analysis, with widespread application foreseen for practical and robust methods. The papers in session 3 illustrate the continuing maturation of segmentation models and algorithms as applied to anatomical images. As this area matures, it is interesting to note that segmentation methods are becoming increasingly anatomically specific, with models tuned to stable anatomical features such as major brain sulci. In this same vein, one may also observe, as in the first paper, that effective medical segmentation may need to make use of a collection of empirical procedures, rather than relying on an algorithm derived from a single overarching principle.

Session 4 is something of a hybrid. The first two papers, dealing with image quality, concern detection and estimation tasks given a statistical model of an image. The mathematical difficulties here often limit one to using unrealistic models of signal and background, and the extension to more realistic statistical models, as discussed in the first paper, represents a real advance. The second paper concerns the approximation of ML and MAP estimates of object parameters that are nonlinear functions of the observed noisy image data, a topic of importance in applications such as quantitation in nuclear medicine. The last two papers also focus on statistical models of low-level data, but not in the context of image quality *per se*. The fourth paper deals with the implications for PET reconstruction of realistic *non*-Poisson models of projection data, and the third paper with new mixture models for clustering, for example, the types of multidimensional data acquired in MR imaging, with implications for segmentation.

The maturation of PET and SPECT and the advent of fMRI have introduced new statistical information processing problems concerning the analyses of activation and functional data in neuroscientific and clinical studies. This is the direct concern of the first three papers in session 6, which address the fascinating challenges of inferences from spatiotemporal functional data. The last paper in this session introduces a statistical method to derive a model of normality from sets of SPECT brain images.

Magnetic resonance is the theme of papers in the last session. In addition to fMRI, the cornucopia of new imaging methods stemming from this modality continues unabated twenty-six years after the first crude MR images were generated at Stony Brook. Just one example: the amazing capability of MR to "tag" tissue parcels has generated a set of image tracking problems useful to cardiac MR, and the first two papers represent recent advances in this area. The latter two papers, dealing with motion correction and volume measurement, address important practical concerns of MR imaging.

IPMI has been lauded as a unique forum for the interchange of ideas in medical image processing and analysis. The editors, naturally, concur, and feel duty bound to add their own observations. IPMI is unique in format, of course, with its (in)famous unlimited discussion periods raging into the night. One could characterize IPMI as a vortex that draws in ideas from our sister communities in applied mathematics, physics, electrical engineering, computer science, and statistics to fertilize advances specific to medical imaging, but this could also be said of other meetings. More than other meetings, however, IPMI demands that contributions pay attention to the real constraints that arise in medical imaging practice. Aesthetic, self-consistent theories, of, say, anatomical image segmentation are challenged if these cannot possibly adapt to the ambiguities of the heterogeneous and complex anatomy of the human body. Latitude is necessary, of course, and the demands of medical practice are not enforced to the point of commercial viability (Is the new reconstruction algorithm too slow to be clinically practical?) or validation extensive enough for government approval (Has the promising new segmentation method been rigorously tested on a large patient population?). These areas are properly addressed in other meetings. These freedoms, suitably tempered by adherence to constraints, thus frame the unique role of IPMI.

New Haven                                                                  James S. Duncan
Stony Brook                                                                  Gene R. Gindi

March, 1997

# Acknowledgments

The XVth IPMI conference was made possible by the efforts of a number of dedicated people. The organizers would first like to thank profusely the Scientific Committee, whose timely, critical reviews ensured that the conference was scientifically first-rate. Second, we thank the many researchers who submitted manuscripts for consideration and regret that we had to turn down a significant number.

IPMI97 would truly not have been possible without the constant help and indulgence of Carolyn Meloling at Yale University. She single- handedly dealt with all of the mailings, organized the paper submissions and reviews, and was constantly there to help with the numerous details related to organizing this meeting. In addition, we appreciate the help and advice of Paul Saunders and Dick Stark from Green Mountain College.

We also gratefully acknowledge the support and encouragement of Debbie Brown and Kathy Duncan over the past several years, especially in some of the IPMI "crunch" times.

Finally, we most gratefully acknowledge and appreciate the financial support of the following organizations:

**Department of Diagnostic Radiology, Yale University**
**Department of Radiology, University of Stony Brook**
**The Whitaker Foundation**
**The Faculty of Engineering, Yale University**
**Belgium Nuclear Research Centre (SCK-CEN), Mol, Belgium**

# Francois Erbsmann Prize

Francois Erbsmann, one of the founders of IPMI, died tragically soon after the first IPMI. In his honor a cash award is given at each meeting for the best paper presented by a young scientist making his or her first IPMI presentation. At the 1995 IPMI meeting in Brest, France, the following awards were made:

**Erbsmann Prize Winner (best paper):**
Maurits Konings, University Hospital Utrecht

Honorable Mention: Gary Christensen, Washington University
Honorable Mention: Paul Hemler, Stanford University

Congratulations to these young scientists on their outstanding efforts.

# The IPMI Board

Yves Bizais
Harrison Barrett
Randy Brill
Alan Colchester
Stephen Bacharach
Frank Deconinck
Robert DiPaola
James Duncan
Michael Goris
Doug Ortendahl
Stephen Pizer
Andrew Todd-Pokropek
Max Viergever

# Conference Committee

## Chair
James Duncan, Yale University, USA

## Co- Chair
Gene Gindi, University of Stony Brook, NY, USA

## Scientific Committee

| | |
|---|---|
| Nicholas Ayache | INRIA, France |
| Stephen Bacharach | NIH, USA |
| Harrison Barrett | University of Arizona, USA |
| Yves Bizais | Universite de Bretagne Occidentale, France |
| Fred Bookstein | University of Michigan, USA |
| Michael Brady | Oxford University, UK |
| Alan Colchester | University of Kent, UK |
| Robert DiPaola | INSERM, France |
| Jeffrey Fessler | University of Michigan, USA |
| Guido Gerig | ETH Zentrum, Zurich, Switzerland |
| Arthur Gmitro | University of Arizona, USA |
| Eric Grimson | MIT, USA |
| David Hawkes | Guys Hospital, London, UK |
| Karl Heinz Höhne | University of Hamburg, Germany |
| Michael Insana | University of Kansas, USA |
| Nico Karsejjimeier | University Hospital, Nijmegen, The Netherlands |
| Nicholas Lange | Harvard University, USA |
| Richard Leahy | University of Southern California, USA |
| Jorge Llacer | EC Engineering Consultants, USA |
| Charles Metz | University of Chicago, USA |
| Kyle Myers | FDA, USA |
| Doug Ortendahl | Toshiba Corporation, USA |
| Stephen Pizer | University of North Carolina, Chapel Hill, USA |
| Jerry Prince | Johns Hopkins University, USA |
| Hemant Tagare | Yale University, USA |
| Chris Taylor | University of Manchester, UK |
| Andrew Todd-Pokropek | University College, London, UK |
| Max Viergever | Utrecht University, The Netherlands |

# Table of Contents

## 4 Image Quality and the Statistical Character of Measured Data

## 5 Registration/Mapping

## 6 Statistical Models in Functional Neuroimaging

# 7  MR Image Analysis and Processing

# 8  Posters

## 8.1  Segmentation/ Structural Models

## 8.2 Quantitative Image Analysis

## 8.3 Registration/ Mapping/ Tracking

## 8.4 Novel Imaging Methods

# Automatic Construction of Eigenshape Models by Genetic Algorithm

Aaron C.W. Kotcheff and Chris J. Taylor

Wolfson Image Analysis Unit, Department of Medical Bio-Physics, University of Manchester, UK.

**Abstract.** A new approach to the problem of automatic construction of eigenshape models is presented. Eigenshape models have proved to be successful in a variety of medical image analysis problems. However, automatic model construction is a difficult problem, and in many applications the models are built by hand - a painstaking process. Previous attempts to produce models automatically have been applicable only in specific cases or under certain assumptions. We show that the problem can be understood very simply in terms of shape symmetries. The pose and parameterisation of each shape must be chosen so as to produce a model that is compact and specific. We define an objective function that measures these properties. The problem of automatic model construction is thus reduced to an optimisation problem. We show that the objective function we define can be optimised by a Genetic Algorithm, and produces models that are better than hand built ones.

## 1 Introduction

Representation of 2D and 3D shape is a common problem in medical image analysis [8, 12]. Objects in medical images often have no identifying characteristics (e.g. color, texture) other than shape. Eigenshape models are statistical shape models that represent the variability of a set of example shapes in a compact and statistically robust way. 2D and 3D eigenshape models have proved to be successful in a variety of medical image analysis [4, 5] and, more widely, computer vision problems generally [1, 17].

Eigenshape models are built by representing each example shape in a *training set* as a vector in a high dimensional vector space, and performing Principal Component Analysis (PCA) upon this set of vectors [6]. PCA determines the principal axes or *modes of variation* along which the data varies. If the variability is well represented by a few modes then the dimensionality of the data is effectively reduced.

Shape training sets usually come from raw data such as edge detected or hand annotated boundaries. However, the problem of constructing eigenshape models automatically from this data is still unsolved. Although several methods that work in specific cases or under certain assumptions have been published [2, 13–15, 18], no generally applicable principle exists. In addition, many of the methods cannot be extended to 3D shape.

The difficulty arises in the vector representation of shape. A bad representation leads to a model that is non-compact (i.e. does not significantly reduce the dimensionality of the training set) and non-specific (i.e. will generate shapes that are significantly different from those in the training set).

In [6] each shape is represented by a set of closely spaced points along the boundary of the object. The x and y values of each point are then arranged into a column vector. The authors call the resulting eigenshape model a Point Distribution Model (PDM). However, in order to produce a compact model, key points must be placed *by hand* on each example shape so that features identified using high-level knowledge correspond. This process is slow, introduces operator bias and, in medical applications, often requires expert knowledge of the objects being modelled.

In [1] each shape is represented by a set of splines. The control points of the splines are then used to construct the vector representation of each shape. This process is automatic, but uses properties of the specific shape being modelled (each shape has a vertical symmetry axis) and therefore is not generally applicable.

In this paper we show that the problem can be understood in terms of shape symmetries. Shapes are invariant under global pose and local reparameterisation transformations. Specific representations of shapes (e.g. as a set of points or splines) do not show explicit invariance under reparameterisation and thus hide the underlying problem.

In order to find the correct pose and parameterisation we define an objective function that gives a mathematical definition to the desired model properties of compactness and specificity. Once this has been achieved the problem of automatic model construction is reduced to an optimisation problem. Since the objective function is highly non-linear and the configuration space of the problem is high-dimensional, we use a Genetic Algorithm as our optimisation technique.

The advantages of this technique are that it makes no assumptions about the nature of the shapes being modelled, does not need an approximate solution to start with, and will, in principle, find the global minimum of the objective function and therefore the best model.

## 2 Principal Component Analysis of Shapes

In this section we derive a formalism for performing PCA on a training set of example shapes which makes the dependency on shape symmetries explicit. Each shape is represented by a curve in 2 dimensions: $\phi(t) = \{\phi^x(t), \phi^y(t)\}, 0 < t < 1$, which could be closed ($\phi(1) = \phi(0)$) or open ($\phi(1) \neq \phi(0)$). The $\phi(t)$ form an infinite dimensional vector space $\mathcal{V}$ with addition defined by:

$$\phi + \psi = \{\phi^x(t) + \psi^x(t), \phi^y(t) + \psi^y(t)\} , \ 0 < t < 1 , \tag{1}$$

and inner product by:

$$\langle \phi, \psi \rangle = \int_0^1 dt \ (\phi^x(t)\psi^x(t) + \phi^y(t)\psi^y(t)) . \tag{2}$$

A vector in this space will be referred to as a shape vector. It will also be useful to define the mean xy distance between two shapes, $\phi$ and $\psi$:

$$d_{xy}(\phi, \psi) = \int_0^1 dt \left( t\sqrt{(\phi^x(t) - \psi^x(t))^2 + (\phi^y(t) - \psi^y(t))^2} \right) . \tag{3}$$

A training set consists of $n$ shape vectors $\phi_i$, $i = 1, \ldots n$, with mean $\mu$ and $\infty \times n$ centred data matrix:

$$W = [\phi_1 - \mu, \phi_2 - \mu, \ldots \phi_n - \mu] . \tag{4}$$

The analogous covariance matrix $K = WW^T/n$ is infinite dimensional:

$$K = K(s,t) = \frac{1}{n} \sum_{i=1}^n (\phi_i(s) - \mu(s))(\phi_i(t) - \mu(t)) , \tag{5}$$

and cannot be diagonalised numerically. However $W$ only has finite rank, $r \leq n$, therefore a singular value decomposition (SVD) of $W$ exists:

$$W = USV^T , \tag{6}$$

where $U$ is the $\infty \times r$ principal component matrix made up of the eigenshape vectors corresponding to the non-zero eigenvalues of $K$:

$$U = [\xi_1, \xi_2, \ldots \xi_r] , \tag{7}$$

$S$ is the $r \times r$ diagonal matrix

$$S = \text{Diag}(\sqrt{ne_1}, \sqrt{ne_2}, \ldots \sqrt{ne_r}) , \tag{8}$$

where $e_i$ are the non-zero eigenvalues of $K$, V is the $r \times n$ score matrix, and the columns of $U$ and $V$ are orthogonal. $S$ and $V$ can be found by diagonalisation of the $n \times n$, positive definite matrix :

$$K' = \frac{1}{n} W^T W = \frac{1}{n} V S^2 V^T , \tag{9}$$

$$K'_{ij} = \frac{1}{n} \langle \phi_i - \mu, \phi_j - \mu \rangle , \tag{10}$$

and $U$ can then be found by substitution back into (6).

The variation away from the mean along each eigenvector is referred to elsewhere in this paper as a mode of variation or principal component. The variance along each mode is the corresponding eigenvalue. Each shape in the training set is approximated by a shape $\beta$ that is the mean plus a linear combination of the $m$ modes with the largest eigenvalues:

$$\beta = \mu + \sum_{i=1}^m b_i \xi_i . \tag{11}$$

The $b_i$ are the shape model parameters. If the approximation is good for $m < n$ then the effective dimensionality of the training set has been reduced. This approximation is measured by an approximation error $E_{\text{approx}}$ which is defined for a shape $\phi$ as the minimum value of $d_{xy}(\phi, \beta)$ w.r.t. variation of $b_i$.

The mapping from shape vectors in $\mathcal{V}$ to shapes is many-to-one. Each shape is invariant under a group, $G$, of *symmetry transformations* of its corresponding shape vector. These symmetries fall into two categories: global pose transformations,

$$\phi \to \phi' = \begin{pmatrix} s \cos\theta & s \sin\theta \\ -s \sin\theta & s \cos\theta \end{pmatrix} \begin{pmatrix} \phi_x(t) \\ \phi_y(t) \end{pmatrix} + \begin{pmatrix} d_x \\ d_y \end{pmatrix} \tag{12}$$

(rotation through $\theta$, scaling by $s$, translation by $\{d_x, d_y\}$), and local reparameterisation invariance,

$$\phi(t) \to \phi(t') \ , \ t' = s(t) \ , \tag{13}$$

where $s : \{0,1\} \to \{0,1\}$ is a 1-to-1 invertible mapping (diffeomorphism) of the line (for open curves) or the circle (for closed curves). We refer to the parameters determining the pose and parameterisation of a shape generically as *symmetry parameters*.

$\mathcal{V}$ can thus be decomposed locally into a product space $\mathcal{V} = \mathcal{S} \times \mathcal{G}$. $\mathcal{G}$ is the set of all points in $\mathcal{V}$ connected by symmetry transformations in the group $G$ and $\mathcal{S}$ is the set of unique shapes.

The matrix $K'$ is not invariant under transformations in $G$, and hence neither are the principal components. This is easy to visualise, as shown in Fig. 1. which shows a cluster of points in $\mathcal{V}$. Each point is free to move along the manifold $\mathcal{G}$ and thus the distribution of the cluster can be changed completely. This is the fundamental reason that eigenshape models are hard to build automatically: *the principal components of a set of shapes depend crucially upon the choice of symmetry parameters.*

## 3    Possible Approaches

In this section we criticise several possible approaches that could be used for dealing with shape symmetries.

### Invariant Representation

This approach would be to find a shape representation that was invariant under the relevant symmetry transformations. The required representation would be highly nonlinear, e.g. a gradient against curvature plot. This is unsatisfactory for several reasons. One of the strengths of eigenshape models is that linear variations are common in many modelling tasks and this would be lost with a non-linear representation. A non-linear transformation may be time-consuming

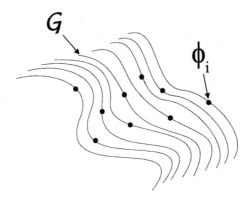

**Fig. 1.** The structure of $\mathcal{V}$. Each shape vector $\phi_i$ is free to move along the manifold $\mathcal{G}$ of points connected by G transformations.

or even impossible to invert, and differential invariants (like gradient vs. curvature plots) are highly sensitive to small variations in the curve and vice-versa, and can be undefined at corners etc. It seems unlikely that a transformation that avoided all these problems could be found.

## Learning Symmetry Transformations

The model could 'learn' about allowed symmetry transformations by including $G$ transformations in the training set. However, in order to generalise sufficiently the training set would have to be enlarged to include several rotated, scaled and reparameterised versions of each base example and the size of the training set would become impractical. In addition, variations in $G$ are intrinsically non-linear and not handled well by PCA.

## Pairwise Correspondence

Correspondence based techniques seek to automate the manual process of identifying common points on each example shape, and are based on the large body of work on correspondence of boundaries [3, 9, 16, 22] and point sets [19–21]. A correspondence is found by optimising a metric that measures the similarity between a pair of shapes. An example is curvature matching - this works well for shapes like hands where the peaks in positive curvature occur at the ends of fingers. Once corresponding points have been located the reparameterisation invariance is fixed and the angle, scale etc. can be determined e.g. using a least squares fit. Although correspondence techniques can work well [13–15], the choice of correspondence metric is arbitrary and often adapted to the problem at hand. Also, since the correspondence metric is optimised over pairs of shapes, global properties of the model are not guaranteed.

# 4   Model Optimisation

We propose an approach based on the idea that the model itself should determine values for symmetry parameters. We are free to choose any value for the symmetry parameters, therefore we choose the values that give the best model. A good shape model should be compact and specific. Our task is to find a measure of model quality that defines these requirements in a more mathematically precise form.

As an example consider the synthetic example shown in Fig. 2. This is a set of shapes with a single linear variation (the semi-circular bump moves along the top of the box). A naive approach to producing an eigenshape model might be as follows:

- Identify a corner of the box (which could be done manually).
- Use an arc-length parameterisation with $t = 0$ at the identified corner.
- Determine the pose parameters by iterative alignment to the mean (see below)

If this process is followed the result is the eigenshape model illustrated in Fig. 2, which shows the $\pm 2\sigma$ variation from the mean along the first three major modes (eigenvectors). With the mean shape vector scaled to unit norm the significant eigenvalues of $K'$ are: (1.1125, 0.3253 ,0.0622, 0.0157, 0.0061, 0.0029, 0.0014). As can be seen, these modes clearly generate illegal shapes. Thus arc-length parameterisation produces a poor model judged by the criteria mentioned above.

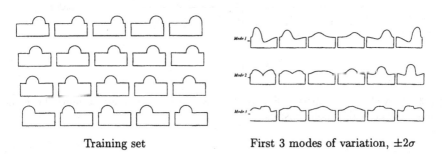

Training set                    First 3 modes of variation, $\pm 2\sigma$

**Fig. 2.** The training set and modes of variation for the synthetic model.

If the same approach is followed but using a parameterisation such that the value of $t$ at each of the 6 'corners' is the same for each example, we get the single mode that we would expect using high-level knowledge. The eigenvalue corresponding to this eigenvector is 2.891.

The algorithm we used for determining the pose parameters above is that discussed in [6] and minimises the sum of the squared distances from the mean to each data point. This is essentially generalised Procrustes analysis in 2 dimensions [11] and is equivalent to minimising the trace of the covariance matrix: $\mathrm{Tr}K = \mathrm{Tr}K' = \sum_i |\phi_i - \mu|^2$. One free parameter is left, the global scale $s$, and it is conventional to set $s$ so that the mean shape has unit norm.

Although the trace of the covariance matrix is a useful objective function in many instances, it is far from ideal when dealing with reparameterisation transformations. The above example demonstrates this well. The trace of $K$ in the first instance is 1.5261, and in the second is 2.891. If we used the trace of the covariance matrix as an objective function the bad parameterisation would be preferred.

Clearly we want an objective function that prefers concentrating the variance into a few modes with large variances. An obvious choice for such an objective function is the determinant of the covariance matrix, $|K|$. It is easy to show (for discrete data vectors) that:

$$\frac{\partial}{\partial \phi_k}|K| = 2|K|K^{-1}\phi_k \ , \tag{14}$$

i.e. that the gradient of $|K|$ is in the same direction as the gradient of the Mahalanobis distance with covariance matrix held constant. Using $|K|$ as an objective function will thus tend to push points towards the larger modes as shown in Fig. 3.

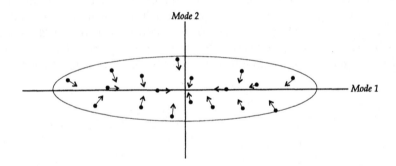

**Fig. 3.** If an objective function $F = |K|$ is used, each point wants to move down the gradient of the Mahalanobis distance.

When the dimension of the vector space (infinite in this case) is greater than the number of examples, the determinant of $K$ vanishes. In this case it is more appropriate to use the determinant of $K'$ since their non-zero eigenvalues are the same. However, zero eigenvalues could still appear during an optimisation since the rank of the data matrix $W$ can change under $G$ transformations of the shapes. If this happens $|K'|$ has degenerate minima and the solution we are looking for is amongst them.

This degeneracy can be broken by artificially enlarging the training set. If our sample set was sufficiently large to begin with, then adding more data points should not have any significant effect on the distribution except to add a small amount of random noise. Adding linearly independent noise is equivalent to adding a small value $\delta$ to each eigenvalue of $K'$. In our experiments $\delta$ was typically set to be less than a pixel at the scale of the original image data.

The objective function that we use thus becomes:

$$F = \ln \det(K' + \delta I) - n \ln \delta \ , \tag{15}$$

where the log is taken to stop rounding errors from dominating $|K'|$ and the final term is added to make the minimum of $F$ zero.

## 5 Optimisation of $F$ by Genetic Algorithm

We wish to find a pose and parameterisation for each shape that minimises $F$. Even if we can find a discrete representation of reparameterisation invariance, the dimensionality of the configuration space for the problem is still very large. In addition $F$ is highly non-linear and likely to have false minima. For this reason we chose a Genetic Algorithm (GA) as the optimisation method. We do not give details of the implementation of the GA here that are not directly relevant to the problem at hand; see e.g. [7, 10] or any good GA review for more details.

### 5.1 Representation of Parameterisation

A parameterisation of a curve is a 1-to-1 $C_\infty$ mapping from the unit line ($0 \leq t \leq 1$) to the curve. We can make a discrete approximation by identifying points on the curve for a small number of discrete values of $t$ ($t_a$, $a = 1 \ldots n_p$) and interpolating between them. This is shown in Fig. 4. Each $t_a$ maps to a point $l_a$ on the curve known as a *landmark* . We will consider only closed curves here but the same techniques can be applied to open curves.

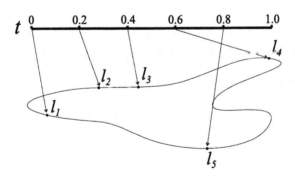

**Fig. 4.** Discrete shape parameterisation (note: $t = 1.0$ maps to $t = 0$).

The parameterisation used to interpolate between values of $t$ is arbitrary but must be used consistently. In all our examples we interpolate between values of $t$ using arc-length parameterisation (if the shape was represented by a set of splines then the cubic spline parametrisation would be more appropriate). This gives a polygonal approximation to any parameterisation, which gets better if we choose to specify more values of t. Each shape must be parameterised independently of the others so a set of independent landmarks must be specified for each shape.

## 5.2 The Chromosome Encoding, Crossover and Mutation

Ideally a chromosome should encode all the $G$ parameters for each example shape. However, our experiments have shown that if pose parameters are encoded onto the chromosome their values get swamped by reparameterisation effects. In order to keep the chromosome as short as possible therefore, we do not include pose parameters. Once the parameterisation is specified, pose parameters are determined using iterative alignment to the mean as described above. Although this method will not find the true minimum of $F$, we have found it to be perfectly satisfactory.

The parameterisation can be encoded on the chromosome by specifying the landmarks for each shape. We take each curve and space $2^D$ points along it, $D$ typically being $\sim 10$. Each landmark can then be specified by $D$ bits on the chromosome. The structure of the chromosome is shown in Fig. 5. If we have n shapes in our data set, the total length of the chromosome is $D \times n_{\mathrm{p}} \times n$ bits.

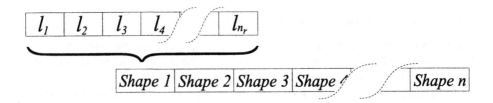

**Fig. 5.** The structure of the chromosome for the GA optimisation

This encoding of the chromosome allows illegal parameterisations. In order for the mapping to be 1-to-1 the landmarks must be ordered consistently around the curve e.g. $l_5$ cannot lie between $l_3$ and $l_4$. The chromosome (Fig. 5) can clearly represent configurations where this can occur, since each landmark can take any value between 0 and $(2^D - 1)$. We impose this constraint by re-ordering the landmarks within each shape section of the chromosome after operations such as mutation or crossover that might permute the landmarks.

## 6 Results

We have applied our method to a selection of model building problems that are typical of those which arise in medical image interpretation (Sect. 6.1 - 6.5). In order to assess the model generated by the GA in each case, control models were also constructed using a manual and/or semi-automatic method. In the manual method common features to each shape (such as fingertips) were identified using high-level knowledge and the parameterisation fixed so that the features corresponded. The semi-automatic method used a manually placed starting point and an arc-length parameterisation around the curve. In all cases the pose parameters were determined using iterative alignment to the mean.

To compare different models we look at the mode variances and the mean approximation error $\bar{E}_{\mathrm{approx}}$. Variances are quoted with the global scale, $s$, set so that the mean shape has unit norm. $\bar{E}_{\mathrm{approx}}$ is the mean over the training set of $E_{\mathrm{approx}}$ for each shape. Since it is measured at the original scale of each example, an $\bar{E}_{\mathrm{approx}}$ of less than 1 pixel is desirable.

## 6.1  Hands

Hands were used as the baseline application to test the system and tune parameters. We used 18 hand shapes which were extracted from test images by thresholding. We set $n_{\mathrm{p}} = 16$ and $D = 11$ giving a chromosome of length 3168 bits. Both manual and semi-automatic models were used as controls. The manual model had a value of $F$ of 19.278, and the semi-automatic model a value of 22.678. The noise parameter $\delta$ was set to $e^{-4}$.

Figure 6 shows graphs plotting the value of $F$ for the best chromosome after every generation against generation number for various values of the GA parameters. These experiments determined the optimal GA parameters to be: population $= 1000$, crossover prob. $= 1.0$ Chrom.$^{-1}$Gen.$^{-1}$, mutation prob. $=$ 0.0001 bit$^{-1}$Gen.$^{-1}$, run length $\geq 1250$ generations.

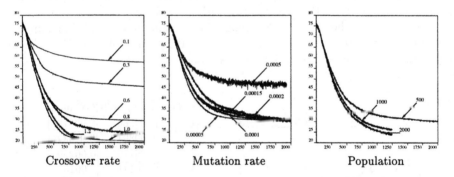

| Crossover rate | Mutation rate | Population |

**Fig. 6.** Value of the objective function for the best chromosome plotted against generation number for different values of the GA parameters. Unless indicted, parameters were: Crossover prob.: 0.6 Chrom.$^{-1}$Gen.$^{-1}$, Mutation prob.: 0.0001 bit$^{-1}$Gen.$^{-1}$, Population: 500

In this case we ran the GA for 3000 generations. The results are shown in Fig. 7. The table gives a comparison of the models generated by the three different techniques and also for a typical random chromosome. There is little difference between the hand built and the GA final indicating that in this case it is probably not possible to do much better than the hand built model. The first 9 modes of the GA model are actually slightly larger than the hand built model, but the approximation error is smaller, indicating that the first 9 modes describe more of the variation of the training set.

The first 4 modes of variation $\pm 2\sigma$

| Mode | GA Random | Semi-automatic | Hand built | GA final |
|------|-----------|----------------|------------|----------|
| 1 | 22.760 | 0.246 | 0.207 | 0.196 |
| 2 | 14.121 | 0.114 | 0.111 | 0.114 |
| 3 | 8.635 | 0.075 | 0.056 | 0.066 |
| 4 | 7.124 | 0.047 | 0.031 | 0.031 |
| 5 | 6.177 | 0.043 | 0.013 | 0.012 |
| 6 | 5.480 | 0.019 | 0.008 | 0.010 |
| 7 | 4.248 | 0.008 | 0.004 | 0.004 |
| 8 | 3.282 | 0.005 | 0.003 | 0.003 |
| 9 | 2.687 | 0.003 | 0.002 | 0.002 |
| F | 79.885 | 22.678 | 19.278 | 19.220 |
| $E_{approx}$ | 24.309 | 1.241 | 0.966 | 0.867 |

Mode variances

**Fig. 7.** The results for the hand models. The modes of variation of the GA model are shown on the left. The table shows the variances of each mode, the value of the objective function, and the 9 mode approx. error for the different models.

## 6.2 Knee Cartilage

The outline of the knee cartilage was manually segmented using Bezier curves from a set of 16 MR images. We set $n_p = 8$ and $D = 9$ giving a chromosome of length 1152 bits. Since the example shapes were quite small the noise parameter $\delta$ was set lower to $e^{-5}$. The GA was run with for 1250 generations.

The results are shown in Fig. 8 compared to a hand built model. The number of modes required to reduce the approx. error to 0.2 pixels is shown. The 6-mode approximation error is smaller for the GA model.

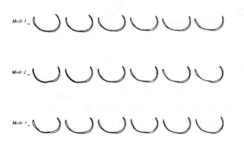

The first 3 modes of variation $\pm 2\sigma$

| Mode | Hand built | GA final |
|------|-----------|----------|
| 1 | 0.04684 | 0.03618 |
| 2 | 0.00897 | 0.01032 |
| 3 | 0.00170 | 0.00259 |
| 4 | 0.00141 | 0.00189 |
| 5 | 0.00121 | 0.00176 |
| 6 | 0.00105 | 0.00096 |
| F | 19.624 | 19.203 |
| $E_{approx}$ | 0.203 | 0.175 |

Mode variances

**Fig. 8.** The results for the cartilage models.

## 6.3 Obturata Foramen

The outline of the obturata foramen was manually extracted from 20 radiographs using Bezier curves. We set $n_p = 10$ and $D = 8$ giving a chromosome of length 1600 bits. Other parameters were as for the knee cartilage, and the results (Fig. 9) are similar.

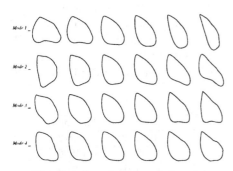

| Mode | Semi-automatic | GA final |
|------|----------------|----------|
| 1 | 0.3289 | 0.3562 |
| 2 | 0.1756 | 0.1843 |
| 3 | 0.0354 | 0.0443 |
| 4 | 0.0152 | 0.0231 |
| 5 | 0.0087 | 0.0079 |
| 6 | 0.0050 | 0.0048 |
| 7 | 0.0034 | 0.0037 |
| F | 35.4185 | 32.44855 |
| $E_{approx}$ | 0.502655 | 0.427876 |

The first 4 modes of variation $\pm 2\sigma$        Mode variances

**Fig. 9.** The results for the obturata models.

## 6.4 Hip Prosthesis

The outline of 30 hip prostheses was extracted from test images using thresholding. We set $n_p = 10$ and $D = 9$ giving a chromosome of length 2700 bits.

As the table in Fig. 10 shows, in this case the GA model was *worse* than a semi-automatically generated model. However the value of the objective function, $F$, was also worse, indicating that the GA simply hadn't converged after 1250 generations. As in the hand model, due to the length of the chromosome, the GA would probably need to run for 2000-3000 generations to improve beyond a hand built model.

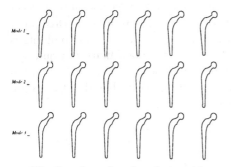

| Mode | Semi-automatic | GA final |
|------|----------------|----------|
| 1 | 0.07320 | 0.05615 |
| 2 | 0.00958 | 0.02215 |
| 3 | 0.00569 | 0.01235 |
| 4 | 0.00314 | 0.00396 |
| 5 | 0.00154 | 0.00066 |
| 6 | 0.00033 | 0.00034 |
| F | 7.665 | 8.028 |
| $E_{approx}$ | 0.9838 | 1.5573 |

The first 3 modes of variation $\pm 2\sigma$        Mode variances

**Fig. 10.** The results for the prosthesis models.

## 6.5 Heart Left Ventricle

The outline of the left ventricle of the heart was manually extracted from 33 echocardiograms. We set $n_p = 16$ and $D = 8$ giving a chromosome of length 4224 bits. The GA was run for 1250 generations.

This was the longest chromosome we tried in any of our experiments. As one might expect, it failed to converge to a model that was better than the hand built one in 1250 generations. However, as can be seen in the table of Fig. 11, even though the objective function $F$ has a significantly higher value, the GA model is quite good, with a 6 mode approximation error only 0.13 pixels higher.

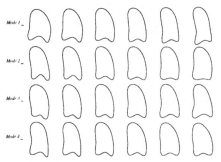

| Mode | Hand built | GA final |
|------|-----------|----------|
| 1 | 0.18810 | 0.39912 |
| 2 | 0.06653 | 0.14576 |
| 3 | 0.03201 | 0.09636 |
| 4 | 0.02286 | 0.07554 |
| 5 | 0.01424 | 0.03528 |
| 6 | 0.01111 | 0.02942 |
| F | 22.603 | 32.817 |
| $E_{approx}$ | 0.8997 | 1.0329 |

The first 4 modes of variation $\pm 2\sigma$      Mode variances

**Fig. 11.** The results for the heart models.

# 7 Conclusion and Discussion

We have shown that optimisation of $|K|$ through explicit reparameterisation of the training set allows good eigenshape models to be generated completely automatically from training data. The practicality of the approach requires further attention - most of the GA runs needed to generate the results for this paper took more that a day to run on a Sun Sparcstation 20. Since model building is a one-time off-line process, this may be acceptable, though matters would get worse for larger training sets and more complicated examples including extension to 3D. We plan to investigate combining GA and gradient-based optimisation methods to achieve more rapid convergence.

# References

1. A. Baumberg and D. Hogg. Learning flexible models from image sequences. In $3^{nd}$ *European Conference on Computer Vision*, pages 299–308, Stockholm, 1994.
2. A. Baumberg and D. Hogg. An adaptive eigenshape model. In D. Pycock, editor, $6^{th}$ *British Machine Vison Conference*, pages 87–96. BMVA Press, Sept. 1995.
3. I. Cohen, N. Ayache, and P. Sulger. Tracking points on deformable objects using curvature information. In G. Sandini, editor, $2^{nd}$ *European Conference on Computer Vision*, pages 458–466. Springer-Verlag, May 1992.
4. T. F. Cootes, A. Hill, and C. J. Taylor. Rapid and more accurate medical image interpretation using active shape models. In $14^{th}$ *Conference on Information Processing in Medical Imaging*, pages (371–372), France, June 1995.

5. T. F. Cootes, A. Hill, C. J. Taylor, and J. Haslam. The use of active shape models for locating structures in medical images. In H. H. Barrett and A. F. Gmitro, editors, $13^{th}$ *Conference on Information Processing in Medical Imaging*, pages 33–47, Flagstaff, Arizona, USA, June 1993. Springer-Verlag.

6. T. F. Cootes, C. J. Taylor, D. H. Cooper, and J. Graham. Active shape models - their training and application. *Computer Vision and Image Understanding*, 61(1):38–59, Jan. 1995.

7. L. Davis. *Genetic Algorithms and Simulated Annealing*. Pitman, 1987.

8. K. Delibasis and P. E. Undrill. Anatomical object recognition using deformable geometric models. *Image and Vision Computing*, 12(7):423–433, Sept. 1994.

9. J. Duncan, R. L. Owen, L. H. Staib, and P. Anandan. Measurement of non-rigid motion using contour shape descriptors. In *IEEE Conference on Computer Vision and Pattern Recognition*, pages 318–324, 1991.

10. D. E. Goldberg. *Genetic Algorithms in Search, Optimisation and Machine Learning*. Addison-Wesley, 1989.

11. C. Goodall. Procrustes methods in the statistical analysis of shape. *Journal of the Royal Statistical Society B*, 53(2):285–339, 1991.

12. A. Hill, T. F. Cootes, C. J. Taylor, and K. Lindley. Medical image interpretation: A generic approach using deformable templates. *Journal of Medical Informatics*, 19(1):47–59, 1994.

13. A. Hill and C. J. Taylor. Automatic landmark generation for point distribution models. In E. Hancock, editor, $5^{th}$ *British Machine Vison Conference*, pages 429–438. BMVA Press, Sept. 1994.

14. A. Hill and C. J. Taylor. A framework for automatic landmark identification using a new method of non-rigid correspondence. *IEEE Transactions on Pattern Analysis and Machine Intelligence*, page (submitted to), 1996.

15. A. Hill and C. J. Taylor. A method of non-rigid correspondence for automatic landmark identification. In $7^{th}$ *British Machine Vison Conference*, pages 323–332. BMVA Press, Sept. 1996.

16. C. Kambhamettu and D. B. Goldgof. Point correspondence recovery in non-rigid motion. In *IEEE Conference on Computer Vision and Pattern Recognition*, pages 222–227, 1992.

17. K. V. Mardia, J. T. Kent, and A. N. Walder. Statistical shape models in image analysis. In *23rd Symposium on the Interface*, pages 259–268. IEEE, Computer Society Press, 1995.

18. A. P. Pentland. Automatic extraction of deformable part models. *International Journal of Computer Vision*, 4(2):107–126, 1990.

19. S. Sclaroff and A. Pentland. A modal framework for correspondence and description. In $4^{th}$ *International Conference on Computer Vision*, pages 308–313, Berlin, May 1993. IEEE Computer Society Press.

20. G. L. Scott and H. C. Longuet-Higgins. An algorithm for associating the features of two images. *Proceedings of the Royal Statistical Society of London*, 244:21–26, 1991.

21. L. S. Shapiro and J. M. Brady. A modal approach to feature-based correspondence. In P. Mowforth, editor, $2^{nd}$ *British Machine Vison Conference*, pages 78–85. Springer-Verlag, Sept. 1991.

22. H. D. Tagare, D. O'Shea, and A. Rangarajan. A geometric criterion for shape-based non-rigid correspondence. In $5^{th}$ *International Conference on Computer Vision*, pages 434–439, June 1995.

# Quadratic Variation of Deformations

Fred L. Bookstein

University of Michigan, Ann Arbor, Michigan 48109 USA

**Abstract.** Hitherto no constitutive formalism of deformations provides a parameterization for the visually obvious features of their transformation grids. This paper notes a property of the thin-plate spline that one may exploit to this end. The bending energy that is minimized by the spline, usually expressed in matrix form, is also the double integral of the output of a nonlinear differential operator, the *quadratic variation* (sum of squared second partial derivatives of displacement), over the whole picture plane. Displaying this integrand as a scalar field over the medical image or template may prove a helpful guide to the interesting regions of a deformation, and the peaks of this field localize and orient a promising set of features for simplistically parameterized deformations that approximate the original.

## 1 Introduction

Lately there has been considerable interest in representations of medical images as deformations of an atlas or of a sample average. Grenander and Miller [1] phrase the mathematics of atlas-matching as a task within the general domain of Grenander's pattern theory. More concretely, there are several different algorithms for fitting geometrically explicit prototypes to images by physical or nonphysical energy-based methods [2, 3]. Another approach [4] estimates a displacement function at a hierarchy of lattice spacings, and still another exploits the hierarchy of Euclidean submanifold dimensions from isolated point data up through surface elements [5] or even volumes [6].

These and similar visualizations usually do not culminate in any summary of the deformation per se for clinical or scientific purposes. Instead, in the overwhelming majority of applications ([5] excepted), the deformation serves only as a sort of tensor-valued "covariate" normalizing pixel or voxel coordinates to ease their later processing without any further reference to the deformation thus normalized out. If features of the deformation are mentioned at all, they have been found by eye, as places where the grid seems "most bent." While the eye seems to pull out such foci of distortion quite intuitively from two-dimensional grids, we have no idea what criteria our neural circuitry is using, or to what sorts of transformations it is relatively more or less sensitive, and we have no effective means of extracting the same information from the analogous structures in 3D.

My own work over the last ten years has emphasized the duality between one representation of shape variability (the approximation to Kendall shape space for landmarks via its tangent manifold, see below) and a convenient visualization of the same variation as deformation, namely, the thin-plate spline. But the relation of this approach to more conventional image-processing concerns has always been problematic. In the usual parlance, the approximation of an image is a simpler image (that is, one more robustly parameterized) that comes close to the target image in some precisely characterized way. At present we lack techniques that supply parameterizations of deformation any simpler than the full set of points and derivative constraints driving the spline. For instance, subsetting the point list does not seem to be associated with visual decompositions of the corresponding grids in the same way that gray-scale scenes can often be usefully "approximated" by a finite set of Gaussian blobs.

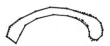

two group means, full outlines

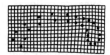

mean normal to mean schizophrenic

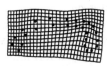

mean normal to mean schizophrenic, x 3

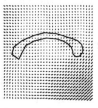

splined shifts, Procrustes coordinates

**Figure 1.** Biometric summaries of a morphometric data set originating in midsagittal brain MRI. Upper left, the Procrustes superposition of normal and schizophrenic averages for a 26-semilandmark outline of the corpus callosum in the midsagittal plane (see text). Upper right, deformation from the normal to the syndromal average, drawn as a conventional thin-plate spline grid. Lower left, grid for a threefold magnification of the shape difference vector in Procrustes space, from which now clear features emerge. Lower right, grid displacement vectors from the thin-plate spline above. The "obvious" features of the grid, which cannot be recovered from a cursory study of these vectors, are produced by careful study of their first and second derivatives.

There is a divergence between the space over which the deformation is displayed and that supporting the actual parametrizations of these deformations, which cannot be regionalized if they are to be of any statistical use. But for the deformation formalism of which I am fondest, the thin-plate spline, a differential operator permits, by theorem, the conversion of one of these representations to the other: the reversion from the representation of bending energy as a quadratic form in the point coordinates to its representation as the integral of quadratic variation. The applications here demonstrate how this reversion immediately simplifies findings that otherwise require strenuous manipulations to disclose.

The data for my main example are not images, but the results of manual processing: a set of hand-digitized outlines of the corpus callosum in midsagittal MRI of 12 doctors and 13 schizophrenics imaged in the Department of Psychiatry, University of Michigan. Each outline is represented as a 26-vertex polygon. All vertices correspond under spline relaxation from their average, but the selection of locations on that average outline, while sensible, is arbitrary [7].

The problem of visualization I am posing is conveyed simply in Figure 1. The representation at upper left is the now-standard *Procrustes superposition* of the two group average callosal shapes. (This superposition and the closely related sense of shape averaging to which it leads will both be defined presently.) While these coordinates, augmented by information about covariance, have precisely the correct multivariate statistics of "shape," as a guide to the eye about where the groups differ they are not at all helpful. The contrasts they so plainly suggest are wholly artifacts of that global superposition rule. At upper right is an equivalent presentation: the thin-plate spline from the solid to the dashed outline at the left. At lower left the grid has been magnified threefold, for legibility. It is now clear to the viewing eye that there has been a strong displacement of the arch at center-right (the *isthmus* of the form) upwards and to the right in the patient subsample, and also apparent shrinkage of the left-hand bulb, which corresponds to the anatomical substructure named *genu*.

The problem posed here is to generate this obvious and intuitive cluster of features objectively, without "looking." The spirit of the task is similar to that of the Chapel Hill group's longstanding attempt to supply a formalism matching our intuitive visual apprehension of image "objects," obvious "parts" of the single image. This paper supplies an analogous formalism capable of producing some of the obvious "parts" of deformations like these.

## 2   Two standard techniques of biometrical shape space

The following material has been published in many different versions elsewhere, both for 2D and for 3D data sets, and will only be summarized here.

### 2.1   The thin-plate spline

Consider, first, the task of interpolating in some principled way between two paired sets of points. Let $U$ be the function $U(r) = r^2 \log r$, and let $P_i = (x_i, y_i)$, $i = 1, \ldots, k$, be $k$ points in the plane. Writing $U_{ij} = U(|P_i - P_j|)$, build up matrices

$$K = \begin{pmatrix} 0 & U_{12} & \ldots & U_{1k} \\ U_{21} & 0 & \ldots & U_{2k} \\ \vdots & \vdots & \ddots & \vdots \\ U_{k1} & U_{k2} & \ldots & 0 \end{pmatrix}, \quad Q = \begin{pmatrix} 1 & x_1 & y_1 \\ 1 & x_2 & y_2 \\ \vdots & \vdots & \vdots \\ 1 & x_k & y_k \end{pmatrix},$$

and

$$L = \begin{pmatrix} K & Q \\ Q^t & O \end{pmatrix}, \ (k+3) \times (k+3)$$

where $O$ is a $3 \times 3$ matrix of zeros. Write $H = (h_1 \ldots h_k \ 0 \ 0 \ 0)^t$ and set $W = (w_1 \ldots w_k \ a_0 \ a_x \ a_y)^t = L^{-1}H$. Then the thin-plate spline $f(P)$ having heights (values) $h_i$ at points $P_i = (x_i, y_i)$ is the function $f(P) = \sum_{i=1}^{k} w_i U(P - P_i) + a_0 + a_x x + a_y y$. This function $f(P)$ has three crucial properties:

1. $f(P_i) = h_i$, all $i$: $f$ interpolates the heights $h_i$ at the landmarks $P_i$.

2. The function $f$ has minimum **bending energy** of all functions that interpolate the heights $h_i$ in that way: the minimum of

$$\iint_{\mathbf{R}^2} \left( \left(\frac{\partial^2 f}{\partial x^2}\right)^2 + 2 \left(\frac{\partial^2 f}{\partial x \partial y}\right)^2 + \left(\frac{\partial^2 f}{\partial y^2}\right)^2 \right),$$

where the integral is taken over the entire picture plane.

3. The value of this bending energy is $(8\pi)^{-1} H_k^t L_k^{-1} H_k$, where $L_k^{-1}$, the *bending energy matrix*, is the $k \times k$ upper left submatrix of $L^{-1}$, and $H_k$ is the initial $k$-vector of $H$, the vector of $k$ heights.

In the application to two-dimensional landmark data, we compute two of these splined surfaces, one ($f_x$) in which the vector $H$ of heights is loaded with the $x$-coordinate of the landmarks in a second form, another ($f_y$) for the $y$-coordinate. The resulting map $(f_x(P), f_y(P))$ is now a deformation of one picture plane onto the other which maps landmarks onto their homologues and has the minimum bending energy of any such interpolant. For the extension to outline data, we minimize the bending energy (in its matrix formulation) over the set of assignments of correspondences over a set of outlines [8]. The callosal data here exemplify that extension, as previously explained in [7].

## 2.2 Procrustes distance and Procrustes coordinates

In a seemingly unrelated development, consider the problem of formulating a *shape distance* between configurations of labeled points in the Cartesian plane. By "shape distance" we mean a function of the pair of point sets that is invariant against the usual Cartesian operations that do not change shape (the similarity group of rotations, translations, and changes of scale applied to either point set separately). If we further require that this distance function be a "submersion" of the original Cartesian metric—that circles around points in the original space correspond to forms at equal distance from the central form in the shape space, etc.—then Kendall [9] shows that there is essentially only one formula, the *Procrustes metric*, that works. For shapes written as vectors $(z_i)_1^k$ of complex numbers with $\Sigma_i z_i = 0$ and $\Sigma_i z_i \bar{z}_i = 1$, this metric $\rho(z^1, z^2)$ is $\cos^{-1} |\Sigma_i z_i^1 \bar{z}_i^2|$. Under this metric the set of all labelled shapes of $k$ landmark points in two dimensions forms a Riemannian manifold, the *Kendall shape manifold*, of dimension $2k - 4$. The Procrustes metric is very nearly equal to the sum of squared deviations $\Sigma_i \|z_i^1 - \beta z_i^2\|$ for $\beta = \exp(i \arg \Sigma_i z_i^1 \bar{z}_i^2)$, where $\|z\| = z\bar{z}$.

Multiplication by $\beta$ rotates the centered and scaled form $z^2$ so as to minimize the sum of squared deviations from the centered and scaled form $z^1$.

Corresponding to any data set $\{z^j\}$ showing biologically reasonable amounts of shape variation, there is a *Procrustes average shape* $Z$, the shape having minimum summed squared distance to the original shapes of the data set. Consider, now, the set of coordinates that arise when each of the original forms is fitted to the sample average by its own superposition: the real and imaginary parts of the points $\beta_j z_i^j$, where $\beta_j = \Sigma_i Z_i \bar{z}_i^j$ is the $j$th superposition multiplier. The geometry of this operation is equivalent to projecting the same set of shapes, construed now as points of the Kendall shape manifold, normally onto the *tangent plane* to that manifold at the average shape $Z$. The formula for Procrustes distance between two shapes $\beta_1 z^1$, $\beta_2 z^2$ after this projection is the usual Euclidean sum of squares: $\rho^2(z^1, z^2) = \Sigma_i \|\beta_1 z_i^1 - \beta_2 z_i^2\|$. These *Procrustes shape coordinates* represent a linearization of the original shape manifold that, although redundant ($2k$ coordinates for a $(2k-4)$-dimensional tangent space), is adequate for most multivariate statistical purposes. For instance, the outlines in Figure 1 are averages of these coordinates by group. The shape difference here is statistically significant at about the $p \sim .02$ level, and so its investigation may be worth a bit more of our time.

# 3 The distribution of quadratic variation

This now-standard biometric technology of shape, which combines Procrustes methods with the thin-plate spline, is capable of supplying a fine summary diagram (Figure 1) of the signal in which we are interested, a signal the component features of which are easily apprehended by the untrained viewing eye; but the associated biometric machinery offers no equivalent of the feature space within which that eye is browsing for candidate features. In the two-dimensional context of the example here, this incompatibility is not so crippling, since understanding the grid features of Figure 1 is visually immediate and unthinking. But in the extension to three-dimensional problems, even though both the computation and the biometrical analysis of shape variation are understood as fully as they are in two dimensions, the corresponding "intuitive" analysis of a deformation grid seems to be out of reach.

This section introduces a candidate differential operator for this specific purpose, and shows how it works for our running two-dimensional example of the callosal outline and some other data sets already analyzed by the biometric toolkit. For a three-dimensional problem the formulation would be identical except that visualization would require multiple slices or a volume representation, not the simple graphics here. (Likewise, the extension to incorporate variable scale is immediate.)

At the lower right in Figure 1 is a representation of the usual callosal data using yet another graphical system. Instead of connecting up the lines of the grid, we connect the two images of each point, pre- and post-deformation, in the Procrustes superposition. Displayed this way, the figure looks compellingly like a displacement vector field; but in fact it does not have the mensural properties of such a field. Any feature analysis of this picture must be independent of the overall similarity transformation by which the second form was put down over the first. (It is the violation of this principle that renders the currently popular method of "probabilistic atlases" so badly flawed. I will return to this issue in the discussion.) The steady growth in magnitude of the displacement vector toward the lower right could be substantially attenuated in a different registration, and thus is not relevant to the signal we seek. Similarly, the precise locations of the "fixed points" of this transformation, inside splenium and genu, are dependent on registration, and so likewise cannot be taken as features.

The largest-scale feature possible for any deformation grid is its global affine term, its "behavior at infinity." In the biometric approach there is an explicit subspace for the affine term [10]. For the callosal data, the groups do not differ in their mean projections into this subspace. For small variations of registration, the remaining information is described in an appropriately invariant fashion by the *second* derivatives of the displacement field. It is thus appropriate to turn our attention to those derivatives, directly.

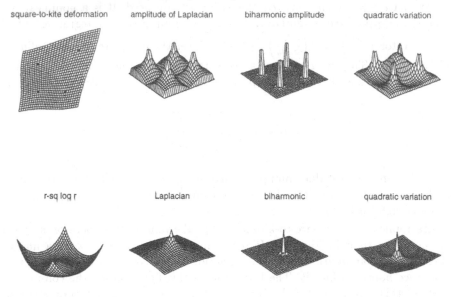

**Figure 2.** Amplitude of some candidate differential operators for displacement fields like that at the lower right in Figure 1. (upper row) The simplest nonlinear spline, a square-to-kite warp. (lower row) Kernel of the thin-plate spline: the function $r^2 \log r$. All vertical scales are arbitrary.

In the literature of medical image analysis, the most familiar second-order differential operator is the Laplacian $\frac{\partial^2}{\partial x^2} + \frac{\partial^2}{\partial y^2}$. We might imagine, for instance, attempting the equivalent of a "Laplacian pyramid" for the displacement field there, applied to the separate Cartesian coordinates of the displacements in Figure 1 and then summed in root-mean-square. But a straightforward initial computation for the simplest possible nonlinear spline, the canonical four-point "square-to-kite" example [11], stops us in our tracks. The transformation in question is drawn out as a grid at the upper left in Figure 2. As shown to its immediate right, the Laplacian of the thin-plate spline varies in a most unpromising fashion. For instance, it is exactly zero in the center of this transformation, although that ought to be the "loudest" signal for this clearly unitary feature. In terms of its zero-crossings, the square-to-kite transformation looks like it has an orthogonal pair of edges intersecting at the center—not a particularly useful representation of this feature!

The biharmonic of the square-to-kite map, as approximated via the grid, is a sum of $\delta$-functions at the landmarks driving the spline. While in one sense this is a "correct" set of features—those that are actually parameterizing the map—it is not really the analysis we are seeking. We want a somewhat different operator that will draw our attention to the whole configuration of four landmarks, not to their locations separately.

We have already encountered the expression we need. It is a nonlinear operator, the **quadratic variation.** The spline minimizes the integral output of the operator $\left(\frac{\partial^2}{\partial x^2}\right)^2 + 2\left(\frac{\partial^2}{\partial x \partial y}\right)^2 + \left(\frac{\partial^2}{\partial y^2}\right)^2$ over the complete (doubly infinite) picture plane. This integrand has a geometric meaning that is intuitively quite accessible: it is a norm for the complete matrix of second derivatives of the map,

$$H = \begin{pmatrix} \frac{\partial}{\partial x}\frac{\partial f}{\partial x} & \frac{\partial}{\partial x}\frac{\partial f}{\partial y} \\ \frac{\partial}{\partial y}\frac{\partial f}{\partial x} & \frac{\partial}{\partial y}\frac{\partial f}{\partial y} \end{pmatrix}$$

where $f$ is the vector-valued mapping conveyed by the grid. In fact, our integrand is the sum of the forms tr $H^t H$ over the components $x$, $y$ of the displacements at lower right in Figure 1.

As applied to our square-to-kite prototype the value of this operator is shown at the upper right in Figure 2. It represents a compromise between a nugget effect at each landmark and an accumulation in the center of the feature, just where we hoped to find it. The lower row of this figure shows the component parts of this expression for the kernel of this spline, the fundamental solution $r^2 \log r$. Its Laplacian, second column, is too broad (analytically it's the function $\log r$). The biharmonic, of course, is a $\delta$-function (third column). The quadratic variation (last column) compromises between the $\delta$-function and the logarithmic dependence. Under appropriate boundary conditions (which do not obtain for this naked kernel), the spline minimizes the volume under this surface when it is computed out to infinity in every direction—but the greatest contribution to that volume is right here in the vicinity of the data. In the upper right panel in Figure 2, the emergence of that "heap" of quadratic variation in the center, exactly where the ridge of medialness would be emerging if this were a search for an "object," is quite reassuring.

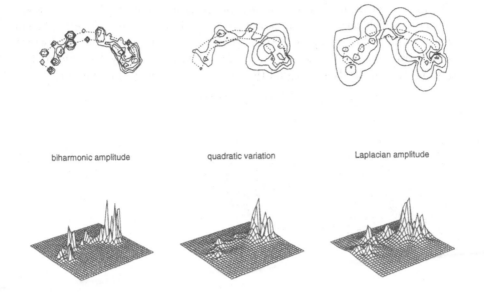

Figure 3. Outputs of the same three operators for the group comparison of callosal outlines, Figure 1. In the contour plots, above, contours are at 5%, 10%, 20%, and 50% of the maxima found in these coarse grids; in the perspective plots, below, vertical ranges are normalized.

Figure 3 shows this same trinity of differential descriptors for the data of Figure 1. On this (arbitrary) grid, the Laplacian of the displacement image $I$ can be approximated as the familiar picture-processing expression (now a complex number; we will tacitly take its amplitude) $4I - \Sigma I_a$, where $a$ is the list of four subscript shifts $(0, \pm 1), (\pm 1, 0)$. The biharmonic is the iterate of that form, $4(4I - \Sigma I_a) - \Sigma(4I - \Sigma I_a)_a = 20I - 8\Sigma I_a + 2\Sigma I_b + \Sigma I_{2a}$, where $b$ is the subscript list $(\pm 1, \pm 1)$. The quadratic variation incorporates the squares of the elements of the Laplacian, plus other terms for the mixed derivatives: on the grid, it is the expression

$$(2I - I_{-1,0} - I_{1,0})^2 + (2I - I_{0,-1} - I_{0,1})^2 + (I_{-1,-1} + I_{1,1} - I_{1,-1} - I_{-1,1})^2/4.$$

Even computed in this far-from-optimal, grid-dependent way, the biharmonic operator, left column, looks like "beads on a string"—a landscape of $\delta$-functions. At the left, in genu, its contours surround discrete peaks at the semilandmarks separately; at the right, in splenium, where the net deformation is quite a bit higher, the contours of biharmonic amplitude follow around the curve with remarkable delicacy. The quadratic variation, at center, seems the most helpful of these three candidates. It shows two clear peaks, one on the lower arc of isthmus and one in the bulb of splenium itself, corresponding to the clear visual features of that part of the grid in Figure 1. Two more features lie near the other end of the form, a peak inside genu and another peak at the upper left of the arch, a region to which our attention had not previously been called. The Laplacian surface, at far right, is similar to the surface of quadratic variation, with which it shares two terms, but it is less concentrated, which is to say, less informative regarding the localization of signal that actually obtains in this example.

schizophrenia landmark data I (k=13)

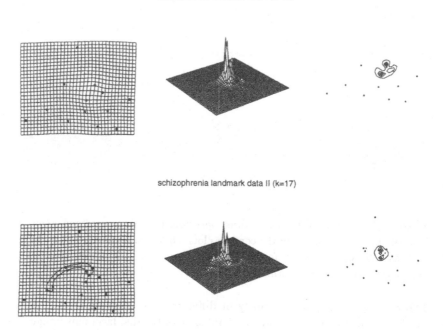

schizophrenia landmark data II (k=17)

**Figure 4.** The quadratic signal for two data sets grids for which were previously published as analyzed by eye.

The display of quadratic variation in this way generally confirms the features claimed for deformations in earlier, visually intuitive reports. At upper left in Figure 4 is the grid of the original 13-landmark analysis of schizophrenia by DeQuardo et al. [12]. The usual observation is to the effect that "the eye is led directly to the nature of the shape difference here" (the increase in separation of the two landmarks at right center). The plot of quadratic variation (now with contours at $\pm.2, .4, .6, .8$ of its maximum) shows indeed that the deformation is concentrated along that segment and in the triangle to its right, which overlies the quadrigeminal cistern of the cerebral ventricular system. In the lower row of that same figure is a reanalysis of 17 landmarks from the same images from which the outlines of corpus callosum were extracted for the separate analysis of Figure 1 (see [13]). The quadratic variation very clearly indicates that the interesting part of the grid is in the crook of corpus callosum at isthmus, almost exactly where we have found it by the landmark-free analysis in Figure 3.

In these last two examples, the emergence of nearly equivalent peaks of quadratic variation at adjacent landmarks strongly suggests the summary of the deformation by a single corresponding relative displacement of each toward or away from the other. Those adjacent pairs are clearly the features "responsible" for the deformations observed. Then we could have seen them as well in the directional expansion of the grid between them, the expression of the first (not the second) derivative of the displacement field. But in the first example, Figure 3, the quadratic variation does not show paired peaks in this way, and the perception of "thrust into isthmus" that arises in Figure 1 is not a matter of grid line spacing, but of the strong *gradient* of that spacing. We can extract a simple parameterization of the observed change, nevertheless, by decomposing the sum of squares $\left(\frac{\partial^2 f}{\partial x^2}\right)^2 + 2\left(\frac{\partial^2 f}{\partial x \partial y}\right)^2 + \left(\frac{\partial^2 f}{\partial y^2}\right)^2$ further. For real and imaginary parts separately, this expression is the sum of squares of entries of the matrices $H$ of second derivatives introduced before. Then, grid point by grid point, it is also the sum of squares of the two eigenvalues of $H$ as we have been approximating it on the grid. One way to generate actual features of the observed deformation, then, is by inspecting the associated tensor field of *eigenvectors* of the same Hessian form, in combination with a reassessment of Figure 1, which conveys the first derivatives of the same coordinates. (These tensors should not be confused with a similar-looking field, the principal axes of the affine derivative [11]. Spatial gradients of those fields are more difficult to read than these representations, which directly visualize their derivatives.)

In Figure 5, the peak of the total quadratic variation, Figure 3, can be here seen to arise from approximately equal components in the two Cartesian directions, at coordinates (20,15) in the contour plots. That is, the principal feature of this landscape is shared between the components: the strong gradient from southwest to northeast of very low *lower* eigenvalue. As is clearest in the lower left eigenvector plot, these represent a consistent gradient of quadratic "slowing," strong deceleration of the shift of the isthmus along the (.6, .8) unit vector in this region of the plane. Just to the lower right of this region, around coordinates (24,13) in the contour plots, is another peak of quadratic variation, this one of larger eigenvalue *positive*. Both coordinates, then, have a saddle in this vicinity, corresponding to the (directional) emergence of the region of expansion in the bulb of splenium. Both coordinates go on to indicate the correction of this acceleration, but the horizontal deceleration is more marked, corresponding to the greater propinquity of the outline in that direction. Finally, there is a local peak at the far left of the grid, the region of genu. Both eigenvalues are (mildly) positive, as the grid shows an isolated center of contraction. Here the quadratic variation plot is conveying nearly the same information as the Laplacian of Figure 3.

Putting these features together, we infer that the grid in Figure 1 can be approximated, *within the region of the form*, by the display in Figure 6. This simulation was produced in Bill Green's public program package **edgewarp** [14], which uses an extended feature set incorporating directional constraints on derivatives alongside repositioning of single points. The grid at right in Figure 6 is remarkably similar in its larger features to the actual thin-plate spline relating these callosal outlines, Figure 1. Its shifts are taken from the Procrustes shift grid and its gradients from the orientations of the eigenvectors in Figure 5 and the signs of the eigenvalues. While I produced Figure 6 by free play in **edgewarp,** the process can perhaps be automated to some extent once we have more experience converting the landscape of quadratic variation to a list of sculpting elements.

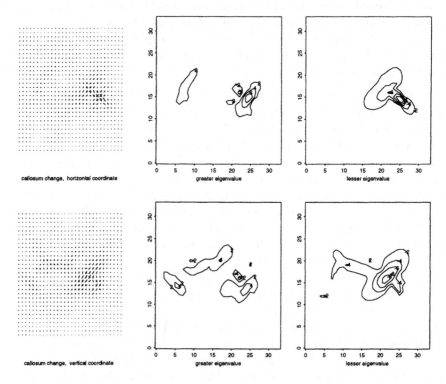

**Figure 5.** Decomposition of the quadratic variation into its four contituent eigenvalues (contours center and right) and corresponding eigenvectors (orthogonal crosses at left) for the callosal outline data. Upper row, horizontal Cartesian component; lower row, vertical Cartesian component. The quadratic variation is the sum of squares of these four eigenvalues. Eigenvectors are scaled to absolute eigenvalue. Contours are plotted at ± .2, .4, .6, .8 of the maximum absolute value of any eigenvalue. The features that were visually obvious in Figure 1 are the principal features here: jointly negative second derivatives directional toward the upper right in the isthmus, derivatives of mixed sign toward the body of splenium, and gentle peak of both derivatives in genu (a local minimum).

## 4  Discussion

*Critique of the approach via "probabilistic atlases."* The emergence of features of deformation from a consideration of its derivatives sheds considerable light on the limitations of a technique recently put forward for the "automatic" detection of anatomical abnormalities, the *probabilistic atlases* of Evans implemented for cortical data by Toga's group at UCLA [3]. In this approach, the population standard deviation of vectors analogous to those at the lower right in Figure 1 is computed, and regions of candidate deformations are declared anomalous if their associated displacements lie beyond some a-priori fractile of the normative distribution, perhaps .1%.

But this diagram is not the appropriate representation for the signal sought. The displacements that are plotted by Evans or Toga are dependent on a single choice of superposition case by case. This choice, although it can be managed objectively, nevertheless alters all the statistics of the resulting displacements in a manner confounding noise of registration with variation in each part of the scene being registered. The anomalies to which the Evans–Toga approach is currently being turned are quite local (a finger-sized depression in the cortical surface, or the deviation of the midplane induced by a unilateral tumor). They would be much more sensitively detected, then, by operators with local support, which in this case are the derivatives of the displacement field, not its vector values over the grid.

Effects that involve local expansion will likely be detected by the quadratic variation here because it incorporates the Laplacian quite explicitly at centers of local expansion. By contrast, effects that involve the systematic displacement of a structure together with elastic responses of neighboring tissues will best be detected by the deceleration of the shift field, as shown here in the region of isthmus. The Evans–Toga publications did not consider derivatives of the displacement field they studied and hence did not investigate whether the coordinate-free analysis of second derivatives at some suitable spatial scale might have detected the tumor or the fingering with a considerable stronger signal strength than their coordinate-dependent displacement method. Neither did they attempt to locate the center of the tumor by studying the grid in its actual vicinity; their attention was limited to the displacement of the midline, a displacement at some distance.

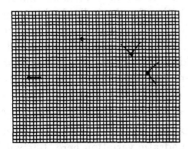 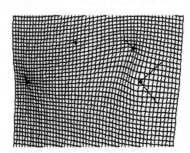

**Figure 6.** Simulation of the grid in Figure 1 by a simplistic combination of sculpting features corresponding to the information in Figure 5. The principal features of the grid have been recovered in this simple parametrization.

*Yes, the quadratic variation is nonlinear in its data.* The elegance of the formalism of *scale space* and its apparent match to certain aspects of visual psychology have focused the attention of the medical image community upon *linear* differential operators. Quadratic variation is clearly not of that class. Because it involves squares of derivatives, its value does not sum over sums of deformations. Its connection to linear methods is only by way of biometric shape space, the coordinates of which drive the spline that minimizes the integral of this quantity over the whole picture plane.

There is no reason to believe that the visual system operates linearly in the processing of the deformation grids, like those in Figure 1, whose features we are trying to automate. The eye certainly does not process these features isotropically, for instance—the same deformation looks indescribably different on a grid rotated 45° [10, Fig. 8]—and the upper right and lower left displays in Figure 1 cannot be "read" as multiples of one another even when the reader has been told explicitly that that is how they were constructed.

From another point of view, linearity, while an elegant part of the scale-space armamentarium of algorithms, does not itself characterize the associated steps that explicitly extract image features, absent which steps we have not accomplished anything biometrically worthwhile. The typical "object" of a scale-space analysis of an image is identified with a local maximum signal on a ridge of medialness. Both of these qualifications—finding a ridge, finding a maximum along it—are *explicitly* nonlinear operators whose implementation in fact requires the same three orders of differentiation that underlie the gridded computations here. Thus I do not believe the presence of the matrix multiplication in the formula $\mathrm{tr} H^t H$ for quadratic variation should be considered any sort of defect or lapse.

*Relation to other grid protocols.* All the demonstrations of quadratic variation here use a field that has been explicitly minimized by the deformation engine responsible for the grids we wish to decompose. It will be of great interest to see how far this formalism can be extended to deformations produced by other energy functionals [2, 3, 4]. I suspect that those fields will be a great deal more fractal than these explicitly smoothest alternatives. Such a fractal character, of course, would render nearly impossible, either for the individual case or for differences between groups, the search for exactly those features that are the concern of this paper. In particular, grids computed by the viscous-fluid methods of the Miller school typically show extensive eddies and regions of high curl that almost certainly *cannot* be put to any subsequent quantitative purpose. (Hardly any known developmental or pathological procedures inject curl into an image!)

Empirical grids based on elasticity minimize an energy that is the sum of squares of *first* derivatives. These will pick up the presence of "sources" and "sinks" rather like the Laplacian part of the quadratic variation here, but will also yield signals over large regions of the image in which, as far as the grid is concerned, "nothing is happening"—where the grid is uniform but anisotropic. Davatzikos et al. [2] report one aspect of the field of those first derivatives, its trace. The quadratic variation is sensitive to the spatial derivatives of this quantity, along with many other forms of deformation.

**Acknowledgement.** Preparation of this chapter was supported by NIH grants DA–09009 and GM–37251 to Fred L. Bookstein.

# References

1. Grenander, U., and M. Miller. Representations of knowledge in complex systems. *Journal of the Royal Statistical Society* B56:549–603, 1994.
2. Davatzikos, C., M. Vaillant, S. M. Resnick, J. L. Prince, S. Letovsky, and R. N. Bryan. A computerized approach for morphological analysis of the corpus callosum. *Journal of Computer Assisted Tomography* 20:88–97, 1996.
3. Thompson, P., and A. Toga. A surface-based technique for warping three-dimensional images of the brain. *I.E.E.E. Transactions on Medical Imaging* 15:402–417, 1996.
4. Collins, D. L., T. Peters, and A. Evans. An automated 3d non-linear image deformation procedure for determination of gross morphometric variability in human brain. Pp. 180–190 in R. Robb, ed., *Visualization in Biomedical Computing*. SPIE *Proceedings*, vol. 2359, 1994.
5. Cutting, C., D. Dean, F. Bookstein, B. Haddad, D. Khorramabadi, F. Zonnefeld, and J. McCarthy. A three-dimensional smooth surface analysis of untreated Crouzon's disease in the adult. *Journal of Craniofacial Surgery* 6:444–453, 1995.
6. Joshi, S. C., M. Miller, G. Christensen, A. Banerjee, T. Coogan, and U. Grenander. Hierarchical brain mapping via a generalized dirichlet solution for mapping brain manifolds. Pp. 278–289 in R. Melter et al., eds., *Vision Geometry IV*. SPIE *Proceedings*, vol. 2573, 1995.
7. Bookstein, F. L. Landmark methods for forms without landmarks. *Computer Vision and Image Understanding*, in press, 1997.
8. Green, W. D. K. The thin-plate spline and images with curving features. Pp. 79–87 in K. V. Mardia et al., eds., *Proceedings in Image Fusion and Shape Variability Techniques*. Leeds University Press, 1996.
9. Kendall, D. G. 1984. Shape-manifolds, procrustean metrics, and complex projective spaces. *Bulletin of the London Mathematical Society* 16:81–121.
10. Bookstein, F. L. Biometrics, biomathematics, and the morphometric synthesis. *Bulletin of Mathematical Biology* 58:313–365, 1996.
11. Bookstein, F. L. *Morphometric Tools for Landmark Data*. Cambridge University Press, 1991.
12. DeQuardo, J. R., F. Bookstein, W. D. K. Green, J. Brumberg, and R. Tandon. Spatial relationships of neuroanatomic landmarks in schizophrenia. *Psychiatry Research: Neuroimaging* 67:81–95, 1996.
13. Bookstein, F. L. Biometrics and brain maps: the promise of the Morphometric Synthesis. Pp. 203–254 in S. Koslow and M. Huerta, eds., *Neuroinformatics: An Overview of the Human Brain Project. Progress in Neuroinformatics*, vol. 1. Hillsdale, NJ: Lawrence Erlbaum, 1996.
14. Bookstein, F. L., and W. D. K. Green. Edgewarp: A flexible program package for biometric image warping in two dimensions. Pp. 135–147 in R. Robb, ed., *Visualization in Biomedical Computing 1994*. S.P.I.E. *Proceedings*, vol. 2359.

# The Softassign Procrustes Matching Algorithm

Anand Rangarajan[1], Haili Chui[1] and Fred L. Bookstein[3]

[1] Departments of Diagnostic Radiology and Electrical Engineering
Yale University
[2] Institute of Gerontology
University of Michigan, Ann Arbor

**Abstract.** The problem of matching shapes parameterized as a set of points is frequently encountered in medical imaging tasks. When the point-sets are derived from landmarks, there is usually no problem of determining the correspondences or homologies between the two sets of landmarks. However, when the point sets are automatically derived from images, the difficult problem of establishing correspondence and rejecting non-homologies as outliers remains. The Procrustes method is a well-known method of shape comparison and can always be pressed into service when homologies between point-sets are known in advance. This paper presents a powerful extension of the Procrustes method to point-sets of differing point counts with correspondences unknown. The result is the softassign Procrustes matching algorithm which iteratively establishes correspondence, rejects non-homologies as outliers, determines the Procrustes rescaling and the spatial mapping between the point-sets.

## 1 Introduction

One of the most commonly encountered problems in medical imaging is image matching: the process of superimposing one image onto another such that an appropriate measure of goodness of match is minimized. The plethora of image matching methods span the spectrum from matching user specified *landmarks* to directly matching image intensities (see [19] for an excellent review). When we restrict the focus to feature matching methods, the problem difficulty changes considerably depending on whether we have well defined landmarks or merely unlabeled features. The essential difficulty in feature matching methods lies in the problem of establishing correspondences or homologies. When we have landmarks, the correspondence between landmarks in one image and the other are usually known in advance. All that is required is to find a suitable spatial mapping (rigid, similarity, affine, non-rigid) between the two sets of landmarks. On the other hand, when we merely have two sets of unlabeled point features, the problem of correspondence is acute [2]. In addition, when the two *point-sets* are of different point count, we are saddled with the problems of outlier (non-homology) rejection as well as the problem of discovering homologies.

The Procrustes method of shape comparison arose as a way of superimposing point-sets with known correspondence [8]. Drawing on the insight that shape can be represented as point-sets with size removed, the Procrustes method first sought to normalize the two point sets prior to superimposition. The normalization operation essentially consisted of centering and scaling each point-set such that the centroid shifted to the (common) origin and the sums of squared distances of the points was unity. The normalization operation annihilates translation and scale factors. Consequently, the search for a similarity transformation that aligns the point-sets can be restricted to a search for rotation alone. (Note that non-rigid operations such as thin-plate splines can be subsequently used to discover localized regions of dissimilarity between the point-sets [4]). The obvious question that arises at this juncture is: What happens to the Procrustes method when we do not know the correspondence between the point-sets?

The present paper answers this question and provides an algorithm for determining the correspondences or homologies and rejecting outliers or non-homologies. We see this as a powerful extension of the Procrustes method, capable of radically extending the scope of application of Procrustes methods in medical imaging. Central to our approach is the iterative combination of the search for correspondence, the spatial mapping and Procrustes rescaling. Correspondence is parameterized via a binary *match matrix* that assigns points in one set to points in the other and discards non-homologies as outliers. Parameterized in this manner, the search for correspondence is tantamount to solving *the linear assignment problem* [12]. The *softassign*, a new technique that first arose in the statistical physics and neural computation literature [14, 12] has been shown to find the optimum solution to the assignment problem. Using the softassign, our algorithm essentially alternates between solving for correspondences, the spatial mapping and Procrustes rescaling.

## 2 The Procrustes method revisited

The modern Procrustes literature began with Kendall's great 1984 paper on the relation between the Procrustes formalism and differential geometry in the large [11]. The recipe for calculating the standard Procrustes distance formula involves centering and scaling each form (point-set) such that the sums of squared distances of each point-set is unity and then evaluating the Euclidean distance between the point-sets after superimposing the two forms [8]. Kendall noted that this standard formula for Procrustes distance is only an approximation to the correct quantity, which is $\arccos |\sum_i z_i \bar{z}'_i|$ when 2-D shapes are written as complex vectors $z_i$ (and $z'_i$) with $\sum_i z_i = 0$ and $\sum_i z_i \bar{z}_i = 1$. Kendall shows how this metric arises naturally from the construal of shapes as equivalence classes of point-sets of the plane under the operation of the similarity group (the same rotations, translations, and rescalings we have been pursuing here all along), and, furthermore, how it is the *only* such metric that satisfies certain reasonable symmetries arising from the symmetries of Euclidean distance in the original Cartesian image space. For more on the resulting smooth Riemannian manifold, which is quite a remarkable geometric object see [17].

In this Kendall formulation, which is now standard in all other applications of Procrustes methods, Procrustes distance is not determined as the sum of squares of the Euclidean distances between the two centered and scaled point-sets. While it happens to agree (approximately) with the minimum sum of squares over the operation of the similarity group, it is defined in a way independent of the selection of an element of that group. It is interesting to consider how the combinatorial context taken in this paper constrains the elegance of this more general mathematical setting.

The present paper has extended the Kendall metric, in its approximate form, to a distance function over the *union* of a sequence of these shape manifolds, one for each different count of matching points. When we change the count of outliers, we change manifolds. Other approaches to this problem have worked only in one of these manifolds at a time. For instance, [9] and [5] deal with the closely related problem of minimizing metrics within linear subspaces of the tangent space to the space of these shapes. The uniqueness of this paper lies in the combinatorial extension of the Procrustes method in order to handle the problems of determining correspondences and rejecting outliers.

## 3 Combining the search for correspondence and the spatial mapping

In its most basic form, the Procrustes distance requires us to center and scale each set of points so that the sum of squared distances of all points in each point-set is unity and then compute a similarity transformation between them. Then the Procrustes average shape and Procrustes residuals can be evaluated. How does this situation change when we do not have information about the homologies or point-to-point correspondences between the two point-sets? The Procrustes distance presupposes correspondence. When the homologies are unknown, we cannot even carry out the first step in the Procrustes distance calculation, namely the centering and scaling of each point-set. The reason: Ignorance of correspondence also implies ignorance of point outliers which hampers the centering and scaling of each point-set. Unfortunately, determining the correspondence beforehand is not easy if not impossible. In order to solve this chicken and egg problem, we embark on a joint formulation of the Procrustes distance and correspondence.

### 3.1 Theory

Denote the point-sets by $X_i \in \mathcal{R}^2$, $i = 1, 2, ..., N_1$ and $Y_j \in \mathcal{R}^2$, $j = 1, 2, ..., N_2$ respectively. $N_1$ and $N_2$ are the numbers of points in the sets $X$ and $Y$ respectively. When $N_1 = N_2 = N$ and the correspondences are known, the Procrustes distance between $X$ and $Y$ (after computing a similarity transformation between $X$ and $Y$) is:

$$D_{\text{Procrustes}}(X, Y) = \sum_{i=1}^{N} \|\frac{(X_i - \mu_X)}{\sigma_X} - R(\theta)\frac{(Y_i - \mu_Y)}{\sigma_Y}\|^2. \tag{1}$$

where

$$\theta = \arctan \left( \frac{\sum_{i=1}^{N} [X_i^c(2)Y_i^c(1) - X_i^c(1)Y_i^c(2)]}{\sum_{i=1}^{N} [X_i^c(1)Y_i^c(1) + X_i^c(2)Y_i^c(2)]} \right) \tag{2}$$

and

$$X_i^c = \frac{X_i - \mu_X}{\sigma_X}, \text{ and } Y_i^c = \frac{Y_i - \mu_Y}{\sigma_Y}.$$

The numbers inside the parenthesis [$X(1)$ or $X(2)$] denote the abscissa and ordinate of the point-set. In (1), $\mu_X$ and $\mu_Y$ are the centroids of the two point-sets $X$ and $Y$ respectively and $\sigma_X$ and $\sigma_Y$ are the sums of squared distances of each point-set from the centroid.

$$\mu_X = \frac{\sum_{i=1}^{N} X_i}{N}, \ \mu_Y = \frac{\sum_{i=1}^{N} Y_i}{N}, \ \sigma_X^2 = \sum_{i=1}^{N} \|X_i - \mu_X\|^2 \text{ and } \sigma_Y^2 = \sum_{i=1}^{N} \|Y_i - \mu_Y\|^2. \tag{3}$$

When the correspondence and the similarity transformation relating the two point-sets are unknown, we can combine the estimation of all of these parameters in the following manner:

$$E(M, \theta, t, s) = \sum_{i=1}^{N_1} \sum_{j=1}^{N_2} M_{ij} \left( \| \frac{\sqrt{s}(X_i - \mu_X)}{\sigma_X} - t - R(\theta) \frac{(Y_j - \mu_Y)}{\sqrt{s}\sigma_Y} \|^2 - \alpha \right)$$

$$\text{subject to } \sum_{i=1}^{N_1} M_{ij} \leq 1, \ \sum_{j=1}^{N_2} M_{ij} \leq 1, \text{ and } M_{ij} \in \{0, 1\}. \tag{4}$$

Equation (4) describes an optimization problem from which the transformation parameters—rotation matrix $R(\theta)$, translation $t$, scale $s$ and the two centroids $\mu_X$ and $\mu_Y$—can be obtained by minimization. (Ignore for the moment the estimation of the two "variance" parameters $\sigma_X$ and $\sigma_Y$.) However, (4) also sets up an optimization problem on the point correspondences. A set of correspondence variables $\{M_{ij}\}$—a *match matrix*—has been defined such that:

$$M_{ij} = \begin{cases} 1 \text{ if point } X_i \text{ corresponds to point } Y_j \\ 0 \text{ otherwise,} \end{cases}$$

$M$ is a correspondence match matrix which indicates when homologies have been found. If $M_{ij}$ is one, feature "$i$" in slice 1 and feature "$j$" in slice 2 are homologies. The constraints on $M_{ij}$ enforce one-to-one correspondence between homologies and also robustness [3]: a point feature in one image may have no corresponding homology and should be discarded as an outlier. The parameter $\alpha > 0$ controls the degree of robustness: as $\alpha$ is increased, less points in both sets are rejected as outliers. (Finer control over robustness is possible by having two parameters, one for each set.) While estimation of $\alpha$ is obviously an important problem, we do not address this issue here. This technique is closely related to the robust statistics approach based on M-estimators and influence functions [3].

Before describing our approach to solving for correspondence, it is worth examining the spatial mapping in (4). In (4), $\mu_X, \mu_Y, \sigma_X, \sigma_Y, t, s$ and $\theta$ constitute the spatial mapping parameters. Since the correspondence matrix $M$ is also unknown, Equation (3) for the centroids and the variances cannot be used. While we can differentiate (4) and solve for the centroids, our first aim is to simplify (4) itself. To this end, we begin with the following Ansatz: the centroids and variances in (4) are set using a weighted mean and variance formula:

$$\mu_X = \frac{\sum_{i=1}^{N_1} \sum_{j=1}^{N_2} M_{ij} X_i}{\sum_{i=1}^{N_1} \sum_{j=1}^{N_2} M_{ij}},$$

$$\mu_Y = \frac{\sum_{i=1}^{N_1} \sum_{j=1}^{N_2} M_{ij} Y_j}{\sum_{i=1}^{N_1} \sum_{j=1}^{N_2} M_{ij}},$$

$$\sigma_X^2 = \sum_{i=1}^{N_1} \sum_{j=1}^{N_2} M_{ij} \|X_i - \mu_X\|^2,$$

$$\sigma_Y^2 = \sum_{i=1}^{N_1} \sum_{j=1}^{N_2} M_{ij} \|Y_j - \mu_Y\|^2 \tag{5}$$

The intuition behind this Ansatz will become clearer as we proceed. Having set the four parameters—the centroids and the variances—we now estimate the translation $t$ and the scale $s$ parameters.

Differentiating (4) w.r.t. the translation parameter $t$ and setting the result to zero, we get

$$t = \sum_{i=1}^{N_1} \sum_{j=1}^{N_2} M_{ij} \left[ R(\theta) \frac{(Y_j - \mu_Y)}{\sqrt{s}\sigma_Y} - \frac{\sqrt{s}(X_i - \mu_X)}{\sigma_X} \right] = 0. \tag{6}$$

Equation (6) directly follows from the Ansatz for the centroids. Similarly, differentiating (4) w.r.t. the scale parameter $s$ and setting the result to zero, we get

$$s^2 = \frac{\sum_{i=1}^{N_1} \sum_{j=1}^{N_2} M_{ij} \|X_i - \mu_X\|^2 \sigma_Y^2}{\sum_{i=1}^{N_1} \sum_{j=1}^{N_2} M_{ij} \|Y_j - \mu_Y\|^2 \sigma_X^2} = 1 \tag{7}$$

Equation (7) directly follows from the Ansatz for the variances. We have shown that the translation and scale parameters can be removed from the objective function since they are annihilated by the centroids and variances. From (6) and (7), we may simplify the objective function in (4):

$$\min_{M,\theta} E(M,\theta) = \sum_{i=1}^{N_1} \sum_{j=1}^{N_2} M_{ij} \left( \|\frac{(X_i - \mu_X)}{\sigma_X} - R(\theta)\frac{(Y_j - \mu_Y)}{\sigma_Y}\|^2 - \alpha \right)$$

$$\text{subject to } \sum_{i=1}^{N_1} M_{ij} \leq 1, \ \sum_{j=1}^{N_2} M_{ij} \leq 1, \text{ and } M_{ij} \in \{0,1\}. \tag{8}$$

The match matrix $M$ is actually a correspondence matrix. Assume for the moment that the correspondences $M_{ij}$ and the rotation matrix $R(\theta)$ are known. It is easy to show that the Ansatz for the centroids and the variances reduces to the Procrustes centroids and variances in (3). In addition, the objective function in (8) reduces to the Procrustes distance measure between the point-sets $X$ and $Y$.

Merely showing that the Procrustes distance emerges when we set the correspondence and the rotation matrices is not enough. We need an algorithm for the simultaneous estimation of the correspondence and rotation matrices as well as the the centroids and variances since they are functions of the match matrix.

The above optimization problem in (8) contains two interlocking optimization problems—one on the rotation between the two point-sets and the other on the point-to-point feature correspondences. When the correspondences are known, a constrained *least squares* problem results from which the rotation matrix can be obtained. When the rotation is known, we obtain a *linear assignment* problem [1] for the correspondences. (The presence of outliers makes our problem slightly different from the traditional linear assignment problem, but for the most part we ignore the technical distinction between the two.) While polynomial time linear assignment algorithms exist in the literature, we'll describe a new algorithm that is better suited to interact with the constrained least squares solution for the rotation. The result is a two stage algorithm which alternates between solving for the rotation and the correspondence match matrix.

The main difficulty in jointly solving for the rotation and the correspondence lies in the seemingly disparate natures of the two problems, one continuous, the other combinatorial. Our approach is designed to overcome this problem. First, ignore the effect of outliers on the match matrix in (8). The match matrix then becomes a *permutation matrix* with binary entries and all rows and columns summing to one. Then we invoke the Birkhoff-von Neumann theorem which states that "the set of $(N \times N)$ doubly stochastic matrices is the convex hull of the set of $(N \times N)$ permutation matrices" [12]. (A doubly stochastic matrix is a square matrix with all positive entries and rows and columns summing to one.) In other words, permutation matrices (or the permutation group) are the vertices of an $N$ dimensional doubly stochastic polytope. Consequently, the linear assignment problem can be solved by linear programming and related interior-point methods which relax the constraint that the match matrix entries be binary and merely require them to be positive. Due to the linear objective, the solution always occurs at a vertex of the doubly stochastic polytope—a permutation matrix. Following the Birkhoff–von-Neumann theorem, we relax the match matrix constraints from permutation matrix constraints to doubly stochastic matrix constraints. (When outliers are included, the above description is slightly modified). Doubly stochastic matrix constraints require positivity of each match matrix entry with rows and columns summing to one. We enforce the row and column constraints using Lagrange parameters and the positivity constraint via a *barrier function* [13]:

$$F(M,\theta,\kappa,\lambda) = \sum_{i=1}^{N_1} \sum_{j=1}^{N_2} M_{ij} \left( \|\frac{(X_i - \mu_X)}{\sigma_X} - R(\theta)\frac{(Y_j - \mu_Y)}{\sigma_Y}\|^2 - \alpha \right) \quad (9)$$

$$+ \sum_{i=1}^{N_1} \kappa_i \left( \sum_{j=1}^{N_2+1} M_{ij} - 1 \right) + \sum_{j=1}^{N_2} \lambda_j \left( \sum_{i=1}^{N_1+1} M_{ij} - 1 \right) + \frac{1}{\beta} \sum_{i=1}^{N_1+1} \sum_{j=1}^{N_2+1} M_{ij} \log M_{ij}.$$

In (9), $\kappa$ and $\lambda$ are two Lagrange parameters enforcing the row and column constraints respectively and $\beta > 0$ is a control parameter of an $x \log x$ *entropy* barrier function [14, 20] which enforces the positivity constraint. We have transformed the original mixed continuous-combinatorial optimization problem into a nonlinear optimization problem.

The entropy barrier function used above can be formally derived using the *saddle-point* approximation—a well known technique in statistical physics [10, 20]. The details are beyond the scope of this paper.

## 3.2 The Softassign Procrustes Algorithm

Moving on to the development of the algorithm, first note that all quantities in (9) are continuous valued. We now derive an algorithm which alternates between finding the spatial mapping and the correspondences.

Fixing the rotation for the moment, we can solve for the match matrix $M$ in the free energy of (9). Minimizing (9) w.r.t. $M$, we get

$$M_{ij} = \exp \left[ -\beta \left( \| \frac{(X_i - \mu_X)}{\sigma_X} - R(\theta) \frac{(Y_j - \mu_Y)}{\sigma_Y} \|^2 - \alpha + \kappa_i + \lambda_j \right) - 1 \right] \quad (10)$$

In (10), $\beta$ is held fixed and we have yet to determine the two Lagrange parameters $\kappa$ and $\lambda$. The exponentiation in (10) keeps all the match matrix entries positive and is a consequence of using the $x \log x$ barrier function. Solving for the two Lagrange parameters using a gradient ascent approach is likely to be slow and inefficient. Fortunately, the row and column constraints in (8) and (10) can be efficiently solved using a remarkable theorem due to Sinkhorn [16]: A doubly stochastic matrix is obtained from any square matrix with positive entries by the simple process of alternating row and column normalizations. (Once again, the presence of outliers leads to minor modifications to Sinkhorn's theorem.) While it may appear that Sinkhorn's theorem is unrelated to the two Lagrange parameters $\kappa$ and $\lambda$, this is not the case. Solving for the Lagrange parameters (alternating between solving for $\kappa$ and then $\lambda$ rather than steepest ascent) is *identical* to Sinkhorn's algorithm [14]. With $\beta$ held fixed, the exponentiation in (10) followed by Sinkhorn's algorithm yields a doubly stochastic matrix as expected. Slowly increasing $\beta$ results in a permutation matrix and the optimal solution to the linear assignment problem [12, 14]. Since the exponentiation and Sinkhorn's algorithm at fixed $\beta$ is central to our approach, we refer to this as the softassign.

Fixing the correspondence match matrix, we can solve for the rotation. The rotation matrix is updated using closed form solutions at each temperature with the match matrix held fixed. Differentiating (8) w.r.t. $\theta$ and setting the result to zero, we get

$$\theta = \arctan\left(\frac{\sum_{i=1}^{N_1}\sum_{j=1}^{N_2} M_{ij}\left[X_i^c(2)Y_j^c(1) - X_i^c(1)Y_j^c(2)\right]}{\sum_{i=1}^{N_1}\sum_{j=1}^{N_2} M_{ij}\left[X_i^c(1)Y_j^c(1) + X_i^c(2)Y_j^c(2)\right]}\right) \tag{11}$$

where

$$X_i^c = \frac{X_i - \mu_X}{\sigma_X}, \text{ and } Y_j^c = \frac{Y_j - \mu_Y}{\sigma_Y}.$$

The numbers inside the parenthesis [$X(1)$ or $X(2)$] denote the abscissa and ordinate of the point-set. Having specified the rotation update, we turn to the estimation of the centroids and variances. Differentiating (8) w.r.t. $(\mu_X, \mu_Y)$ and setting the result to zero, we obtain

$$\sum_{i=1}^{N_1}\sum_{j=1}^{N_2} \frac{M_{ij}}{\sigma_X}\left[\frac{(X_i - \mu_X)}{\sigma_X} - R(\theta)\frac{(Y_j - \mu_Y)}{\sigma_Y}\right] = 0$$

$$\sum_{i=1}^{N_1}\sum_{j=1}^{N_2} \frac{M_{ij}}{\sigma_Y}\left[\frac{(X_i - \mu_X)}{\sigma_X} - R(\theta)\frac{(Y_j - \mu_Y)}{\sigma_Y}\right] = 0 \tag{12}$$

It is straightforward to show that the Ansatz for the centroids in (5) is one solution to (12). (Showing that it is a minimum is also straightforward.) The same approach does not work for the variances, however. We think that it is difficult to construct an objective function on the centroids *and* the variances such that the Procrustes distance emerges as a minimum. Due to this inability to specify a global optimization problem on all relevant parameters, the Ansätze for the variances in (5) remain.

As the deterministic annealing parameter $\beta$ is increased, the match matrix entries "harden"—they approach binary values. Outlier rejection occurs in the limit when $\beta \to \infty$ with the outliers becoming binary valued. We do not have a proof of convergence (to a local minimum) for the softassign Procrustes algorithm. The presence of the Ansätze for the centroids and the variances makes it difficult to prove convergence. Variable and constant definitions can be found in Table 1.

**The Softassign Procrustes Algorithm**
**Initialization:** $\theta$ to zero, $\beta$ to $\beta_0$ and $\hat{M}_{ij}$ to $1 + \epsilon_{ij}$
Center and scale each point-set as in the Procrustes method.
**Begin A: Deterministic Annealing.** Do A until $\beta \geq \beta_f$
    **Begin B:** Do B until $M$ converges or # of iterations > $I_0$
        **Begin C: Centroids, Variances and Rotation matrix update.**
        Update $\mu_X$, $\mu_Y$, $\sigma_X$, $\sigma_Y$ using the Ansatz in (5)
        Update $\theta$ using analytical solution in (11)
    **End C**
    **Begin D: Softassign.**
        $Q_{ij} \leftarrow -\|\frac{(X_i - \mu_X)}{\sigma_X} - R(\theta)\frac{(Y_j - \mu_Y)}{\sigma_Y}\|^2 + \alpha$

$$M_{ij}^0 \leftarrow \exp(\beta Q_{ij})$$

**Begin E: Sinkhorn.** Do E until $\hat{M}$ converges or # of iterations
$> I_1$

Update $\hat{M}$ by normalizing the rows:

$$\hat{M}_{ij}^1 \leftarrow \frac{\hat{M}_{ij}^0}{\sum_{j=1}^{N_2+1} \hat{M}_{ij}^0}$$

Update $\hat{M}$ by normalizing the columns:

$$\hat{M}_{ij}^0 \leftarrow \frac{\hat{M}_{ij}^1}{\sum_{i=1}^{N_1+1} \hat{M}_{ij}^1}$$

**End E**
**End D**
**End B**
$$\beta \leftarrow \beta_r \beta$$
**End A**

**Table 1.** Variable and constant definitions for the softassign Procrustes matching algorithm

| | |
|---|---|
| $\beta$ | control parameter of the deterministic annealing method |
| $\beta_0$ | initial value of the control parameter $\beta$ |
| $\beta_f$ | maximum value of the control parameter $\beta$ |
| $\beta_r$ | rate at which the control parameter $\beta$ is increased |
| $\{\epsilon_{ij}\}$ | small positive random variable |
| $\{M_{ij}\}$ | match matrix variables |
| $\{\hat{M}_{ij}\}$ | match matrix variables including the outliers |
| $\{Q_{ij}\}$ | $\{-\|\frac{(X_i-\mu_X)}{\sigma_X} - R(\theta)\frac{(Y_j-\mu_Y)}{\sigma_Y}\|^2 + \alpha\}$ |
| $I_0$ | maximum # of iterations allowed at each value of the control parameter, $\beta$ |
| $I_1$ | maximum # of iterations allowed for Sinkhorn's method (back and forth row and column normalizations) |

## 4  Results

We have applied the softassign Procrustes matching algorithm to the problem of autoradiograph alignment [15]. Primate autoradiographs of functional (metabolic) activation were obtained using the 2-DG method developed by [18]. Alignment of sequential pairwise sections is the first stage of reconstructing a 3-D high resolution functional map of the primate brain.

Slices 379-385 (left parietal and temporal cortex) are shown in Figure 1. First we run a Canny edge detector [6] on each slice. The edge detector is a single scale (Gaussian filter with width $\sigma$) edge detector incorporating hysteresis and non-maximum suppression. The edge detector outputs are shown in Figure 2. The point sets $X$ and $Y$ are obtained from the edge images. Since many thousands of points result, the points are first clustered in order to reduce the point count. The degree of clustering was chosen to yield approximately 200 points in each point-set, as shown in Figure 3.

Having obtained the point sets, we now execute the softassign Procrustes algorithm. Exactly as described above, the point-sets are first centered and scaled as in the original Procrustes algorithm. The parameter values were: $\beta_0 = 10\sqrt{N_1 N_2}$, $\beta_{max} = 1000\sqrt{N_1 N_2}$, $\beta_r = 0.93$, $\alpha = 0$. The maximum number of iterations in each Sinkhorn step was 30. We allowed a maximum of two iterations at each temperature.

The results are shown in Figure 5. Initial conditions are shown in Figure 4. The x's and o's indicate the coordinate locations of the edge (point) features. Note that a subset of the x's and o's do not match. The method has discarded them as outliers. The matrix $M_{ii}$ has all zero rows (columns) corresponding to the outliers. all zero. All experiments used exactly same parameters. Despite the much larger rotation between some slices, the softassign Procrustes algorithm had no difficulty aligning the point-sets and discarding outliers in the process. The method is not restricted to merely aligning adjacent pairwise sections. The results shown in Figure 5 and summarized in Table 2 were obtained with an eye towards averaging of forms. Incorporating correspondence and outlier rejection in Procrustes averaging is a natural extension of our approach.

**Table 2.** Procrustes matching parameters

| Slices | Rotation | X-Centroid | Y-centroid | X-Variance | Y-Variance |
|--------|----------|------------|------------|------------|------------|
| 379 and 380 | -3.3 | [-0.0011 , 0.0013] | [-0.0039,0.0093] | 0.8996 | 0.8789 |
| 384 and 385 | 9.7 | [-0.0022 , 0.0020] | [-0.0044 , 0.0056] | 0.8556 | 0.8577 |
| 379 and 385 | 5.3 | [0.0009, 0.0024] | [-0.0034,0.0063] | 0.8957 | 0.8704 |
| 380 and 384 | 1.7 | [-0.0022,0.0068] | [0.0005, -0.0030] | 0.8838 | 0.8750 |
| 379 and 384 | 3.0 | [0.0012,0.0022] | [-0.0002,0.0022] | 0.8977 | 0.8618 |
| 380 and 385 | 9.7 | [-0.0011, 0.0078] | [-0.0025,0.0014] | 0.8624 | 0.8545 |

## 5  Discussion and Extensions

This paper has extended the Procrustes distance measure to a distance function over the union of point-sets with different point counts. Previous work [9], [5] deal with the related problem of minimizing metrics within linear subspaces of the tangent space to the space of these shapes. In this approach there is no combinatorial problem, only a geometric one, the solution to which emerges directly from the nesting of a projection operation inside a linear approximation of the Procrustes step. These and related algorithms have no equivalent to the notion of "outlier" that gives the softassign Procrustes algorithm its power. And this, in turn, leads to the distinction between the two classes of Procrustes parameters in the alternating algorithm here. Translation and rotation could be incorporated in the minimizing algebra of alternations, but variance could not be. This is because translation and rotation deal with the same relation between two forms that the matching function is attempting to minimize, but the scaling step is a function of only one form at a time–it has nothing to do with the actual least-squares superposition–and thus cannot be imputed to one form by any computation based in the other. The scale $\sigma_X$ of a form $X$ is *not* the minimizer of any summed squared interlandmark distance. [4] One can continuously pass from one form to a matched form by a smooth curve in one of these shape manifolds, along which arc-length is approximated by the Procrustes distance formula; but one *cannot* continuously pass from one form to a form having one landmark more or fewer. The sum-of-squares jumps *discontinuously* from 1 to $\frac{(N+1)}{N}$, and needs to be reset by a jump. That is, the Kendall shape metrics of different point counts are incommensurate. The Ansätze of this paper are all entailed in the embedding of the shape manifold in the original picture space, where the structural difference between variance and the other two parameters is not so clear. At their mathematical foundation, however, translation and rotation pertain to similarities over the same manifold; they are thus quite different from scaling, which links manifolds of different point count.

For an extension of constructions like these to the production of averaged forms, correlations between forms and their causes or consequences, and the like, one can speculate on a variety of approaches. All define the average as a form showing the least summed squared Procrustes distance to the forms of the sample–the Fréchet mean–but they would differ in the combinatorics of that average. In one approach, once the forms are matched they are modeled as combinations of isolated points and curves, and averaged in that hybrid Procrustes space by the method of [9], which matches outline arcs rather than outline samples and thus ignores point counts along curves. That is, outliers would be estimated, when appropriate, as linear interpolants of the points of curves nearest to them, and then treated by the standard (noncombinatorial) Procrustes tactics. In a second approach, the standard Procrustes averaging algorithm would be applied (fit all forms to one form, average the fitted values, and iterate), modified for use in our context of correspondence and outlier estimation: the only points that could be "averaged" are those that were never considered to be outliers in any step of the averaging [7]. (While our initial foray into averaging [7] estimated spatial mappings and correspondences during the averaging step, it did not include the crucial Procrustes centering and rescaling steps.) If this new algorithm resulted in a nonempty point-set, that would be "an average"; of course, we have no idea how many averages exist for any set of outlines in this approach. In a third possibility, one would average the matrices $M$ to supply a weighted Procrustes average, where the weighting is by tendency to be an outlier. We have no data sets yet to which these speculations can be turned, but expect this to be a topic of an IPMI 1999 submission.

## Acknowledgments

Anand Rangarajan and Haili Chui are supported by a grant from the Whitaker Foundation. Fred Bookstein is supported by NIH grants DA–09009 and GM–37251. The former grant is jointly supported by the National Institute on Drug Abuse, the National Institute of Mental Health, and the National Institute on Aging as part of the Human Brain Project.

# References

1. D. P. Bertsekas and J. N. Tsitsiklis. *Parallel and Distributed Computation: Numerical Methods*. Prentice-Hall, Englewood Cliffs, NJ, 1989.
2. P. J. Besl and N. D. McKay. A method for registration of 3-d shapes. *IEEE Trans. Patt. Anal. Mach. Intell.*, 14(2):239–256, Feb. 1992.
3. M. Black and A. Rangarajan. On the Unification of Line Processes, Outlier Detection and Robust Statistics with Applications in Early Vision. *Intl. J. Computer Vision*, 19(1):57–91, 1996.
4. F. L. Bookstein. *Morphometric tools for landmark data: Geometry and biology*. Cambridge University Press, 1991.
5. F. L. Bookstein. Landmark methods for forms without landmarks: Localizing group differences in outline shape. In A. Amini, F. L. Bookstein, and D. Wilson, editors, *Proc. of the Workshop on Mathematical Methods in Biomedical Image Analysis*, pages 279–289. IEEE Computer Society Press, 1996.
6. J. Canny. A Computational Approach to Edge Detection. *IEEE Trans. on Pattern Analysis and Machine Intelligence*, 8(6):679–698, Nov. 1986.
7. S. Gold, A. Rangarajan, and E. Mjolsness. Learning with preknowledge: clustering with point and graph matching distance measures. *Neural Computation*, 8(4):787–804, 1996.
8. C. Goodall. Procrustes methods in the statistical analysis of shape. *J. R. Statist. Soc. B*, 53(2):285–339, 1991.
9. W. D. K. Green. The thin-plate spline and images with curving features. In K. V. Mardia, C. A. Gill, and I. L. Dryden, editors, *Proceedings in image fusion and shape variability techniques*, pages 79–97. Leeds University Press, 1996.
10. J. Hertz, A. Krogh, and R. G. Palmer. *Introduction to the Theory of Neural Computation*, volume 1 of *A Lecture Notes volume in the Santa Fe Institute Studies in the Sciences of Complexity*. Addison–Wesley, New York, 1991.
11. D. G. Kendall. Shape-manifolds, Procrustean metrics and complex projective spaces. *Bulletin of the London Mathematical Society*, 16:81–121, 1984.
12. J. J. Kosowsky and A. L. Yuille. The invisible hand algorithm: Solving the assignment problem with statistical physics. *Neural Networks*, 7(3):477–490, 1994.
13. D. Luenberger. *Linear and Nonlinear Programming*. Addison–Wesley, Reading, MA, 1984.
14. A. Rangarajan, S. Gold, and E. Mjolsness. A novel optimizing network architecture with applications. *Neural Computation*, 8(5):1041–1060, 1996.
15. A. Rangarajan, E. Mjolsness, S. Pappu, L. Davachi, P. Goldman-Rakic, and J. Duncan. A Robust Point Matching Algorithm for Autoradiograph Alignment. In K. H. Hohne and R. Kikinis, editors, *Fourth International Conference on Visualization in Biomedical Computing*, Lecture Notes in Computer Science, LNCS 1131, pages 277–286. Springer, New York, NY, 1996.

16. R. Sinkhorn.   A relationship between arbitrary positive matrices and doubly stochastic matrices. *Ann. Math. Statist.*, 35:876–879, 1964.
17. C. Small. *The Statistical theory of shape.* Springer-Verlag, 1996.
18. L. Sokoloff, M. Revich, C. Kennedy, M. H. DesRosiers, C. S. Patlak, K. D. Pettigrew, O. Sakurada, and M. Shinohara. The C14-deoxyglucose method for the measurement of local cerebral glucose utilization: theory, procedure, and normal values in the conscious and anesthetized albino rat. *J. Neurochem.*, 28:897–916, 1977.
19. P. Van den Elsen. *Multimodality matching of brain images.* PhD thesis, Utrecht University, Utrecht, Netherlands, 1993.
20. A. L. Yuille and J. J. Kosowsky.   Statistical physics algorithms that converge. *Neural Computation*, 6(3):341–356, May 1994.

**Figures**

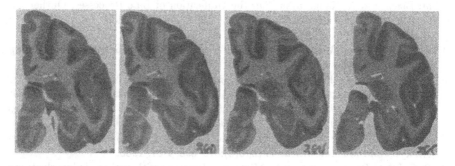

**Fig. 1.** Slices (a) 379 (b) 380 (c) 384 and (d) 385 of primate autoradiographs of functional (metabolic) activation. The coronal slices correspond to the left parietal and temporal cortex. After digitization, the slices were sampled down into $\simeq$ 475x350 pixels each with a resulting spatial resolution of $\simeq$ 100$\mu$m.

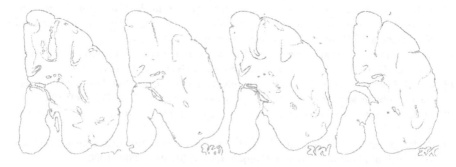

**Fig. 2.** Canny edge images corresponding to the autoradiograph slices of Figure 1. Note the number of edges that are not in common in (a) - (d). While we have not dwelled on the instability of edge detection, it is yet another reason for our strong emphasis on robustness.

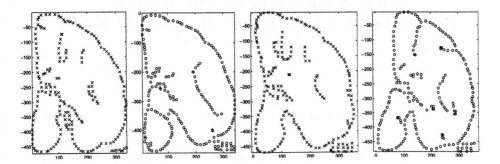

**Fig. 3.** Point-sets corresponding to the edge images. There were approximately 200 points in each point-set.

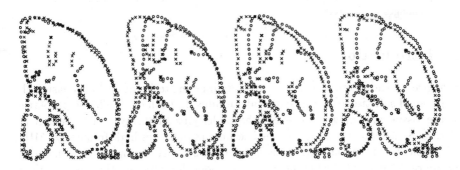

**Fig. 4.** Initial Condition

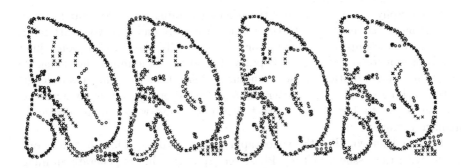

**Fig. 5.** Final solution found by the method. Again note the number of (mostly internal) x's and o's that do not match but remain isolated during overlay. These have been rejected as outliers and play no role towards the final stages of the algorithm.

# Acoustic and Elastic Imaging to Model Disease-Induced Changes in Soft Tissue Structure

Pawan Chaturvedi, Michael F. Insana and Timothy J. Hall

University of Kansas Medical Center
Kansas City, KS 66160-7234, USA

**Abstract.** Ultrasonic techniques are presented for the study of soft biological tissue structure and function. Changes in echo waveforms caused by microscopic variations in the elastic properties of tissue can reveal disease mechanism, in vivo. On a larger scale, elasticity imaging describes the macroscopic elastic properties of soft tissues. We present an analysis framework and preliminary results for studying disease-induced changes in soft tissue using these two acoustic techniques to investigate structural changes at different scales.

## 1   Introduction

Sonography and elastography are two body imaging techniques that measure the response of soft tissue to a mechanical stimulus. In both cases, elastic properties of the tissue are imaged to reveal the underlying anatomy and to search for disease. Sonography is an established technique that uses high-frequency (MHz) vibrations to probe the variations in small-scale elastic properties. Conversely, elastography is a new technique currently under development that uses static or very low-frequency vibrations (Hz) to probe the variations in large-scale elastic properties. Together, the two techniques describe important material properties over a broad size range that are useful for discovering and modeling disease mechanisms in soft biological tissues.

Sonography is a spatial map of the echoes generated as a broad-band pulse of high-frequency sound energy travels through tissue. Sound energy is scattered at sites of acoustic impedance fluctuations. [1] Specifically, the tissue response function is proportional to the second spatial derivative of the impedance along the direction of wave motion. Tissue structures of size near the central wavelength of the probing sound pulse scatter the most sound energy, although structures between 1 $\mu$m to 1 mm will interact with ultrasound waves in the diagnostic frequency range.

It is well known that the sonographic image structure does not map one-to-one with the tissue structure. Phase sensitive transducers generate an image speckle pattern that is characteristic of both the tissue and the imaging system. Therefore, sonography does not provide detailed information about tissue

---

[1] Specific acoustic impedance is the ratio of acoustic pressure to particle velocity, $z = p/u$. For plane waves of sound, the square of the acoustic impedance reduces to the ratio of mass density to adiabatic compressibility, $z^2 = \rho/\kappa$.

structure. However, echo formation is a linear process that can be inverted using signal processing techniques to recover information about the underlying tissue structure [1]. By carefully selecting the size of the analysis volume element, an accurate statistical description of the average size, number, shape, and impedance of scattering structures in the volume element can be obtained and displayed as parametric ultrasound images. The methods of *quantitative ultrasound* (QUS) have been used to describe the internal microstructure of ocular lesions [2], myocardial infarctions [3], and renal vasculature [4], in vivo.

Information about large-scale elastic properties, from 1 mm to 10 cm, is available with elastic imaging techniques. For example, acoustic elastography is a technique that compares ultrasound echoes recorded before and after tissue compression [5]. Tissue displacements at each location are calculated using time-delay correlation techniques, and the gradient of the displacement field yields a strain image. If the stress field applied by the compressor is known, an elastic modulus (stiffness) image can be computed from the constitutive equations of continuum mechanics. Alternatively, shear waves generated by low-frequency external vibrations ($<1$ KHz) are detected by Doppler ultrasound [6] or magnetic resonance angiography (MRA) techniques [7] and processed to form strain images. Others have used natural body movements, such as pulsatile blood flow, to measure tissue stiffness [8].

All of these techniques describe the macroscopic stiffness of tissue, the same property involved in one of the oldest and most successful diagnostic procedures — palpation. A physician's hand displaces the surface of a patient's body while the finger tips sense for variations in the internal stress field that indicate the presence of a stiff region. Cancerous tumors are often 10 to 100 times stiffer than the surrounding tissue [9]. This very large object contrast is responsible for the success of the self examination for breast cancer. While palpation is only sensitive to lesions near the surface of the skin, elastic imaging provides a quantitative measure of stiffness deep into the body.

Tissue models are important as basic research tools for understanding how normal tissue architectures are altered with disease. In addition, it is essential to understand the statistical properties of the object to evaluate the sensitivity and specificity of these techniques for detecting altered structures and for developing object priors for Bayesian estimation. The purpose of this paper is to outline a method we are developing for modeling the internal structure of normal and diseased soft tissues using quantitative ultrasound and elastography. Examples of measurements in kidney tissues are discussed throughout the paper.

## 2 Mechanics of Tissue Morphology

The cells of a biological organ system may be divided into two classes: parenchyma is the functioning element and stroma is the supporting structural framework. Both elements are modified with age and disease in a well-defined and characteristic manner that is the basis for the histological definitions of disease.

The stroma is a network of collagen and elastin fibers [10] that has an acoustic impedance much higher than the surrounding cells. On the scale that ultrasound is sensitive, these networks are the principal sources of acoustic scattering. Since the sound energy interacts at the scatterer surface normal to the direction of wave propagation, ultrasound is not sensitive to the *connections* among the collagen and elastin fibers. It is most sensitive to tissue microstructure — the same level of information provided by histology but for the perfused living tissues of the body. On this microscopic scale, tissue can be modeled as an inhomogeneous continuum that contains both randomly and periodically positioned sound scatterers. Incoherent scattering occurs due to the randomly positioned structure and is characterized by the form factor matrix of the acoustic impedance [1]. Coherent scattering occurs due to the periodic impedance structure and is characterized by the phase coupling matrix of the acoustic impedance [11]. Both incoherent and coherent scattering are parts of the tissue response function.

On the scale of a centimeter, tissue is a homogeneous, linear, viscoelastic continuum. It is homogeneous at this scale because the mass density and compressibility converge to average values within tolerable errors [12]. Most soft tissues exhibit linear stress-strain curves for strains less than 2%. Tissues are viscoelastic since there is stress relaxation when they are deformed and held, and their stress-strain curves exhibit hysteresis for cyclic deformation.

It should be clear that while the microscopic and macroscopic structures of tissue are related, the information about the structure provided by sonography (via quantitative ultrasound techniques) and elastography are largely uncorrelated. For example, the sonogram of an object consisting of a circular lesion is nearly uniform as seen from Fig. 1a, while the elastogram (Fig. 1b) shows an internal structure. This phantom contained a random distribution of independent graphite fibers embedded in gelatin. The sonogram is uniform, except at the interfaces between regions where there exists a phase relationship between scattering sites, because the concentration and size of graphite fibers is uniform. However the gelatin matrix is a weakly scattering, collagenous network that is connected over a long range. The gelatin in the targets was stiffer than the gelatin in the background. Fig. 1 exemplifies how both imaging techniques are needed to probe the microstructure of graphite fibers and the macrostructure of the collagenous network in the sample.

The normal structure of living tissues is remodeled when it is subjected to stress, as every weight lifter and mountain climber knows. Environmental changes like hypoxia, trauma, and disease disturb the normal homeostasis of the body. The cells of the tissues respond by changing their mass, metabolism, and intra- and extracellular structure.

Often the remodeling is beneficial. In some cases, however, tissue remodeling is detrimental and requires medical intervention to prevent death. For example, when renal functional mass is reduced because of trauma, disease, substance abuse or natural aging, so is the number of filtering units or glomeruli. The remaining glomeruli enlarge to compensate for the loss. However, glomerular hypertrophy damages the capillary lumen, producing sclerotic lesions and hy-

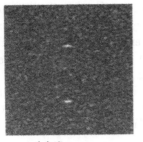
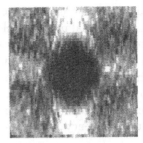

(a) Sonogram        (b) Elastogram

**Fig. 1.** Sonogram and elastogram of a phantom containing a circular lesion that is approximately 3 times stiffer than the background. The central dark area in the elastogram shows a lesion that is approximately 8 mm in diameter. The bright regions are the artifacts caused by stress concentration.

pertension, which further accelerates parenchymal loss. The result is end-stage renal disease (ESRD) that requires dialysis or transplantation to maintain homeostasis. ESRD may be preventable once its mechanisms are understood and if the hypertrophy and hypertension can be controlled. Ultrasonic analysis of the microstructure is the only technique to monitor the evolution of glomerular hypertrophy and sclerosis in kidneys, in vivo. Elastography can follow the vascular remodeling from chronic hypertension that stiffens the tissue. The analyses together show how microscopic disease develops into a process that affects the entire organ. The unique capability of acoustic and elastic imaging methods is their ability to provide morphometric information over the time course of a process without interfering with the progression.

## 3   Quantitative ultrasonic analysis

Since microstructural changes frequently occur early in the progression of a disease, observing changes in scatterer size provides valuable information about the evolution of the disease. Recently, the average scatterer size $D$ has been used to monitor microscopic changes in tissue histology [2, 4]. $D$ is estimated by first normalizing the rf echo data to eliminate instrumentation dependent properties, and then comparing the tissue response function thus obtained from the experiment against empirical models [13]. Estimation is performed in two steps to permit us to use a linear data model,

$$\mathbf{X} = \mathbf{HR} + \mathbf{N} \tag{1}$$

$\mathbf{X}_{M \times 1}$ is the Fourier transform of the rf echo data, $\mathbf{R}_{M \times 1}$ is the Fourier transform of the tissue response and is a nonlinear function of $D$, $\mathbf{N}_{M \times 1}$ is the Fourier transform of a signal independent noise process, and $\mathbf{H}_{M \times M}$ is the sensitivity function that maps the object space to data space. For a linear space-invariant system, $\mathbf{H}$ is a diagonal matrix, yielding a system of uncoupled equations.

Fundamental to the procedure for determining $D$ described above is the assumption that scattering from the target is incoherent. In general, however, both coherent and incoherent components contribute to the rf echo data. From solutions to the inhomogeneous wave equation, it can be shown that the total acoustic backscatter coefficient for a scattering volume $V$ illuminated by a plane wave of spatial frequency $k = 2\pi f/c$ is given by [1]

$$
\sigma_b(k) = \frac{k^4 H^2(k)}{16\pi^2 V} \left[ \int_V \int_V \langle\gamma_1\rangle\langle\gamma_2\rangle \, \exp\left\{-i\mathbf{K}\cdot(\mathbf{r}_1 - \mathbf{r}_2)\right\} \, dv_1 \, dv_2 \right.
$$

$$
+ \int_V \int_V b_\gamma(\mathbf{r}_1, \mathbf{r}_2) \left\{ \langle(\gamma_1 - \langle\gamma_1\rangle)^2\rangle\langle(\gamma_2 - \langle\gamma_2\rangle)^2\rangle \right\}^{1/2}
$$

$$
\left. \times \exp\left\{-i\mathbf{K}\cdot(\mathbf{r}_1 - \mathbf{r}_2)\right\} \, dv_1 \, dv_2 \right] . \tag{2}
$$

In Eq. (2), $\mathbf{r_1}$ and $\mathbf{r_2}$ are the position vectors of two locations in the medium, and $\gamma = \gamma_\kappa + \gamma_\rho$ represents the fluctuation in compressibility $\kappa$ and density $\rho$, with $\langle.\rangle$ denoting the ensemble mean. $\sigma_b(k) \propto |X(k)|^2$ in Eq. (1).

The first term is the coherent scattering contribution and the second term is the incoherent scattering contribution. By assuming that the medium contains $N$ small, discrete, acoustically identical scatterers, and the medium inside the scatterers is uniform, we can show that [11]

$$
\sigma_b(k) \approx \frac{k^4 H^2(k)}{16\pi^2 V} \left[ \langle\gamma_o\rangle^2 \, \mathbf{w}^t \, \underline{\mathbf{C}} \, \mathbf{w} + V^2 \left(\langle\gamma_o^2\rangle - \langle\gamma_o\rangle^2\right) \, \mathbf{w}^t \, \underline{\mathbf{F}} \, \mathbf{w} \right] , \tag{3}
$$

where $\langle\gamma_o\rangle$ and $\langle\gamma_o^2\rangle$ are the mean and mean squared fluctuations in acoustic impedance per scatterer, $\mathbf{w}$ is a column vector of the volume fractions occupied by the scatterers, $\underline{\mathbf{C}}$ is the *inter-scatterer* phase coupling matrix whose diagonal terms are all zero, and $\underline{\mathbf{F}}$ is the diagonal acoustic form factor matrix representing *intra-scatterer* coupling $(F(k) = \langle|R(k)|^2\rangle$ for estimating $D$ from Eq. (1)).

In the absence of phase coherence, $\sigma_b(k)$ cannot exhibit frequency dependence stronger than $k^4$, as seen from Eq. (3). $k^4$ dependence is characteristic of Rayleigh scattering observed for sparse distributions of randomly positioned small scatterers. However, as the concentration of scatterers in the volume increases, the random medium becomes more ordered, and in some cases results in a stronger frequency dependence of the backscatter coefficient. Such behavior has been observed experimentally by Waag and Campbell [14] and by Chen and Zagzebski [15]. For example, Chen and Zagzebski showed that a gel phantom containing $42\mu m$ glass spheres that occupy 50% of the total volume, when probed with a 3.5 MHz transducer, exhibits $k^{4.6}$ dependence of the backscatter coefficient. For these conditions, Eq. (3) predicts $k^{4.92}$ dependence of the backscatter coefficient.

This scattering formulation is ideally suited to renal diseases that result in a loss of glomeruli. Glomeruli are the primary source of scattering at frequencies below 5 MHz [4]. The loss of glomeruli reduces the number density of scatterers, but it also increases the size of the remaining glomeruli as the kidney attempts to maintain functional capacity. Such changes, and their effect on the frequency dependence of the backscattered signals, are conveniently modeled by Eq. (3). Eq. (3) also provides a mechanism for testing the validity of the assumption of a random medium that is central to the idea of determining average scatterer size.

The algorithm we employ to estimate $D$ performs a mean squared error (MSE) comparison between the tissue response estimated from Eq. (1), and an empirical tissue response model, as shown in Fig. 2. The choice of estimator for computing the tissue response $R(k)$ depends on the available prior information. When little prior information is available, the maximum likelihood (ML) estimator is used for estimating the tissue response $R(k)$. $R(k)$ is obtained by taking the ratio of the rf data $X(k)$ to the transducer sensitivity function $H(k)$; equivalently, the form factor $F$ is estimated using $\hat{F}(k) \propto \langle|X(k)|^2\rangle/|H(k)|^2$ [13]. $|X(k)|^2$ is the power spectral density (PSD), and is estimated with a periodogram. The ML estimate is asymptotically unbiased, but results in unacceptably high variance for thin C-scan slices (Fig. 3) and for noisy data segments. High noise level is particularly troublesome in imaging applications since it degrades target visibility. For example, reconstruction from a 1-mm thick C-scan slice of a simulated kidney phantom depicted in Fig. 4a is shown in Fig. 4b for 20 dB electronic SNR. The excessive image noise renders the phantom structure almost indistinguishable.

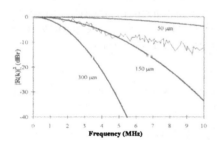

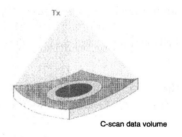

**Fig. 2.** Measured (jagged curve) and modeled (smooth curves) form factors for dog kidney data.

**Fig. 3.** Geometry of a C-scan measurement. Tx indicates the transducer position.

One way to reduce noise in the image is by incorporating additional prior knowledge. Such prior information could be available in several forms. For a Gaussian tissue response function, we can use an autoregressive (AR) model to estimate the PSD since we know that the spectrum does not have any sharp valleys. Use of an AR model results in the image shown in Fig. 4c. Another way to use prior information is by forming a maximum a posteriori (MAP) estimate from the knowledge of the statistics of the estimated parameter. Under

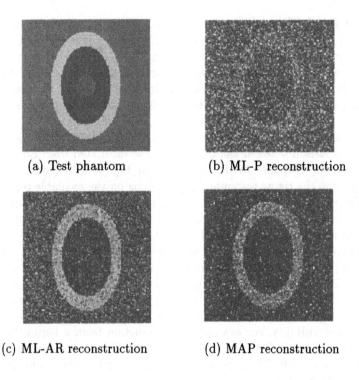

(a) Test phantom        (b) ML-P reconstruction

(c) ML-AR reconstruction        (d) MAP reconstruction

**Fig. 4.** Scatterer size images of a simulated test phantom with ML and MAP estimators. $D = 100\mu$m for the background, $D = 200\mu$m for the outer ring simulating renal cortex, $D = 50\mu$m for the inner region simulating renal medulla, and $D = 75\mu$m for the central circular region. "P" refers to the periodogram PSD estimate, and "AR" refers to an autoregressive PSD model.

the assumption of Gaussian noise, it is straightforward to show that the MAP estimate of the tissue response at frequency $k$ is

$$\hat{R}(k) = \frac{H(k)^* X(k) + \eta(k)\bar{R}(k)}{|H(k)|^2 + \eta(k)} \quad , \tag{4}$$

where $\bar{R}(k)$ represents the prior knowledge about $\langle R(k)\rangle$, and $\eta(k)$ is the weight assigned to the prior knowledge. We have shown that $\eta(k) = c_1/|H(k)|^2$, where $c_1$ is a constant, is an appropriate choice for our application [16].

By assuming that the object is uniform with $D = 100\mu$m throughout the image plane, the MAP estimate shown in Fig. 4d is obtained. Although a large reduction in the noise is apparent in both Figs. 4c and 4d, it is at the cost of an increased bias in the estimates. If our primary task is to improve detectability, biased estimates are acceptable as long as the contrast is preserved, which is clearly the case in Figs. 4c and 4d. Whether such a bias is tolerable for any given situation will depend on the specific task. For example, if we are using the actual size estimates as the indicator of a disease [17], it may be necessary to have unbiased estimates.

Histological analysis shows that there is a wide distribution of glomerular diameters in a kidney. This object distribution provides yet another source of bias in the estimates. As seen from Eq. (3), the presence of scatterers of different sizes in the volume modifies the backscatter coefficient such that it is a weighted sum of the contributions from all sizes. The weights are determined by the volumes of the scatterers; larger scatterers contribute more backscattered energy than small scatterers. Therefore, an average scatterer size estimated from the data will be biased high compared to the true mean for an object containing a wide distribution of scatterers.

To test the hypothesis, we constructed a gel phantom with two targets. In a $200 \times 185$ pixel image (Fig. 5), the background contained 90-212 $\mu$m diameter glass spheres. A circular target "A" (radius 9.5 mm) containing 90-106 $\mu$m glass spheres was centered at pixel location (100,50) in the image. Another target "B" (same radius) contained 150-180 $\mu$m glass spheres and was located 33 mm (80 pixels) below and approximately 6.25 mm (25 pixels) to the right of target "A." A 5 MHz transducer with 60% full-width-at-half-maximum bandwidth was used to capture the data at an electronic SNR of 25 dB. The rf data was attenuation-corrected. The ML reconstruction with a periodogram PSD estimate computed from a 10$\mu$sec (256 samples) slice of the phantom is shown in Fig. 5. The means for the three regions are: $\mu_b = 148.0\mu$m for the background (true mean 138.3 $\mu$m), $\mu_A = 93.8\mu$m for target A (true mean 97.7 $\mu$m), and $\mu_B = 161.7\mu$m for target B (true mean 163.1 $\mu$m). While both targets, with their narrow size distributions, provide a small negative bias, the background, with its broad size distribution shows a significant *positive* bias, as predicted by Eq. (3). As a result of large variance and the positive bias in the background (making $\mu_b \approx \mu_B$), target B is only faintly visible in the image.

Object variability reduces target detectability for two reasons. Besides biasing the estimates in such a way that contrast between the target and the background is reduced, it also results in a larger estimation variance. Many renal diseases, e.g., glomerulosclerosis that precedes ESRD, affect different glomeruli to different extents at any given time (see Section 5). Therefore, glomerular sizes in the diseased parts of a kidney also have an abnormally broad distribution. Results of the experiment described above indicate that use of only the mean of the scatterer size estimate may not be optimal for discriminating between normal and diseased tissues under these circumstances. Rather, use of the variance in conjunction with the mean may provide a more effective diagnostic technique.

# 4 Elastography

The previous section showed how QUS provides information about changes in elastic properties of the tissue at the microscopic level. Changes in macroscopic elastic properties, frequently associated with sclerosis and the formation of lesions and tumors, can be detected through elastic imaging. Elastography is a new imaging technique in which strain images are formed by computing the have unbiased estimates.

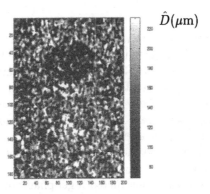

$\hat{D}(\mu m)$

**Fig. 5.** Scatterer size image of the phantom obtained with the ML-P reconstruction used for investigating the effect of object variability. The dark region at (100,50) is target A, and the bright region at (125,135) is target B.

axial displacement field for the object before and after a small amount of compression [5]. Correlation analysis is employed to estimate the displacement, and the strain image is obtained by taking a gradient of the axial displacement. Due to the different amounts of strain experienced by regions with unequal stiffness, elastography provides an image of the large scale elastic properties of the object. Throughout this paper, we will use the word elastogram to refer to strain images, with the understanding that elastic modulus images are possible from the knowledge of applied stress.

An example of an elastogram was shown in Fig. 1b. The object consisted of a cylindrical inclusion with circular cross-section embedded in a homogeneous background. The dark regions represent small strain (stiff media), and the bright regions indicate high strain (soft media). For detecting this large-scale isoechoic lesion that is stiffer than the background, the elastogram is clearly superior to the sonogram. However, there are two important features of the image that warrant discussion. First, although the lesion was circular, its image appears in the shape of a "diamond." Strain analysis using finite-element techniques reveals that when an object with a circular inclusion is compressed from the top, the strain profile for the *object* also exhibits the distortion in lesion shape. Another feature of the strain image is the appearance of "wings" that protrude vertically and horizontally from the stiff lesion. These wings caused by stress concentration are also present in the object strain profile. We observed that these artifacts are more pronounced for two-dimensional geometries (infinite cylinders) than for three-dimensional geometries (spheres), as seen later in this section.

An important part of forming the elastograms is the pre-processing required to maximize the signal-to-noise ratio (SNR) in the images. For small strains, linear axial stretching of the signal by the nominal applied strain is a commonly used technique for improving the correlation estimates [18]. On average, linear stretching compensates for the axial motion. Unfortunately, non-axial motion cannot be compensated for in the same manner. Moreover, for a complex target, stretching the entire image by the average results in over-stretching of the stiff regions and under-stretching of the soft regions, even when the applied strain is small. Therefore, a mechanism to adaptively stretch or compress the signal both laterally and axially is often desirable, and sometimes necessary.

For example, a strain image of a simulated phantom consisting of two small spherical lesions is shown in Fig. 6c. The lesions, 4 and 2 mm in diameter, are three times stiffer than the surrounding medium and are centered on the axis of the phantom (Fig. 6a). Linear stretching was employed to improve displacement estimates obtained from the correlation analysis. A comparison with the object strain depicted in Fig. 6b indicates that the reconstruction suffers from high noise. In fact, the smaller lesion is almost invisible.

To correct the compressed signal both laterally and axially, we have developed a technique based on the sum absolute difference (SAD) algorithm that was recently used for speckle-tracking [19]. The algorithm determines the displaced location of an $m \times n$ kernel region in the uncompressed image $U$ by computing the sum of absolute differences between the original kernel and all matching regions belonging to a search area in the compressed image $C$:

$$s_{AD}^{ij} = \sum_{p=1}^{m} \sum_{q=1}^{n} |C_{p,q} - U_{p+i,q+j}| \quad , \tag{5}$$

where $i, j$ are the coordinates of a matching region in image $C$. The position $i, j$ that yields the smallest value of $s_{AD}$ represents the new position of the kernel. By adaptively correcting $C$ to eliminate axial and lateral motion, we achieve better correlation estimates. For example, a reconstruction of the two-lesion phantom shown in Fig. 6a when SAD algorithm is used for adaptive stretching is shown in Fig. 6d. The lower noise compared to the image of Fig. 6c results in higher detectability of the lesions. The smaller lesion as well as the artifacts of the object strain are more visible in the image shown in Fig. 6d.

We also tested these elastographic methods by probing an excised dog kidney cast in a uniform block of gelatin. Fig. 7 shows an unoptimized sonogram and two elastograms of the kidney. Fig. 7b was obtained for 2% preloading, and 7c was obtained with 6% preloading. The sonogram and elastograms provide different information about the object. While the sonogram probes impedance variations in renal microstructure, elastograms provide information about macroscopic variations in elastic properties. This example also illustrates how changes in microscopic properties accumulate to manifest themselves at the macroscopic level. Collecting ducts in the center of the kidney appear hypoechoic in the sonogram, and they appear softer in the elastogram (Fig. 7b). However, the elastogram also shows that the cortex is softer than the outer medulla region, a feature not seen in the sonogram. For larger preloading, the soft regions stiffen and the contrast is lost (Fig. 7c).

Experiments described in this section demonstrate the potential of elastography for detecting tumors and investigating renal histology, in vivo. Alterations of elastic properties at the microscopic and macroscopic levels depend on the type, severity and progression of disease. By developing the proposed soft-tissue

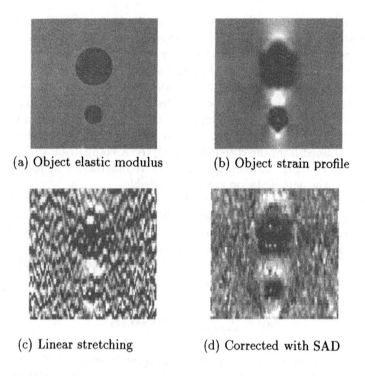

(a) Object elastic modulus      (b) Object strain profile

(c) Linear stretching      (d) Corrected with SAD

**Fig. 6.** Elastograms of a 2-lesion phantom: (c) and (d) are the reconstructions of (b) with different processing strategies.

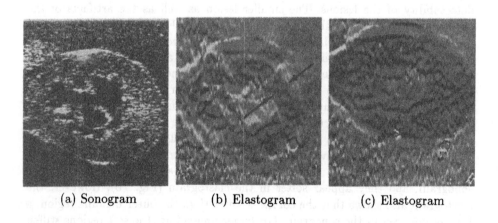

(a) Sonogram      (b) Elastogram      (c) Elastogram

**Fig. 7.** Sonogram and elastograms of a dog kidney. (b) 2% pre-compression; (c) 6 % pre-compression. Arrows in (b) indicate the stiff region of the cortex.

model, wherein QUS and elastography are used in tandem, we hope to be able to study a variety of diseases from their initial stages to the terminal stage.

In the next section, we briefly describe how a mathematical model of progressive renal diseases can be used to form object priors for Bayesian estimation of parameters using QUS.

## 5 Renal Disease Model for Obtaining Object Priors

Experiments and analysis described in Section 3 indicated that scatterer size image contrast and target visibility can be improved with Bayesian estimation. To construct accurate priors, which are essential for the success of Bayesian analysis, and to predict estimation performance, we need a reliable model of the object variability. A quantitative model of the progression of disease provides us with information on how a disease process alters the statistical properties of the object, such as the mean and the variance.

Based on our understanding of the mechanisms participating in progressive renal disease, we have developed a set of three coupled differential equations to model the dynamics of renal disease [17]. These equations describe the time progression of three state variables $s$ (severity of sclerosis), $g$ (glomerular size) and $n$ (number of sclerosed glomeruli) based on the experimental observation of a subtotal nephrectomy (sNPX) rat model [20]. Using the disease model, we were able to predict distributions of glomerular size and sclerosis similar to the distributions observed experimentally. For example, distributions of $s$ and $g$ 12 weeks post-sNPX are shown in Fig. 8.

Distributions of $s$ and $g$ (Fig. 8) indicate that the mean glomerular size first increases and then decreases with the progression of sclerosis. The variance of glomerular size follows a similar pattern. It is also known that sclerosis is accompanied by the deposition of excessive amounts of extra-cellular matrix in the mesangium of the glomerulus, resulting in an increase in the collagen and, therefore, in the integrated backscatter coefficient (IBC) from the glomeruli. These phenomena provide valuable prior information for performing Bayesian estimation, and indicate that a combination of mean glomerular size, variance of glomerular size and IBC may provide a more accurate framework for investigating renal disease. The excessive accumulation of extra-cellular matrix in the mesangium may also result in the stiffening of glomeruli, which would manifest itself at the organ level as the disease progresses. Therefore, elastography may be vital for monitoring disease-induced changes late in the progression of the disease. Although preliminary results presented in the previous section are encouraging, detailed investigation is necessary to verify these hypotheses.

## 6 Conclusions

We propose a framework for studying diseases of soft tissues at many scales to model their progression. While QUS is capable of detecting changes in elas-

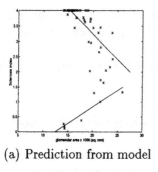
(a) Prediction from model

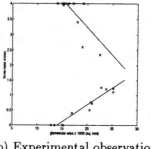
(b) Experimental observation

**Fig. 8.** Distributions of glomerular surface area $g$ and sclerosis index $s$ 12 weeks after subtotal nephrectomy. $s = 0$ represents no sclerosis and 4 represents 100% sclerosis on a 0-4 linear scale. (a) Theoretical prediction, (b) Experimental observation.

tic properties of tissue at the microscopic level, elastography provides information about macroscopic changes in the elastic properties. In a kidney, QUS provides information about histological changes in the glomeruli affected by disease, whereas elastography may be useful for monitoring more advanced renal disease. Elastography also provides high-resolution images of tumors and hard lesions in soft tissues. Valuable information about object priors used with Bayesian estimation is obtained from a theoretical model of disease progression. Together, these techniques may provide a powerful tool for modeling and measuring the progression of many soft tissue diseases.

## Acknowledgment

This work was supported by NIH grants R01 DK43007, P01 CA64597 (through the University of Texas) and the Clinical Radiology Foundation.

## References

1. M.F. Insana, and D.G. Brown, "Acoustic Scattering Theory Applied to Soft Biological Tissues," in *Ultrasonic Scattering in Biological Tissues*, edited by K.K. Shung and G.A. Thieme, CRC Press, Boca Raton, pp. 75-124, 1993.
2. E.J. Feleppa, F.L. Lizzi, D.J. Coleman, and M.M. Yaremko, "Diagnostic spectrum analysis in ophthalmology: a physical perspective," *Ultrasound Med. Biol*, vol. 12, pp. 623-631, 1986.
3. J.E. Perez, J.G. Miller, M.R. Holland, S.A. Wickline, A.D. Waggoner, B. Barzilai, and B.E. Sobel, "Ultrasonic tissue characterization: integrated backscatter imaging for detecting myocardial structural properties and on-line quantitation of cardiac function," *Am. J. Card. Imaging*, vol. 8, pp. 106-112, 1994.

4. M.F. Insana, J.G. Wood, and T.J. Hall, "Identifying acoustic scattering sources in normal renal parenchyma in vivo by varying arterial and ureteral pressures," *Ultrasound Med. Biol.*, vol. 18, pp. 587-599, 1992.

5. J. Ophir, I. Cespedes, H. Ponnekanti, Y. Yazdi, and X. Li, "Elastography: A Quantitative Method for Imaging the Elasticity of Biological Tissue," *Ultrason. Imaging,* vol. 13, pp. 111-134, 1991.

6. K.J. Parker, S.R. Huang, R.A. Muslin, R.M. Lerner, "Tissue Response to Mechanical Vibrations for Sonoelasticity Imaging," *Ultrasound Med. Biol.*, vol. 16, pp. 241-246, 1990.

7. R. Muthupillai, D.J. Lomas, P.J. Rossman, J.F. Greenleaf, A. Manduca, R.L. Ehman, "Magnetic Resonance Elastography by Direct Visualization of Propagating Acoustic Strain Waves," *Science*, vol. 269, pp. 1789-1936, 1995.

8. M. Tristan, D.C. Barbosa, D.O. Cosgrove, D.K. Nassiri, J.C. Bamber, and C.R. Hill, "Ultrasonic Study of In Vivo Kinetic Characteristics of Human Tissues," *Ultrasound Med. Biol.*, vol. 12, pp. 927-937, 1986.

9. A.P. Sarvazyan, A.R. Skovoroda, S.Y. Emelianov, J.B. Fowlkes, J.G. Pipe, R.S. Adler, R.B. Buxton, P.L. Carson, "Biophysical Bases of Elasticity Imaging," *Acoustical Imaging*, vol. 21, pp. 223-240, 1995.

10. A. Viidik, "Mechanical Properties of Parallel-fibered Collagenous Tissue," (Chapter 17, pp. 237-255) and "Interdependence between Structure and Function in Collagenous Tissues," (Chapter 18, pp. 257-280), in *Biology of Collagen*, edited by A. Viidik and J. Vuust, Academic Press, New York, 1980.

11. P. Chaturvedi, and M.F. Insana, "A Generalized Acoustic Backscatter Model with Implications on Tissue Characterization," *under preparation*, 1997.

12. Y.C. Fung, *A First Course in Continuum Mechanics*, second ed., Prentice Hall, Englewood Cliffs, NJ, 1977.

13. M.F. Insana, and T.J. Hall, "Parametric ultrasound imaging from backscatter coefficient measurements: image formation and interpretation," *Ultrasonic Imaging*, vol. 12, pp. 245-267, 1990.

14. J.A. Campbell, and R.C. Waag, "Ultrasonic Scattering Properties of Three Random Media with Implications for Tissue Characterization," *J. Acoust. Soc. Am.* vol. 75, pp. 1879-1886, 1984.

15. J.F. Chen, and J.A. Zagzebski, "Frequency Dependence of Backscatter Coefficient Versus Scatterer Volume Fraction," *IEEE Trans. Ultrason., Ferroelec., Freq. Control*, vol. 43, pp. 345-353, 1996.

16. P. Chaturvedi and M.F. Insana, "Bayesian and Least Squares Approaches to Ultrasonic Scatterer Size Image Formation," *IEEE Trans. Ultrason., Ferroelect., Freq. Contrl.*, vol. 44, no. 1, 1997.

17. P. Chaturvedi, and M.F. Insana, "A Mathematical Model for Progression of Renal Diseases," *J. Theor. Biol.*, in print, 1997.

18. M. Bilgen, and M. F. Insana, "Deformation Models and Correlation Analysis in Elastography," *J. Acoust. Soc. Am.*, vol. 99, pp. 3212-3224, 1996.

19. L.N. Bohs, and G.E. Trahey, "A Novel Method for Angle Independent Ultrasonic Imaging of Blood Flow and Tissue Motion," *IEEE Trans. Biomed. Imaging*, vol. 38, pp. 280-286, 1991.

20. Y. Yoshida, T. Kawamura, M. Ikoma, A. Fogo, and I. Ichikawa, "Effects of antihypertensive drugs on glomerular morphology," *Kidney Int.*, vol. 36, pp. 626-635, 1989.

# 2D Intravascular E.I.T. Using a Non-iterative, Non-linear Reconstruction Algorithm

M.K. Konings, C.J. Bouma, W.P.Th.M. Mali, and M.A. Viergever

Department of Radiology - Image Sciences Institute
PO Box 85500, AZU-E.01.334, NL-3508 GA Utrecht,
the Netherlands.

**Abstract.** We developed an Intravascular Impedance Catheter (2D-IIC) together with a non-iterative, non-linear reconstruction algorithm, capable of assessing a series of 2D discretized images of the impedance distribution of the arterial wall.

The 2D-IIC uses a differential measurement technique based on our early version of the IIC [1], but features two new elements: asymetrically placed electrodes and a rotational motion of the catheter around its longitudinal axis. This transforms the original 1D technique into a tomographic 2D imaging device. Because of these extensions however, the Finite Element or Boundary Element calculations that solve the forward problem in Newton-like reconstruction algorithms would be prohibitively time-consuming.

In this paper we first decribe the 2D-IIC, and subsequently formulate a new, non-linear, algorithm solving the inverse problem non-iteratively. This algorithm exploits the algorithmic possibilities offered by the differential measurement technique and combines the Clausius-Mosotti approximation for field distortion with a modified Boundary Element method. Furthermore we provide a mathematical foundation for the validity of this method when applied to the 2D-IIC, and describe more generally its applicability to E.I.T.-techniques that involve a differential measurement.

## 1 Introduction

Over the last two decades, a number of intravascular therapeutic devices (e.g. balloon angioplasty catheters, atherectomy, stents) have been developed in order to reduce the need for classical surgery in the treatment of atherosclerotical circulation failure. Despite the many advantages, the outcome of an intravascular therapeutical intervention remains highly unpredictable, since both mechanical and pathophysiological properties of a specific lesion on the arterial wall strongly depend on the material composition of that lesion, which may content fibrotic tissue, calcium crystals, thrombocytes and lipid deposits in all possible combinations. Especially detection and localisation of lipid pools is of relevance before and during intravascular therapy: recent studies [2] show that the presence of a lipid pool in the atherosclerotic vessel wall is a risk factor for acute occlusion of bloodvessels.

At present, there is no reliable in vivo method available to show the presence of these pools: For example, X-ray angiography only reveals the location of a stenosis, not its material composition. The Intravascular Ultrasound catheter (IVUS) offers a transaxial view of the vessel wall. With respect to the composition of plaques, however, it reliably discriminates only calcium [3].

In [1] we described an early version of an Intravascular Impedance Catheter (IIC) capable of measuring a 1D electrical impedance distribution in an array of cylinder-symmetrical voxels around the longitudinal catheter axis. Because fat and calcium have a high specific electrical resistivity compared to other possible plaque compounds [4], a high local electrical impedance value is a suitable indicator for the presence of a lipid pool or calcium crystals in a plaque. Once a plaque of high electrical impedance has been detected, IVUS can be used to determine whether or not calcium was responsible for the high impedance value. While the 1D technique is capable of detecting major lipid pools, it falls short for clinical investigations, since it has been shown that even small, haemodynamically insignificant, fatty lesions are potentially dangerous.

In this paper we show that a substantial improvement in accuracy can be reached by the following two alterations (described in section 3):

First: If the 3D-shape of the arterial lumen is known from e.g. X-ray (from different angles) or Intravascular Ultrasound, this information can be used to split up each of the original cylindersymmetrical, annular voxels in two parts: an inner part between catheter body and lumen boundary, having a known resistivity (viz. that of blood), and an outer part outside of the lumen of which the resistivity is to be assessed.

Second: The accuracy of the assessment of the material composition of the vessel wall improves significantly if the electrodes are no longer cylindersymmetrical and the catheter is connected to a motor forcing it to rotate around its longitudinal axis, thus introducing an angular dependency of the measurements. This transforms the original non-rotating 1D technique (IIC) into a tomographic imaging device (2D-IIC).

By nature, however, reconstructing the impedance distribution from measured potential differences is a highly non-linear, ill-posed problem that is usually solved by means of an iterative algorithm, in which during each iteration the potential distribution has to be computed. The above mentioned two alterations imply that the forward calculation is far more complicated and cannot be based on rotational symmetry, as was the case in [1]. Instead a Finite Element (FEM) or Boundary Element (BE) method has to be used. This makes an iterative algorithm time-consuming.

*The purpose of this paper is the introduction of a fast, non-iterative, non-linear algorithm that reconstructs a 2D map of the impedance distribution from the measured intravascular electrical potentials on basis of the lumen contour as detected with IVUS or X-ray.*

This non-iterative algorithm (described in section 4) is a modification of the BE-method that exploits the specific mathematical possibilities that result from the differential measurement scheme used for the IIC. This opens the possibility of almost real-time detection of lipid pools, using diagnostic catheters along with therapeutical catheters during e.g. a balloon angioplasty session.

## 2 Catheter Hardware and Measurement Method

At present, cardiac impedance catheters (conductance catheters) are used clinically to measure the volume of the ventricle during the cardiac cycle. These catheters have a number of electrodes (usually eight), some of them being used as excitation electrodes connected to current sources to create a current density field in the ventricle, which gives rise to a distribution of the electric potential that depends on the impedances surrounding the catheter.

One of the main premises to make this technique work is that the catheter remains at a *fixed position* during the measurement, thereby leaving the global

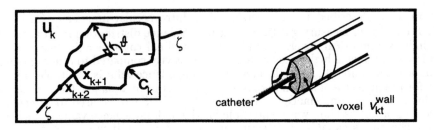

**Fig. 1.**

Schematic of the catheter in an artery, showing coordinate system and voxel discretization. In this example $N_{ang} = 3$. See text.

geometrical order of all surrounding impedances the same. In case of an intravascular diagnostic catheterization however, a diagnostic catheter is pulled back through the arterial lumen, and its position to its environment changes continuously. Therefore, cardiac impedance catheters cannot be used for intravascular measurements.

In [1] we described a new catheter, the Intravascular Impedance Catheter (IIC), with a different electrode configuration, capable of performing a differential measurement procedure, as is explained below.

The IIC contains only three measurement electrodes (me1,me2, and me3), which are placed equidistantly, separated by a small electrode spacing $\mu_{me} = 1.0$mm. These measurement electrodes are cylindersymmetrical band-electrodes. The necessary current field is created by the combination of one excitation electrode on a guiding catheter, and one skin-electrode on a distal part of the patient. Whereas in the case of the cardiac impedance catheter there is a fixed distance between the excitation and the measuring electrodes, in the case of the IIC there is no a priori knowledge available concerning the current field within the arterial segment of interest, except that the sources may be considered to be "far away" with respect to the dimensions of this arterial segment.

During the pull-back manoeuvre, the catheter travels through the arterial lumen. Let point P be a fixed point on the catheter, located on its central longitudinal axis, coinciding with the midpoint of electrode me2. Let $\zeta$ denote the trajectory (i.e. the curved line segment) along which point P travels during the pull-back manoeuvre, and let $x$ denote the displacement of this point P along $\zeta$. In the following, the displacement of the catheter is defined to be the displacement $x$ of this reference point P, which is measured from outside the patient by a device [5] through which the catheter is fed, located at the spot where the catheter enters the patient. Along the trajectory $\zeta$ a series of $N_{pos}$ equidistant catheter positions $x_k$ is defined ($k \in \{1, \ldots, N_{pos}\}$), separated by a distance $\delta x = x_{k+1} - x_k$. At each catheter position $x_k$, both the potential difference $\phi_k^{(me12)}$ between me1 and me2, and the potential difference $\phi_k^{(me23)}$ between me2 and me3 are measured *simultaneously*.

From a mathematical point of view, in the case of intravascular impedance assessment we have to deal with the following *inverse problem*: given this limited number of measured potential differences, calculate the conductivity distribution.

Inverse problems generally suffer from non-uniqueness, instability, or a combination. In [1] we showed that a unique solution is obtained by using the following spatial discretization:

Let $z_1$, $z_2$, and $z_3$ be spatial cartesian coordinates, and let $\bar{z} = (z_1, z_2, z_3)^T$ be a vector pointing to point $(z_1, z_2, z_3)$ in 3D space. Let $\mathcal{L}$ be a layer in the immediate environment of the catheter: point $\bar{z}$ is in $\mathcal{L}$ if and only if the distance $r_{\mathcal{L}}$ between point $\bar{z}$ and the catheter axis is smaller than some constant $r_{\mathcal{L}}$. This distance $r_{\mathcal{L}}$ is chosen such that, roughly, the vascular wall is within $\mathcal{L}$, but the surroundings of the artery are not. A more specific description of the value of $r_{\mathcal{L}}$ is given later on. We divide this tube-shaped layer into $N$ annular voxels $v_k$ ($k \in \{1, \ldots, N\}$) of constant width $\delta x$, and consider the $\sigma(\bar{z})$ within each $v_k$ to be constant and equal to $\sigma_k$.

Furthermore, we showed that it is possible to formulate a reconstruction algorithm of sufficient stability using such a set of voxels, if electrode configuration and measurement procedure are such that, for each position $x_k$, some parameter $m_k$ can be calculated from the measured potentials $\phi_k^{(me12)}$ and $\phi_k^{(me23)}$ having the following properties (p1) and (p2):

(p1): The value of $m_k$ depends only on the conductivity distribution in a compact volume around point P on the catheter. This compact volume lies within $\mathcal{L}$, and will be referred to as 'sensitivity area'. (A more quantitative definition is given in section 4).

(p2): $m_k$ is insensitive to the intensity of the excitation current density field around point P.

Subsequently we showed that these conditions are met by the normalized differential measurement procedure, in which $m_k$ is defined as:

$$m_k = 2 \frac{\phi_k^{(me12)} - \phi_k^{(me23)}}{\phi_k^{(me12)} + \phi_k^{(me23)}} \tag{1}$$

Owing to the subtraction in eq.(1), the sensitivity of $m_k$ for the value of $\sigma(\bar{z})$ decays strongly as a function of the distance $|\bar{z}_k - \bar{z}|$, viz. typically as a $|\bar{z}_k - \bar{z}|^{-4}$-function, in which $\bar{z}_k$ is the 3D position vector of point P when the catheter is at position $x_k$. Because of this, choosing $r_{\mathcal{L}} = 3r_{cath}$ is sufficient to concentrate over 90% of the sensitivity of the measurement within $\mathcal{L}$, in which $2r_{cath}$ is the diameter of the catheter. These $m_k$ values constitute the input for the reconstruction algorithm. By nature, the subtraction in eq.(1) is suited to detect inhomogeneities in the $\sigma$-distribution. If $\sigma_k$ is constant for all $k$, the $m_k$ would be zero. More generally, on basis of the $m_k$-values, only the differences of the $\sigma_k$ with respect to some reference $\sigma_0$ may be reconstructed; this global offset $\sigma_0$ remains unknown.

In the search for fatty intravascular lesions, it is desired to detect deviations from a healthy physiological situation. A healthy segment of artery features a high degree of translational invariance along the $x$-axis, except for bifurcations and physiological tapering. Therefore, for the specific case of intravascular diagnosis at hand, we are interested in the detection of boundaries between areas of different $\sigma_k$, rather than the values of the $\sigma_k$ themselves.

We therefore introduce the difference variables $s_k$:

$$s_k = \sigma_k - \sigma_{k-1} \tag{2}$$

A drawback of the above defined voxel discretization is a poor spatial resolution: only major fatty lesions are detected, because the layer $\mathcal{L}$ contains the vessel wall, as well as the blood-filled volume between catheter and the vessel wall. By definition, we are interested in subvoxel-information, viz. the specific impedance in the vessel wall. This results in artifacts: Since the specific resistivity of a non-fatty, non-calcified, atherosclerotic lesion ( 300 to 800$\Omega$cm ) is still higher than that of blood ($250\Omega$cm), variations in lumen diameter cause non-zero $m_k$, although no fat or calcium may be present. This is the subject of the next section.

# 3 Resolution Enhancement

In order to distinguish variations in vessel wall composition from effects caused by diameter variations, we introduce two modifications to the original IIC concept: the incorporation of lumen contour information in the reconstruction algorithm, and the introduction of angular dependency of the measurement using a rotating catheter.

## 3.1 Incorporation of lumen contour information

Let $\mathcal{L}_{blood}$ denote that part of $\mathcal{L}$ that is filled with blood, and let $\mathcal{L}_{wall}$ denote the rest of $\mathcal{L}$. Each of the original voxels $v_k$ is divided into two new voxels: $v_k^{blood}$ and $v_k^{wall}$. Within each of these new voxels the conductivity is assumed to be constant and equal to $\sigma_k^{blood}$ and $\sigma_k^{wall}$ respectively. Although blood conductivity depends on its velocity [6] and hence varies as function of time during the cardiac cycle, this has no influence on the $m_k$-values, since blood conductivity variations are global, and have the same effect as fluctuations of the strength of the excitation current (i.e. multiplication of $\phi^{(me12)}$ and $\phi^{(me23)}$ with some coefficient that is the same for both electrode pairs), whereas the $m_k$-values are based on potential differences measured *simultaneously*. Therefore the $m_k$-values depend on the $\sigma_k^{wall}$ alone, and thus a unique $s_k^{wall}$-distribution can be reconstructed from the measured $m_k$-values, in which $s_k^{wall} = \sigma_k^{wall} - \sigma_{k-1}^{wall}$.

If the 3D-shape of the lumen is known by means of some other imaging modality, e.g. IVUS, then size and shape of the voxels $v_k^{wall}$ are known. In order to create a coordinate frame in which the shape of the $v_k^{wall}$ voxels are to be expressed, we define a set of flat planes $U_k$, such that for each $k$, the plane $U_k$ intersects with the trajectory $\zeta$ at point $x_k$, and that the trajectory is perpendicular to $U_k$ at $x_k$. Within each plane $U_k$, we define a 2D polar coordinate system $(r, \vartheta)$ having point $x_k$ as origin. For each $k$, we define the closed contour $C_k$ as the intersection of the plane $U_k$ with the boundary surface between $\mathcal{L}_{blood}$ and $\mathcal{L}_{wall}$, known from IVUS. Each contour $C_k$ may be described by the function $r_k^{Lum}(\vartheta)$, which gives the distance from point $x_k$ to the contour $C_k$ when travelling along a straight line with direction $\vartheta$.

In [1], the reconstruction solving the $s_k$ from the $m_k$ was performed by a Newton-like iterative algorithm, in which during each iteration the forward calculation was done using a simple first-order approximation exploiting the cylinder symmetry and translational invariance of the $v_k$ voxels. Since the $v_k^{wall}$ voxels do not have this cylinder symmetry and translational invariance, the forward problem needs a more general approach, like a Finite Element (FEM) or Boundary Element (BE) method. This makes the forward calculation considerably more time-consuming, and furthermore requires a 3D (FEM) or 2D (BE) mesh based on the shape of $\mathcal{L}_{wall}$.

In chapter 4 we will show that for the specific problem of assessing the $s_k^{wall}$-values from IIC measurements, it is possible to formulate an explicit expression for $s_k^{wall}$, using a modified Boundary Element approach that exploits the specific advantages of the differential measurement procedure. The use of this explicit expression avoids the disadvantages of an iterative scheme.

## 3.2 Rotating catheter

Size and shape of the sensitivity area around point P depend on catheter diameter and electrode width. For example, if the catheter would be very thin, and would lie parallel against one side of the wall, most of the vascular wall would be outside the sensitivity area, except for that portion of the wall that is in the immediate neighbourhood of the catheter. In order to improve spatial resolution, we exploited this phenomenon and designed a rather thick catheter, filling up a substantial part of the lumen, and covered the cylinder-symmetrical electrodes with a layer of isolating material, leaving only a limited angle of the total circumference of each electrode uncovered. (See fig. 1). Thus we created a constellation of three rectangular measuring 'windows' of identical shape, facing the same direction; i.e. the windows me2 and me3 would coincide exactly with window me1 if translated along the catheteraxis by a distance $\mu_{me}$ and $2\mu_{me}$ respectively.

In combination with a rotational motion of the catheter around its longitudinal axis, this transforms the original 1D technique (IIC, uncovered electrodes) into a 2D imaging device (2D-IIC). Let $\vartheta$ denote the angle of rotation of the catheter around its longitudinal axis. At each position $x_k$ of the catheter along $\zeta$ during the pull-back manoeuvre, the catheter makes one complete rotation around its axis, during which, at each angle of rotation $\vartheta_t$ out of a series of $N_{ang}$ rotation angles ($t \in \{1 \dots N_{ang}\}$), potential differences $\phi_{kt}^{(me12)}$ and $\phi_{kt}^{(me23)}$ are measured. For each combination of $k$ and $t$, this constellation of three measuring windows is in the immediate neighbourhood of a different part of the vessel wall, since for each $t$ the measuring windows face another direction.

Furthermore, for each combination $(k,t)$, we define $m_{kt}$ as

$$m_{kt} = 2\, \frac{\phi_{kt}^{(me12)} - \phi_{kt}^{(me23)}}{\phi_{kt}^{(me12)} + \phi_{kt}^{(me23)}} \tag{3}$$

Owing to the shape of the measuring windows, the sensitivity of $m_{kt}^{diff}$ decays typically as a $| \bar{z}_{kt} - \bar{z} |^{-4}$-function, where $\bar{z}_{kt}$ is the position of the center of mass of the uncovered part of electrode me2, whilst the catheter is situated according to the indices $(k,t)$. Because $\bar{z}_{kt}$ is located near the catheter wall, whereas $\bar{z}_k$ is located at the central axis of the catheter, $| \bar{z}_{kt} - \bar{z} |^{-4}$ decays steeper than $| \bar{z}_k - \bar{z} |^{-4}$ (from the 1D IIC) for $\bar{z}$ outside the catheter. Therefore, the volume containing 90% of the sensitivity is significantly smaller than was the case with the original IIC. (In subsection 4.3 this is explicified more quantitively). This enables a spatial discretization of higher resolution than was the case with the original 1D-IIC. In order to define this new set of voxels, let for each $k$, the space inside $\mathcal{L}_{wall}$ between the planes $U_k$ and $U_{k+1}$ be divided into subvolumes by the introduction of a set of planes $T_{kt}$ (with $t$ running from 1 to $N_{ang}$) that are perpendicular to $U_k$, in such a way that all planes $T_{kt}$ intersect at point $x_k$, and that the angle between $T_{kt}$ and $T_{k,t+1}$ equals $2\pi/N_{ang}$ for all $t$. ($T_{k,N_{ang}+1} \equiv T_{k,1}$).

We now define the final voxels $v_{kt}^{wall}$ as follows: $v_{kt}$ is the subvolume of $\mathcal{L}_{wall}$ bounded by $U_k$, $U_{k+1}$, $T_{kt}$, and $T_{k,t+1}$. Within each $v_{kt}^{wall}$ the conductivity is assumed to be constant and equal to $\sigma_{kt}^{wall}$. On basis of the measured $m_{kt}$ and the given geometry of the voxels $v_{kt}$, the reconstruction algorithm (section 4) calculates the $s_{kt}^{wall} = \sigma_{kt}^{wall} - \sigma_{k-1,t}^{wall}$.

# 4    Non-iterative Non-linear Reconstruction Algorithm

In this section we will show that for the specific problem of reconstructing the
$s_{kt}^{wall}$-values from the measured $m_{kt}$-values, it is possible to formulate an explicit
expression for $s_{kt}^{wall}$, using a modified Boundary Element approach that exploits
the specific advantages of the differential measurement procedure. These explicit
expressions are non-linear functions of the measured data, and enable a direct
calculation of the $s_{kt}^{wall}$ without the need of an iterative scheme. As will be
explained below, this approach is based on the Clausius-Mosotti approximation
of the secondary electrical field.

In the following, we will first describe the modified Boundary Element method,
and derive an explicit expression for the discretized intravascular electrical field.
(subsection 4.1).

Subsequently, we will the derive the explicit expression for $s_{kt}^{wall}$ on basis of
the differential measurement.

## 4.1    Non-iterative method: Modified Boundary Element method

Consider the general case of an isotropic, Ohmic, conductive environment with
given conductivity distribution $\sigma(\overline{z})$, in which $\overline{z}$ is a three-dimensional spatial
coordinate. The continuity equation for the current density, relating the potential
distribution $\phi(\overline{z})$ to $\sigma(\overline{z})$, reads:

$$\nabla \cdot (\sigma(\overline{z})\nabla\phi(\overline{z})) = 0 \qquad (4)$$

Equation (4) holds for any volume $\Omega$ containing any $\sigma(\overline{z})$-distribution, provided
that no electrical free charges or current sources are present in that volume. For
E.I.T. this means that $\Omega$ should not contain any excitation electrodes.

As for experiments, one measures potential differences between electrodes,
rather than the $\phi(\overline{z})$-distribution itself; therefore the electrical field $\overline{E}(\overline{z}) = -\nabla\phi(\overline{z})$ is the relevant entity to be solved in the forward problem concerning eq.(4). Using $\overline{E}(\overline{z}) = -\nabla\phi(\overline{z})$ and $\nabla \cdot (a\overline{B}) = a\nabla \cdot \overline{B} + \overline{B} \cdot \nabla a$ for any
scalar $a$ and vector $\overline{B}$, and knowing that, for biological materials, $\sigma(\overline{z})$ is always
non-zero and positive, it follows from eq.(4) that:

$$\nabla \cdot \overline{E}(\overline{z}) = -\frac{\nabla\sigma(\overline{z})}{\sigma(\overline{z})} \cdot \overline{E}(\overline{z}) \qquad (5)$$

The left side of (5) equals the left side of the electrostatic Maxwell-equation
$\nabla \cdot \overline{E}(\overline{z}) = \rho(\overline{z})$, in which $\rho(\overline{z})$ is an electrostatic charge density distribution.
Therefore, we may infer the following interpretation of (5): Given some $\sigma(\overline{z})$-
distribution, and a corresponding $\overline{E}(\overline{z})$ field as result of solving (4), this $\overline{E}(\overline{z})$
field is equal to the electrostatical field arising from a $\rho(\overline{z})$-distribution, with
$\rho(\overline{z})$ numerically equal to $\frac{\nabla\sigma(\overline{z})}{\sigma(\overline{z})} \cdot \overline{E}(\overline{z})$

From the discretization it follows that $\nabla\sigma(\overline{z}) = 0$ inside each voxel. Thus the
equivalent charge distribution $\rho(\overline{z})$ contains only surface charges at boundaries
between voxels. This is the basis of the BE-method.

Generally, given some known $\rho(\overline{z})$-distribution, the resulting electrostatic
$\overline{E}(\overline{z})$-field is calculated by solving Poissons equation:

$$\overline{E}(\overline{z}) = \int d^3z' \frac{\rho(\overline{z'})(\overline{z} - \overline{z'})}{|\,\overline{z'} - \overline{z}\,|^3} \qquad (6)$$

Thus we have that $\overline{E}(\overline{z})$ depends on these surface charges (eq. (6)), whereas the density of a surface charge itself is proportional to $\overline{E}(\overline{z})$ (eq.(5)). This 'self-reference' of $\overline{E}(\overline{z})$ reflects the non-linear character of eq.(4).

In the BE method, this selfreference is avoided by taking the following three steps:

(i) The boundaries between voxels are divided into a 2D-mesh of triangular surfaces,

(ii) The potential is assumed to be constant within each triangular surface,

(iii) For each triangular surface, only the effect that the charges at such a surface have on other surfaces is calculated.

The BE-method solves the discretized potential distribution for a given set of voxels having known conductivities. This is done by solving a set of linear equations, that result from combining eq.(5) and (6), and applying the steps (i) to (iii). The number of equations is equal to the number ($N_{tria}$) of triangular surfaces.

In this paper, however, we aim at a method for solving the $s_{kt}^{wall}$-values non-iteratively. In the following, we will show that this can be done by altering the BE-method in such a way that the number of equations is lowered from $N_{tria}$ to the number of voxels in $\Omega$.

To this aim we apply the Clausius-Mosotti equation [7] in order to replace the combination of the surface charges at the various sides of a voxel by a single charge dipole at the center of the voxel, as follows:

Consider one single voxel $\lambda$ (in which $\sigma(\overline{z}) = \sigma_\lambda$) in a homogeneous environment (with $\sigma(\overline{z}) = \sigma_0$), and some applied external field $\overline{E}_0(\overline{z})$. Let the voxel $\lambda$ be small enough with respect to the distances to the sources of the applied field $\overline{E}_0(\overline{z})$ to allow the following assumption (A):

(A): If $\sigma_\lambda = \sigma_0$, the field may be considered to be constant within the voxel $\lambda$.

Let $\overline{E}_0^\lambda$ denote this field: if $\sigma_\lambda = \sigma_0$, $\overline{E}_0(\overline{z}) = \overline{E}_0^\lambda$ for all $\overline{z} \in \lambda$. This implies that the total of the surface charges at the boundaries of $\lambda$ is zero (eq.(5), BE).

We now replace the combination of the surface charges at the various sides of a voxel by a single charge dipole $\overline{p}_\lambda$ at the center of the voxel. The relation between $\overline{p}_\lambda$, $\sigma_\lambda$ and $\overline{E}_0^\lambda$ is given by the Clausius-Mosotti formula:

$$\overline{p}_\lambda = 3V_\lambda \frac{\sigma_\lambda - \sigma_0}{\sigma_\lambda + 2\sigma_0} \overline{E}_0^\lambda \tag{7}$$

in which $V_\lambda$ is the volume of voxel $\lambda$.

The electrical field caused by such a dipole is given by the standard dipole formula:

$$\overline{E}(\overline{z}) = \frac{3\hat{r}_{(\overline{z}\overline{z}_\lambda)}(\overline{p}_\lambda \cdot \hat{r}_{(\overline{z}\overline{z}_\lambda)}) - \overline{p}_\lambda}{|\overline{z} - \overline{z}_\lambda|^3} \tag{8}$$

in which $\overline{z}$ is any point outside $\lambda$, $\overline{z}_\lambda$ is the center point in $\lambda$, and $\hat{r}_{(\overline{z}\overline{z}_\lambda)}$ is a unit vector pointing in the direction from $\overline{z}$ to $\overline{z}_\lambda$.

If the environment of $\lambda$ is not a homogeneous $\sigma_0$-distribution but contains other voxels with $\sigma \neq \sigma_0$, this method may still be used as long as assumption (A) is valid, in which $\overline{E}_0^\lambda$ now is the sum of the primary excitation field and the secondary fields from voxels other than $\lambda$. Let the excitation sources be so remote from the volume of interest $\Omega_{ROI}$ (as is the case with the IIC excitation), that we may write their effect on $\Omega_{ROI}$ as some applied primary field $\overline{E}_\Omega$ that is constant within $\Omega_{ROI}$.

Furthermore, let $N_\Omega$ denote the number of voxels in $\Omega_{ROI}$ having a conductivity different from $\sigma_0$, and let these voxels be numbered from 1 to $N_\Omega$. Let $n$ and $n'$ be indices ($n, n' \in \{1 \ldots N_\Omega\}$) referring to specific voxels, and define ($\alpha$) and ($\beta$) (with $\alpha, \beta \in \{1, 2, 3\}$) as indices referring to one of the three components in a vector like $\overline{E}_n = (E_n^{(1)}, E_n^{(2)}, E_n^{(3)})^T$.

We now may combine eq.(7) with eq.(8), resulting in eq.(9), provided the following assumption (B) is valid:

(B): the conductivity $\sigma(\overline{z})$ is constant everywhere *outside* the region of interest $\Omega_{ROI}$.

$$E_n^{(\alpha)} = E_\Omega^{(\alpha)} + \sum_{\substack{n'=1 \\ n' \neq n}}^{N_\Omega} \frac{3\hat{r}_{nn'}^{(\alpha)} \left( \sum_{\beta=1}^{3} E_{n'}^{(\beta)} c_{n'} \hat{r}_{nn'}^{(\beta)} \right) - E_{n'}^{(\alpha)} c_{n'}}{|\,\overline{z}_n - \overline{z}_{n'}\,|^3} \tag{9}$$

in which

$$c_{n'} = 3V_{n'} \frac{\sigma_{n'} - \sigma_0}{\sigma_{n'} + 2\sigma_0} \tag{10}$$

Thus $E_n^{(\alpha)}$ is a linear function of the entries $E_{n'}^{(\beta)}$, and eq.(9) represents a set of linear equations.

In order to introduce a more compact notation for eq.(9), we will look upon the various $E_n^{(\alpha)}$-values as belonging to one set, and combine all these $E_n^{(\alpha)}$-values into one $3N_\Omega$-dimensional vector $\mathbf{E}$, having elements $\mathbf{E}_i$, with $i = 3n + \alpha$. Thus every value of $i$ corresponds to exactly one combination of $n$ and $\alpha$.

Similarly, we define the vector $\mathbf{G}$ containing the constant global excitation field in $\Omega_{ROI}$ as: $\mathbf{G}_i = \mathbf{E}_\Omega^{(\alpha)}$ and, using $j = 3n' + \beta$, define the matrices $\mathcal{C}$ and $\mathcal{W}$ according to:

$$\mathcal{C}_{ij} = \delta_{nn'} \delta_{\alpha\beta} c_{n'} \tag{11}$$

and

$$\mathcal{W}_{ij} = \frac{3\hat{r}_{nn'}^{(\alpha)} \hat{r}_{nn'}^{(\beta)} - \delta_{\alpha\beta}}{|\,\overline{z}_n - \overline{z}_{n'}\,|^3} \tag{12}$$

in which $\delta_{nn'}$ is a Kronecker delta.

We may now rewrite eq.(9) in matrix notation:

$$\mathbf{E} = \mathbf{G} + \mathcal{W}\mathcal{C}\mathbf{E} \tag{13}$$

The matrix $\mathcal{W}$ depends only on shape and position of the voxels; whereas the matrix $\mathcal{C}$ contains only conductivity information. This separability into $\mathcal{W}$ and $\mathcal{C}$ enables an explicit expression for the $c_{n'}$:

Since $\mathcal{C}$ is diagonal, we may solve its elements $\mathcal{C}_{ii}$ from eq.(13) as follows (eq.(14)):

$$\mathcal{C}_{ii} = \frac{[\mathcal{W}^{-1}(\mathbf{E} - \mathbf{G})]_i}{\mathbf{E}_i} \tag{14}$$

provided that $\mathbf{E}_i$ is non-zero (this is assumption C). Since $\mathcal{C}_{ij} = \delta_{nn'} \delta_{\alpha\beta} c_{n'}$, we have that for each $n$, the value of $\mathcal{C}_{ii}$ is independent of the direction ($\alpha$). Therefore, the sheer presence of any non-zero $\overline{E}$-field in voxel $n$ is sufficient to guarantee that some value of $\alpha$ exists for which $\mathbf{E}_i$ is non-zero, thus satisfying assumption C. This equation represents a direct method for retrieving the $c_{n'}$-values (and hence the $\sigma_{n'}$-values ) from a given $\mathbf{E}$.

This method however can not be used for the specific case of the Intravascular impedance Catheter at hand: the assumptions (A) and (B) impose strict limitations on its validity. The fact of the matter is that generally these assumptions are not valid. For instance, (B) is not valid since if some part in the human body is defined to be the region of interest $\Omega_{ROI}$, the conductivity outside $\Omega_{ROI}$ will be non-homogeneous due to the rest of the body. Then theoretically the matrices and vectors in eq.(14) should involve all voxels outside $\Omega_{ROI}$ as well, resulting in unbounded matrix dimensions.

At this point it is a natural step to investigate whether a satisfactory approximation can be obtained by replacing these unbounded matrices with matrices that involve only voxels within some volume $\Omega_{calc}$ (with $\Omega_{ROI} \subset \Omega_{calc}$) of finite dimensions. The dimensions of $\Omega_{calc}$ will depend on the desired accuracy of the calculation of the second term $\mathcal{WCE}$ in (13).

In the following subsection (4.2) we show that generally no such $\Omega_{calc}$ exists for which a certain accuracy of the approximation can be guaranteed. In subsection 4.3 however we will show that when applying the above described non-iterative method to new variables (viz. $m_{kt}$ and $s_{kt}^{wall}$) based on the normalized differential measurement procedure, such a $\Omega_{calc}$ does exist, leading to results of satisfactory accuracy. In (4.3) we will also show how to satisfy assumption (A).

## 4.2 Approximation matrices: General case

In order to decide whether or not a certain $\Omega_{calc}$ is large enough to produce a satisfactory accuracy, a suitable criterion is the following:

$$\|(\mathcal{W}_\infty \mathcal{C}_\infty \mathbf{E}) - (\mathcal{W}_{\Omega_{calc}} \mathcal{C}_{\Omega_{calc}} \mathbf{E})\|_{\Omega_{ROI}} < f \, \|(\mathcal{W}_\infty \mathcal{C}_\infty \mathbf{E})\|_{\Omega_{ROI}} \qquad (15)$$

in which $f$ is some small number ($f \in [0,1]$) indicating the allowed error fraction, and $\|\cdot\|_{\Omega_{ROI}}$ is the 2-norm of a vector, taking in account only those elements of the vector that belong to region $\Omega_{ROI}$:

$$\|\mathbf{X}\|_{\Omega_{ROI}} = \sqrt{\sum_{\substack{all\ i\ with \\ \overline{z}_i \in \Omega_{ROI}}} (X_i)^2} \qquad (16)$$

for any vector $\mathbf{X}$.

Furthermore, in eq.(15) $\mathcal{W}_\infty$ refers to the original $\mathcal{W}$ in which $\Omega$ is set to infinite dimensions in order to include all possible voxels, and $\mathcal{W}_{\Omega_{calc}}$ is defined according to:

$(\mathcal{W}_{\Omega_{calc}})_{ij} = (\mathcal{W}_\infty)_{ij}$ if both $\overline{z}_i$ and $\overline{z}_j \in \Omega_{calc}$,
$(\mathcal{W}_{\Omega_{calc}})_{ij} = 0$ otherwise.

In words: if eq.(15) holds, the relative error in $\mathcal{WCE}$ caused by the use of the approximation matrices on basis of volume $\Omega_{calc}$ instead of infinity, does not exceed $f$.

Using that the 2-norm $\|\mathcal{Y}\|$ of any symmetrical $N \times N$-matrix $\mathcal{Y}$ is approximated [8] by

$\|\mathcal{Y}\| \leq \max_{(1 \leq i \leq N)} \sum_{j=1}^{N} |\mathcal{Y}_{ij}|$, and defining the volume $\Omega_{calc}$ as a sphere of radius $u_{calc}$, we now estimate the lefthand side of eq.(15) by a volume integral over the righthand side of eq.(9), writing $u$ for $\mid \bar{z}_n - \bar{z}_{n'} \mid$:

$$\|(\mathcal{W}_\infty \mathcal{C}_\infty \mathbf{E}) - (\mathcal{W}_{\Omega_{calc}} \mathcal{C}_{\Omega_{calc}} \mathbf{E})\|_{\Omega_{ROI}} \leq e_{max} \int_{u_{calc}}^{\infty} 4\pi u^2 du \frac{K}{u^3} \qquad (17)$$

in which $K$ is a dimensionless quantity whose range is limited to $K \in [-\frac{9}{2}, \frac{9}{2}]$, and $e_{max}$ is the largest possible value of the norm of the electrical field vector given a certain excitation, which is also limited.

Nevertheless, the right-hand side of eq.(17) generally is a diverging integral, and hence no finite $\Omega_{calc}$ can be found that is guaranteed to produce a satisfactory approximation, i.e. satisfies eq.(15).

In the following subsection however we will apply the above described non-iterative method on new variables based on the normalized differential measurement (viz. $s_{kt}^{wall}$ and $m_{kt}$ instead of $\sigma_n$ and $\overline{E}_n$ respectively), and show that on basis of these new variables, it *is* possible to provide satisfactory approximations using limited matrices, within error bounds defined by $f$.

## 4.3 Non-iterative method: Applying normalized differential measurement

In the case of the 2D-IIC, potential differences are measured between the electrodes. Because of the small interelectrode spacing, these potential differences produce good approximations of the longitudinal components of the electrical field immediately surrounding the catheterbody. The position of electrode me2 is indicated by $\bar{z}_{kt}$; we denote the electrical field at point $\bar{z}_{kt}$ by $\overline{F}_{kt}$. The region of interest $\Omega_{ROI}$ is the layer $\mathcal{L}_{wall}$ containing the voxels $v_{\kappa\tau}^{wall}$ (section 3), in which $(\kappa, \tau)$ plays the role of the index $n$ from the previous section. (We here write $\kappa\tau$ (with $\kappa \in \{1 \dots N_{pos}\}$ and $\tau \in \{1 \dots N_{ang}\}$) instead of $kt$, in order to distinguish voxel indices from measurement indices). The electrical field at the centerpoint of each voxel $v_{\kappa\tau}^{wall}$ is indicated by $\overline{E}_{(\kappa,\tau)}$.

We will now derive the non-iterative algorithm in three steps: Formulation of the equivalent of $\mathbf{E} = \mathbf{G} + \mathcal{W}\mathcal{C}\mathbf{E}$ in terms of $\overline{F}_{kt}$ (step (I)); introduction of the differential measurement into the algorithm and proof of convergence (step (II)); and introduction of the variables $s_{\kappa\tau}^{wall}$ instead of $\sigma_{\kappa\tau}^{wall}$ (step (III)).

step (I): We combine the $E_{(\kappa,\tau)}^{(\alpha)}$-values into one $3N_{pos}N_{ang}$-dimensional vector $\overline{\mathbf{E}}$, having elements $\mathbf{E}_i$, but now with
$i = 3N_{ang}\kappa + 3\tau + \alpha$.

Analogously we combine the $\overline{F}_{kt}$-values into $\mathbf{F}$, having elements $\mathbf{F}_h$, with $h = 3N_{ang}k + 3t + \alpha$.

Thus $\mathbf{E}$ and $\mathbf{F}$ concern two different spatial volumes, viz. $\mathcal{L}_{wall}$ and $\mathcal{L}_{blood}$. As $\sigma_0$ we choose: $\sigma_0 = \sigma_{blood}$, in which $\sigma_{blood}$ is the specific conductivity of the volume $\mathcal{L}_{blood}$ at the instance of measurement. The global primary excitation field $\overline{E}_\Omega$ is defined as the field that would result if the $\sigma_{\kappa,\tau}$ of all voxels in $\mathcal{L}_{wall}$ would be equal to $\sigma_0$. Because the excitation sources are remote from $\mathcal{L}$ and arteries behave like conducting wires, we consider this field $\overline{E}_\Omega$ to be homogeneous in $\mathcal{L}$, pointing in a direction parallel to the catheter-axis, and having strength $\mid \overline{E}_\Omega \mid = e_0$.

Furthermore, in analogy with $\mathcal{W}$, we define $\mathcal{W}_*$ as the matrix describing the effect that the dipoles in the $(\kappa, \tau)$-voxels have on the electrical field at the $(k, t)$

locations:

$$(\mathcal{W}_*)_{hi} = \frac{3\hat{r}^{(\alpha)}_{(\kappa,\tau)(kt)}\,\hat{r}^{(\beta)}_{(\kappa,\tau)(kt)} - \delta_{\alpha\beta}}{|\,\overline{z}_{\kappa\tau} - \overline{z}_{kt}\,|^3} \tag{18}$$

We now have:

$$\mathbf{F} = \mathbf{G} + \mathcal{W}_*\mathcal{C}\mathbf{E} \tag{19}$$

Combining eq.(19) with eq.(13) yields the following relation between $\mathbf{E}$ and $\mathbf{F}$:

$$\mathbf{F} - \mathbf{G} = \mathcal{W}_*\mathcal{W}^{-1}(\mathbf{E} - \mathbf{G}) \tag{20}$$

Hence we can formulate the equivalent of $\mathbf{E} = \mathbf{G} + \mathcal{W}\mathcal{C}\mathbf{E}$ in terms of $\mathbf{F}$ and $\mathbf{G}$:

$$\mathbf{F} - \mathbf{G} = \mathcal{W}_*\mathcal{C}(\mathbf{G} + \mathcal{W}\mathcal{W}_*^{-1}(\mathbf{F} - \mathbf{G})) \tag{21}$$

step (II): In order to formulate the differential measurement procedure in terms of the vector $\mathbf{F}$, we introduce the matrix $\mathcal{D}$ representing a subtraction between two neighbouring positions along the catheter axis:
$\mathcal{D}\mathbf{X} = \frac{1}{\delta x}\left(\mathbf{X}_{3N_{ang}k+3t+\alpha} - \mathbf{X}_{3N_{ang}(k-1)+3t+\alpha}\right)$ for any vector $\mathbf{X}$.
We now define the 'normalized derivitive' of $\mathbf{F}$ as:

$$\mathbf{M} = \frac{1}{e_0}\mathcal{D}\mathbf{F} \tag{22}$$

The values $m_k$ that result from the normalized differential measurement are closely related to the elements of $\mathbf{M}$, as will be shown lateron.

Applying the operation $\mathcal{D}$ to both sides of eq.(21), dividing by $e_0$, and using that $\mathcal{D}(\mathbf{F} - \mathbf{G}) = \mathcal{D}\mathbf{F}$ because $\mathbf{G}$ is constant, we obtain:

$$\mathbf{M} = \mathcal{D}\mathcal{W}_*\mathcal{C}\frac{\mathbf{G}}{e_0} + \mathcal{D}\mathcal{W}_*\mathcal{C}\mathcal{W}\mathcal{W}_*^{-1}(\mathbf{F} - \mathbf{G}) \tag{23}$$

In order to show that it is possible to define a useful approximation volume $\Omega_{calc}$ on basis of eq.(23), we first introduce two abbreviations: $\mathbf{U} = \frac{1}{e_0}\mathbf{G}$ and $\mathbf{A} = \mathcal{W}\mathcal{W}_*^{-1}(\mathbf{F}-\mathbf{G})$. The vector $\mathbf{U}$ is constant and independent of the excitation current density.

Since $\mathcal{C}$ is diagonal and $\mathbf{A}$ is a vector, we have that $\mathcal{C}\mathbf{A} = \mathcal{A}\mathbf{C}$, in which $\mathbf{C}_i = \mathcal{C}_{ii}$ and $\mathcal{A}_{ii} = \mathbf{A}_i$, thus interchanging the roles of diagonal matrix and vector. Similarly we have $\mathcal{C}\mathbf{U} = \mathcal{U}\mathbf{C}$.

Applying this to eq.(23), we obtain:

$$\mathbf{M} = \mathcal{D}\mathcal{W}_*(\mathcal{U} + \mathcal{A})\mathbf{C} \tag{24}$$

In analogy with eq.(15) from the previous subsection, $\Omega_{calc}$ should meet the following criterion:

$$\|(\mathcal{D}\mathcal{W}_*)_\infty(\mathcal{U}+\mathcal{A})_\infty\mathbf{C} - (\mathcal{D}\mathcal{W}_*)_{\Omega_{calc}}(\mathcal{U}+\mathcal{A})_{\Omega_{calc}}\mathbf{C}\|_{\Omega_{ROI}} < f \,\|(\mathcal{D}\mathcal{W}_*)_\infty(\mathcal{U}+\mathcal{A})_\infty\mathbf{C}\|_{\Omega_{ROI}} \tag{25}$$

We write $u = |\,\overline{z}_n - \overline{z}_{n'}\,|$, and estimate the left-hand side of eq.(25) by a volume integral, but now over the elements of the matrix $(\mathcal{D}\mathcal{W}_*)$ instead of $\mathcal{W}$:

$$\|(\mathcal{D}\mathcal{W}_*)_\infty(\mathcal{U}+\mathcal{A})_\infty\mathbf{C} - (\mathcal{D}\mathcal{W}_*)_{\Omega_{calc}}(\mathcal{U}+\mathcal{A})_{\Omega_{calc}}\mathbf{C}\|_{\Omega_{ROI}} \leq e_{max}\int_{u_{calc}}^{\infty} 12\pi u^2 du \frac{K}{u^4} \tag{26}$$

in which the integral *does* converge, and the right-hand side expression is finite and equal to

$12\pi e_{max}K/u_{calc}$. Therefore for every non-zero $\|(\mathcal{DW}_*)_\infty(\mathcal{U}+\mathcal{A})_\infty\mathbf{C}\|_{\Omega_{ROI}}$ and $f \in \langle 0,1]$, it is possible to guarantee the validity of inequality (25) by choosing a finite $u_{calc}$ that is large enough, thus putting a limit to the error that is caused by the fact that assumption (B) is not valid. Following similar arguments it can be shown that the error due to the invalidity of assumption (A) may be limited as well on basis of the differential measurement, by choosing the appropriate ratio $\delta x/r_{cath}$.

In section 2 we showed that as a natural consequence of using the $m_k$-data as basis for the reconstruction, only the conductivity differences $s_k$ can be obtained, since any offset may be added to the $\sigma_k$-values without having an effect on the $m_i$. Because of this, $\mathcal{DW}_*$ cannot be inverted as such. This inversion however is necessary for calculating $\mathbf{C}$ from eq.(24).

step (III): The problem caused by the fact that $\mathcal{DW}_*$ can not be inverted, is solved by realizing that the $s_{\kappa\tau}^{wall}$ are the values to be retrieved by the non-iterative algorithm. We write

$$\mathbf{C} = \mathbf{C}_0 + \mathcal{J}\mathbf{S} \tag{27}$$

in which $\mathbf{C}_0$ is a vector of which all the elements $(\mathbf{C}_0)_i$ have the same value $(\mathbf{C}_0)_i = c_0$. This constant $c_0$ represents an offset in the conductivity distribution. Furthermore the matrix $\mathcal{J}$ is a summation matrix, defined as:

$$(\mathcal{J}\mathbf{X})_i = \sum_{\kappa'=1}^{\kappa} \mathbf{X}_{3N_{ang}\kappa'+3\tau+\alpha}$$

Thus $c_0$ follows from the $\sigma_{\kappa\tau}$-values for at position $\kappa = 1$, which is the starting point of the measured trajectory $\zeta$. This starting point has to be chosen such that it is situated at a locally unstenosed, healthy segment of the artery, so that $c_0$ is known, viz. the $c_0$ of normal arterial wall.

Substitution of eq.(27) in (24) yields:

$$\mathbf{M} = [\mathcal{DW}_*(\mathcal{U}+\mathcal{A})\mathcal{J}]\,\mathbf{S} + \mathcal{DW}_*(\mathcal{U}+\mathcal{A})\mathbf{C}_0 \tag{28}$$

This substitution does not alter the range over wich the matrix has to be evaluated.

Since the offset vector $\mathcal{C}_0$ is known, we can subtract $\mathcal{DW}_*(\mathcal{U}+\mathcal{A})\mathbf{C}_0$ from the measured $\mathbf{M}$ to obtain the 'corrected' $\mathbf{M}'$ vector: $\mathbf{M}' = \mathbf{M} - \mathcal{DW}_*(\mathcal{U}+\mathcal{A})\mathbf{C}_0$.

We now obtain the final result:

$$\mathbf{S}_i = \left[[\mathcal{DW}_*(\mathcal{U}+\mathcal{A})\mathcal{J}]^{-1}\mathbf{M}'\right]_i \tag{29}$$

Since both $\mathcal{A}$ and $\mathbf{M}$ depend on the measured data, the $\mathbf{S}_i$ are non-linear functions of these data. The matrix $[\mathcal{DW}_*(\mathcal{U}+\mathcal{A})\mathcal{J}]$ can be inverted.

Ideally, the catheter would contain a multitude of electrodes, measuring potential differences in two directions at the catheter wall, from which the $\mathbf{M}_i$ values follow directly.

For practical reasons (section 3), however, the 2D-IIC contains only three window electrodes, producing signals from which the $\mathbf{M}_i$-values in the direction $(\alpha) = (1)$ (parallel to the catheteraxis) follow directly from the $m_{kt}$-values, and the other $\mathbf{M}_i$-values are estimated.

# 5 Conclusions

We designed a new Intravascular Impedance Catheter (2D-IIC) suited for performing 2D intravascular E.I.T., and showed that using this 2D-IIC, the spatial resolution is improved with respect to that of the 1D-IIC. Furthermore we introduced a non-iterative, non-linear algorithm, of which the applicability is restricted by the assumptions concerning field homogeneity and sparseness of voxels having deviating impedances (assumptions (A) and (B) in section 4). Generally, in E.I.T., these assumptions prevent application of the algorithm, *unless* the following three conditions are met:

(1) Only the boundaries between regions of different $\sigma$ are of interest; global offsets in the $\sigma$-distribution may remain unknown.

(2) A normalised differential measurement method is used.

(3) The primary stimulus field is (approximately) constant in the region of interest.

We showed that these three conditions are met in case of detection of fatty intravascular lesions using the 2D-IIC; the non-iterative method reconstructs a 2D intravascular impedance map within seconds, as we showed in in-vitro experiments.

In other fields of bio-electrical measurements, the concept of the spatial derivative of the electrical field is used as well, e.g. in the case of the surface Laplacian [9], which is a concept related to the differential measurement used in the 2D-IIC.

Therefore, the non-iterative algorithm of section 4 may be of use in other applications of E.I.T., provided that they are aimed at detection of boundary surfaces between different tissues having different $\sigma$, rather than at the assessment of absolute $\sigma$-values.

**ACKNOWLEDGEMENTS** - This research is supported by the Technology Foundation of the Netherlands (STW).

## REFERENCES

1) M.K. Konings, W.P.Th.M. Mali, M.A. Viergever, "Design of a robust strategy to measure intravascular electrical impedance", In: Y. Bizais, C. Barillot, R. di Paola (eds): Information Processing in Medical Imaging, Kluwer Academic Publishers, pp. 1-12, june 1995.

2) V. Fuster, L. Badimon, J.J. Badimon, J.H. Chesebro, "The pathogenesis of coronary artery disease and the acute coronary syndromes", New Engl. J. Med., vol.326, No.4 pp.242-250 & No.5 pp.310-318, 1992.

3) E.J. Gussenhoven, C.E. Essed, C.T. Lancee, F. Mastik, P. Frietman, N. Bom; "Arterial wall characteristics determined by intravascular ultrasound imaging: an in vitro study", J Am Coll Cardiol 14, pp.947-952, 1989.

4) C.J. Slager, A.C. Phaff, C.E. Essed, N. Bom, J.C.H. Schuurbiers, P.W. Serruys, "Electrical impedance of layered atherosclerotic plaques on human aortas", IEEE Trans. Biomed. Eng. 39, pp.411-419, 1992.

5) F.C. VanEgmond, W. Li, E.J. Gussenhoven, C.T. Lancee, "Catheter Displacement Sensing Device", Thoraxcentre Journal vol.6/2, Rotterdam, 1994.

6) K.R. Visser, R. Lamberts, H.H.M. Korsten, W.G. Zijlstra, "Observations on blood flow related electrical impedance changes in rigid tubes", Pfluegers Arch. , vol.366 : 289-291, 1976.

7) J.D. Jackson, "Classical Electrodynamics", 2nd edition, J. Wiley, New York, 1975.

8) G.H. Golub, C.F. van Loan, "Matrix Computations", John Hopkins, 1989.

9) T.F. Oostendorp, A. van Oosterom, "The Surface Laplacian of the Potential: Theory and Application", IEEE Trans. Biomed. eng., vol.43, no.4: 394-405, april 1996.

# Optimal Data Types in Optical Tomography

M. Schweiger[1] and S. R. Arridge[2]

[1] Dept. of Medical Physics, University College London, UK
[2] Dept. of Computer Science, University College London, UK

**Abstract.** This paper addresses the problem of image reconstruction in optical tomography with respect to the measurement types used. We demonstrate the difficulty of the simultaneous reconstruction of absorption and diffusion images, by using both a simple circular case with embedded inhomogeneities, and a complex neonatal head model, and show that improvements are possible by combining suitable measurement types. We analyse the potential ability of the reconstruction program to separate absorption and scattering features by plotting the error norm as a function of absorption and scattering coefficient in the single-perturbation case for a number of different measurement types.

## 1 Introduction

Near-infrared imaging, or Optical Tomography (OT), is potentially a powerful tool to noninvasively obtain spatially resolved data of the optical parameters of tissue, from which physiologically relevant information such as local oxygenation can be calculated. Primary applications of this new imaging modality are the monitoring of cerebral blood and tissue oxygenation of newborn and preterm infants [1,2] to prevent death or permanent brain damage caused by asphyxiation during birth, functional mapping of brain activation during physical or mental exercise [3], and imaging of the breast to detect tumours [4].

The principal problem of OT is the dominance of scattering in the near-infrared wavelength range which causes light to propagate diffusely in tissue and thus prohibits the application of direct reconstruction methods using the Radon transform. Our approach, as reported previously [5, 6], uses an iterative reconstruction scheme, including a diffusion model as the forward model of light transport. The forward problem is solved using the finite element method (FEM) which provides a high degree of flexibility for the definition of the surface geometry and internal tissue boundaries.

### 1.1 Measurement Geometry and Data Types

Data acquisition for OT is not limited to steady-state attenuation measurements. Time-of-flight systems using an ultra-short pulsed laser as a light source and time-resolved detectors allow the boundary measurement of the temporal intensity response function with a resolution of a few picoseconds [7]. Frequency domain systems use a radio frequency modulated light source and measure the phase shift and modulation amplitude of the transmitted light [8]. While the data acquisition equipment for the steady-state, temporal and frequency domain are quite different, the methods are related from the theoretical viewpoint: the time-of-flight method includes the steady-state case via the integral over time of the detected light, and is related to the frequency domain case via its Fourier transform. It is therefore sufficient to consider the problem of OT in the temporal domain.

The aim in OT is to reconstruct the spatial distribution of the optical parameters of the tissue in the imaging plane from a set of boundary measurements within this plane. Let $\Omega$ be the domain under consideration, with surface $\partial\Omega$. We consider $s$ source positions $\zeta_i \in \partial\Omega$ ($i = 1...s$) and $m_i$ measurement positions $\xi_j \in \partial\Omega$ for each source $i$ ($j = 1...m_i$), resulting in a total number of measurements $n = \sum_{i=1}^{s} m_i$. The data acquisition system provides the temporally resolved flux intensity $\Gamma_i(\xi_j, t)$ for each source-detector pair $(i, j)$. From $\Gamma$ we extract a number of characteristic functionals $M$ to be used in the reconstruction. Some possibilities are:

$$\text{integrated intensity:} \quad M_{ij} = E = \int_0^\infty \Gamma_i(\xi_j, t)dt, \tag{1}$$

$$\text{time-gated intensity:} \quad M_{ij} = \bar{E}(T) = \int_0^T \Gamma_i(\xi_j, t)dt, \tag{2}$$

$$\text{n-th temporal moment:} \quad M_{ij} = \langle t^n \rangle = E^{-1} \int_0^\infty t^n \Gamma_i(\xi_j, t)dt, \tag{3}$$

$$\text{n-th central moment:} \quad M_{ij} = c_n = E^{-1} \int_0^\infty (t - \langle t \rangle)^n \Gamma_i(\xi_j, t)dt, \tag{4}$$

$$\text{normalised Laplace transform:} \quad M_{ij} = L(s) = E^{-1} \, \mathrm{L}(\Gamma_i, s)$$
$$= E^{-1} \int_0^\infty e^{-st} \Gamma_i(\xi_j, t)dt \ . \tag{5}$$

Additional features could be chosen, such as the logarithmic slope of the temporal decay of $\Gamma$, the peak intensity, etc. However, we aim to chose features that satisfy two conditions: robustness of the experimental measurements with respect to systematic errors such as fluctuations of the source power, detector sensitivity, or fibre coupling losses, and secondly the ability of the forward model to generate the corresponding data efficiently. Both conditions are satisfied for measurement types (3), (4) and (5), since these are normalised and therefore not dependent on absolute intensity measurements, and they can be calculated directly by our forward model without the need of explicitly generating the temporal profile of $\Gamma$ [9]. We will thus restrict the following discussion largely to these three measurement types. The time-gated intensity, $\bar{E}$, could also be normalised by $E$, but the forward model cannot efficiently generate the corresponding data.

# 2  Forward Model

Light transport in biological tissue in the near-infrared (NIR) wavelength range is dominated by scattering, and the unscattered component at a penetration depth of several centimetres is negligible. Some authors have suggested to use time-gating techniques, whereby only the first arriving photons contribute to the measurement, which have undergone only a few scattering events and have not deviated significantly from the straight line path, thus reducing the image reconstruction to a Radon transform approximation. Due to loss in signal-to-noise ratio (SNR) however this technique is restricted to very small optical thicknesses and not generally applicable.

Our approach has been to use the diffusion approximation to the radiative transfer equation:

$$\frac{1}{c}\frac{\partial \Phi(\mathbf{r},t)}{\partial t} - \nabla \cdot \kappa(\mathbf{r})\nabla\Phi(\mathbf{r},t) + \mu_a(\mathbf{r})\Phi(\mathbf{r},t) = q_0(\mathbf{r},t), \tag{6}$$

where $\Phi$ is the isotropic photon density, $q_0$ is an isotropic source distribution and $c$ is the speed of light in the medium. The model is characterised by the two spatially varying absorption and diffusion parameters, $\mu_a(\mathbf{r})$ and $\kappa(\mathbf{r})$, where

$$\kappa(\mathbf{r}) = [3(\mu_a + (1-\bar{f})\mu_s]^{-1}, \tag{7}$$

$\mu_s$ is the scattering coefficient and $\bar{f}$ is the mean cosine of the single scattering angle. The quantity $(1-\bar{f})\mu_s$ is commonly referred to as reduced scattering coefficient, $\mu_s'$.

Equation 6 assumes $\mu_a \ll \mu_s'$ and only weakly anisotropic light propagation. While the former is generally true for biological tissues, the latter is violated near sources and boundaries. However, comparisons of diffusion calculations with experimental results [10,11] and Monte Carlo simulations [12] show that diffusion models provide sufficient accuracy for most applications. Higher precision can be obtained, if required, by using higher order approximations to the transfer equations, at the expense of increased computational effort in the implementation of the model.

The boundary measurement $\Gamma(\xi, t)$ at $\xi \in \partial\Omega$ is related to $\Phi(\mathbf{r}, t)$ by

$$\Gamma(\xi, t) = -c\kappa(\xi)\hat{\mathbf{n}} \cdot \nabla\Phi(\xi, t), \tag{8}$$

where $\hat{\mathbf{n}}$ is the outer normal of $\partial\Omega$ at $\xi$. We use the Robin-type boundary condition

$$\Phi(\xi, t) + 2\kappa A\hat{\mathbf{n}} \cdot \nabla\Phi(\xi, t) = 0, \tag{9}$$

where $A$ is a term to incorporate boundary reflections as a result of a refractive index mismatch at $\partial\Omega$ [13]. A collimated source incident at $\zeta \in \partial\Omega$ is commonly represented by a diffuse point source $q_0(\mathbf{r}) = \delta(\mathbf{r} - \mathbf{r}_s)$ where $\mathbf{r}_s$ is located at depth $1/\mu_s'$ below the surface.

We have implemented the diffusion model ((6) and (9)) by using the finite element method. The domain $\Omega$ is divided into $P$ elements, joined at $D$ vertex nodes. $\mu_a$ and $\kappa$ are assumed piecewise constant. The solution $\Phi$ of (6) is approximated by the piecewise linear function $\Phi^h(\mathbf{r}, t) = \sum_i^D \Phi_i(t) u_i(\mathbf{r}) \in \mho^h$, where $\mho^h$ is a finite dimensional subspace spanned by basis functions $u_j(\mathbf{r})$, $j = 1...D$ chosen to have limited support. The problem of solving for $\Phi^h$ becomes one of sparse matrix inversion for which standard methods such as Cholesky decomposition or conjugate gradient solvers are readily available. The boundary condition (9) is implemented by an extrapolated boundary method [13, 14]. The advantage of the FEM approach is its versatility which makes it applicable to complex geometries and highly inhomogeneous parameter distributions.

The FEM forward model is capable of generating the time-dependent exitance at each point of the boundary, given a source distribution, where the temporal dimension is modelled by a finite difference scheme [5]. From this temporal profile any feature can be extracted. However a computationally more efficient direct method exists for calculating intensity, moment and Laplace transform data which avoids the need for explicit time-sampling and typically reduces the run-time for the forward solver by a factor $\approx 30$, depending on the number of moments required [9].

## 3   Inverse Model

The purpose of the inverse model is the spatial reconstruction of the model parameters $\mu_a(\mathbf{r})$ and $\kappa(\mathbf{r})$ (or alternatively $\mu_s'$) into a discrete solution basis. This may either be directly the element basis of the forward model, a subspace thereof obtained by grouping elements to regions, or an independent basis, e.g. a regular pixel grid. We have previously discussed a number of approaches to solving the inverse problem. By defining an appropriate error norm, it can be expressed as a multidimensional minimisation problem and solved using a modified Newton-Raphson approach:

$$[\mathbf{J}^T(\mathbf{p}^{(k)})\mathbf{J}(\mathbf{p}^{(k)}) + \lambda^{(k)}\mathbf{I}]\Delta\mathbf{p} = \mathbf{J}^T(\mathbf{p}^{(k)})[M - F(\mathbf{p}^{(k)})], \qquad (10)$$

where $\mathbf{p}^{(k)}$ is the solution at the k-th iteration, $\Delta\mathbf{p}$ is the new update ($\mathbf{p}^{(k+1)} = \mathbf{p}^{(k)} + \Delta\mathbf{p}$), $M$ is the measurement vector, $F$ is the forward operator mapping solution $\mathbf{p}$ to boundary measurements according to (8), and $\mathbf{J}$ is the $n \times P$ Jacobian matrix ($\partial F/\partial\mathbf{p}$). $\lambda$ is a relaxation parameter controlled by a Levenberg-Marquardt procedure. Computationally efficient methods to calculate $\mathbf{J}$ have been reported previously [15, 16].

Where the explicit inversion of $\mathbf{J}^T\mathbf{J}$ is not feasible, row action methods such as the algebraic reconstruction technique (ART) can be used:

$$\Delta\mathbf{p} = \lambda^{(k)}\frac{M_i - \mathbf{J}_i \cdot \mathbf{p}^{(k)}}{||\mathbf{J}_i^T||^2}\mathbf{J}_i^T, \qquad (11)$$

where $\mathbf{J}_i$ is the $i$-th row of $\mathbf{J}$. A variation of this method is *Block-ART* where several rows of $\mathbf{J}$ are used simultaneously, i.e. $\mathbf{J}_i$ is matrix of dimension $m \times P$,

$1 \leq m \leq n$). A natural choice for the FEM forward model is to group together all measurements obtained from the same source. In all following examples we use the Block-ART reconstruction kernel.

## 4  Noise Model

The error norm used in the inverse solver is given by

$$\phi = \sum_{i=1}^{n} \frac{(M_i - F_i(\mathbf{p}))^2}{\sigma_i^2} \ . \tag{12}$$

This requires a knowledge of the standard deviation $\sigma_i$ for each measurement $i$. For experimental measurements the error may be calculated directly from the noise in the temporal distribution of the response function. For data generated with the FEM forward solver we require a noise model providing a realistic estimation of $\sigma$ for each measurement type. Such a noise model was discussed previously for the steady-state intensity and temporal moments data types [17]. We found there that

$$\sigma_E^2 = N\beta(1 - \beta), \tag{13}$$

$$\sigma_{\langle t^n \rangle}^2 \approx \sigma_{T_1^n}^2 / N\beta \quad \text{in the limit of large N,} \tag{14}$$

where $N$ is the number of input photons, $\beta$ is the integrated flux density at the measurement position, and $\sigma_{T_1^n}^2$ is the conditional variance for a single photon arriving at time $T$, given by

$$\sigma_{T_1^n}^2 = G^{(\Gamma,2k)}(\xi)/G^{(\Gamma,0)}(\xi) - (G^{(\Gamma,k)}(\xi)/G^{(\Gamma,0)}(\xi))^2, \tag{15}$$

where $G^{(\Gamma,k)}(\xi) = \int_{-\infty}^{\infty} t^k g^{(\Gamma)}(\xi,t)dt$ and $g^{(\Gamma)}(\xi,t)$ is the Green's function of the problem for a given point source. It is straightforward to show that for the Laplace transform we get

$$\sigma_{L_1^n}^2 = G^{(2s)}(\xi)/G^{(\Gamma)}(\xi) - (G^{(s)}(\xi)/G^{(\Gamma)}(\xi))^2, \tag{16}$$

$$\sigma_{L(s)}^2 \approx \sigma_{L_1^n}^2 / N\beta \quad \text{in the limit of large N,} \tag{17}$$

where $G^{(s)}(\xi) = \int_{-\infty}^{\infty} e^{-st} g^{(\Gamma)}(\xi,t)dt$. The error estimates listed above assume $N$ to be the number of photons injected by the source pulse. Often it is desirable to find the error assuming that a constant number of photons has been *received*, which corresponds to an increased measurement time at large source-detector separations, which is often done in practice. We find the modified expressions for $\sigma^2$ by replacing the denominator in (14) and (17) with the number of received photons.

# 5 Error Maps for Single Perturbation

The image reconstruction algorithms produced by us and other groups work generally well when only one of the two model parameters, $\mu_a$ or $\mu'_s$, is being reconstructed, while the other is assumed to be known a priori. In general however both parameters are unknown. Since any error in one parameter will induce an error in the reconstruction of the other parameter, they must necessarily be reconstructed simultaneously. This is a fundamental problem of OT and has so far not been solved satisfactorily. To illustrate this problem we consider the simple problem of a homogeneous circle with parameters $\bar{\mu}_a$ and $\bar{\mu}'_s$ and a single embedded perturbation region. For this case we can explicitly draw the map of error norms as a function of the absorption and scattering parameters of the perturbation region, $\mu'_s$ and $\mu'_s$, given by

$$\phi(\mu_a, \mu'_s) = \sum_{i=1}^{n} \frac{F_i(\mu_a, \mu'_s) - F_i(\bar{\mu}_a, \bar{\mu}'_s)}{\sigma_i^2} \tag{18}$$

These error maps give some insight into the nonlinearity of the inverse problem. The mesh for which the homogeneous reference data $F_i(\bar{\mu}_a, \bar{\mu}'_s)$ and perturbation data $F_i(\mu_a, \mu'_s)$ were generated had a radius of 25 mm, and the reference parameters were $\bar{\mu}_a = 0.025\,\text{mm}^{-1}$, $\bar{\mu}'_s = 2\,\text{mm}^{-1}$. Data were calculated at 16 equally spaced source positions and 16 detector positions, each placed between two sources. We then generated the error maps $\phi(\bar{\mu}_a, \bar{\mu}'_s)$, sampled at 41 $\bar{\mu}_a$ values in the range from $0.0125\,\text{mm}^{-1}$ to $0.0375\,\text{mm}^{-1}$ (vertical axis) and at 41 $\bar{\mu}'_s$ values in the range from $1\,\text{mm}^{-1}$ to $3\,\text{mm}^{-1}$ (horizontal axis).

The first seven graphs of Fig. 1 show error maps for the measurement types $E$, $\langle t \rangle$, $\langle t^2 \rangle$, $c_2$, $c_3$, $L(s = 0.001)$ and $L(s = 0.01)$. Characteristic for all types is an elongated 'valley', while the orientation of the valley differs between measurement types. Specifically, we note the following points:

1. The error behaviour of $E$ and $\langle t \rangle$ is markedly different. This is in agreement with previous investigations on the effect of absorption and scattering perturbations on measurements, where we showed that absorbers and scatterers affect $E$ qualitatively in the same way, i.e. $\partial E/\partial\bar{\mu}_a < 0 \wedge \partial E/\partial\bar{\mu}'_s < 0$, while they act qualitatively different on $\langle t \rangle$: $\partial\langle t \rangle/\partial\bar{\mu}_a < 0 \wedge \partial\langle t \rangle/\partial\bar{\mu}'_s > 0$. Note that the latter condition is not generally true for the point-wise derivative, as $\partial\langle t \rangle_i/\partial\mu'_s(\mathbf{r})$ can locally change sign.

2. For small $s$ the error map of $L(s)$ is similar to that of $\langle t \rangle$. This follows directly from (5). With the approximation $e^{-st} \approx 1 - st$, $L$ can be written as a linear function of $\langle t \rangle$:

$$L(s) \approx 1 - s\langle t \rangle \ . \tag{19}$$

3. On the other hand, for a high value of $s$ the measurement error norm is more sensitive to errors in $\mu'_s$ than $\mu_a$. To understand this we look at the Laplace transform of (6),

$$\left[ \frac{s}{c} + \mu_a - \nabla \cdot \kappa\nabla \right] L(\Phi(t), s) = L(q_0(t), s), \tag{20}$$

where we used $L(\partial\Phi/\partial t, s) = s\, L(\Phi, s)$. With substitution $L(\Phi(t), s) \to \Phi'$, $L(q_0(t), s) \to q_0'$ we obtain the time-independent diffusion equation with the modified absorption parameter $\mu_a' = s/c + \mu_a$. Since the measurement perturbation is essentially proportional to the logarithm of the parameter perturbation [18], a large $s$ reduces the influence of $\mu_a$.

4. Conversely the error norm of central moments is more sensitive to errors in $\mu_a$ than $\mu_s'$.

The shape of the error functions suggests that the simultaneous reconstruction of $\mu_a$ and $\mu_s'$ will be ambiguous for any single measurement type. The reconstruction algorithm will have no problem descending into the valley at some point, but due to the small gradient along the valley the convergence towards the true solution is ill-posed.

In order to overcome this problem we have to use multiple measurement types for the reconstruction. This can be done in two ways: either by simultaneous reconstruction of $\mu_a$ and $\mu_s'$ from a data vector composed of several measurement types, as described in [19], or by iteratively reconstructing each parameter from a different measurement type. For the latter method we seek measurement types whose error functions depend predominantly on one parameter, so that artefacts introduced by errors in the estimate of the other parameter are minimised. Under this aspect, we conclude from the error maps in Fig. 1 that the skew ($c_3$) is a good choice for the reconstruction of $\mu_a$, as its error norm varies with $\mu_a$ significantly more than with $\mu_s'$, while conversely $L(s = 0.01)$ is suitable for the reconstruction of $\mu_s'$.

For the simultaneous reconstruction we require a combination of measurement types for which the sums of the error norms exhibit a clearly defined minimum, to avoid the $\mu_a/\mu_s'$ ambiguity of the single-measure case. The last five graphs of Fig. 1 show error maps for various combinations of measurement types. It is obvious that in some cases the problem is significantly better posed than for single type reconstructions, e.g. for the combinations $\langle t \rangle + c_3$, or $c_3 + L(0.01)$. From the error maps it may be expected that a combination of $E + \langle t \rangle$ or $E + L(0.001)$ produces a good result due to the significantly different error behaviour, but we have not included these cases here as intensity measurements are usually avoided in practical applications due to the above mentioned problems with unnormalised data types.

Finally we would like to note that the application of the Laplace transform to $\Gamma$ simulates time-gating techniques by suppressing late arriving photons. Increasing $s$ will therefore eventually lead to similar problems of poor photon statistics as seen in explicit time-gating during data acquisition. This imposes an upper limit to the value of $s$, both with respect to the signal-to-noise ratio of the data, and the numerical stability of the forward solver. In the FEM forward model, a high $s$ value has to be matched with a sufficiently highly resolved mesh to guarantee the numerical stability of the calculation. For the circular object used here a typical mesh size of the order of 3000 element was used to generate all data except $L(s = 0.01)$, which required a mesh with about twice the number of elements.

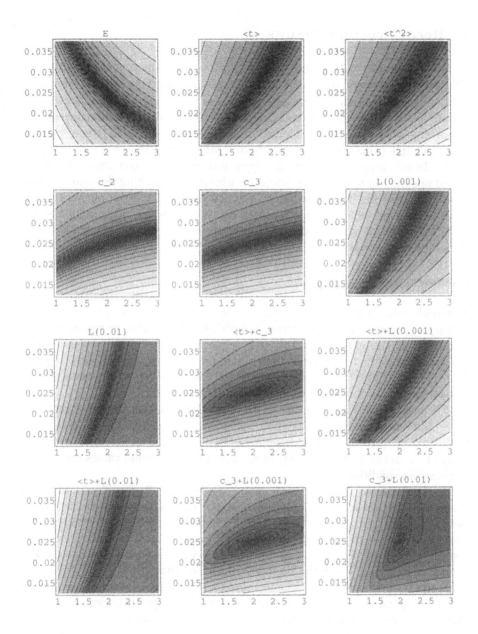

**Fig. 1.** Measurement error norms as a function of global $\bar{\mu}_a$ and $\bar{\mu}_s'$ for different measurement types and combinations thereof. Abscissae: $\bar{\mu}_s'$ (mm$^{-1}$), ordinates: $\bar{\mu}_a$ (mm$^{-1}$).

# 6 Reconstruction Results

To test the reconstruction performance predictions of the previous chapter for different measurement types we carried out test reconstructions from simulated data of objects containing both absorption and scattering inhomogeneities. We present two cases: A simple circular object with three embedded inhomogeneities (absorbing, scattering, and combined absorbing/scattering), and a more complicated example using a mesh derived from a MRI scan of the head of a newborn infant. In all cases we assume that each measurement is composed of $10^4$ received photons. In practice this would be achieved by adapting the source power or integration time corresponding to the attenuation for each source/detector pair. We use the noise model discussed above to generate noise estimates for each measurement and use this to add random Gaussian-distributed noise to the simulated forward data.

## 6.1 Circular Test Object

The mesh radius is 25 mm, and the background parameters are $\mu_a = 0.025\,\text{mm}^{-1}$ and $\mu_s' = 2\,\text{mm}^{-1}$. There are three embedded objects, with increased absorption ($\mu_a = 0.05\,\text{mm}^{-1}$) at the top, with increased scattering ($\mu_s' = 4\,\text{mm}^{-1}$) at the lower right, and combined absorption/scattering ($\mu_a = 0.05\,\text{mm}^{-1}$, $\mu_s' = 4\,\text{mm}^{-1}$) at the lower left. $c_3$ and $L(0.01)$ data are sampled at 16 source and 16 measurement positions equally spaced along the boundary.

Figure 2 shows reconstructions of $\mu_a$ (left column) and $\mu_s'$ (right) column for three different choices of data types: $\mu_a$ from $c_3$ and $\mu_s'$ from $L(0.01)$ (row 2), both from $c_3$, (row 3), and both from $L(0.01)$ (row 4). The first row shows the absorption and scattering targets. In all cases the background values are used as the starting condition.

As we expected from the error maps, the best result is achieved when reconstructing $\mu_a$ from $c_3$ and $\mu_s'$ from $L(0.01)$. In this case a clear distinction between absorption and scattering features is possible. When using only $c_3$ for the reconstruction of both parameters the $\mu_a$ image is essentially the same as in the previous case, while the $\mu_s'$ image has a lower contrast and contains marked artefacts, especially along the boundary. Reconstructing from $L$ only produces the worst results. In this case, in addition to artefacts, the algorithm is no longer able to distinguish between absorption and scattering perturbation, and shows the scattering object as an artefact in the absorption image.

## 6.2 Neonatal Head Model

To demonstrate the potential of OT in a more complex case we created a mesh based on an MRI scan of a neonatal head. The original image was segmented using a standard image processing tool to define regions of the following tissue types: skin, bone, grey and white brain matter.

The segmentation provided the outline information for automatic mesh generation with an adaptive mesh generator [20]. The sagittal diameter of the mesh

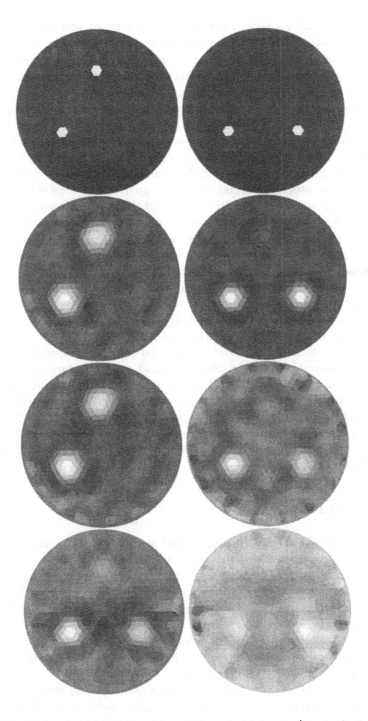

**Fig. 2.** Reconstruction of circular object with embedded $\mu_a$, $\mu'_s$ perturbations. Left column: $\mu_a$, right column: $\mu'_s$. Rows from top to bottom: target, reconstruction from $c_3$ and $L(0.01)$, from $c_3$ alone, from $L(0.01)$ alone.

is 10 cm. For the forward data calculation, the absorption and scattering parameters for each element were set from literature values according to its assigned region. To investigate the ability of the reconstruction algorithm to recover highly localised objects we added to this background distribution regions of increased absorption and scattering, with a contrast between 50 and 200 percent.

We generated data for all 1024 combinations of 32 equally spaced data points and 32 interleaved measurement sites. $\mu_a$ is reconstructed from $c_3$, and $\mu'_s$ from $L(0.01)$, initially assuming a homogeneous distribution of $\mu_a(\mathbf{r}) = 0.022\,\text{mm}^{-1}$ and $\mu'_s(\mathbf{r}) = 1.0\,\text{mm}^{-1}$. These values represent the optical parameters of skin in the model, assuming that these surface characteristics can be determined by other means. No other a priori information is used. In Fig. 3 we show the target distributions (top row) of $\mu_a$ (left) and $\mu'_s$ (right), and the corresponding reconstructions after the 5-th iteration (bottom row). Note that the reconstructions generally cannot recover the absolute values of the high-contrast perturbations, in particular in the centre where the resolution is low. Therefore the greyscale range of the reconstructed images has been adjusted to the solution range. To allow a quantitative assessment of the reconstruction performance we show cross sections through the targets and reconstructions in Fig. 4.

Despite considerable artefact, especially in the boundary, the algorithm has succeeded in identifying the absorption and scattering anomalies, as well as recovering some of the low-contrast background structure, especially in the $\mu'_s$ image. The separation between absorption and scatter features is quite good, although there is some indication that the strong scattering object in the top left region of the mesh appears in the absorption image. In the absorption image we see quite clearly that the resolution is highest towards the boundary, while the strong central perturbation is not well-defined and shows little contrast in the reconstruction. These images represent the best likely to be obtainable in real clinical situations.

## 7    Conclusion

We have discussed the reconstruction problem in OT with emphasis on the simultaneous reconstruction of absorption and scattering. We demonstrated that this can be achieved only by using a suitable combination of measurement types. The best combination of data types available so far seems to be skew ($c_3$) for the reconstruction of $\mu_a$ and the Laplace transform ($L(s)$) with sufficiently high $s$ for the reconstruction of $\mu'_s$. The error maps for these data types show that they predominantly depend on only one parameter, so that artefacts due to errors in the other parameter are minimised. This in turn leads to a good separation between absorption and scattering features.

We find that the reconstruction of complex geometries, in particular in cases with boundary layers such as the presented head model, is significantly more difficult than simple test geometries such as objects embedded in a homogeneous background medium, especially with respect to recovery of absolute quantitation of high-contrast perturbations. To date very little research has been carried out

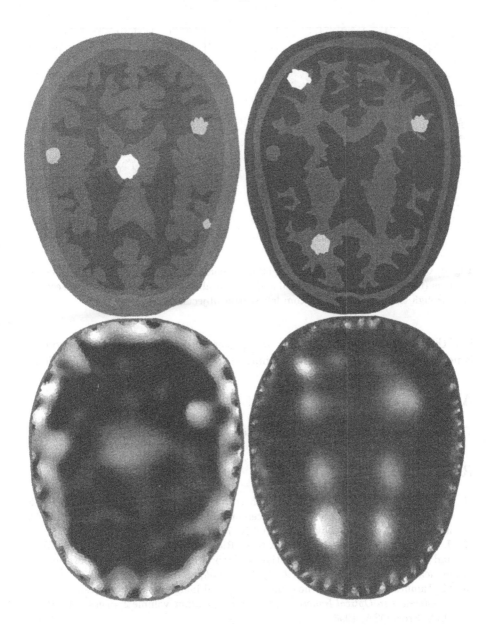

**Fig. 3.** $\mu_a$ and $\mu'_s$ reconstructions of a four-layer neonatal head model with embedded objects. Top left: target $\mu_a$ image, top right: target $\mu'_s$ image, bottom left: $\mu_a$ reconstruction, bottom right: $\mu'_s$ reconstruction. The optical parameters of the target ($\mu_a, \mu'_s$ in mm$^{-1}$) are: skin = (0.022,1.0), skull = (0.025,2.0), grey matter = (0.02,0.55), white matter = (0.01,2.0). The embedded objects are between 0.05 and 0.1 ($\mu_a$) and between 2 and 6 ($\mu'_s$).

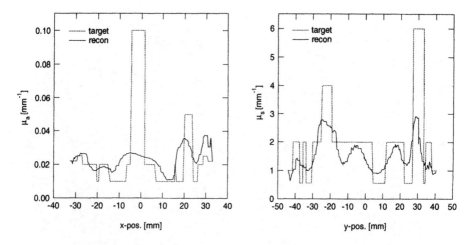

**Fig. 4.** Cross-sections through the target and reconstruction images in Fig. 3. $\mu_a$ cross-sections (left) are through the central and top-left absorption objects, $\mu'_s$ cross sections are through the top left and bottom left scatter objects.

into the reconstruction of complex geometries, and more work on this problem is needed to assess the feasibility of optical tomography in clinical applications.

## Acknowledgements

This work was supported by Action Research.

## References

1. A. D. Edwards, J. S. Wyatt, C. E. Richardson, D. T. Delpy, M. Cope, and E. O. R. Reynolds. Cotside measurement of cerebral blood flow in ill newborn infants by near infrared spectroscopy. *Lancet*, ii:770–771, 1988.
2. J. S. Wyatt, M. Cope, D. T. Delpy, C. E. Richardson, A. D. Edwards, S. C. Wray, and E. O. R. Reynolds. Quantitation of cerebral blood volume in newborn infants by near infrared spectroscopy. *J. Appl. Physiol.*, 68(3):1086–1091, 1990.
3. M. Tamura. Multichannel near-infrared optical imaging of human brain activity. In *Advances in Optical Imaging and Photon Migration*, volume 2, pages 8–10. Proc. OSA, Proc. OSA, 1996.
4. J. C. Hebden, R. A. Kruger, and K. S. Wong. Time resolved imaging through a highly scattering medium. *Appl. Opt.*, 30(7):788–794, 1991.
5. S. R. Arridge, M. Schweiger, M. Hiraoka, and D. T. Delpy. A finite element approach for modeling photon transport in tissue. *Med. Phys.*, 20(2):299–309, 1993.
6. M. Schweiger, S. R. Arridge, and D. T. Delpy. Application of the finite-element method for the forward and inverse models in optical tomography. *J. Math. Imag. Vision*, 3:263–283, 1993.
7. D. T. Delpy, M. Cope, P. van der Zee, S. R. Arridge, S. Wray, and J. Wyatt. Estimation of optical pathlength through tissue from direct time of flight measurement. *Phys. Med. Biol.*, 33:1433–1442, 1988.

8. B. Chance, M. Maris, J. Sorge, and M. Z. Zhang. A phase modulation system for dual wavelength difference spectroscopy of haemoglobin deoxygenation in tissue. volume 1204, pages 481–491. Proc. SPIE, 1990.

9. S. R. Arridge and M. Schweiger. Direct calculation of the moments of the distribution of photon time of flight in tissue with a finite-element method. *Appl. Opt.*, 34(15):2683–2687, 1995.

10. S. J. Madsen, M. S. Patterson, B. C. Wilson, S. M. Jaywant, and A. Othonos. Numerical modelling and experimental studies of light pulse propagation in inhomogeneous random media. In B. Chance and R. R. Alfano, editors, *Photon Migration and Imaging in Random Media and Tissues*, volume 1888, pages 90–102. Proc. SPIE, 1993.

11. J. B. Fishkin and E. Gratton. Propagation of photon-density waves in strongly scattering media containing an absorbing semi-infinite plane bounded by a straight edge. *J. Opt. Soc. Am. A*, 10(1):127–140, 1993.

12. T. J. Farrell and M. S. Patterson. A diffusion theory model of spatially resolved, steady-state diffuse reflectance for the noninvasive determination of tissue optical properties *in vivo*. *Med. Phys.*, 19(4):879–888, 1992.

13. M. Schweiger, S. R. Arridge, M. Hiraoka, and D. T. Delpy. The finite element model for the propagation of light in scattering media: Boundary and source conditions. *Med. Phys.*, 22(11):1779–1792, 1995.

14. J. D. Moulton. Diffusion modelling of picosecond laser pulse propagation in turbid media. M. Eng. thesis, McMaster University, Hamilton, Ontario, 1990.

15. S. R. Arridge. Photon measurement density functions. Part 1: Analytical forms. *Appl. Opt.*, 34(31):7395–7409, 1995.

16. S. R. Arridge and M. Schweiger. Photon measurement density functions. Part 2: Finite element calculations. *Appl. Opt.*, 34(34):8026–8037, 1995.

17. S. R. Arridge, M. Hiraoka, and M. Schweiger. Statistical basis for the determination of optical pathlength in tissue. *Phys. Med. Biol.*, 40:1539–1558, 1995.

18. M. Schweiger, S. R. Arridge, M. Hiraoka, and D. T. Delpy. Application of the finite element method for the forward model in infrared absorption imaging. volume 1768, pages 97–108. Proc. SPIE, 1992.

19. S. R. Arridge and M. Schweiger. The use of multiple data types in time-resolved optical absorption and scattering tomography (TOAST). volume 2035, pages 218–229. Proc. SPIE, 1993.

20. S. R. Arridge and M. Schweiger. Reconstruction in optical tomography using MRI based prior knowledge. In Y. Bizais, C. Barillot, and R. di Paola, editors, *Information Processing in Medical Imaging '95*, pages 77–88. Springer, Berlin, 1995.

# Using Spatial-Temporal Images for Analysis of Gated Cardiac Tomographic Data: The "M-Mode" Revisited

I. Buvat[1], M.L. Bartlett[2], A.N. Kitsiou[2], J.M. Carson[2], G. Srinivasan[2], K.A. Nour[2], C.C. Chen[2], V. Dilsizian[2], S.L. Bacharach[2]

[1] U66 INSERM/CNRS, CHU Pitié-Salpêtrière, 91 Bd de l'Hôpital, 75 634 Paris Cedex 13, France
[2] National Institutes of Health, 9000 Rockville Pike, Bethesda, MD 20892, USA

**Abstract.** Recent advances in SPECT and PET technology permit ECG gating of tomographic cardiac images, allowing simultaneous measurement of 3D cardiac ventricular function with perfusion/metabolism. Extracting indices of regional function from these 4D data sets (3D space + time) remains a challenge. All approaches currently used to quantitate gated tomographic sequences deal *separately* with the spatial and temporal data. As functional information is based on close coupling between spatial and temporal changes, it could be beneficial to produce an image *combining* spatial and temporal information. In this paper we describe a method for producing such spatial-temporal images and, using gated FDG PET data, test the ability of these images to improve visual and quantitative assessment of cardiac function. Other potential schemes to make use of the space-time nature of this new representation are also discussed.

## 1 Introduction

Recent advances in SPECT and PET technology have permitted ECG gating of tomographic cardiac images. ECG tomographic gating of tracers which tag the myocardium permits simultaneous measurement of 3D cardiac ventricular function and perfusion/metabolism. However, extracting indices of regional function from these data sets remains a challenge for several reasons: 1) The data are intrinsically 4 dimensional (3D + time) and ideally, these 4 dimensions should all be taken into account to describe heart motion; 2) SPECT and PET gated images are often noisy; 3) Cardiac motion is complex, involving torsion, dilatation and contraction. Nearly all approaches used to estimate functional indices from gated tomographic sequences deal separately with the spatial and temporal data. For instance, standard 2D image processing tools are typically first applied to the 2 D spatial images for each time point (e.g. [1-4]). The processed images might then be smoothed or fitted along space in the third spatial dimension, and finally along time, using a priori models (e.g. [5]). These approaches may not be the best way to estimate functional information, since such information relates directly to changes in time. In addition, certain of the spatial dimensions behave in relatively constrained ways temporally. It could therefore be beneficial to deal with such spatial dimensions simultaneously with temporal information. Visual analysis corroborates this suggestion, since it is well known that gated cardiac images are best interpreted visually by looking at the image sequence in cine mode, rather than as a set of static 2D/3D images, so that the eye can analyze simultaneously both the spatial and temporal deformations. A method which can represent spatial and temporal information simultaneously might therefore help in both the visual and quantitative analysis of tomographic image sequences. In this paper, we describe a "new" method for simultaneously portraying the spatial and temporal aspects of gated tomographic cardiac data. The method is based loosely on the "M-mode" method used in the early days of echocardiography, and is also similar to the "kymographic" techniques first described over 50 years ago [6], and tried and abandoned nearly 20 years ago in planar nuclear medicine imaging [7]. Because this "new" nuclear M-mode (NMM) representation of gated tomographic sequences permits both the spatial and the temporal information in the data to be portrayed simultaneously, it potentially improves both visualization and quantitative analysis. Preliminary measurements to define the extent of this improvement are made by applying the technique to gated FDG PET images from several subjects. The visual and quantitative results obtained from the NMM representation were compared to those obtained from more conventional methods. Other potentially useful schemes which make use of the space-time nature of the new representation are also discussed.

## 2 Materials and methods

### 2.1 Nuclear M-mode representation

Tomographic gated cardiac image sequences can be viewed as a set of NxT slices, where N is a number of slices encompassing the heart, while T is the number of time points dividing the cardiac cycle. Let us assume, for the sake of simplicity, that the left ventricle (LV) has been reoriented into N short axis slices. Each short axis slice can be divided up into a number of sectors (Fig. 1a). A sector in a slice therefore represents a region of the LV, and the function of that region is determined by following the behavior of this sector with time. A convenient representation of the signal for a particular sector is obtained by calculating the count-profile corresponding to that sector (Fig. 1b). Count-profiles can be obtained for instance by casting the short axis images into cylindrical coordinates (Fig. 1b), or by taking normal profiles to an estimated mid-myocardial surface. Following the sector behavior with time therefore corresponds to looking at the count-profile changes with time. The representation we propose gives a static image that portrays motion by creating an image in which each column is the count-profile at a particular time point, the pixel intensity being the count-profile intensity (Fig. 1c,d). Note that this representation is analogous to the M-mode images which were used in echocardiography prior to the introduction of 2D echo and to a method proposed for planar nuclear images nearly 20 years ago [7]. The nuclear M-mode displays on a single static image how the profile changes in time during the cardiac cycle.

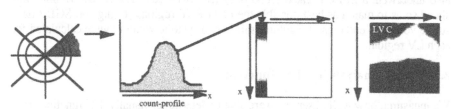

Fig. 1: The different steps used to create NMM images. LV C stands for LV cavity.

The NMM images can be used to distinguish overall motion of the LV from LV contraction, by displaying two NMM images from opposing sectors (with respect to the LV long central axis) at the top and bottom of a composite NMM image (Fig. 2). As will be further described below, the NMM images portray deformation of the myocardial wall with time, possible delays in these deformations, geometric thickening of the wall, and thickening of the wall as indicated by (non-linear) intensity changes due to the partial volume effect. In addition, the separation of the two endocardial surfaces in the opposite NMM images (the interior edges in Fig. 2) portrays regional LV cavity shortening with time.

Fig. 2: Example of opposing NMM representation of gated FDG PET images.

## 2.2  Data

Studies from seven patients (age 54 to 71) with coronary artery disease were used to investigate the value of the NMM representation. Each patient underwent gated F18 fluorodeoxyglucose (FDG) PET imaging at rest after intravenous injection of 185 MBq (5 mCi) FDG, using a GE-Advance PET scanner in 3D mode with scatter and attenuation correction. Slice separation was 4.25 mm and pixel size was 2 mm. The LV volume was resliced into 6 short axis images from the apex to the base. The thickness of each short axis slice therefore depended on LV size, and varied from 9.66 mm to 11 mm. The two extreme slices (apex and base) were excluded from analysis, and only the remaining 4 slices per patient were used.

Each short axis image was divided up into 8 sectors. An initial, manual estimate of the LV center was made on the end-diastolic image and from this estimate an "optimal" center was computed for each time point [8]. The average optimal center location over all time points was used as the fixed LV center for all time points.

The fixed centers were used to cast the LV FDG PET short axis images into cylindrical coordinates. Using this cylindrical coordinate system, count-profiles were calculated and NMM images were created.

To obtain an independent assessment of regional LV function, 4 out of the 7 patients also underwent a SPECT gated blood pool (SGBP) study. The SGBP volume was sliced so as to match as best possible the FDG PET regions. Using the SGBP data, stroke volumes (end diastolic volume minus end systolic volume) were calculated for each LV region.

## 2.3  Visual analysis of LV function

We measured how well observers were able to determine, visually, LV function from the NMM images compared to the standard cine display. LV function was visually analyzed independently by 6 observers using both approaches. First, all four slices for a given patient were presented in cine mode display, so that the observer could assess regional LV function using the following scale: 0-Normal, 1-Mildly hypokinetic, 2-Severely hypokinetic, 3-Akinetic or dyskinetic, 4-Undetermined. The observers were shown two sets of cine mode displays simultaneously: one with an overlaid grid dividing the short axis image into 8 sectors, each image normalized to its own maximum, and one without grids (i.e. conventional cine mode display), normalized to the maximum of the time series. The image sequences from the 7 patients were presented in random order.

Second, NMM images of patients different from those included in this study were presented to the observers as a "training" set, for them to gain experience with reading NMM images (the observers were already familiar with reading cine images). After training, the NMM images of the 7 patients described above were presented to the observers as a set of static images, each NMM image corresponding to a sector in a short axis slice. Again, the data from each patient were presented in random order, and each NMM image was displayed normalized to its own maximum. The observers were asked to score LV function using the same scoring system as above.

## 2.4 Automatic quantitative analysis of the LV function

Several approaches could be used to automatically estimate functional parameters from the NMM images, such as methods based on image segmentation or model fitting. Ideally, these methods would employ some of the constraints known to exist in the temporal direction. In this section, we present the details of one particular method, but other possible approaches (currently under investigation) will be briefly described in the discussion section.

Each FDG PET NMM image was analyzed using three stages : 1) calculating a set of isodensity lines in the NMM image; 2) identifying the isodensity line that separates background from wall; 3) deriving functional indices. Each stage employed temporal constraints.

**Temporal Constraints.** It is known that many features of the time behavior of global LV volume (such as stroke volume, ejection fraction, etc) can be very accurately described by the first 2 Fourier harmonics of the time data [9]. However, it is not known whether a limited number of harmonics could also adequately describe the temporal changes occurring on a *regional* basis (i.e. sector by sector). To investigate this, we studied 3 patients with gated SPECT blood pool imaging. The GBP images were sliced and sectored in exactly the same way as used for FDG images. The changes in endocardial motion observed on the NMM images should therefore produce whatever changes in blood pool activity that occurred in the GBP images. The volume curves derived from each of the 96 GBP sectors were filtered using 1, 2, 3 and 4 Fourier harmonics. Amplitude, local time to minimum volume, ejection fraction, and stroke volume were computed from each filtered regional volume curve. The parameters computed from regional volume curves described by a 1 harmonic fit were significantly different from those computed from the 2, 3 or 4 harmonic fits. However, aside from increased noise, there was little change in any of the 4 parameters whether 2, 3 or 4 harmonics were used. We conclude that, in terms of the above 4 parameters, the endocardial border in NMM images can be tracked in the temporal direction by a 2 harmonic function. This considerably constrains the edge tracking problem and reduces noise significantly.

**Calculating a set of isodensity lines on the NMM images.** First, for each time point (i.e. each column), the location of the maximum pixel value was determined, giving a crest line from the left to the right of the image, dividing up the image into two NMM parts (Fig. 3): above the crest line was the temporal change of the count-profile from the center of the cavity to the mid-myocardium going through the endocardium; below the crest line was the temporal change of the count-profile from the mid-myocardium to the epicardium and beyond. To ensure regularity, the crest line was fitted using 2 Fourier harmonics. The maximum pixel intensity on crest line was determined and defined the FDG uptake, UT, for that sector. Using this uptake value, a set of n/2 values was calculated, $v_1$ to $v_{n/2}$, ranging from 0 to UT by step of UT*2/n, where n was the total number of points in each count profile. A set of n/2 isodensity lines was then derived. Each isodensity line corresponding to value $v_k$ was defined as the line which, for each time t (each column), passed through the pixel with the value closest to $v_k$. The isodensity lines were fitted using 2 Fourier harmonics. The isodensity lines were obtained only by considering pixels on the endocardial side of the crest line (i.e. above the crest line). Each isodensity line defined two regions R1 and R2. R1 was above the isodensity line and R2 was the region located between the isodensity line and the crest line (Fig. 3).

The main hypothesis used to automatically analyze the NMM image is that, for a particular sector, the background activity inside the cavity is uniform in space (along the x direction) and does not change significantly with time (along the t direction, see Fig. 1c), so that there is an isodensity line in the NMM image that separates a cavity region with uniform activity in the spatio-temporal domain from a wall region. The challenge therefore lies in identifying this isodensity line, which will be called the background-wall edge (BWE) among all the isodensity lines that are calculated. Note that this choice may not have to be absolutely accurate. The BWE need not be a true representation of the endocardial border - it must simply vary temporally in the same way that the border does.

**Identifying the isodensity line separating background from the wall.**
Above the BWE, activity should be fairly uniform (apart from noise perturbations) *both* in x and t directions and no structures should be seen. Pixel intensity should thus vary randomly around a value corresponding to the cavity activity both in x and t directions. However, it is well known that tomographic reconstruction and volume reslicing introduce correlated noise in space. On the other hand, as tomographic reconstruction and reslicing are performed independently for each time point, there is a priori *no* autocorrelation of noise in time. Therefore, to test the randomness of signal variation around the unknown cavity activity in the NMM image, it seems reasonable to give a greater weight to randomness along time than to randomness along space. For each isodensity line, the hypothesis that signal above the isodensity line (region R1) corresponded to background was tested as follows. First, the values of pixels in R1 were ordered in a so called feature vector, row by row, i.e. time dimension varying faster than space dimension (Fig. 3). The randomness of the signal variation in the feature vector was tested using the distribution-free change point test [10]. Briefly, this test assumes that initially, the distribution of values in the feature vector has one median, and that at some point there is a shift in the median of the distribution. H0 is the hypothesis that there is no change in the median, i.e. that the signal distribution in the feature vector is homogeneous, while H1 is the hypothesis that there is a change. The test assesses the likelihood that a

change occurred in the sequence of values in the feature vector and whether the change exceeds the fluctuations expected due to chance.

The hypothesis that signal in R1 follows a random distribution around its median (i.e. corresponds to cavity activity) was tested using the feature vector calculated for each isodensity line. The BWE was then defined as the isodensity line corresponding to the greatest $v_k$ value for which one could accept the hypothesis that the variations in the feature vector were random, and that no change of trend occurred in that vector.

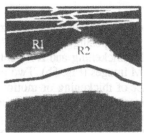

Fig. 3: Crest line and isodensity line on an NMM image. The scanning process used to calculate the feature vector is shown in white.

Other methods taking advantage of the space-time behavior could be used to identify the BWE or describe its motion. Some of these will be described further in the discussion section.

**Deriving functional indices.** Several methods can be used to derive functional indices on preprocessed images, supposedly free of background and/or noise. In this paper, we have used an approach derived from an hybrid method recently described [8], which has been shown to be more reliable than methods based on geometry only, or on counts only.

A profile across the LV wall can be approximately modeled by a square wave, convolved with the point spread function of the detector (Fig. 4a). Using this model, even after convolution by the system PSF, if there were no background, the activity under half of the profile would be exactly equal to the true uptake UT times half the true wall thickness. Therefore, after background removal, half the wall thickness can be estimated by the integral of counts N under half the profile divided by the uptake. Assuming that the BWE separates wall from background activity, the integral of counts between the BWE and the crest line was calculated for each line (each time point), and given the uptake UT estimated as previously described, the corresponding half thickness of the wall at each time point, d(t), was deduced (Fig. 4b).

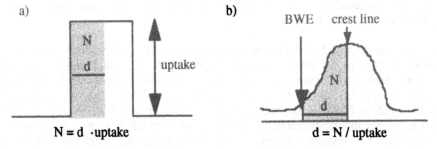

Fig. 4: Square wave model and method used to estimate the functional index SH.

d(t) was then fitted using 2 Fourier harmonics, giving d'(t) and an index related to the shortening of the cavity was deduced as:

SH = d'(ES) - d'(ED), where ES and ED stand for end-systole and end-diastole respectively.

## 3 Results

### 3.1 NMM images

Fig. 5 shows an example of a gated FDG short axis image series displayed conventionally (Fig. 5a) and in "opposing sector" NMM format (Fig. 5b). When only static display is available, thickening and LV contraction are much easier to perceive on the opposing NMM images (Fig. 5b). Two pieces of information on the NMM images can give evidence of thickening or motion: 1) the deformation of the wall with time, i.e. in the horizontal direction (see, for instance, sectors 1, 2, 3); and 2) the brightness changes (see for instance sector 8). Although the brightness does not show up well on the printed images (in either 5a or b), the use of a different intensity scale, especially color display instead of gray scale, can make the brightness change with time much more visible. Finally, even when the magnitude of contraction is normal, delays or asynchronies in contraction are readily apparent in the NMM images as shifts in time of the occurrence of the maximal thickening or motion - i.e. by right/left shifts in the NMM image. Such temporal "phase shifts" are often very difficult to see from cine images.

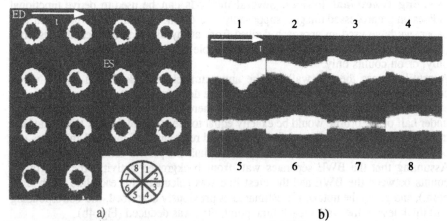

Fig. 5: a: Conventional static display of a gated FDG short axis image series. b: Corresponding NMM display.

Typical examples of NMM images for normal, akinetic, and dyskinetic sectors are shown in Fig. 6. An NMM image corresponding to a normal sector (Fig. 6a) exhibits both wall deformation (close to a sinusoidal shape) and brightness enhancement at ES (around the middle column of the NMM image). An akinetic region yields an NMM image which displays a straight line (Fig. 6b), i.e. no wall deformation, without noticeable brightness change from left to right (i.e. during the cardiac cycle). A dyskinetic region gives an NMM image displaying thinning and/or outward motion of the endocardium during systole (Fig. 6c), as well as a decrease in brightness around ES.

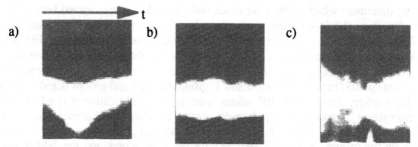

Fig. 6: Typical examples of NMM images: a: Normal region; b: Akinetic region; c: Dyskinetic region.

## 3.2 NMM image visual analysis

A total of 224 regions (4 slices x 7 patients x 8 sectors) were scored by the 6 observers, using the cine mode display and the NMM display. The distribution of the 1344 scores (224 regions x 6 observers) is given in Fig. 7 for both display modes.

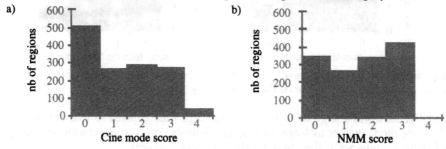

Fig. 7: Distribution of the scores given using cine mode display (a) and NMM display (b).

More regions were called normal using the cine display (38%) than using the NMM display (25%). There was a general trend of more severe defects when interpreting NMM images compared to the cine images. There were only 2 undetermined answers when reading the NMM imagescompared to 32 when reading the cine.

After excluding the undetermined answers, there was a consensus between the 6 observers for 46 regions (21%) when using the cine display. The scores given by the 6 observers were within one point for 94 regions (42%), and the scores disagreed by more than one point for 84 regions (37%). When using the NMM representation, the scores given by the 6 observers were in perfect agreement for 61 regions (27%), were within one point for 118 regions (53%) and differed by more than 1 in 45 regions (20%). The corresponding kappa values measuring the agreement between observers were .35±.01 and .51±.01 for cine mode and NMM display respectively, showing better agreement among the observers when interpreting NMM images.

Four observers performed the cine mode and NMM image reading twice at a ten day interval. For the conventional cine mode display, and all readers lumped together, identical scores between the 2 reading sessions were given in 621 regions (69%), scores differed by 1 in 231 regions (26%), and scores differed by more than one in 44 regions (5%). For the NMM display, identical scores between the 2 reading sessions were given in 636 regions (71%), scores differed by 1 in 208 regions (23%) and scores differed by more than 1 in 52 regions (6%).

To try determine which of the cine mode and the NMM scores agreed best with the LV function, the independent measurements of the LV function provided by the SGBP stroke volume values were correlated with the scores. The mean SGBP stroke volume values for the different groups as called from the reading are shown in Fig. 8. For the cine reading, the mean SGBP stroke volume values were significantly different (p<.05) between groups 0 and 1, groups 0 and 2 and groups 0 and 3. For the NMM reading, the mean SGBP values were significantly different (p<.05) for all combinations of groups, except between group 1 (Mild hypokinetic) and group 2 (Severe hypokinetic). The empirical correlation ratios, a crude indicator of separation between the groups, were .342 and .347 for the cine scores and the NMM scores respectively, and the corresponding Fisher-Snedecor test values were 14.09 (ddl=3;81) and 15.77 (ddl=3;89) respectively, showing a slightly better agreement between SGBP values and NMM scores than between SGBP values and cine scores.

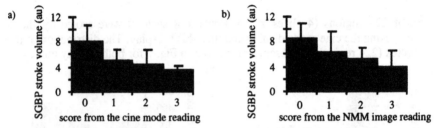

Fig. 8: Mean SGBP stroke volume values for the different groups, as called from the cine mode reading (8a) and from the NMM image reading (8b).

Finally, there was a large difference in the average time required to read the studies. The cine mode images took approximately 1.9 times longer to read (with an average of about 4.7 min per 4 slice study for the cine mode images).

## 3.3 Automatic quantitative analysis of NMM image

All gated image sequences were processed using the automatic procedure described in section 2.4. Fig. 9 shows the 9 lowest level ($v_1$ to $v_9$) Fourier fitted isodensity lines derived from the analysis of sector 3 of the study presented in Fig. 5.

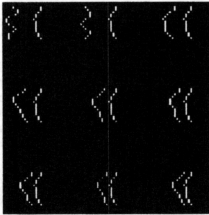

Fig. 9: 9 lowest level isodensity lines derived from the analysis of sector 3 in Fig. 5.

The two lowest level isodensity lines (top row, left and center) present shapes without any pronounced spatio-temporal trend, and the signal intensity $v_1$ to $v_2$ are therefore likely to correspond to cavity activity level. From isodensity line 3, the line starts fitting a regular spatio-temporal deformation, matching the expected wall deformation. The challenge therefore lies in identifying the isodensity line with the lowest value belonging to the wall (i.e. the BWE). This line should indeed mark the edge between wall activity and cavity activity. The method described above to identify the BWE was by testing the spatio-temporal randomness of the signal above it using the feature vector.

Examples of feature vectors for isodensity lines in the cavity or belonging to the wall are given in Fig. 10. The corresponding change point test values for these two feature vectors were 1.42 and 7.07, yielding the acceptance of the null hypothesis (no change in the sequence of events) for the first feature vector, and the rejection of this null hypothesis for the second feature vector. This second vector indeed clearly shows that there is a change in the spatio-temporal behavior of the data at some point. This change in the feature vector means that R1 is not pure background, and that this isodensity line therefore touches or crosses the wall. The BWE is defined as the isodensity line with the highest value (i.e. closest to the crest line) that satisfies the null hypothesis of random signal fluctuations in R1.

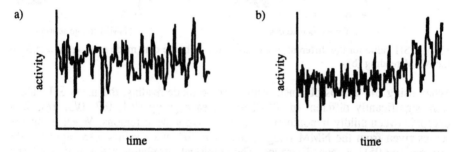

Fig. 10: Feature vector for an isodensity line in the cavity (a) and for an isodensity line belonging to the wall (b).

As the functional index derived from the NMM images depends on the choice of the BWE, the sensitivity of the SH value on the choice of the BWE was studied. Fig. 11 gives an example of the curve of the SH value as a function of the isodensity line that is chosen to separate regions R1 and R2 for a normal sector.

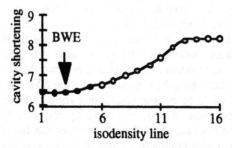

Fig. 11: SH value as a function of the isodensity line taken as the background-wall edge.

For this region, the location of the BWE as given by the test is represented by the arrow. The value of the SH index calculated from the 5 isodensity lines marked as filled circles varied by less than 3%, showing that the choice of the exact BWE is not crucial in deriving this index of LV function.

The automatic quantitative analysis was performed on all NMM images, yielding a set of 224 SH values. Only those regions for which there was a consensus between at least 4 observers were considered when studying the relationship between the index SH and the scores. The mean and standard deviations of SH for the different regions as determined from the cine mode reading are shown in Fig. 12a. The same analysis was repeated by considering only those regions for which at least 4 observers agreed when reading the NMM images (Fig. 12b).

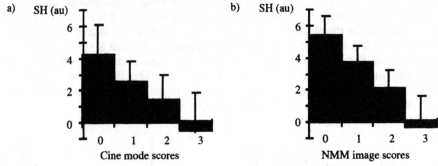

Fig. 12: SH value for the different groups as called from the cine mode reading (a) and from the NMM reading (b)

When using the groups obtained from the cine mode reading, the mean SH values were significantly different (p<.05) between each group (0/1, 0/2, 0/3, 1/3, 2/3) except between mildly hypokinetic and severe-hypokinetic regions. When using the scores given from the NMM images, the mean SH index values were significantly different (p<.05) between all groups. The empirical correlation ratios were .544 and .712 for the grouping based on the cine scores and on the NMM scores respectively, corresponding to Fisher-Snedecor test values of 57.3 (ddl=3;144) and 138.9 (ddl=3;168) respectively. These quantitative results show that the SH index was more closely related to the scores given from the visual analysis of the NMM images than to the scores derived from the visual analysis of the cine.

Finally, ROC curves measuring the ability of SH to distinguish normal (score 0) from abnormal (scores 1, 2 or 3) regions were created, as well as ROC curves showing the ability to separate contracting (scores 0, 1 and 2) from akinetic/dyskinetic (score 3) regions. To derive the ROC curves, the scores given by the observers were taken as the gold standard to determine the actual nature of the regions, and only those regions for which at least 4/6 observers agreed were considered. For separating normal from abnormal regions, the ROC curve areas were .91±.02 and .96±.02 when using the cine scores and the NMM scores respectively as the gold standard, and when separating contracting from akinetic/dyskinetic regions, the corresponding areas were .89±.03 and .96±.02 respectively. When separating normal from abnormal regions, the difference between the two ROC areas was not significant. When separating contracting from akinetic/dyskinetic regions, the area under the curve obtained by using the NMM scores as the gold standard was significantly greater than the area under the curve obtained by using the cine scores as the gold standard (p<.05), suggesting that quantitative shortening (SH) could be better determined visually from the NMM images than from the cine images.

## 4 Discussion

Ideally, when analyzing gated tomographic data sets, all four dimensions should be dealt with simultaneously, and any special constraints which might be present in a particular dimension or combination of dimensions taken advantage of. Unfortunately, 4D analysis tools are not yet readily available. Instead, usually spatial and temporal features are analyzed independently, typically first analyzing spatial features using edge detection or model fitting, either in 2D, by processing the pile of 2D slices that constitutes the 3D volumes, or (more rarely) directly in 3D [5]. It is only after the spatial features have been extracted at each time point that functional indices are derived from the temporal information. The NMM representation described in this paper is an attempt to synthesize spatial and temporal information into a single image, facilitating simultaneous processing in space and time, and permitting temporal constraints to be combined with spatial ones (e.g. the low order harmonic motion of the endocardial border).

We first investigated whether this new NMM representation could help observers visually assess cardiac function. Typical examples (Fig. 5 and 6) showed the value of NMM representation: normal, mildly or severely hypokinetic, and akinetic/dyskinetic regions yield typical patterns in the NMM images, suggesting that this representation could help analyze cardiac function both qualitatively and quantitatively. The NMM images portray, in a single image, several kinds of information that can give evidence of impaired cardiac function: brightness change, magnitude of deformation of the wall (both overall motion and thickening) during the cardiac cycle, and information as to when in the cycle such motion occurred.

Despite the much greater familiarity of the readers with cine display, the NMM scores were slightly better correlated with the GBP regional stroke volume values than were the scores given on the cine images. Inter (but not intra) observer variability was also lower with NMM than with cine mode. In addition, the SH index was more closely related to the NMM scores than to the cine scores. This suggests that the NMM scores are closer to the truth than the cine mode scores. Moreover, the fact that more severe defects were called on the NMM image reading than on the cine mode reading might imply that the NMM images allow more subtle defects to be detected visually, but this remains speculative.

Lastly, the time required to visually interpret the NMM images was much shorter than that needed to assign scores from the cine mode display. Therefore, NMM images could potentially increase the throughput of reading sessions in addition to yielding a more reproducible assessment of the cardiac function.

In conventional approaches, the spatial and temporal analyses are separated. Functional parameters are usually measured by spatial image segmentation techniques (geometry-based methods) [2], by count-based methods [1, 11, 12], by spatial model fitting [3], or more recently, by hybrid methods combining counts and geometric considerations [8]. The NMM representation could conceivably make all these techniques more robust, especially with respect to noise, by allowing a more appropriate inclusion of temporal constraints. The segmentation in NMM space by using isodensity lines, as described above, is one example of how one might make simultaneous use of signal intensity (isodensity line level), geometry (isodensity line location), and time (isodensity line shape). The method of choosing an appropriate isodensity line to separate background from wall also illustrates a way in which spatial and temporal information may be integrated in NMM analysis. The feature vector describes spatio-temporal background homogeneity and can be tested for randomness to determine from which isodensity line R1 is not pure background. That is, a unique feature of the temporal behavior of noise could be incorporated into the NMM model. It has been previously shown that combining brightness changes with geometry results in an index which more accurately describes wall motion [8] than an index based on geometry alone or an index based on brightness alone. Therefore an index derived from a hybrid method has been used in this study. Our preliminary results showed that this index could distinguish, on the average, between normal, mildly-hypokinetic, moderately-hypokinetic, or akinetic/dyskinetic regions.

As previously mentioned, other image processing approaches, normally used only in a pure spatial or pure temporal domain, might also be used to good effect when applied to the NMM domain. For example the square wave model of myocardial profiles allows absolute measurement of myocardial thickening [3], but has been shown [13] to be clinically impractical due to excessive sensitivity to noise and background. Introducing new time constraints by means of NMM representation could reduce this sensitivity, perhaps making the method robust enough for clinical use. Time constraints could also be used to directly perform endocardial edge detection in 2D, finding that curve in the NMM space which is best constrained by the combination of 2 harmonics in the time direction, and using spatial criteria in the x direction (e.g. derivatives of the profiles, or maximum brightness).

Although the NMM representation was applied to FDG gated PET images in this paper, it could be applied to any SPECT/PET metabolic or perfusion tomographic gated data (e.g. Tl201 gated SPECT), as well as to gated blood pool SPECT images (an extension of Groch's [7] planar approach), or even to gated MR images, with potential benefit for both visual and quantitative analysis of these data. The NMM representation provides a number of new opportunities to revisit conventional approaches used to characterize regional cardiac function, using regional ejection fraction, wall thickening, etc. The NMM representation is still not completely satisfactory as it does not deal with spatial connectivity of regions. This difficulty may well prove tractable, and in any case, we feel that the NMM is a valuable step towards a real spatio-temporal analysis and processing of the data.

## 5 Conclusion

A reassessment of some older methods of portraying spatial-temporal data has led to a new method for representing tomographic gated cardiac image sequences. This "nuclear M-mode" representation portrays, in a single static image, how a cardiac region contracts in space and time. Preliminary results using FDG gated PET and SPECT gated blood pool studies suggest that the visual assessment of the regional LV function may be more accurate when performed using NMM images compared to conventional cine mode display. This representation might also increase the throughput of the reading sessions. Taking into account space-time constraints to derive quantitative LV functional indices was shown to be feasible and yielded promising results for distinguishing between normal and abnormal contraction. Further studies will be necessary to confirm these preliminary results and to explore how conventional data analysis schemes might be applied to NMM images in order to take full advantage of the space-time constraints underlying the data.

# References

1. K. Yamashita, N. Tamaki, Y. Yonekura, H. Ohtani, H. Saji, T. Mukai, H. Kambara, C. Kawai, T. Ban and J. Konishi: Quantitative analysis of regional wall motion by gated myocardial positron emission tomography: validation and comparison with left ventriculography. J. Nucl. Med. 30, 1775-1786 (1989)

2. K.T.A. Yang and H.D. Chen: A semi-automated method for edge detection in the evaluation of left ventricular function using ECG-gated single-photon emission tomography. Eur. J. Nucl. Med. 21, 1206-1211 (1994)

3. G. Porenta, W. Kuhle, S. Sinha, J. Krivokapich, J. Czernin, S. S. Gambhir, M. E. Phelps and H. R. Schelbert: Parameter estimation of cardiac geometry by ECG-gated PET imaging: validation using magnetic resonance imaging and echocardiography. J. Nucl. Med. 36, 1123-1129 (1995)

4. K.A. Williams and L.A. Taillon: Gated planar technetium 99m-labeled sestamibi myocardial perfusion image inversion for quantitative scintigraphic assessment of left ventricular function. J. Nuc. Cardiol. 2, 285-295 (1995)

5. G. Germano, H. Kiat, P.B. Kavanagh, M. Moriel, M. Mazzanti, H.T. Su, K.F. Van Train and D.S. Berman: Automatic quantification of ejection fraction from gated myocardial perfusion SPECT. J. Nucl. Med. 36, 2138-2147 (1995)

6. J.S. Barata: La radiokymographie cardiovasculaire. Presse Méd. 14, 277-279 (1939)

7. M.W.Groch, G.K. Lewis, P.H. Murphy, E.G. DePuey and J.A. Burdine: Radionuclide kymography for the assessment of regional myocardial wall motion. J. Nucl. Med. 19, 1131-1137 (1978)

8. I. Buvat, M.L. Bartlett, A.N. Kitsiou, V.Dilsizian and S.L. Bacharach: A "hybrid" method for measuring myocardial wall thickening from gated PET/SPECT images (in press). J. Nucl. Med. (1997)

9. S.L. Bacharach, M.V. Green, D. Vitale, G. White, M. A. Douglas, R.O. Bonow and S.M. Larson: Optimum Fourier Filtering of Cardiac Data: A minimum error method. J. Nucl. Med. 1176-1184 (1983)

10. S. Siegel and N.J. Castellan: The change-point test. In: Nonparametric statistics for the behavioral sciences. New York: McGraw-Hill 1988, pp. 64-71

11. C. Marcassa, P. Marzullo, O. Parodi, G. Sambuceti and A. L'Abbate: A new method for non-invasive quantitation of segmental myocardial wall thickening using Technetium-99m 2-methoxy-isobutyl-isonitrile scintigraphy - results in normal subjects. J. Nucl. Med. 31, 173-177 (1990)

12. T. Mochizuki, K. Murase, Y. Fujiwara, S. Tanada, K. Hamamoto and W.N. Tauxe: Assessment of systolic thickening with Thallium-201 ECG-gated single-photon emission computed tomography: a parameter for local left ventricular function. J. Nucl. Med. 32, 1496-1500 (1991)

13. M.L. Bartlett, I. Buvat, J.J. Vaquero López, D. Mok, V. Dilsizian and S.L. Bacharach: Measurement of myocardial wall thickening from PET/SPECT images: comparison of two methods. J. Comput. Assist. Tomogr. 20, 473-481 (1996)

# Automated Segmentation of Brain Exterior in MR Images Driven by Empirical Procedures and Anatomical Knowledge

Andrew J. Worth, Nikos Makris, James W. Meyer, Verne S. Caviness, Jr. and David N. Kennedy

Center for Morphometric Analysis, Neuroscience Center, Massachusetts General Hospital, CNY-6, Building 149, 13th St., Charlestown, MA 02129-2000, USA.
http://neuro-www.mgh.harvard.edu/cma/cma.homepage.html
Email: andy@cma.mgh.harvard.edu

**Abstract**. This work demonstrates encouraging initial results for increasing the automation of a practical and precise MR brain image segmentation method. The intensity threshold for segmenting the brain exterior is automatically determined by locating the choroid plexus. This is done by finding peaks in a series of histograms taken over regions specified using anatomical knowledge. Intensity inhomogeneities are accounted for by adjusting the global intensity to match the white matter peak intensity in local regions. The results from 20 different brain scans (over 1000 images) obtained under different conditions are presented to validate the method which was able to determine the appropriate threshold in approximately 80% of the data.

## 1.    Introduction

### 1.1.    Significance

Magnetic resonance imaging provides a highly efficacious means for observing brain anatomy. Morphometric analysis provides quantitative measures of location, volume, shape and homogeneity of component brain structures. This type of analysis in conjunction with neuropsychological, neurological, and psychiatric observations and coupled with functional neuroimaging can then be used to aid in answering broad classes of questions about brain structure and function for both normal subjects and patient populations [1, 2]. For example, quantitative brain measurements have contributed to the study of developmental language disorders and autism [3], Alzheimer's disease [4-7], dyslexia [8, 9], attention deficit hyperactivity disorder [9-12], schizophrenia [13], multiple sclerosis [14, 15], Huntington's disease [16], and obsessive compulsive disorder [17].

**Segmentation is the Bottleneck.** In order to provide quantitative neuroanatomical measurements, the first step is to classify voxels as belonging to gray matter, white matter, cerebral spinal fluid (CSF), etc. and to delineate regions of these tissues in each brain slice image. The next step is to identify subregions as specific neuroanatomical structures. This task is difficult because it requires detailed anatomical knowledge and careful scrutiny of large amounts of data. This procedure accomplished manually is very tedious and therefore becomes prone to errors.

Segmentation is a bottleneck to further volumetric analysis [18], cerebral cortical subparcellation [19], and anatomic shape analysis [20].

While determination of absolute "accuracy" is problematic since there is no gold standard, there are many advantages of automating segmentation compared with performing the task manually. The main ones are: improved repeatability, improved reliability, and decreased variability. Results will be more repeatable because automated methods will always produce the same answer given he same data. Reliability will increase because errors that occur due to fatigue are eliminated. We have shown that inter-segmentor variability can decrease by automating the determination of thresholds while intra-segmentor reliability remains high [21]. Therefore consistency will improve both within and across morphometric studies. In addition to this, automatic routines act as a completely unbiased observer. Also, the availability of the analysis will increase since a computer program that can perform a given method is more portable and reproducible than a person. The decrease in human time necessary to perform a given segmentation task will allow a trade-off between the amount of time necessary for a study and the completeness of the morphometric analysis because more complete segmentations can be performed at the same cost. The use of automation can then lead to new classes of questions whereas previously the time commitment would have been prohibitive.

## 1.2. Task Definition

Much of the MR brain segmentation research focuses on assigning voxels to gray matter, white matter, and CSF classes. While this can be sufficient for applications such as 3D visualization, it is not adequate for undertaking *quantitative* neuroanatomical studies which hope to uncover correlations between brain structure and function or disease. Beyond classifying each voxel in the entire brain scan, a specific label must be assigned to the voxel regions that represent the corresponding neuroanatomical structure. Furthermore, it can be desirable to subdivide these structures and even to parcellate gray matter and white matter into meaningful units [19]. Also, each structure has its own specific problems arising from its characteristic intensities, shape, position, and its neighboring structures. A *complete* segmentation is desirable because it is not always clear which neuroanatomical structures may be of interest in advance. For instance, Filipek et al. segment cortical gray matter, subcortical white matter, lateral, third and fourth ventricles, caudate, putamen, globus pallidus, hippocampus-amygdala complex, thalamus, brainstem, cerebellum cortex and cerebellar central mass [22] .

In order to produce statistically significant results, the segmentation boundary in the image must precisely represent the boundary of the anatomical structure even if the information present in the image is corrupted or missing. Since practical MR image data often comes from a variety of sources and has variable scan quality, the procedures which convert raw image data into useful statistics must be robust. They must also be reliable enough to allow the quantitative comparison of brain volumes across multiple studies. And finally, the entire procedure must use only a reasonable amount of time and effort.

These constraints pose significant difficulties for the currently available methods to satisfy without human intervention. Therefore, while the ultimate goal is completely automatic MR brain segmentation, the interim and more practical goal of the research described here is to increase reliability and repeatability while decreasing variability and cost. We seek to automate the segmentation and identification tasks which are necessary to precisely measure neuroanatomical structures of interest. In this paper, the specific structure of interest is the exterior of the brain.

### 1.3. Previous and Related Work

There is currently no completely automatic method for segmenting a given neuroanatomical structure or even separating gray and white matter that has been shown to work with the precision of a human expert on large numbers of brain scans. For surveys on segmentation of brain images, see [23-26]. For a general image processing reference (and specifically for finding peaks in histograms as described below) see [27].

There are many descriptions of manual or semi-automatic methods in the literature (for a survey involving schizophrenia, see [28]). Some recent work includes [11, 29-31]. While there are no completely automatic methods which can precisely segment a complete set of specific neuroanatomical structures, there are a number of recent techniques that provide solutions and produce good results for specific problems [32-39]. Due to its cost in time and effort, many demonstrations are presented in the literature but a thorough validation is rarely performed. In this work, we attempt to present favorable results using a significant amount of practical data.

## 2. Method

### 2.1. Overview

This paper focuses on increasing the automation of segmentation of the exterior of the brain. In the sections below, we describe the currently established segmentation method, the techniques developed to automate part of the segmentation task, and finally, how the automated results are incorporated into the segmentation method. The remaining sections in the paper describe and discuss the results of applying this method to 20 test brains.

### 2.2. Positional Normalization and Cropping

In studies performed at the Center for Morphometric Analysis, coronal T1-weighted volumetric MR scans are used because they provide good contrast for the visualization of brain anatomy. The first step in their quantitative analysis is to normalize the position of the brain in 3D. This is done by trained experts who reposition the scan using the midpoints of the decussations of the anterior and posterior commisures ("AC" & "PC") and the midsagittal plane at the level of posterior commisure. The repositioned scans are then resliced into a normalized coronal scan which is used for subsequent analyses. This translation and rotation places the brain in the orientation of the Talairach coordinate system [40, 41].

The next step is to manually crop the normalized scan. In this step, the slice range where brain tissues are seen is determined by examining representative coronal and sagittal images. The horizontal and vertical extents of the brain are also determined using these images. All data outside of these locations are ignored and subsequent analysis is performed on the cropped and positionally normalized data.

## 2.3. Established Segmentation Method

The goal of the this paper is to automate part of the general semi-automated segmentation method which has already been established. This method involves a skilled operator using a computer program to produce outlines around each neuroanatomical structure of interest by choosing appropriate isointensity contours and making manual refinements and corrections [18, 22]. Corrections can become necessary when the data is too noisy, has low contrast, is skewed by intensity gradients, has extensive partial volume voxels (when a voxel includes multiple tissue types resulting in an intermediate intensity), or because part of the structure is too small to make a sufficient appearance. Moreover, manual drawing is always necessary when there is no contrast difference between neuroanatomical structures because they are composed of similar tissues.

Specifically, we seek to automate the segmentation of the exterior boundary of the brain. This border is defined as the outermost edge of the cortex that underlies the pia mater. This boundary should include all gray matter and exclude all dura mater, meninges, and other cerebral extra-cerebral CSF and tissues. The optic chiasm is also considered to be outside of the brain. The expert segmentor produces outlines for the cerebral exteriors using isointensity contours in the coronal view. However, sagittal and axial views are also inspected to resolve spatial ambiguities regarding the extent of the brain. First the screen is brightened so that the low range of intensities becomes visible. An intensity value is chosen such that the isointensity contour produced is definitely outside of the brain. Then, the intensity is increased to "tighten" the outline around the hemispheres. Lastly, meninges and connections with other tissues must be removed by manually drawing outlines that exclude them from the final exterior outline. Each cerebral hemisphere is extracted independently. When corpus callosum is present, it is necessary to separate the hemispheres by manually drawing along the midline. At the frontal-temporal junction, if the contour encompasses the entire hemisphere, but the white matter between the lobes is not continuous, it is necessary to separate them as well.

After segmentation, the final step in a quantitative brain volume study is to calculate the volumes of the structures of interest. This is done by counting the number of voxels that belong to each structure as prescribed by the outlines. The outline voxels themselves are considered to belong half inside and half outside of the structure.

## 2.4. Rationale: Choroid Plexus Indicates Brain Exterior Threshold

The method described above involves many different judgments by the segmentor. The most significant is the determination of the intensity threshold which defines the majority of the outline – i.e. how "tight" to make the exterior border around the brain. To automate this decision, we base our method on the observation (described in an unpublished report [42]) that since the choroid plexus is composed of tissues and fluids which are similar to those found in the subarachnoid space (dura and pia mater, vessels, and cerebral spinal fluid), the MR signal intensity should also be similar. Figure 1 shows the choroid plexus as it appears in a T1-weighted coronal slice. Since the subarachnoid space separates the exterior of the brain from the exterior CSF and since this area should have an MR intensity that is between CSF and gray matter, a border may be placed at this location using an isointensity contour

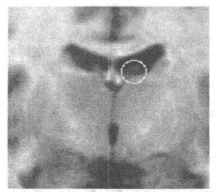

**Fig. 1:** Choroid plexus (circled) as seen in a coronal T1 MR image.

defined by the intensity of the choroid plexus. However, because there is usually a drift in intensity both between and across slices, this threshold must be adjusted for each local slice region. The next section describes the series of automatic procedures necessary to determine the intensity of the choroid plexus and how this intensity is locally adapted for use in each slice.

## 2.5. Determination of Automated Exterior Threshold

Before it is possible to determine the intensity of the choroid plexus, approximate global thresholds for gray matter, white matter, and CSF must be determined. This is done by finding the peaks in a histogram of the entire brain. After classifying all voxels using global thresholds determined using the peaks, a histogram of the ventricles is taken so that accurate thresholds may be determined within the CSF. The new thresholds allow a more accurate classification of voxels, and a second histogram taken over CSF voxels finally contains a peak for the choroid plexus. These steps are now described in detail.

**Take Global Histogram.** In order to get a general idea of the intensity values for gray matter, white matter and CSF, a histogram is taken over the intracranial region defined by a series of boxes accounting for Talairach atlas sections "B" through "H" which are completely inside the skull [40]. Only the data in these "intracranial boxes" is considered so that when a histogram is taken, it will represent primarily brain tissues and CSF and will not be influenced by other non-brain tissues with similar intensities. This atlas technique is accurate enough for the central brain regions and it is only necessary that *most* of the non-brain intensities be excluded so that they do not have a significant effect on determining the peaks in the histogram. To emphasize the homogeneous tissue intensities, voxels that are part of strong edges are excluded (as measured by their Sobel edge magnitude, see [27]).

**Find Peaks in Histogram.** The derivative of the histogram is taken by convolving it with the derivative of a Gaussian and then the peaks are found by locating negative-going zero crossings. Very small peaks in the original histogram do not survive in the derivative of the histogram (the derivative never actually goes below zero) since the derivative of a Gaussian convolution kernel also smoothes the result by an amount that depends on the standard deviation of the Gaussian. This standard deviation is determined from the width of the histogram; it is calculated as 0.04 times the difference between the intensities at 10% and 90% of the cumulative histogram. Other slightly larger peaks are ignored if their area is less than 1/30th of the total area of the histogram. This incorporates *a priori* knowledge about the occurrence of these primary tissues of interest.

The method for determining intensity model parameters using histograms and their derivatives works well even for a wide variety of brain scan data sets obtained at different times from different scanners under different protocols: in an initial study, the correct peaks were identified in a representative slice in 59 out of 79 brains scans attempted and the failures occurred in very noisy and large intensity gradient data which was far worse than the data used in the current study [21].

**Set Global Thresholds and Label Voxels**. After finding the peaks in the histogram, the lowest intensity peak is assumed to be CSF, the second to highest peak is gray, and that the highest peak found is white matter. Next, the gray-white and CSF-white matter thresholds are calculated by taking the intensity midway between their respective peaks:

$$CSFG_{thresh} = (CSF_{mean} + WM_{mean})/2,$$
$$GW_{thresh} = (GM_{mean} + WM_{mean})/2.$$

This "mid-peak histogram method" was devised because the regions over which histograms are taken are often too small to provide significant estimates of the variances of the tissue intensities. Using only the peaks makes the procedure repeatable and robust.

The next step is to use these global thresholds to classify each voxel in the whole data set as belonging to the following classes: "CSF", "gray", "white", and "other".

**Find Real CSF peaks, Calculate New Thresholds, Reclassify Voxels**. Next, a histogram is taken over only those voxels which are classified as CSF. Also, by defining a box around the center of the brain, only ventricle CSF will be included in this histogram. This box is defined to be half of the horizontal width of the cropped data (in the coronal view) and vertically extends from the level of the anterior commisure (AC) to one third of the distance between the AC and the top of the brain. Only the coronal slices between and including the AC and posterior commisure (PC) are in this box to minimally include CSF-gray partial volume voxels (since the main axes of the lateral ventricles in these slices are perpendicular to the coronal plane). Peaks are found in this histogram as was done previously and again CSF is assumed to be the lowest intensity peak. A new CSF threshold is calculated to be midway between this new CSF peak and the previously determined gray peak. This new threshold allows a more accurate classification of every voxel.

**Find Choroid Plexus Intensity**. With this new voxel classification, a more accurate histogram can be taken over CSF voxels in the ventricle box (defined above). This histogram should include choroid plexus because choroid plexus is found inside the ventricles at an intensity that is between CSF and gray matter but closer to CSF intensities. The last (highest intensity) peak found in this histogram (using the previously described zero-crossing method) is assumed to represent choroid plexus intensities. This intensity value is the desired global value for defining isointensity contours to outline the brain exterior. Figure 2 shows an example of the peaks and histogram after this step. The small bump in the middle of the histogram in Figure 2

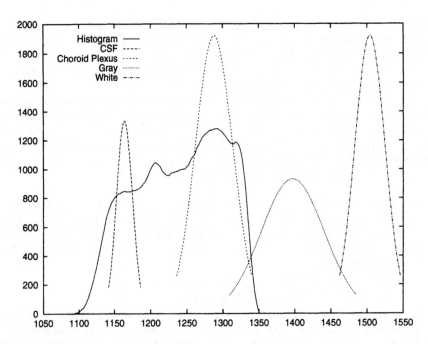

**Fig. 2:** Plot showing a smoothed histogram taken over voxels classified as CSF in the ventricle region. The 4 peaks shown correspond (from left to right) to ventricle CSF, choroid plexus, gray matter, and white matter. Peaks heights are arbitrary. The gray and white peaks were obtained from an earlier histogram (not shown).

is ignored since it is the highest intensity peak in the ventricle histogram that corresponds to choroid plexus.

**Adjust Global Exterior Intensity for Each Slice.** Due to intensity drift in the image data, the global intensity which defines the cerebral exterior outline must be adjusted in each half of the brain in each slice. This is done by locally finding the white matter peak in this region of each slice. First, the brain region is located by finding the largest connected region of voxels classified as "gray" and "white" that is in the middle of the left (or right) half of the image. Peaks are found in a histogram taken over this brain region and the highest intensity peak is assumed to be white matter. The local threshold for the brain exterior is calculated as:

$$lExterior = \frac{(gExterior - gCSF)}{(gW - gCSF)} \times (lW - gCSF) + gCSF,$$

where "l" means local and "g" means global. The result is a threshold that can be used to segment the exterior of the brain. If there were any problems (i.e. if no local white matter peak could be found), then the global threshold is used. The "localness" of this calculation can range from one threshold per slice to a continuous field of thresholds (one for each voxel).

## 2.6. Incorporation of Automated Results

The intensity threshold results are provided to the segmentor as the first step towards segmenting each slice. The threshold is available as a button which generates intensity contours over the entire slice at that intensity. The segmentor then incorporates this pre-calculated intensity contour into the normal segmentation method. If the pre-calculated thresholds are accurate, this saves time because it obviates the need to pick an intensity and adjust it by hand. However, the automated threshold provides no assistance where the boundary needs to be hand-drawn or if the pre-calculated threshold is incorrect.

# 3. Results

## 3.1. Data

The coronal MR brain slice images in this study are obtained using T1-weighted "spoiled GRASS" (SPGR, GE MRI Systems), "FLASH" or "MP-RAGE" (Siemens MRI Systems) images. The segmentation task becomes easier with increasing scan quality and resolution, and by using multispectral images [26]. However, we focus on segmentation using only a single structural image because this data provides a good balance between contrast, spatial resolution, and scanning time, and is routinely available. Furthermore, since the problem is defined as the detailed segmentation of specific neuroanatomical structures, the difficulties which we overcome here are still important when using less noisy and multispectral data.

Scans were typically acquired at the NMR Center of the Massachusetts General Hospital with a 1.5 Tesla General Electric Signa. Contiguous 3.0 mm three-dimensional coronal T1-weighted SPGR images of the entire brain were attained with the following parameters: TR = 50 msec, TE = 9 msec, flip angle = 50 degrees, field of view = 24 cm., matrix = 256x256, and averages = 1. Some scans were acquired using a similar protocol at the McLean Hospital. The scans were taken of twelve females and eight males who were roughly divided between controls and patients. The patients were diagnosed with obsessive compulsive disorder, Trichotillomania, schizophrenia, or with stroke.

Figure 3 shows an example of using the automated threshold to segment the brain exterior. The initial outlines produced with this threshold (b) must usually be edited to obtain the desired final outline (c). This manual drawing can be to add a boundary that is not present (e.g. the right/left division), remove meninges (e.g. at the upper right of the slice), or possibly to include some brain material that was missed (not shown).

## 3.2. Complete Evaluation of One Brain

In order to evaluate the effectiveness of the automatic threshold determination method, the exterior was segmented in a single brain with and without using the automated threshold. After the global thresholds were determined, only one local threshold was calculated for each slice, and this was taken over only the right half of the image (the left half of the brain) to explore the sensitivity of this method to gradients within each slice. The resulting average overlap (number of pixels in both outlines divided by 1/2 the sum of the number of pixels in each) was measured to be 94% and 93% for

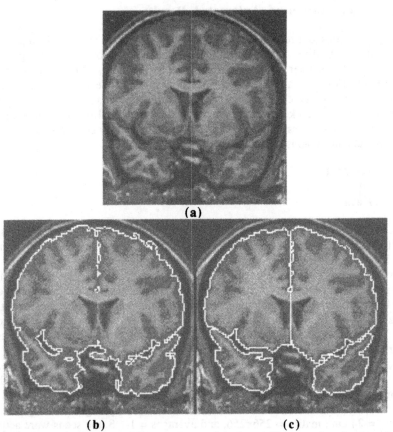

**Fig. 3:** Example Results. The raw image (a) the outlines produced using the resulting threshold (b), and the final image after being edited by the expert segmentor (c).

the left and right exteriors (respectively). This indicates that the segmentor performed basically the same segmentation with and without using the automated threshold and that there was little effect of left-to-right gradients within the slices. The amount of time necessary for segmenting without the automatic threshold was 91 minutes and 73 minutes when using the automated threshold. This is a time savings of about 20%.

## 3.3.  Appraisal of 20 Brains

After the complete segmentation of one brain scan, it became clear that the other scans had similar results. In order to save time by not performing the complete segmentation, 20 scans were evaluated by estimating the number of changes that would be needed to finish the segmentation. This was done by giving two scores for each brain: the percentage of slices where the intensity was correctly chosen, and (in these slices) the percentage of the outlines that were useful. Using all 20 scans, the intensity threshold was correctly chosen for approximately 80% of the images. Because hand drawing needs to be done in most slices (as can be seen in Figure 3 above) the outlines in each slice are approximately 80-95% useful. By multiplying the usefulness of each correctly thresholded slice by the percentage of useful slices in each scan, and by assuming that the image slices where the threshold was *not* chosen correctly contain no useful outlines (which is not the case), in the 20 scans we obtained an average "usefulness" of 74%. In fact, many of the scans where the threshold was slightly miscalculated do contain useful outline information, so this number is slightly low.

Three of the scans had intensity thresholds chosen correctly for every slice image. In the majority of the other scans, around 95% of the outlines were correct using the automatic threshold and a few scans were as low as 16% correct. The worst scan had a large intensity gradient. Most of the errors occurred at the anterior and posterior slice extremes. This is understandable since the method adapts the local threshold to the white matter peak which becomes increasingly effected by partial volume as the folds of the cortex pass in and out of the slice acquisition plane in the extreme slices.

A number of brain scans were not able to be segmented at all by this method because the algorithm was not able to determine the location of the initial global peaks. This occurred in very noisy data with large intensity inhomogeneities or in data where there was very little grey-white contrast (i.e. these two peaks began to merge together). A numerical measurement of how close the automatic threshold comes to the intensity chosen by the expert segmentor presents difficulties due to the hand drawing which is usually necessary. It is also not clear that the expert segmentor's result should always be treated as the correct answer since that segmentor's state of alertness and amount of training is unknown.

## 4. Discussion

Theoretically driven approaches found in the literature can claim to segment MR brain images fully automatically only if they solve a less demanding problem than the one defined herein. No method can be used for precise segmentation unless it adequately deals with, among other things: parameter estimation, missing boundary completion, partial voluming, and intensity inhomogeneities. These problems may not fit well into the theoretical formalism or else they may make the method intractable. As an alternative to such theoretically-driven approaches, we pursue the more empirical direction taken in the present work. We seek to directly address the most significant problems by incorporating as much available information as is necessary (as have, for instance [38, 39, 43, 44]). This brute force or *ad hoc* strategy usually results in solutions that are detailed, complicated and thereby difficult to understand and evaluate. The only certain way to judge the effectiveness of any approach is by the results, and therefore a thorough validation is necessary even lacking a true "gold standard". Our emphasis here is to automate an established, precise segmentation procedure and not to develop abstract segmentation methods.

However, we also seek to encourage the development of rigorous ways of flexibly incorporating various kinds of information for segmentation. Since one of the fundamental problems of all image segmentation methods is to continue to produce acceptable results as problems become more demanding, the utility of this paper to the general image processing community is to add evidence for the importance of dealing directly with problems by using deep domain specific knowledge. This paper provides an example of the application of *structural knowledge* (expectations about tissue response in MR such as histogram peak sizes and knowing which peak to use in which situation; templates located relative to landmarks such as the intracranial boxes and knowing where to find the choroid plexus), and *procedural knowledge* (specific sequence of successive region of interest refinements), along with image processing and pattern recognition methods (locating peaks using the derivative of a Gaussian; and excluding edge voxels from influencing threshold determination).

## 5. Conclusion

Semi-automated methods are currently the only way to perform a complete volumetric analysis and (with the appropriate controls and testing) are the only way to insure that the segmentation boundary in the image precisely represents the boundary of the anatomical structure of interest. This is due to the following reasons: practical MR image data often comes from a variety of sources and has variable scan quality; the information which should be in the scan is often corrupted or missing; painstaking, precise segmentation of MR images requires a lot of time and effort; a great deal of scans are needed to make a study's result significant; and also that completely automatic approaches have not yet been shown to produce sufficiently accurate segmentation results in all situations.

We have contributed to the automation of MR brain segmentation by demonstrating an improvement to an existing method for undertaking quantitative neurological studies using MR images. The methods presented in this paper provide an automatic determination of thresholds to segment the exterior of the brain in MR images. We will continue this effort by determining region shapes (such as the intracranial boxes mentioned above) and parameter settings from previously segmented brain data sets. We will also extend this method to other neuroanatomical structures and will combine the entire package in a system which will produce precise, reliable results with minimal human intervention.

**Acknowledgment** This work was supported in part by grant NS 27950 and NS 24279 from the National Institute of Neurologic Disorders and Stroke and also in part by the Fairway Trust. We thank the anonymous reviewers for their helpful comments. The authors would also like to thank Julie M. Goodman, Elizabeth A. Hoge, Mark R. Patti, Jason A. Tourville, Jill M. Goldstien, Larry J. Sideman, and Pauline A. Filipek for their valuable contributions to the segmentation methods described herein.

## References

1.  V. S. Caviness, Jr., P. A. Filipek, and D. N. Kennedy, "Magnetic resonance technology in human brain science: A blueprint for a program based upon morphometry," *Brain Dev*, vol. 11, pp. 1-13, 1989.
2.  V. S. Caviness, Jr., P. A. Filipek, and D. N. Kennedy, "Quantitative magnetic resonance imaging and studies of degenerative diseases of the developing human brain," *Brain-Dev.*, no. 14 Suppl, pp. S80-5, 1992.
3.  P. Filipek, C. Richelme, D. Kennedy, J. Rademacher, D. Pitcher, S. Zidel, and V. C. Jr., "Morphometric analysis of the brain in developmental language disorders and autism," *Ann Neurol.*, vol. 32, p. 475, 1992.

4.  M. Ashtari, J. Zito, B. Gold, J. Lieberman, Borenstein, and P. Herman, "Computerized volume measurement of brain structure," *Invest Rad*, vol. 25, pp. 798-805, 1990.

5.  C. Jack, F. Sharbrough, C. Twomey, G. Cascino, K. Hirschorn, W. Marsh, A. Zinsmeister, and B. Scheithaure, "Temporal Lobe Seizures: Lateralization with MR Volume Measurements of the Hippocampal Formation," *Radiology*, pp. 423-429, 1990.

6.  P. Scheltens, D. Leys, F. Barkhof, and e. al., "Atrophy of the medial temporal lobes on MRI in probable Alzheimer's disease and normal ageing: Diagnostic value and neuropsychological correlates," *J. Neurol Neurosurg Psychiatry*, vol. 55, pp. 967-72, 1992.

7.  J. Seab, W. Jagust, S. Wong, M. Roos, B. Reed, and T. Budinger, "Quantitative NMR measurements of hippocampal in Alzheimer's disease," *Mag Res Med*, vol. 8, pp. 200-8, 1988.

8.  R. Duara, A. Kushch, K. Gross-Glen, and e. al., "Neuroanatomic differences between dyslexic and normal readers on MRI scans," *Arch Neurol*, vol. 48, pp. 410-16, 1991.

9.  G. Hynd, M. Semrud-Clikeman, A. Lorys, and e. al., "Brain morphology in developmental dyslexia and attention deficit disorder," *Arch Neurol*, vol. 47, pp. 919-26, 1990.

10. G. Hynd, M. Semrud-Clikeman, A. Lorys, and e. al., "Corpus callosum morphology in attention deficit disorder (ADHD): Morphometric analysis of MRI," *J Learn Disab*, vol. 24, pp. 121-46, 1991.

11. F. X. Castellanos, J. N. Giedd, W. L. Marsh, S. D. Hamburger, A. C. Vaituzis, D. P. Dickstein, S. E. Sarfatti, Y. C. Vauss, J. W. Snell, N. Lange, D. Kaysen, A. L. Krain, G. F. Ritchie, J. C. Rajapakse, and J. L. Rapoport, "Quantitative brain magnetic resonance imaging in attention-deficit hyperactivity disorder," *Archives of General Psychiatry*, vol. 53, pp. 607-616, 1996.

12. P. A. Filipek, M. Semrud-Clikeman, R. J. Steingard, P. F. Renshaw, D. N Kennedy, and J. Biederman, "Volumetric MRI Analysis Comparing Attention-Deficit Hyperactivity Disorder and Normal Controls," *Annals of Neurology*, in press.

13. M. E. Shenton, R. Kikinis, F. A. Jolesz, S. D. Pollak, M. LeMay, C. G. Wible, H. Hokama, J. Martin, D. Metcalf, M. Coleman, and et al., "Abnormalities of the left temporal lobe and thought disorder in schizophrenia," *N-Engl-J-Med.*, vol. 327, no. 9, pp. 604-12, 1992.

14. D. Wicks, P. Tofts, D. Miller, and e. al., "Volume measurement of multiple sclerosis lesions with magnetic resonance images: A preliminary study," *Neuroradiology*, vol. 34, pp. 475-9, 1992.

15. J. Simon, R. Schiffer, R. Rudick, and R. Herndon, "Quantitative determination of MS-induced corpus callosum atrophy in vivo using MR imaging," *AJNR*, vol. 8, pp. 599-604, 1987.

16. G. J. Harris, G. D. Pearlson, C. E. Peyser, E. H. Aylward, J. Roberts, P. E. Barta, G. A. Chase, and S. E. Folstein, "Putamen volume reduction on magnetic resonance imaging exceeds caudate changes in mild Huntington's disease," *Ann-Neurol.*, vol. 31, no. 1, pp. 69-75, 1992.

17. H. Breiter, P. Filipek, D. Kennedy, and e. al., "Pronounced white matter abnormalities in patients with obsessive compulsive disorder," in *Paper presented at Boston Society of Neurology and Psychiatry*, 1992, .

18. D. N. Kennedy, P. A. Filipek, and V. S. Caviness, Jr., "Anatomic segmentation and volumetric calculations in nuclear magnetic resonance imaging," *IEEE Transactions on Medical Imaging*, vol. 8, no. 1, pp. 1-7, 1989.

19. J. Rademacher, A. Galaburda, D. Kennedy, P. Filipek, and V. C. Jr., "Human cerebral cortex: Localization, parcellation and morphometry with magnetic resonance imaging," *J Cog Neurosci.*, vol. 4, pp. 352-74, 1992.

20. D. Kennedy, P. Filipek, and V. C. Jr., "Fourier shape analysis of anatomic structures," in *Recent Advances in Fourier Analysis and its Applicaitons, NATO ASI Series.* Dordrecht, The Netherlands: Kleuwer Academic Publishers, 1990, pp. 17-287.

21. A. J. Worth, N. Makris, M. R. Patti, J. M. Goodman, E. A. Hoge, V. S. Caviness, Jr. , and D. N. Kennedy, "Precise Segmentation of the Lateral Ventricles and Caudate Nucleus in MR Brain Images using Anatomically Driven Histograms," *IEEE Transactions on Medical Imaging*, (submitted).

22. P. A. Filipek, C. Richelme, D. N. Kennedy, and V. S. Caviness, Jr., "The young adult human brain: an MRI-based morphometric analysis," *Cereb-Cortex.*, vol. 4, no. 4, pp. 344-60, 1994.

23. L. O. Hall, A. M. Bensaid, L. P. Clarke, R. P. Velthuizen, M. S. Silbiger, and J. C. Bezdek, "A comparison of neural network and fuzzy clustering techniques in segmenting magnetic resonance images of the brain," *IEEE Transactions on Neural Networks*, vol. 3, no. 5, pp. 672-82, 1992.

24. J. C. Bezdek, L. O. Hall, and L. P. Clarke, "Review of MR image segmentation techniques using pattern recognition," *Medical Physics*, vol. 20, no. 4, pp. 1033-1048, 1993.

25. A. P. Zijdenbos and B. M. Dawant, "Brain segmentation and white matter lesion detection in MR images," *Critical Reviews in Biomedical Engineering*, vol. 22, no. 5-6, pp. 401-65, 1994.

26. L. P. Clarke, R. P. Velthuizen, M. A. Camacho, J. J. Heine, M. Vaidyanathan, L. O. Hall, R. W. Thatcher, and M. L. Silbiger, "MRI segmentation: Methods and applications," *Magnetic Resonance Imaging*, vol. 13, no. 3, pp. 343-368, 1995.

27. J. C. Russ, *The image processing handbook*, 2nd ed. Boca Raton, Florida: CRC Press, Inc., 1995.

28. S. Chua and P. McKenna, "Schizophrenia – a Brain Disease? A Critical Review of Structural and Functional Cerebral Abnormalidy in the Disorder," *British Journal of Psychiatry*, vol. 166, pp. 563-582, 1995.

29. R. G. Petty, P. E. Barta, G. D. Perlson, I. K. McGilcrist, R. W. Lewis, A. Y. Tien, A. Pulver, D. D. Vaughn, M. F. Casanova, and R. E. Powers, "Reversal of Asymmetry of the Planum Temporale in Schizophrenia," *American Journal of Psychiatry*, vol. 152, no. 5, pp. 715-721, 1995.

30. M. S. Buchsbaum, T. Someya, C. Y. Teng, L. Abel, S. Chin, A. Najafi, R. J. Haier, J. We, and W. E. Bunney, "PET and MRI of the Thalams in Never-Medicated Patients with Schizophrenia," *American Journal of Psychiatry*, vol. 153, no. 2, p. 191–199, 1996.

31.  J. N. Giedd, J. W. Snell, N. Lange, J. C. Rajapakse, B. J. Casey, P. L. Kozuch, A. C. Vaituzis, Y. C. Vauss, S. D. Hamburger, D. Kaysen, and J. L. Rapoport, "Quantative Magnetic Resonance Imaging of Human Brain Development: Ages 4-18," *Cerebral Cortex*, vol. 6, pp. 1047-3211, 1996.

32.  A. P. Zijdenbos, B. M. Dawant, and R. A. Margolin, "Inter- and Intra-Slice Intensity Correction in MR Images," *Proc Information Processing in Medical Imaging*, vol. 14, pp. 349-350, 1995.

33.  P. H. Bland and C. R. Meyer, "Robust three-dimensional object definition in CT and MRI," *Medical Physics*, vol. 23, no. 1, pp. 99-107, 1996.

34.  W. M. Wells, W. E. L. Grimson, R. Kikinis, and F. A. Jolesz, "Adaptive Segmentation of MRI Data," *IEEE Transactions on Medical Imaging*, vol. 15, no. 4, pp. 429-442, 1996.

35.  J. C. Rajapakse, J. N. Giedd, and J. L. Rapoport, "Statistical approach to segmentation of single-chhannel cerebral MR images," *IEEE Transactions on Medical Imaging*, (in press).

36.  E. A. Ashton, M. J. Berg, K. J. Parker, J. Weisberg, C. Chang Wen, and L. Ketonen, "Segmentation and feature extraction techniques, with applications to MRI head studies," *Magnetic Resonance in Medicine*, vol. 33, no. 5, pp. 670-7, 1995.

37.  A. Lundervold and G. Storvik, "Segmentation of brain parenchyma and cerebrospinal fluid in multispectral magnetic resonance images," *IEEE Transactions on Medical Imaging*, vol. 14, no. 2, pp. 339-349, 1995.

38.  C. Tsai, B. S. Manjunath, and R. Jagadeesan, "Automated segmentation of brain MR images," *Pattern Recognition*, vol. 28, no. 12, pp. 1825-37, 1995.

39.  M. Sonka, S. K. Tadikonda, and S. M. Collins, "Knowledge-Based Interpretation of MR Brain Images," *IEEE Transactions on Medical Imaging*, vol. 15, no. 4, pp. 443-452, 1996.

40.  J. Talairach and P. Tournoux, *Co-Planar Stereotaxic Atlas of the Human Brain*: New York: Thieme Medical Publishers, Inc., 1988.

41.  P. Filipek, D. Kennedy, and V. Caviness, "Volumemetric analysis of central nervous system neoplasms based on MRI," *Pediatric Neurology*, vol. 7, pp. 347-51, 1991.

42.  N. Makris, "Theoretical segmentation mechanism for identifying periventricular structures in the human central nervous system," Boston University, Department of Biomedical Engineering, BE 515 Term Paper, Boston, MA, (unpublished report) Spring 1995.

43.  M. E. Brummer, R. M. Mersereau, R. L. Eisner, and R. R. J. Lewine, "Automatic detection of brain contours in MRI data sets," *IEEE Transactions on Medical Imaging*, vol. 12, no. 2, pp. 153-66, 1993.

44.  A. J. Worth and D. N. Kennedy, "Segmentation of magnetic resonance brain images using analogue constraint satisfaction neural networks," *Image and Vision Computing*, vol. 12, no. 6, pp. 345-354, 1994.

# Automated 3D Segmentation Using Deformable Models and Fuzzy Affinity

Timothy N. Jones and Dimitris N. Metaxas

Department of Computer and Information Science
University of Pennsylvania, Philadelphia, PA, 19104-6389, USA

**Abstract.** We have developed an algorithm for segmenting objects with closed, non-intersecting boundaries, such as the heart and the lungs, that is independent of the imaging modality used (e.g., MRI, CT, echocardiography). Our method is automatic and requires as initialization a single pixel/voxel within the boundaries of the object. Existing segmentation techniques either require much more information during initialization, such as an approximation to the object's boundary, or are not robust to the types of noisy data encountered in the medical domain. By integrating region-based and physics-based modeling techniques we have devised a hybrid design that overcomes these limitations. In our experiments we demonstrate across imaging modalities, that this integration automates and significantly improves the object boundary detection results. This paper focuses on the application of our method to 3D datasets.

## 1  Introduction

Automatic internal organ segmentation from various imaging modalities is a very important yet open research problem. Over the past several years a variety of boundary and region-based segmentation methods have been developed. 2D and 3D boundary-based techniques such as snakes [8] and Fourier-parameterized models [15] start with a deformable boundary and attempt to align this boundary with the object boundary, typically using gradient features and often balloon forces [4]. The solution to these systems generally involves minimizing an energy functional which quantifies the shape of the model and image information near the boundary of the model. To avoid becoming stuck in local minima, most model-based techniques require that the model be initialized near the solution or supervised by an interactive interface or some higher-level reasoning entity. In [10], a modified snake model is presented which reparameterizes the model depending on the local topology, potentially avoiding some of the problems in previous designs. However, this method does not explicitly address the issue of noise in the image and requires well-defined boundaries, as is the case with front propagation methods [9].

Region-based techniques such as region growing [1] assign membership to objects based on homogeneity statistics. The advantage here is that image information inside the object is considered as well as on the boundaries. However, there is no provision in the region-based framework for including the shape of the region in the decision making process, which can lead to noisy boundaries and holes in the interior of the object.

Like several other recent approaches [2],[3], [13], [16], our design integrates the model-based and the boundary and region-based techniques into a hybrid framework. In [2], the model-based and region-based techniques are set in a game-theoretic setting where each represents a "player." The segmentation process proceeds in an iterative fashion, where at each iteration each player updates their strategy based on the results from both players in the previous iteration. The idea is that each player will pull the other away from noise and local minima, while pushing it toward the solution. In [3], a framework is presented in which the solution is in the form of a maximum matching of region, gradient, and curvature terms. The high-level matching functional is a product of individual feature matches, which maximizes the correlation of the individual features. In [13], the probabilistic deformable model energy functional is augmented such that in certain locations within the interior of objects, where the straightforward image (gradient) energy cannot be computed, a gradient-based energy is used such that the model boundary is driven in the direction of the boundary of the object in the priors. In [16], a unifying framework is derived which generalizes the deformable model, region growing, and prior matching approaches and presents a new energy functional which represents them. By combining the model-based and region-based techniques, these approaches offer greater robustness than either technique alone. However, most still require significant initialization to avoid local minima. Furthermore, most of the above approaches use prior models for their region-based statistics, which we would rather avoid to increase usefulness in situations where a comprehensive set of priors may not be available.

Our approach is based on the integration of region-based and physics-based boundary estimation methods. Starting from a single voxel within the interior of an object, we make an initial estimate of the object's boundary using the techniques of fuzzy affinity [14] and clustering. A deformable surface model is then fitted to the extracted boundary data to fill in the missing boundary data and to override the spurious boundary data due to image noise. This is achieved by generalizing the formulation of our deformable models [11] to incorporate simple domain-specific knowledge. In our particular application, we use knowledge of the fact that the detected organ boundaries are closed curves [6] and the number of detected voxels on these boundaries will be significantly larger than the number of voxels which lie on false boundaries detected with our above clustering method.

The elastic properties of the model help it to override small patches of noise, while the domain knowledge attenuates the rest. Once the deformable model achieves an equilibrium, we refine the extracted boundary by using forces computed from the intensity gradient. The above two step boundary extraction process is recursively applied, by using the result of the deformable model fit to refine and improve the affinity statistics, which are then used to better initialize the deformable model. We have found that our 3D shape estimation results are better than those in 2D since both the clustering and the 3D model fitting use information across slices as well.

In our experiments we demonstrate that the interplay between these two methods automates and significantly improves the segmentation results, independent of the imaging modality used.

## 2 Boundary Estimation Using Fuzzy Affinity

We describe the region-based process by which we initially estimate the organ boundary that is then used to initialize the deformable model to further improve the organ boundary estimation. Unlike gradient and threshold-based methods, which are not robust with respect to noise within the object boundaries, our method combines both intensity and gradient information to better estimate those boundaries. In addition, in the following section we present the integration of the boundary segmentation results with the deformable model fitting method to further improve the organ segmentation.

Fuzzy affinity is the assignment of a probability (real number between 0 and 1) to two voxels belonging to the same object. Pairs of voxels which have an affinity of 0 definitely do not belong to the same object, while an affinity of 1 indicates that the voxels definitely do belong to the same object. This probability is a function which is based on the eucledian distance between the voxels and the image features in the neighborhoods of the voxels. Typical features used are the intensities of the voxels and the gradient of the voxel intensities.

In [14], the following general model of fuzzy affinity is proposed:

$$u_k(c, d) = h(u_a(c, d), f(c), f(d), c, d) , \qquad (1)$$

where $c$ and $d$ are the image locations of the two voxels, $u_a$ is an adjacency function based on the distance between the two voxels, and $f(i)$ is the intensity of voxel $i$. A simplified, shift-invariant version which was used in [14] is the following:

$$u_k(c, d) = \begin{cases} u_a(c, d) \ ( \ w_i h_i(f(c), f(d)) + w_g h_g(f(c), f(d)) \ ) & \text{if } c \neq d \\ 1 & \text{otherwise} \end{cases} , \qquad (2)$$

which is a linear combination of fuzzy intensity, $h_i$, and fuzzy gradient, $h_g$, affinities, with weights $w_i$ and $w_g$ whose sum is unity. For our purposes the location of voxels is unimportant, so we do not include the $c$ and $d$ terms in the affinity functional. Instead, we use three features to compute the affinity:

- the distance between the voxels (the adjacency)
- the average intensity of the voxels
- the intensity gradient between the voxels

The adjacency function, $u_a$, is a 4-neighbor test in 2D and a 6-neighbor test in 3D. For voxels $c$ and $d$ with n-dimensional coordinates $c_1, c_2, \ldots, c_n$ and $d_1, d_2, \ldots, c_n$:

$$u_a = \begin{cases} 1 \text{ if } \sqrt{\sum_{i=1}^{n}(c_i - d_i)^2} \leq 1 \\ 0 \text{ otherwise} \end{cases} , \qquad (3)$$

where $h_i$ and $h_g$ are functions which rate the affinities between the two voxels based on intensity and intensity gradient magnitude, respectively:

$$h_i(f(c), f(d)) = e^{-\frac{1}{2}[\frac{\frac{1}{2}(f(c)+f(d))-m_i}{s_i}]^2},$$

$$h_g(f(c), f(d)) = e^{-\frac{1}{2}[\frac{|f(c)-f(d)|-m_g}{s_g}]^2}. \tag{4}$$

Here $h_i$ assigns a higher affinity to two voxels whose average intensity is similar to the intensity of other voxels believed to be in the object. From these other voxels, the intensity mean and standard deviation, $m_i$ and $s_i$, are computed. $h_g$ assigns a lower affinity to two voxels whose difference in intensity is similar to that of other voxels believed to be in the object. From these voxels, the gradient magnitude mean and standard deviation, $m_g$ and $s_g$, are computed.

The derivation of the above equations is as follows. Let $f_{cd} = \frac{1}{2}(f(c) + f(d))$ be the average intensity of the two voxels. Let $\Delta = \frac{f_{cd} - m_i}{s_i}$ be the difference between the average intensity of the two voxels and the mean intensity of voxels in the object, $m_i$, normalized by the standard deviation, $s_i$, of the intensity of voxels in the object. The skew of the difference, $Sk = \frac{1}{2}\Delta^2$, is defined in such a way as to decouple the difference from the dimensionality of the values. What we seek is a function $h_i$ which maps $Sk : 0 \to n$ to $1 \to 0$, that is, the affinity $h_i$ is inversely proportional to the skew of the difference between the voxel intensities and the intensities of other voxels in the object. The exponential, $e^x$, satisfies this requirement when $x = -Sk$. The equation for $h_g$, the gradient component, is derived in a similar manner. Figure 1 shows a plot of the affinity function for a sample image.

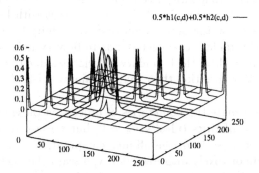

0.5*h1(c,d)+0.5*h2(c,d) ——

**Fig. 1.** plot of affinity function, $u_k$, for sample image ($w_i = w_g = 0.5$, $m_i = 100.7$, $s_i = 4.7$, $m_g = 2.3$, $s_g = 1.9$)

Previous approaches [14] for estimating the $m_i$, $s_i$, $m_g$, and $s_g$ parameters of the other voxels believed to be in the object include thresholding or user-selection. Our approach uses an iterative feedback mechanism, where the voxels used for these statistics are updated based on the shape of the deformable model. Initially, we apply this method only to the voxels in the local neighborhood of the user-provided starting voxel, which gives an initial approximation to voxels which are known to be within the object boundaries.

The optimal distribution for the intensity and gradient weights $w_i$ and $w_g$, respectively (see (2)), depends on the properties of the object being segmented as well as the imaging modality. We initially use an equal distribution ($w_i = w_g = 0.5$) and in the following sections we propose methods for automatically tuning the distribution based on a specific imaging situation, where the default may fail because of excessive or minimal gradient information or intensity homogeneity.

In [14] the fuzzy affinity function is used to produce the connectedness of all pixels to the starting pixel. The result is then thresholded to yield the segmented object. The problem with the fuzzy connectedness approach in our experiments has been that noisy images with deteriorated gradients can cause the connectedness to "leak" into non-object pixels such that boundary information is lost [7]. In the following section we develop a method in which we utilize the fuzzy affinity in a novel way to estimate the object boundaries.

## 2.1 Affinity Clustering

Our aim is to automatically determine based on the theory of fuzzy affinity a reliable estimate of the organ boundary that will be used to initialize the deformable model. To overcome the often incorrect object boundary estimation caused by the above mentioned leaking problem in the fuzzy connectedness approach, we do not use voxels with high connectedness ratings in the model fitting stage. Instead of trying to identify voxels inside the object, we identify the voxels that lie outside the object by considering those voxels with low connectedness ratings. This is based on the observation that the affinity between voxels along the exterior of the boundary of objects tends to be very low. Of course, we lose information at points where the boundary deteriorates due to noise, but we consider this a far better situation than that of gaining misleading information in noisy areas.

We therefore estimate the boundaries of objects as those areas where there are voxels with low affinities (ideally $u_k = 0$, but we use $u_k \leq 0.1$ to account for noise). To filter noise from the affinity computations, we extract the connected components of voxels with low affinity, discard the ones with small area as likely noise[1], and retain the rest as potential boundary regions. Each region is assigned a unique identifier which is used later by the knowledge-based noise suppression rules. Figure 2 shows a 2D cross section of an MRI image of the left ventricle along with its gradient magnitude and boundary pixels estimated from the affinity data.

---

[1] It is worth noting that the estimated boundaries will always have a closed boundary [6]

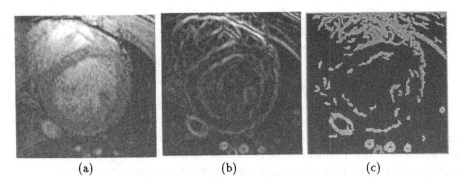

**Fig. 2.** (a) MRI slice of left ventricle, (b) its gradient magnitude, (c) its estimated boundaries

# 3 Deformable Models

We summarize our recently developed physics-based framework for deformable models [11] and describe the integration of affinity data into the framework.

Our model is a 3D superellipsoid with local deformations. The finite element method is used to compute the local displacements by dividing the model into small regions called elements. Between the nodal points within the model, the displacement is approximated using a small number of interpolating polynomials called shape functions.

Points on the model move under the influence of externally applied forces. The Lagrangian dynamics provides us with a set of equations describing this motion while considering mass, damping, and a deformation strain energy. The simplified Lagrange equations we use in estimation problems [11] are:

$$\dot{\mathbf{q}} + \mathbf{K}\mathbf{q} = f_q , \tag{5}$$

where $\mathbf{q}$ contains the nodal deformations, $\mathbf{K}$ is the stiffness matrix and $\mathbf{f_q}$ are the generalized external forces. We experimentally select the material parameters which compose the stiffness matrix, $\mathbf{K}$. However, this process can also be automated by integrating our recent work in elastically adaptive models [12] which can be done in a straightforward manner.

## 3.1 External Force Calculation

In the model fitting stage we apply generalized forces $\mathbf{f_q}$ to the nodes of the model to estimate and segment the boundary of the organ. These generalized forces are computed from 2D or 3D data forces $\mathbf{f}$ as demonstrated in [11]. A potential function is defined

$$P(x, y, z) = \|\nabla(G_\sigma * I)\| , \tag{6}$$

where $G_\sigma$ is a Gaussian smoothing filter of width $\sigma$ and $I$ is the original image. Based on this potential we define a 3D force

$$\mathbf{f} = \beta \nabla P \; , \tag{7}$$

where $\beta$ controls the strength of the force.

One problem with this approach is that the nodes have to be close enough to the real solution so that they neither get stuck in local minima nor become influenced by gradients at boundaries other than at the object of interest. A partial solution to this problem is the so called "balloon force" [5] which constantly pushes nodes along their normal, $\mathbf{n}$, away from the center of the model.

$$\mathbf{f} = \alpha \, \mathbf{n}(x) - \beta \frac{\nabla P}{\|\nabla P\|} \; , \tag{8}$$

where $\alpha$ controls the strength of the balloon force and $\beta$ controls the strength of the opposing potential force.

When using a balloon force, the nodes are initialized inside the object so that the balloon force pushes them toward the solution. Local minima can still be a problem in noisy images where there is too much gradient information inside the object.

### 3.2 Integration of Affinity Information into Deformable Model Framework

Our solution to the model fitting problem is to localize the nodes without the use of the image gradient information, and instead to use the affinity information described in Sect. 2. The boundary estimation step yields regions of connected voxels likely to lie on the object boundary. Noisy images may cause non-boundary regions to be present inside the object, and multiple objects may cause non-boundary regions to be present outside the object. Our clustering operation eliminates much of the noise inside the object, so we proceed to fit the model "from the inside" by initializing the nodes inside the object and applying balloon forces to them to drive them toward the true boundary (see Fig. 3). Instead of using gradient forces to deform the model nodes, we apply forces from voxels within the estimated boundary regions. When a node is pushed into an estimated boundary region, the region "pushes back" on the node with an opposing force. The goal is to have the nodes come to a stop at the object boundary. See Fig. 4 for a diagram of the forces applied to model nodes.

When the object to be segmented is non-convex, some additional steps need to be taken to ensure alignment of the model boundary with the object boundary in the concave regions. The balloon forces we use are initially radial, that is, they are directed along a straight line from the center of the model toward the node. In concave regions, we need to use instead a force which is directed along the normal to the model boundary at the node. Another approach to handling concavity is to adaptively add nodes to the model in the concave regions. This gives the model more deformation flexibility and allows it to fit more accurately

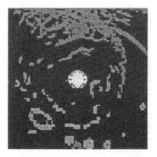

**Fig. 3.** initialized model with potential data

with the object boundary. This is accomplished by dividing the finite elements of the model mesh and by inserting new nodes. This last approach has produced the best results in our experiments.

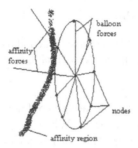

**Fig. 4.** depiction of forces applied to model nodes

Once the model has reached equilibrium, as shown in Fig. 5, the entire process is repeated in a feedback loop where we use the voxels covered by the model to generate more accurate statistics for the affinity function. This yields an even better affinity-based boundary potential which we use to achieve a better model fit. During each iteration the fit of the model to the object boundary is improved, and the statistics used to generate the affinity function are optimized. Our experiments show that 2-3 iterations of the two phases result in a very convincing boundary.

**Segmenting Complex Images** For particularly noisy images, or objects that contain "holes" such as tumors, not all of the estimated boundary regions lie on the true object boundary. If there are enough false regions inside the object, the nodes may get stuck in local minima (see Fig. 6). It is here that we use the domain-specific knowledge to overcome the noise. The goal of the rules is to assign a confidence to all regions, and ignore those regions with a low confidence.

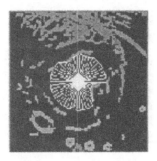

**Fig. 5.** model localized to potential data

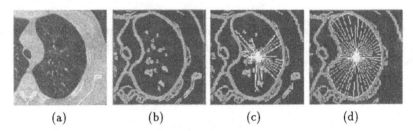

(a)           (b)           (c)           (d)

**Fig. 6.** (a) CT slice of lung, (b) its estimated boundaries, (c) model stuck on false boundary regions, (d) model localized after skipping false regions

One simple yet effective rule is to assign confidence to a region proportional to the number of model nodes near it. When the confidence of a few regions becomes strong enough, we discard the other regions that have a low confidence. While some of the noise suppression rules depend on the specific object being segmented, some are general enough to be stated in terms of the model alone without regard to the target object. We have previously stated, that the objects we are segmenting have simple closed (Jordan) boundaries. Given this, we know that if the model boundary at any point violates this property, then the data we are fitting it to must be corrupted. Whenever a model node, $n$, becomes attracted to a potential boundary region of the image, and its immediate neighbors continue to advance such that they "cross over" $n$ and form a cusp in the model boundary, the data which $n$ is attracted to must be bad since this topology could not occur in the real object. Consequently, the offending potential boundary region is discarded.

Another possible noise suppression technique is based on continuity. If we know that we are segmenting an object which has a specified continuity, say $C^2$, then we can discard potential boundary regions when they attract model nodes and induce high curvature into the model boundary.

It is noteworthy that our segmentation is truly 3D at all stages. This presents several advantages over the reconstruction approach of first segmenting individual 2D slices, stacking them on top of one another, and interpolating between them to obtain a surface. The shape of the surface elements represent more accurately that of the data in the fully 3D case. In the stacking approach, the shape of the surface elements is purely a geometric artifact (e.g., the top and bottom will probably be flat). While this may not be much of an issue when using a large number of elements, the shape discrepancy could lead to inaccurate measurement results such as volume computations when using a coarser mesh. In addition to the time savings of skipping the reconstruction step, the fully 3D approach allows for faster application of computational geometry measurements during the fitting process. For example, if it were desirable to track the volume of the model as it is being fitted to the data or to detect collisions between multiple models, it would be extremely expensive to stop at each iteration to reconstruct and triangulate the surface for these computations. In the fully 3D approach (where triangular elements are native), these computations can be run against the model directly, saving an expensive preprocessing step.

## 3.3 Improved Estimation of $w_i$ and $w_g$

One simple method for automatically selecting the weight distribution in the affinity calculation (see Sect. 2) is to match the image against a catalog of previously segmented objects (priors). The weights for the object with the best match would be used.

Another, adaptive, method is one in which the weights are initially 0 for the intensity and 1 for gradient. The gradient is used as the initial feature as it is often the most striking in image segmentation. Once we estimate the initial boundary by clustering the voxels based on their respective affinities computed above (see Sect. 2.1), we initialize a deformable model (see following sections) to further refine the estimated boundary and to update the boundary voxel affinities. At each iteration of the model fitting process, the quality of the gradient information at voxels near the nodes is evaluated, and if it is poor (i.e., gradient information is missing at many voxels), the gradient weight is lowered and the intensity weight is raised. Placing this in functional form we have

$$w_i = 1 - w_g$$
$$w_g = \beta \prod_{i=1}^{n} \nabla f(m(i)) , \qquad (9)$$

where $\beta$ is a normalizing coefficient, $n$ is the number of nodes in the model, $m(i)$ is the voxel nearest the model node $i$, and $\nabla f$ is the gradient magnitude at a voxel. Based on these new weights, we recompute the object boundaries and refit the model based on the previously described process.

## 4 Gradient-Based Fine Tuning

Once the balloon forces and affinity forces have reached equilibrium and the nodes of the model have come to rest, the model is considered localized to the estimated boundaries of the object. Because we took a conservative approach to selecting the boundary regions to avoid noise in the interior of the object, there are likely to be parts of the object boundary for which we have no affinity data. Consequently, at the end of the localization phase, the positions of the model nodes along these areas are interpolated from areas where there is affinity data. Unless the true shape of the object happens to match the finite element shape functions we use for the interpolation, there is likely to be some minor misalignment at this point.

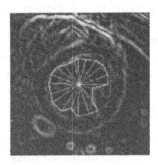

**Fig. 7.** final fit to gradient data

To resolve this error, we switch to a gradient-based potential to push the nodes toward the true object boundary. Because many of the nodes will have been localized at the true object boundary (assuming reasonable affinity data), the problems of local minima should not be a problem. The nodes which were correctly localized will not move far, and the "floating" nodes along parts of the boundary where there was no affinity data will be constrained by the deformation strain forces of the model from the well-localized nodes. Figure 7 shows the LV model fitted to the gradient map after being localized with the affinity data.

## 5 Results

We have tested our combined, automated approach to organ segmentation using region-based and physics-based modeling techniques on several datasets from MRI, CT, and echocardiography. The results have been very promising, yielding a convincing estimation of organ boundary while requiring no interaction or detailed initialization from the user. Spatial limitations constrain our presentation of results to a few cases from MRI, CT, and echocardiography, but similar results have been verified on many others. For viewing ease, 2D cross sections of 3D models and datasets are displayed throughout the paper.

Figure 2(a) shows an MRI slice of a human heart. Figure 2(c) shows the estimated boundaries of the left ventricle produced in the initial iteration of our algorithm using affinity data. A deformable model was initialized on the image in Fig. 3. Forces were applied to the nodes of the model as described in Sect. 3 until it reached equilibrium as shown in Fig. 5. Finally, the gradient forces were applied as described in Sect. 4 and the final results after two iterations are shown in Fig. 7.

Figure 6(a) shows a CT slice of a human lung. Figure 6(b) shows the estimated boundaries, which contain some false boundary regions. Once a model is initialized to the boundary data and becomes stuck on the false boundaries as shown in Fig. 6(c), we apply the noise suppression rules described in Sect. 3.2. The final fit after one iteration is shown in Fig. 6(d).

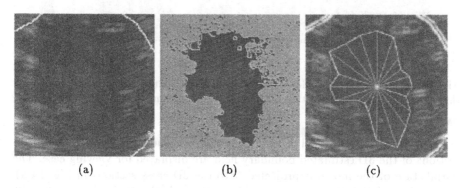

(a)            (b)            (c)

**Fig. 8.** (a) echo slice of left ventricle, (b) boundary potential, (c) fitted model with gradient data

An echocardiography image from a human heart is shown in Fig. 8. The original data is in Fig. 8(a). The white curves near the corners of the image are an artifact of the imaging hardware and did not affect the results of the algorithm. The estimated boundary data is shown in Fig. 8(b). The final fit after three iterations is shown in Fig. 8(c). Note the high quality of the estimated boundary data as compared to the gradient data shown in the final fit.

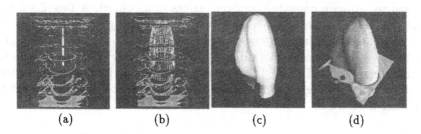

(a)          (b)          (c)          (d)

**Fig. 9.** (a) initial 3D lung model with cross sections of boundary potential, (b) midway through fit, (c) final fit, (d) fitted model with cross section of original CT data

A view of the 3D model of the lung is shown in Fig. 9. 2D cross-sections of the 3D estimated boundary field are displayed for viewing ease. The initial state of the model is projected onto the 2D cross sections in Fig. 9(a). A snapshot of the fitting process midway through the fit is shown with the same cross sections in Fig. 9(b). A view of the final 3D model is shown in Fig. 9(c). A cross section of the original CT data is shown with the final 3D model in Fig. 9(d).

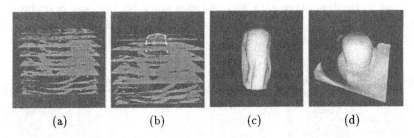

(a)                    (b)                    (c)                    (d)

**Fig. 10.** (a) initial 3D LV model with cross sections of boundary potential, (b) midway through fit, (c) final fit, (d) fitted model with cross section of original CT data

A view of the 3D model of the left ventricle is shown in Fig. 10. 2D cross-sections of the 3D estimated boundary field are displayed for viewing ease. The initial state of the model is projected onto the 2D cross sections in Fig. 10(a). A snapshot of the fitting process midway through the fit is shown with the same cross sections in Fig. 10(b). A view of the final 3D model is shown in Fig. 10(c). A cross section of the original CT data is shown with the final 3D model in Fig. 10(d). Deformations in the ventricle wall are due to the fact that our segmentation does not include the papillary muscle.

## 6   Conclusions

In this paper we have shown how the boundary-based and region-based segmentation techniques can be combined to yield good results with very little initialization or interactive supervision. The fuzzy affinity concept is reviewed and used to estimate possible boundary regions of an object. A two-phase segmentation method is presented which consists of localizing a deformable model to the estimated boundary regions and fine-tuning the model fit by adding gradient forces once the model is localized. Results of the algorithm on human heart and lung organs from 3D MRI, CT, and echocardiography images are presented. The algorithm is undergoing further verification on other organs and using data from other modalities.

## Acknowledgments

The authors are grateful for the contribution of data from Dr. Eric Hoffman of the University of Iowa and Drs. Leon Axel and Ivan Salgo of the University of Pennsylvania, and for discussions with Drs. Gabor Herman and Jayaram Udupa of the University of Pennsylvania. This work has been supported by NSF Career Award NSF-9624604 and a grant from the Whittaker Foundation.

# References

1. D.H. Ballard and C.M. Brown. *Computer Vision*. Prentice Hall, 1982.
2. Amit Chakraborty and James S. Duncan. Integration of boundary finding and region-based segmentation using game theory. In Y. Bizais et al., editor, *Information Processing in Medical Imaging*, pages 189–201. Kluwer, 1995.
3. Amit Chakraborty, Marcel Worring, and James S. Duncan. On multi-feature integration for deformable boundary finding. In *Proc. Intl. Conf. on Computer Vision*, pages 846–851, 1995.
4. I. Cohen, L.D. Cohen, and N.J. Ayache. Using deformable surfaces to segment 3-d images and infer differential structures. *CVGIP: Image Understanding*, 56(2):242–263, 1992.
5. Laurent D. Cohen. On active contour models and balloons. *CVGIP: Image Understanding*, 53(2):211–218, 1991.
6. G.T. Herman. Oriented surfaces in digital spaces. *CVGIP: Graphical Models and Image Processing*, 55:381–396, 1993.
7. Timothy N. Jones and Dimitris N. Metaxas. Segmentation using deformable models with affinity-based localization. In *Proc. First Joint Conf. of CVRMed II and MRCAS III*, 1997.
8. Michael Kass, Andrew Witkin, and Demetri Terzopoulos. Snakes: Active contour models. *Intl. J. of Computer Vision*, 1(4):321–331, 1988.
9. R. Malladi, J.A. Sethian, and B.C. Vemuri. Shape modeling with front propagation: A level set approach. *Pattern Matching and Machine Intelligence*, 17(2), 1995.
10. Tim McInerney and Demetri Terzopoulos. Topologically adaptable snakes. In *Proc. Intl. Conf. on Computer Vision*, 1995.
11. D. Metaxas. *Physics-Based Deformable Models: Applications to Computer Vision, Graphics and Medical Imaging*. Kluwer-Academic Publishers, 1996.
12. Dimitri N. Metaxas and Ioannis A. Kakadiaris. Elastically adaptive deformable models. In *Proc. European Conf. on Computer Vision*, 1996.
13. Rémi Ronfard. Region-based strategies for active contour models. *Intl. J. of Computer Vision*, 13(2):229–251, 1994.
14. Jayaram K. Udupa and Supun Samarasekera. Fuzzy connectedness and object definition. In *Medical Imaging*, 1995.
15. Marcel Worring, Arnold W.M. Smeulders, Lawrence H. Staib, and James S. Duncan. Parameterized feasible boundaries in gradient vector fields. *Computer Vision and Image Understanding*, 63(1):135–144, 1996.
16. S.C. Zhu, T.S. Lee, and A.L. Yuille. Region competition: Unifying snakes, region growing, and bayes/mdl for multi-band image segmentation. In *Proc. Intl. Conf. on Computer Vision*, pages 416–423, 1995.

# Segmentation of Medical Image Objects
# Using Deformable Shape Loci

Daniel Fritsch, Stephen Pizer, Liyun Yu, Valen Johnson[†], and Edward Chaney

Medical Image Display and Analysis Group
The University of North Carolina at Chapel Hill

[†]Institute of Statistics and Decision Sciences, Duke University

**Abstract.** Robust segmentation of normal anatomical objects in medical images requires (1) methods for creating object models that adequately capture object shape and expected shape variation across a population, and (2) methods for combining such shape models with unclassified image data to extract modeled objects. Described in this paper is such an approach to model-based image segmentation, called *deformable shape loci* (DSL), that has been successfully applied to 2D MR slices of the brain ventricle and CT slices of abdominal organs. The method combines a model and image data by warping the model to optimize an objective function measuring both the conformation of the warped model to the image data and the preservation of local neighbor relationships in the model. Methods for forming the model and for optimizing the objective function are described.

## 1. Introduction

A variety of model-directed methods have been developed to address the increasing clinical need for more reliable and automatic means for segmenting objects in medical images. One popular class of models incorporates some form of *a priori* information about characteristics of the object boundary, requiring (for example) that the extracted boundary be sufficiently smooth [9]. Another class of techniques attempts to model *a priori* object information in the form of some kind of local consistency constraint(s) on the image intensities, requiring (for example) that the local intensities within a segmented object vary smoothly from pixel to pixel [10]. More powerful methods exhibit some combination of the two approaches [3,4], wherein both boundary-based and regional intensity properties of the object are taken into account during the modeling process. In all cases, the model serves to constrain the final segmentation, which is driven by certain measurements obtained from the unclassified image.

A shortcoming, we believe, of many such methods is their lack of use of important, global properties of object shape and their failure to recognize the importance of measurement scale during model construction and during the segmentation process wherein the model is combined with image information. For example, models based on only small-scale, local boundary information are unable to take advantage of higher order figural information that manifests itself at multiple, object-relevant scales [14]. Without such figural information, such methods often require that the model be initialized very close to the actual object boundary (to avoid convergence to undesired local extrema) and are notoriously sensitive to image disturbances, such as intensity noise and blurring.

A more complete representation of shape – one that recognizes the object and its component figures as a unit – can serve as a powerful basis for automatic segmentation of anatomical objects in medical images. Measures of medial strength called medialness [8,14,17] capture figural shape directly from the image intensities, and do so in a way that exhibits great insensitivity to image disturbances such as intensity and boundary noise, and blurring [15]. In addition, medial loci (called *cores*) extracted using medialness permit the specification of inter-figural relations and stably allow for determination of figural boundaries [12].

In this paper we report on a method of modeling such *figural* aspects of object shape in order to create models which can then be applied to an unclassified image to robustly locate and segment similar objects. This method has in common many of the attractive features of other deformable loci (active contour) methods [13], but introduces and integrates several particular strengths. Some of these strengths include the following:

1. A rich prior model of object shape based on the formality of Markov random fields and related statistical methods.
2. A means for incorporating more stable information into the model fitting process.

## 1.1 Bayesian Approaches to Model-Based Image Segmentation

Many of the model-based approaches to image segmentation may be cast in a Bayesian framework, wherein the model prescribes a prior distribution on allowable shape deformations and wherein the likelihood function describes how well measurements derived from the image accord with a given geometric state of the model. Given such a framework, the problem becomes one of how to (a) model and encode shape information in the prior term in a way that adequately captures normal object shape and its variabilities and that (b) permits the model to be combined with the image (via the likelihood term) through appropriate choice of image information consistent with the model representation.

In the classical papers on deformable, or active, contours, an initial contour is deformed to optimize an objective function (log posterior) that is the sum of an image energy (log likelihood) term, measuring the degree to which the contour matches the image data, and an internal energy (log prior) term, measuring the degree to which the contour is smooth [9]. The prior is intended to measure the degree to which the contour has the location, size, orientation, and shape of the family of objects that are to be extracted, e.g., of a particular organ. Wilson [20] and Pizer [17] have argued that such shape properties are captured more richly by a linked locus of medial and boundary sites than by a locus of only linked boundary sites. With such a locus, the agreement of the locus with the image, i.e., the log likelihood involves not only the boundariness at the boundary sites but also the medialness at the medial sites, where medialness measures the degree to which the medial site behaves as being medial between a pair of boundaries. Also, the log prior measures the variation of the inter-site links from a model. The relations defining the objective function are as follows:

Objective function (log posterior)
$$= \text{log likelihood} \qquad\qquad + \text{ log prior}$$
$$= k_{image} \times \textit{Image Energy} \qquad\qquad + k_{internal} \times \textit{Internal Energy}$$
$$= k_{bound} \times \textit{Boundariness Summed Over Boundary Sites} + k_{med} \times \textit{Medialness Summed Over Medial Sites}$$
$$+ -k_{internal} \times \textit{Sum Of Variation Of Site Links From Model} \quad (1)$$

where the $k$'s are constants that weight the relative importance of the image measurement terms ($k_{bound}$ and $k_{med}$) and the model term ($k_{internal}$). The method we have implemented involves creating a model, consisting of linked medial and boundary sites, from a training image and deforming the model to optimize the objective function.

## 2. Theory of Deformable Shape Loci

Here we lay out the basic principles for deformable shape loci (DSL) and describe the construction of the prior (or internal energy term) and the likelihood function (or image energy term) and the means for combining each to permit segmentation of an object via optimization of the posterior (the objective function). In the sections to follow, we first describe how we encode figural aspects of object shape in a prior model (Section 2.1). We then discuss the construction of the likelihood function (Section 2.2), which uses image measurements as to both figural (medial) features and boundary features to allow for the stable extraction of objects from unclassified images via optimization of the posterior (Section 2.3).

## 2.1 The Prior: Modeling Normal Object Shape

Shape may be (loosely) defined as the set of measurable geometric properties of an object that remain unchanged, i.e., that are invariant to, a given set of geometric operations; for example, translation, rotation, and magnification. Object shape, as we consider it in this paper, has three important aspects:

1. Figural shape: includes a description of the track of the middle of a figure and the variation in width of the object along that track (medial axis).
2. Inter-figural shape: relative position, size, and orientation of component figures.
3. Boundary shape and boundary location relative to figural location and size.

Each of these aspects of object shape are represented, in a model, by relationships between coarsely samples medial sites and boundary sites, as illustrated in Fig. 1.

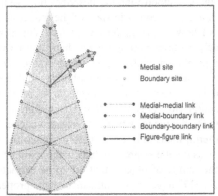

**Fig. 1.** A medial-boundary DSL model for a teardrop figure with a protrusion subfigure.

There are two essential aspects to these models: (1) The discrete, sparse set of points, the *template sites*, at which certain image features are to be measured, and (2) the local relations between these sites, the *template links*, which serve to constrain the possible deformations that the template can undergo when it is applied to an image.

**Specifying Template Sites in the Prior.** The template sites for our DSL models consist of an orderly arrangement of points at which certain important image features are to be measured when the template is applied to an unclassified image. In general, these image features may be considered to be either multilocal (figural) or local (boundary), which are captured by medial measurements or boundary measurements, respectively. Each component figure of an object to be modeled is represented by a set of linked medial sites, sampled from the core of that figure in a training image. The medial sites establish both the center positions and local widths of the figure and specify a set of scaled *medialness* measurement apertures, each of which responds most strongly to centers of objects of similar width. In turn, each medial site is associated with two or more boundary sites to which we associate a scale value proportional to the scale of the linked medial site. The scale values at the boundary sites serve to establish the width of *boundariness* measurement apertures.

**Specifying and Using Template Links in the Prior.** Our objective function (Eq. 1) has a log prior term that measures the shape between a deformed model and the model itself. This measure is expressed in terms of differences in the links illustrated in Fig. 1 as the model deforms. The shape difference measure has a basis in the theory of Markov random fields and Gibbs priors [20], but for the purposes of this paper, we will take the pragmatic point of view that, except for the multiplicative constant ($k_{internal}$ in Eq. 1), the log prior term is simply the sum over the links of the norm-squared of the difference of each link in the deformed model from the same link in the model:

log prior =

$$-k_{internal}\left( \sum_{l_k \in MM\,links}\left\|l_k-l_k^{model}\right\|^2 + \sum_{l_k \in MB\,links}\left\|l_k-l_k^{model}\right\|^2 + \sum_{l_k \in BB\,links}\left\|l_k-l_k^{model}\right\|^2 + \sum_{l_k \in FF\,links}\left\|l_k-l_k^{model}\right\|^2 \right). \quad (2)$$

Using Fig. 1 as an example, the links labeled *MM* are the medial-medial links; those labeled *MB* are the medial-boundary links; those labeled *BB* are the boundary-boundary links; and those labeled *FF* are the figure-figure links. The remainder of this section covers two issues. The first is the process by which one specifies the links in the model. The second is the measure of link difference which we use in the above formula to calculate the prior term in the objective function.

The $k^{th}$ link connects two neighboring template sites, $i$ and $j$. The model loci, and thus the links, are established through interaction by a user who understands the shape in question and thus is able to specify which figures are of importance in the model. These figures might include not only portions of the anatomical object to be extracted but also those containing the object of interest (e.g., the whole abdomen when the object of interest is the liver), those in objects neighboring the object of interest (e.g., the gall bladder when the object of interest is the liver), or those made from the gap between the object of interest and a boundary of a neighboring object (e.g., the chest wall when the object of interest is the liver). For each figure that is to appear in the model, a medial locus (core) must be extracted, and we provide tools for aiding the model definer to do this. We also provide tools that, given a figure's medial locus, calculate associated boundary points automatically in the training image. These tools are described further in the sub-section to follow. Finally, the figure-figure links are determined by the model definer by defining which figure is a child of which parent figure.

In the program we have implemented to deform a model locus by optimization of the objective function, the norm of a link difference that we use is the same for each link type. Each link $l_k$ is a vector in scale space specifying both

1) the vector $\bar{v}_k$ in image space (2D in this paper) that indicates the change of location between the $i^{th}$ and $j^{th}$ positions $\bar{x}_i$ and $x_j$, and

2) a pair of scales, $\sigma_i$ and $\sigma_j$, indicating the change in widths between the $i^{th}$ and $j^{th}$ positions.

The difference between a link's position and width of changes in the model and the corresponding pair of changes in the deformed model, is measured by the magnitude of the difference between the two scale space vectors. This difference is computed from a scale space distance function $d_{SS}$ on two scale space points and a scale space cosine function $\cos_{SS}$ on two scale space vectors, both of which are defined in Wilson [20]:

$$\begin{aligned}
\left\|l_k-l_k^{model}\right\|^2 &= d_{SS}{}^2\left[(\bar{x}_i,\sigma_i),(\bar{x}_j,\sigma_j)\right] + d_{SS}{}^2\left[(\bar{x}_i^{model},\sigma_i^{model}),(\bar{x}_j^{model},\sigma_j^{model})\right] \\
&\quad - 2d_{SS}\left[(\bar{x}_i,\sigma_i),(\bar{x}_j,\sigma_j)\right] \times d_{SS}\left[(\bar{x}_i^{model},\sigma_i^{model}),(\bar{x}_j^{model},\sigma_j^{model})\right] \\
&\quad \times \cos_{SS}\left[(\bar{x}_i,\sigma_i)-(\bar{x}_j,\sigma_j),(\bar{x}_i^{model},\sigma_i^{model})-(\bar{x}_j^{model},\sigma_j^{model})\right]
\end{aligned} \quad (3)$$

This formulation provides invariance under the operations of translation and zoom (magnification) of the template, but relaxes the requirement for rotation invariance due to the angle-preserving term in the $\cos_{SS}$ function. We are investigating means, using 3-neighbor, triangular cliques, of restoring rotational invariance.

**Automating the Formation of and Editing of the DSL Model.** In this section, we briefly describe how we make use of existing algorithms and programs for extraction of the medial loci called cores to permit efficient construction of object shape templates on a training image. Core extraction can be initiated, under user control, by the specification of an approximate middle and width of a figure in question. From such a "stimulus" point, a nearby point on the track in scale space that is the core is first found, and then the core itself is tracked. We have been able to compute figural cores in a variety of imaging modalities and for a variety of objects in a few to tens of seconds.

Given a set of extracted cores, one for each of the figures which comprise the object in question, each figural core is first coarsely sampled to yield the set of linked medial sites. We currently use a user-specified, equidistant spatial sampling of the core. The linked medial sites serve to establish a model for the global figural shape, and thus capture figural width and positional changes. For each medial site, there exist a pair of opposing boundary points (called medial involutes) to which we establish links to that medial site. These boundary points become the boundary sites in the model. These medial-to-boundary site links model the expected location of the boundary relative to the stable figure, and thus provide for stable boundary localization in the model fitting process. Finally, the adjacent figural boundary sites are linked. These boundary-boundary site links serve to establish a model for expected boundary shape. These connections also serve to define the coarsely sampled boundary contour that will be used to produce the segmentation of a figure after posterior optimization.

At any point in the automated model building stage, the user may wish to edit the site configurations. To facilitate user interaction, we have developed a model editing tool which incorporates the processes for automatic model generation discussed above and which allows for insertion, deletion, and movement of sites and links. The model building tool communicates with a relational database stored on a centralized server for convenient access, storage, and management of model data.

## 2.2 The Likelihood Function: Capturing Image Information on Shape

Just as the measurement of shape change of the deformed template from the model template, producing the internal energy (prior), is intended to have built-in invariances to translation, rotation, and magnification, so should the image energy (likelihood) function, so that the segmentation can be unaffected by overall translations, rotations, and magnifications of objects in the image space. That is, for a given mapping of the model template to a given image, producing a posterior value, that posterior value should not change if the same transformation is applied to both the template and the image. Such measurement invariances can be obtained if (1) the measurement at a given site is based on a differential invariant (e.g., gradient magnitude), and (2) such a measurement is obtained with a Gaussian aperture that scales in size in proportion to object zoom [16] (see also Lindeberg [11] for a detailed discussion of Gaussian scale space and differential invariants).

In the construction of the likelihood function we make use of two types of features, boundaries and middles, each of which is measured using scale-space differential invariants. The log likelihood function in our method is a weighted sum of the log of boundariness measurements at the $N_b$ boundary sites, $(b_i, \sigma_{b_i})$, and the log of medialness measurements at the $N_m$ medial sites, $(\vec{m}_i, \sigma_{m_i})$:

$$\text{log likelihood} = k_{bound} \sum_{i=1}^{N_b} \log B(\vec{b}_i, \sigma_{b_i}) + k_{med} \sum_{i=1}^{N_m} \log M(\vec{m}_i, \sigma_{m_i}), \qquad (4)$$

where the weights, $k_{bound}$ and $k_{med}$, on the boundariness and medialness hyper-parameters which can be estimated from training data [20].

**Medialness at Sites on the Medial Locus.** Medialness at a point and width is intended to accumulate boundariness contributions at a distance from the point equal to the width and in normal directions associated with rays emanating from the point. Magnification invariance requires that the scale of measurement of these boundariness contributions are proportional to the width; this leads to medialness values that are produced from boundariness measurements at a significant scale when the object has significant width. This large scale, together with the accumulation of multilocal boundariness contributions, has the property of producing a measurement that is much more stable against a variety of image disturbances than boundariness at the somewhat smaller scale at which it is typically measured. Fig. 2 illustrates this effect, which is proven at length in Morse [15], for a simple object in a noise-free image and in the same image with a significant amount of additive noise. The effect is that an objective function optimization that includes medialness stabilizes the computation as compared to methods that only use boundariness information at a small, object-width-independent scale. In effect, when we perform optimization of the posterior in the model fitting process, the boundary locus localization is guided by the more stable medial locus localization.

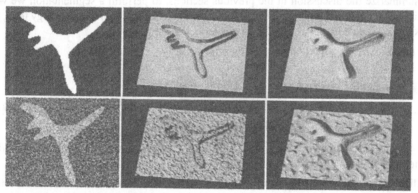

**Fig. 2.** Effects of image disturbances on boundariness and medialness. Top row, left to right: Original image and graphs of boundariness (gradient magnitude) and medialness (at optimal scale). Bottom row, left to right: Image with additive noise and graphs of boundariness and medialness.

The medialness function that we have used is related to the maximum over orientation of the second derivative of the image at medial position $\vec{m}$ and scale $\sigma_m$,

$$M(\vec{m}, \sigma_m) = \sigma_m^2 L_{\vec{p}\vec{p}} = -\sigma_m^2 \vec{p}' D^2 Lp = -\sigma_m^2 \lambda,$$  (5)

where $L$ is the scale-space representation of the original image,

$$L(\vec{m}, \sigma_m) = I(\vec{m}) \otimes G(\vec{m}, \sigma_m),$$  (6)

where $G$ is a unit-normalized Gaussian kernel of standard deviation $\sigma_m$. In equation 5, $D^2 L$ is the 2x2 matrix of second-order spatial derivatives of $L$, $D^2 L\vec{p} = \lambda\vec{p}$, and $\lambda$ is the largest magnitude eigenvalue of $D^2 L$.

**Boundariness at Sites on the Boundary Locus.** Boundariness, at a smaller scale than that typically used for medialness measurement, is needed to guide each boundary point from its position relative to the medial locus in the model to the position which the image information indicates. This allows the boundary locus to reflect details while limiting its ability to deviate, relative to the figural width, from the location predicted by the model. In our method boundariness measurements are computed at an image location $b$ that is linked to a single medial point $\vec{m}$. The boundariness is computed at a scale $\sigma_b$ that is a fixed fraction of the scale $\sigma_m$ of the medial point to which it is linked. The boundariness $B(b, \sigma_b)$ is computed as a directional derivative of the image intensity in the direction of the link $\vec{u} = b - \vec{m}$,

$$B(\vec{b}, \sigma_b) = \vec{u} \cdot \nabla L(\vec{b}, \sigma_b),$$  (7)

where $\vec{u}$ is a unit vector and $\nabla L(b, \sigma_b)$ is the image space gradient of the intensity at position $\vec{b}$ and scale $\sigma_b$.

## 2.3 Optimizing the Posterior: Segmentation via Deformable Shape Loci

This section describes the process whereby the DSL model (the log prior or internal energy component) is combined with the image information (the log likelihood or image energy component) such that the deformation of the model template results in a segmentation of a modeled object in an unclassified image (a relative maximum in the log posterior or objective function). Specifically, we describe how our method uses large-scale, figural information captured by the medial locus to allow for the stable localization of the model in the image and for the subsequent local optimization of the posterior to allow for segmentation.

To summarize the discussion in the previous sections, to perform a segmentation we wish to optimize an objective function, the log posterior, that consists of an image energy term, the log likelihood, and a model or internal energy term, the log prior:

log posterior = log likelihood + log prior

$$
= k_{bound} \sum_{i=1}^{N_b} \log B(\vec{b}_i, \sigma_{b_i}) + k_{med} \sum_{i=1}^{N_m} \log M(\vec{m}_i, \sigma_{m_i})
$$

$$
- k_{internal} \left( \sum_{l_k \in MM \, links} \left\| l_k - l_k^{model} \right\|^2 + \sum_{l_k \in MB \, links} \left\| l_k - l_k^{model} \right\|^2 + \sum_{l_k \in BB \, links} \left\| l_k - l_k^{model} \right\|^2 + \sum_{l_k \in FF \, links} \left\| l_k - l_k^{model} \right\|^2 \right), \quad (8)
$$

where the hyper-parameters, $k_{bound}$, $k_{med}$, and $k_{internal}$, can be estimated from training data obtained from human observers [20].

**Initialization of the DSL Model for Object Localization.** Like most deformable contour methods, we require that the model be initially positioned "close" to the object to be segmented in order to avoid convergence to an incorrect local maximum during the optimization process. Because we use a prior that reflects shape richly and explicitly recognizes figural middles and widths as important descriptors of shape, we believe our method has advantages over many other approaches. Use of multiscale and multilocal information, in the form of the medial sites and their figural width information, makes it possible to stably find (localize) approximate object locations, orientations, and sizes.

Initialization of a model to a candidate image containing an object to be segmented occurs in three stages (Fig. 3). In the first stage, the model template is mapped to the image space of the candidate image using a coarse registration of the training image and the candidate image to establish the approximate location of the object in question. In the second stage, an optimization procedure is initiated which attempts to fit the collection of medial sites to their respective positions in the candidate image via maximization of the sum of the medialness in the candidate image at the template medial sites as a function of a global translation, rotation, and scaling applied to the template. This process is the same as the registration method proposed and implemented by Fritsch [7,8] and, due to the invariance properties built into the prior, does not change the value of the prior from its model "mean". Due to the use of relatively large-scale medial information, this stage is remarkably robust in the presence of small-scale image disturbances (e.g., boundary and/or intensity noise) and exhibits a region of convergence for translation on the order of the average scale (half-width) of the figures comprising the object. In the third stage of initialization, each of the individual figures is allowed to deform rigidly with zoom in order to optimize the same functional as with global initialization. This step allows for any small adjustments in the position, orientation, and size of the figures relative to the global object shape. In the case where the figures comprising an object are linked, this stage can produce small changes in the prior term as figure-subfigure links are deformed from the model mean. We have found that initialization, using a strategy called simplex optimization [18], takes on the order of a few seconds per modeled figure.

134

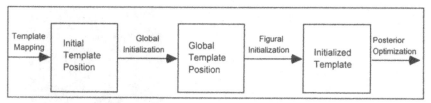

**Fig. 3.** Schematic of the DSL model localization process.

Fig. 4 illustrates the initialization procedure on an axial MR image of a brain ventricle. Fig. 4a shows a sample model for a ventricle consisting of two unlinked figures (for simplicity, no figural hierarchy nor cross-figural links have been defined). In Figs. 4b-e, a warped image with the model template (shown in the form of the segments connecting the boundary sites) in various stages of initialization is shown. This image was generated by warping the image from which the model was generated (Section 3.1 describes the warping procedure).

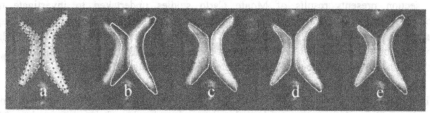

**Fig. 4.** Initialization of the model's global parameters on a warped image. (a) Original model superimposed on training image. (b) Initial mapping of the model to an image. (c) Model after global initialization. (d) Model after the left figural initialization. (e) Model after right figural initialization.

**Local Optimization of the DSL for Object Segmentation.** Once an object in localized and the template is initialized, the template links are allowed to deform locally, via movement of the individual template sites, in order to optimize the objective function. Again, we take advantage of the stability properties of the relatively large-scale medial sites by first performing sequential, local optimization over all medial sites with associated boundary sites moving in concert so as to maintain the deformation energy (link difference) in the medial-boundary links at its post-initialization level. This allows the template links for each individual figure to deform based on the most stable features, medialness at the medial sites, and thus to adjust to slight variations in figural shape from the prior mean.

Following this step, all of the template sites are allowed to move, in a sequential fashion, in an attempt to locally optimize the objective function. During this stage the boundary sites, which have been approximately aligned with the image features by the initialization process and by the previous step, move toward regions of high boundariness subject to the stabilizing constraints imposed by the prior links in the model. Fig. 5 shows a plot of the log posterior versus iteration (over all sites) and the final configuration of the linked boundary sites after the last iteration. Typically, convergence toward a maximum in the log posterior occurs in a number of iterations on the order of 10-20, and on an ordinary workstation the entire optimization process takes on the order of tens of seconds to several minutes (depending on the total number of sites in the model). Again, we use simplex optimization [18] to optimize each point as a function of its scale space position.

135

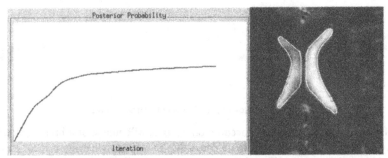

**Fig. 5**. Left: Plot of the posterior probability versus iteration over all sites for the model in Fig. 6a applied to the image in Fig. 6e. Right: Final configuration of the boundary after the 20th iteration.

## 3. Results

This section presents results of Monte Carlo studies undertaken to investigate the effectiveness of the segmentation method and to test its robustness in the presence of image disturbances (Section 3.1). Also presented are recent results demonstrating the applicability of this method to clinical MR and CT images (Sections 3.2-3.3), including a discussion of how object hierarchies may be used to facilitate object localization (Section 3.3).

### 3.1 Monte Carlo Investigations

We have performed a pair of pilot studies to examine the robustness of the method under increasing object deformation and under increasing levels of intensity noise. The methodologies and results of these studies are described below.

**Deformation.** To be clinically useful, a model-based segmentation method must be able to handle the normal variability seen in object shape across a population of patients. To test the robustness of our method in the presence of such variability, we have devised a method for deforming, in a random way, a test object in an image on which we have defined a model template. We take the model image and define a warping on that image which displaces a set of fixed reference points by a random distance drawn from a uniform bivariate normal distribution with standard deviation $\sigma_{warp}$. Given the reference points and their respective randomly perturbed positions, we apply Bookstein's [2] thin-plate-spline warping algorithm to produce a new image containing a warped version of the test object. The same warping function is applied to the model template to generate "truth" in the warped images.

Following initialization and optimization of the model to each of the warped images (see Fig. 6 for examples), the final template is compared to the warped model to give a measure of segmentation quality. We currently use the mean distance between the model template and warped template boundary points as our error measure. Results of this study are shown in the plot in Fig. 7. Note that rather "large" warps still lead to subpixel mean errors. Moreover, the outliers with the higher errors for any level of warp have most of their error at figural ends, where we have not yet implemented measures of figural endness to attract the boundary.

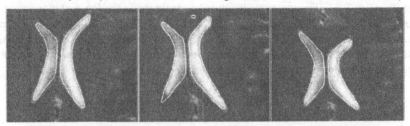

**Fig. 6.** Boundaries resulting from optimization of the objective function in warped images. The standard deviations for the warps were 2, 4, and 8 pixels for the left, center, and right images, respectively.

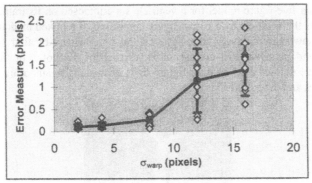

Fig. 7. Mean segmentation error (in pixels) plotted as a function of warp.

**Noise.** We make the claim that our methods are able to robustly handle image disturbances because of the stabilizing effects of large-scale, medial measurements. To illustrate this robustness, we have repeated the experiment above using increasing amounts of additive, Gaussian-distributed white noise. A sample warped image near the mean in the middle group in Fig. 7 (with $\sigma_{warp} = 8$) was used as the unclassified test image. Shown in Fig. 8 are the final optimized boundaries for representative samples from the Monte Carlo runs. Even with noise levels much greater than one would expect to find in clinical images, the method is able to yield segmentations of the ventricle with sub-pixel errors (Fig. 9).

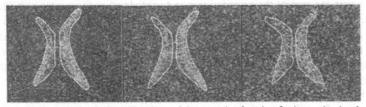

Fig. 8. Boundaries resulting from optimization of the posterior function for increasing levels of noise (SNR ~ 6, 3, and 1.5 from left to right).

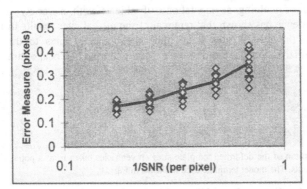

Fig. 9. Mean segmentation error plotted as a function of noise for a warp of 8 pixels.

## 3.2 Use of a Model with Inter-Figural Links on Clinically-Variable Ventricles

The simple, two-figure model of the ventricle used to produce the results in the preceding section made no use of inter-figural links. Hence, except during the global initialization stage, each of the figures was allowed to deform independently during the optimization process. We have recently begun to investigate the use of models that include such inter-figural links, and to take advantage of figural hierarchies wherein the most "stable" figures are used to establish the approximate location of less-stable subfigures.

Fig. 10 shows a five-figure model for a ventricle superimposed on its training image. The model represents the ventricle by a parent figure comprised of a linked medial and boundary locus running down the relatively large-scale central portion, and by four subfigures with linked medial and boundary loci corresponding to each of the horns of the ventricle. In addition, we have defined a set of inter-figural links connecting neighboring boundary sites on the subfigures and the parent figure.

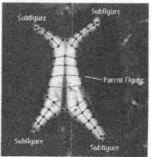

**Fig. 10.** A five-figure model of a ventricle superimposed on its training image.

This model was applied to a series of axial MR images, taken at approximately the same slice depth in the head, from a population of patients using a *hierarchical* localization scheme. First, the template sites for only the parent figure were matched to the images in order to optimize the sum of the boundariness and medialness at these sites as a function of global translation, rotation, and scaling. Following this initial mapping, each of the subfigures was placed relative to the parent figure such that the inter-figural link differences were zero, and each of the sites for the subfigures were then optimized over the individual figural parameters of translation, rotation, and scaling. Finally, sequential optimization over all template sites was performed to yield the results shown in Fig. 11.

A hierarchical approach provides for more flexible localization, as each of the subfigures is allowed to adjust for differences in size, position, and orientation relative to the larger scale, more stable parent figure. As Fig. 11 demonstrates, a model generated from a single training image is capable of yielding segmentations of objects with a variety of subtle shape differences. Experience has shown that removal of the medial sites results in few successful segmentations, as the medial sites help guide the boundary sites to their approximate locations in the initialization stage and provide stability during the local optimization stage.

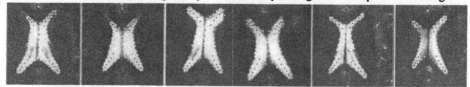

**Fig. 11.** Final position of the deformed template sites on ventricles taken from a population of images from different patients. The model template used is shown in Fig. 10.

### 3.3 Variants: Using External and Hierarchical DSL Models

We are investigating the possibility of using external structures, such as indentations, neighboring objects, and the spaces between objects, as means for defining models. When gaps between the anatomical object to be segmented and a neighboring object are narrow, the use of the gaps to guide the segmentation by the correspondingly narrow medialness apertures can avoid problems of inter-object interference. A recent example of such an approach applied to a liver in an axial CT slice through the abdomen is demonstrated in Fig. 12. In this study, an external model created on a characteristic slice. The model consists of four figures corresponding roughly to the gap between the liver and the chest wall, the gap between the liver and the kidney, the anterior tip of the liver (the only internal structure used), and a structure identified as the gall bladder. A boundary was defined by choosing a set of connections between certain boundary sites in the model and is shown superimposed on the adjacent CT slices from the same scan, above and below the model slice, in the left and right image in the top row of Fig. 12. The optimization process was applied to the full model on all slices and the resulting boundary is shown for each of the three images in the bottom row of Fig. 12.

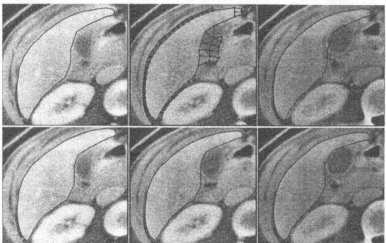

**Fig. 12.** Segmentation results from a 2D external model of the liver. Top row shows 3 adjacent CT slices through the liver with the defined boundary in the initialized model superimposed (full model is shown on the middle training image). Bottom row shows the same slices with the optimized model boundary superimposed.

As a final example, we present an application of a DSL approach utilizing multiple objects organized in an object hierarchy. Similar to the use of figural hierarchies (for multi-figure objects), where subfigures are located relative to more stable parent figures, this approach seeks to utilize the most stable objects to establish the relative location of other objects. In this example, a model was constructed on an axial CT slice through the abdomen on five objects: the entire abdomen cross section, each of the kidneys, the vertebra, and the spinal cord where the linked boundary loci are shown in Fig. 13. Using the strategy outlined below, the hierarchy of object models was fit to another slice (from the same CT scan) approximately 1.6 cm away from the model slice.

Because the model of the abdomen contains the largest-scale information in its medial sites, and hence is little-affected by the presence of smaller-scale image structure, the localization approach is first applied to the template sites in only the abdomen template. The shift, rotation, and scaling needed to match the abdomen template is then applied to all of the models such that the initial position of each of the sub-objects (kidneys, vertebra, and spinal cord) is defined relative to the abdomen. Next, the localization process is applied to all of the sites in the kidneys, vertebra, and spinal cord and they move as a collection to optimize the image energy as a function of their overall position, orientation, and scaling. This establishes the approximate location of the group of sub-objects. Finally, the localization process is applied to each of the individual sub-objects, after which the local optimization process commences. In the current implementation, we have defined no inter-object links which could potentially constrain the shape of a sub-object conditional upon the shape and position of a parent object. How to introduce such inter-object links and how to most effectively make use of hierarchies of object models is a subject of ongoing work.

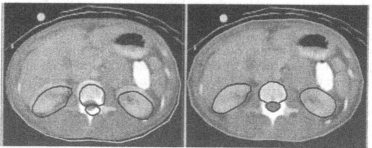

**Fig. 13**. Use of an object hierarchy to segment structures in an axial CT slice through the abdomen. (a) Original configuration of object models (on an unclassified image). (b) Final template configurations following hierarchical object localization and local object posterior optimization.

## 4. Discussion and Conclusion

We have described a method which takes a deformable loci approach to segmentation but uses a prior richly describing shape in terms of both figural and boundary aspects, and an image energy that stabilizes by its use of medialness that has a scale significant relative to figural width and yet sensitively locates the boundary using smaller-scale measurement of boundariness. The model is formed through a user's appreciation of what are the stable figures of the shape of a target object, so the model formation involves interaction, aided by core-extracting methods. On the other hand, the segmentation of the object for a new patient is intended to be fully automatic in most cases. When applied to relatively high contrast objects such as the ventricle in MR brain images, the method has been shown to produce subpixel accuracy in the presence of deformations of the model and large amounts of intensity noise. It has also been shown able to follow quite a range of normal clinical variation in ventricle shape.

We believe that the method has additional advantages to be explored in future research:
1. The locality of the links allows it to localize shape anomalies or locations in which the intensity relations in a clinical image deviates from what is expected.
2. The locality of the model allows one to designate the intensity properties reflecting boundariness as a function of boundary site. Thus luminance change polarity, intensity range, contrast range, and the choice of type of edge: e.g., outline vs. luminance edge vs. texture edge, can be designated with boundary site.

Additional features that we expect to be added in the future include the following:
1. Testing of the method in more challenging clinical situations, with lower signal-to-noise, lengthy regions of boundary dropout, complex backgrounds, etc.
2. Including measurements of figural endness at figural ends in the image energy.
3. Using 3-site in place of 2-site cliques (links), leading to rotational invariance.
4. Measuring variabilities in the model over various training images, and reflecting these variabilities in the hyperparameters (weights) of the objective function.
5. Extending the method to 3D, in which the medial and boundary loci are 2-manifolds. We have developed a method for creating such 3D models from a training image and will report this development in another paper.

## 5. Acknowledgements

The authors gratefully acknowledge the contributions to this research by David Eberly, who has formulated algorithms and mathematics for core extraction, by Allyson Wilson, who developed much of the statistical framework on which this work is based, and by KC Low and Matthew McAuliffe, who have provided much assistance in the development of the segmentation software. We also acknowledge financial support from the NCI Program Project Grant P01 CA47982 and from funds provided by the National Library of Medicine grant 5 RO1 LM05508.

# 6. REFERENCES

1. Blum H and Nagel RN: Shape description using weighted symmetric axis features. *Pattern Recognition* 10, 167-180 (1978).
2. Bookstein FL: Principal warps: Thin-plate splines and the decomposition of deformations. *IEEE Trans Pattern Anal and Machine Intell*, **11**:567-585 (1989).
3. Chakraborty A, Staib L, and Duncan JS: Deformable boundary finding influenced by region homogeneity. *Proc Conf Computer Vision and Pattern Recognition* (CVPR '94), 624-627 (1994).
4. Cootes TF, Hill A, Taylor CJ, and Haslam J: The use of active shape models for locating structures in medical images. *Information Processing in Medical Imaging*, HH Barrett, AF Gmitro eds., Lecture Notes in Comp. Sci., **687**:33-47, Springer-Verlag, Berlin (1993).
5. Eberly D, Gardner RB, Morse BS, Pizer SM, Scharlach C: Ridges for image analysis. *Journal of Mathematical Imaging and Vision*, **4**:351-371 (1994a).
6. Eberly D: A differential geometric approach to anisotropic diffusion. In *Geometry-Driven Diffusion in Computer Vision*, BM ter Haar Romeny (ed.), Kluwer Academic Press: 371-392 (1994b).
7. Fritsch DS, Chaney EL, Boxwala A, McAuliffe MJ, Raghavan S, Thall A, and Earnhart J: Core-based portal image registration for automatic radiotherapy treatment verification, *Int J Radiat Oncol Biol Phys* **33**(5): 1287-1300 (1995).
8. Fritsch DS: Registration of radiotherapy images using multiscale medial descriptions of image structure. Ph.D. dissertation, Department of Biomedical Engineering, University of North Carolina at Chapel Hill (1993).
9. Kass M, Witkin A, Terzopoulos D: Snakes: Active contour models. *Int J Comp Vision* **1**:321-331 (1987).
10. Leahy R, Herbet T, and Lee R: Application of Markov random fields in medical imaging. *Information Processing in Medical Imaging*, 1-14 (1989).
11. Lindeberg T: *Scale-Space Theory in Computer Vision*, Kluwer Academic Publishers, Boston (1994a).
12. McAuliffe MJ, Eberly D, Fritsch DS, Chaney EL, and Pizer SM: Scale-space boundary evolution initialized by cores. *Proc. Fourth International Conference on Visualization in Biomedical Computing*, Hamburg, IEEE Computer Society Press, Los Alamitos, CA (1996).
13. McInerney T and Terzopoulos D: Deformable models in medical image analysis. *Proc Workshop on Math Methods in Biomed Img Anal*, IEEE Cat. # 96TB100056: 171-180 (1996).
14. Morse BS, Pizer SM, and Liu A: Robust object representation through object-relevant use of scale. *Information Processing in Medical Imaging*, HH Barrett, AF Gmitro eds., Lecture Notes in Computer Science, **687**:112-131, Springer-Verlag, Berlin (1993).
15. Morse BS, Pizer SM, Puff DT, and Gu C: Zoom-invariant vision of figural shape: Effects on cores of image disturbances. University of North Carolina technical report TR96-005. To appear in *Computer Vision and Understanding* (1996).
16. Pizer SM, Eberly D, Morse BS, and Fritsch DS: Zoom-invariant vision of figural shape: The mathematics of cores. University of North Carolina Computer Science Technical Report, TRN96-004. To appear in *Computer Vision and. Image Understanding* (1996).
17. Pizer SM, Fritsch DS, Johnson VE, and Chaney EL: Segmentation, registration, and measurement of shape variation via image object shape. University of North Carolina Computer Science Technical Report, TRN96-031 (1996).
18. Press WH, Teukolsky SA, Vetterling WT, and Flannery BP: Numerical Recipes in C: The Art of Scientific Computing, Second Edition. Cambridge University Press, Cambridge (1995).
19. Staib L and Duncan J: Boundary finding with parametrically deformable models. IEEE Transactions on Pattern Analysis and Machine Intelligence 14: 161-175 (1992).
20. Wilson A: Statistical models for shapes and deformations. Ph.D. dissertation, Institute of Statistics and Decision Sciences, Duke University, Durham, NC (1995).

# Mapping the Cerebral Sulci: Application to Morphological Analysis of the Cortex and to Non-rigid Registration

Marc Vaillant and Christos Davatzikos

Neuroimaging Laboratory, Department of Radiology, Johns Hopkins University School of Medicine, 600 N. Wolfe Street, Baltimore MD 21287
email: vaillant@cbmv.jhu.edu, hristos@welchlink.welch.jhu.edu
http://ditzel.rad.jhu.edu

**Abstract.** We propose a methodology for extracting parametric representations of the cerebral sulci from magnetic resonance images, and we consider its application to two medical imaging problems: quantitative morphological analysis and spatial normalization and registration of brain images. Our methodology is based on deformable models utilizing characteristics of the cortical shape. Specifically, a parametric representation of a sulcus is determined by the motion of an active contour along the medial surface of the corresponding cortical fold. The active contour is initialized along the outer boundary of the brain, and deforms toward the deep edge of a sulcus under the influence of an external force field restricting it to lie along the medial surface of the particular cortical fold. A parametric representation of the surface is obtained as the active contour traverses the sulcus. In this paper we present results of this methodology and its applications.

## 1   Introduction

A great deal of attention has been given during the past several years to the quantitative analysis of the morphology of the human brain. Much progress has been made in the development of methodologies for analyzing the shape of subcortical structures [1, 2, 3]. However, the complexity of the cortical shape has been an obstacle in applying these methods to this highly convoluted structure. In this paper we present a methodology for finding a representation of the shape of the deep cortical folds from MR images, which extends our previously reported work [4].

The region between two juxtaposed sides of a cortical fold, called a *sulcus*, is a thin convoluted ribbon embedded in 3D. The cerebral sulci are important brain structures, since they are believed to be associated with functionally distinct cortical regions. In particular, during the development of the brain in the embryo, connections between specific cortical regions and connections between cortical regions and subcortical structures, in conjunction with an overall growth process constrained by the skull, are believed to induce the sharp inward folding of the cortex, resulting in the formation of the sulci. The roots of the sulci often demarcate the boundaries between functionally and structurally different cortical regions [5]. Most notably, the central sulcus is the boundary between its posteriorly located primary somatosensory cortex and its anteriorly located primary motor cortex. Along both sides of the central sulcus is a fairly consistent somatotopic distribution of motor and somatosensory functional regions of the cortex, known as Penfield's homunculus.

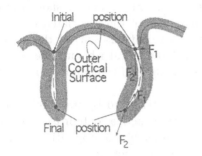

In order to study the cerebral sulci and the distribution of the function along their associated cortical folds, we first need to establish a quantitative methodology for describing the shape of these ribbon-like structures. In this paper we present a methodology for finding parametric representations of the sulcal ribbons.

**Fig. 1.** A 2D schematic diagram of the force field acting on the active contour.

Related to our work is the work in [5], which studies the cortical topography by determining a graph of the sulci. Although some global characteristics of the sulcal shape, including depth and orientation, were considered in [5], no attempt was made to characterize the local geometric structure of the sulci. The latter is the focus of our work. Also related is the work in [6, 7], which determines the medial axis of arbitrary shapes at multiple scales, the work in [8], which is based on manually outlining the sulci and the work in [9, 10] which focuses on segmentation of the sulci.

The method we propose in this paper is a physically-based algorithm utilizing the particular characteristics of the cortical shape. Specifically, our algorithm uses the outer cortical surface as a starting point. Based on the principal curvatures of this surface, we identify the outer edges of the sulcal ribbons. By placing active contours [11, 12] along these edges, which are then let free to move inward following the cortical gyrations, our method obtains a parametric representation of the sulcal ribbons.

Two main applications are considered in this paper. The first is the quantitative morphological analysis of the sulci. In particular, we use the parametric representation of the sulcal ribbons to determine the average shape of a sulcus and the inter-individual variability around this average. Inter-subject comparisons can be readily formulated based on this representation. The second application is in the spatial normalization and registration of brain images, in which a key issue is often obtaining a parametric representation of distinct surfaces which can then be matched based on their geometric characteristics [13, 14, 15, 16]. The sulcal ribbons of distinct cortical folds can be used for this purpose in shape transformation methodologies [16, 15].

# 2 Extraction of the Sulcal Ribbons

## 2.1 Overall Idea

The overall idea behind our algorithm is based on the particular shape of the sulci. Specifically, since a sulcus resembles a thin ribbon embedded in 3D, it can be extracted from an MR volumetric image as an active contour slides along the sulcal groove in between two juxtaposed sides of the associated cortical fold (see Fig. 1). The collection of the deformed configurations of the active contour readily provides a parameterization of the sulcal ribbon. The initial active contour is along the outer cortical surface; its final configuration is along the root of the sulcus.

The inward motion of the active contour is determined by two force fields (see Fig. 1). The first one restricts the motion of the active contour to be along the medial surface of a sulcus. The second one resembles a gravitational force and is responsible for the inward motion of the active contour.

## 2.2 Initial Placement of the Active Contours

As mentioned earlier in the paper, one active contour for each sulcus is initially placed along the outer boundary of the brain. In order to determine this initial configuration of the active contour, we first find a parametric representation of the outer cortical surface using a deformable surface algorithm described elsewhere [17]. A deformable surface, initially having a spherical configuration surrounding the brain, deforms like a contracting elastic membrane attracted by the outer cortical boundary and eventually adapts to its shape.

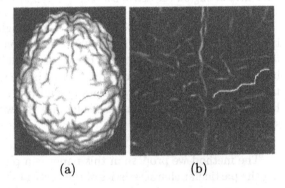

(a)                              (b)

**Fig. 2.** (a) Outer cortical surface with the initial active contour superimposed. (b) Flattened outer cortical map of the minimum (principal) curvature with the initial active contour superimposed.

We determine the outer cortical boundary through a sequence of three operations. A morphological erosion is first used to detach the brain tissue from the nearby dura, skull, and bone marrow. A seeded region growing then extracts the brain tissue. Finally, a conditional morphological dilation recaptures the brain tissue lost in the erosion step. In some cases manual editing of the final result is required, if the erosion step does not fully detach the parenchyma.

Resulting from the deformable surface algorithm is a parametric representation of the outer cortical surface, denoted by $\mathbf{b}(u, v)$, where $(u, v)$ takes values in a planar domain in which the deformable surface is parameterized. The intersections of this surface with the sulcal ribbons are the outer edges of the sulci, and are identified along the outer cortical surface using the minimum (principal) curvature of $\mathbf{b}(u,v)$, which has high value along them [17] (see Fig. 2). On these high curvature curves we then initialize active contours having evenly spaced points. The initial configuration of an active contour will be denoted by $\mathbf{x}(s,0) = \mathbf{x}(s,t)|_{t=0}$. Here, the parameter $t \in [0,1]$ denotes time. As $s \in [0,1]$ sweeps the unit interval, $\mathbf{x}(s,t)$ runs along the active contour at its configuration at time $t$. Equivalently, $\mathbf{x}(s,t)$ and $\mathbf{x}(s,t+\Delta t)$ are two consecutive deformed configurations of the active contour.

## 2.3 External Force Fields

After its initial placement along the outer edge of a sulcus, the active contour slides along the medial surface of the sulcus, in between two opposite sides of a cortical fold, under the influence of its internal elastic forces and two external force fields which are described next.

**Center-of-Mass Force.** The first force field, $\mathbf{F}_1$, acting on the active contour restricts its motion to be on the sulcal medial surface. This force is based on the observation that the points lying on the medial surface of a sulcus satisfy the following condition (see Fig. 3):

$$\mathbf{X} = \mathbf{c}(\mathbf{X})\,, \tag{1}$$

where $\mathbf{c}(\mathbf{X})$ is the center of the cortical mass included in a spherical neighborhood, $\mathcal{N}(\mathbf{X})$, centered on $\mathbf{X}$ [1]. Accordingly, we define the force acting on a point located at $\mathbf{X}$ as

$$\mathbf{F}_1(\mathbf{X}) = \frac{\mathbf{c}(\mathbf{X}) - \mathbf{X}}{\rho(\mathbf{X})}\,, \tag{2}$$

where $\rho(\mathbf{X})$ is the radius of $\mathcal{N}(\mathbf{X})$ and is spatially varying, as described below.

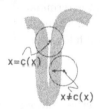

**Fig. 3.** Schematic diagram of the cross-section of a sulcus and its surrounding cortex.

If the cortex had exactly uniform thickness throughout its extent, and if the two juxtaposed sides of the cortical folds were always in contact with each other, then $\rho$ in (2) would be fixed to a value equal to the cortical thickness. In that case, $\mathbf{F}_1$ would be exactly zero on the sulci. However, this is often not the case. In order to account for variations in the cortical and sulcal thickness, we allow $\rho(\mathbf{X})$ to vary throughout the cortex; at each point $\mathbf{X}$, $\mathcal{N}(\mathbf{X})$ adapts its size to encompass the cortical gray matter in its full width. In particular, at each point $\mathbf{X}$, $\rho(\mathbf{X})$ is defined as the radius of the smallest spherical neighborhood intersecting the cortical boundaries on both sides of a cortical fold.

Now consider an active contour point located at $\mathbf{X}$. If $\mathbf{X}$ is exactly on the medial axis of the sulcus then $\mathbf{F}_1(\mathbf{X}) = 0$; in this case $\mathbf{F}_1$ does not affect this point. Otherwise, $\mathbf{F}_1$ moves the point towards the sulcal medial axis (see Fig. 3). After a sequence of incremental movements, the point balances at a position satisfying

---

[1] In the experiments herein, the cortical mass is the indicator function of the cortex, and is obtained at a pre-segmentation step using a fuzzy C-means algorithm, courtesy of Dzung Pham.

(1) (within some preset tolerance factor) where $\mathbf{F}_1$ vanishes. It is important to note that $\rho(\cdot)$ adapts continuously to the cortical thickness during this restoring motion. At equilibrium, the spherical neighborhood balances between the two opposite boundaries of the cortical fold.

**Inward Force.** The second force field, $\mathbf{F}_2$, acting on the active contour is responsible for its inward motion toward the deepest edge of a sulcus. At the active contour's initial configuration $\mathbf{x}(s, 0)$, $\mathbf{F}_2$ at each contour point is in the direction of the inward normal to the outer cortical surface, which is denoted by $\mathbf{F}_N[\mathbf{x}(s, 0)]$. As mentioned earlier, the orientation of the sulci tend to deviate from this normal direction, especially deep in the brain. Accordingly, we adapt $\mathbf{F}_2$ as the active contour moves inward. If $\mathbf{x}(s, t)$ is the position of an active contour point at time $t$, then $\mathbf{x}_t(s, t)$, and $\mathbf{x}_{tt}(s, t)$ respectively represent speed and acceleration components of the active contour's dynamics. These terms effectively provide a directional estimation of the active contour's motion. We now define $\mathbf{F}_2(s, t)$ as

$$\mathbf{F}_2(s, t) = \alpha \mathbf{x}_t + \beta \mathbf{x}_{tt} + \gamma \mathbf{F}_N[\mathbf{x}(s, 0)], \tag{3}$$

where subscripts denote partial derivatives.

The first two terms in (3) give rise to damping and inertial influences which have the effect of averaging the previously traveled direction of the active contour with the initial inward direction. This actively adapts the inward force to the shape of the sulcus.

Under the influence of the two force fields, $\mathbf{F}_1$ and $\mathbf{F}_2$, the active contour deforms elastically, sliding along the medial surface of a sulcus towards its deepest edge. The inward trajectory of each active contour point is terminated when the magnitude of the total force acting on it becomes less than a threshold $\zeta \in [0, 1]$. This typically occurs at the bottom parts of the cortical folds where $\mathbf{F}_1$ and $\mathbf{F}_2$ have almost opposite directions (see Fig. 1).

## 2.4 Refinement of the Sulcal Surface

The collection of the deformed configurations of the active contour constitute a surface, parameterized by $\mathbf{x}(s, t)$. This surface tends to be smooth along one family of isoparametric curves, the one obtained by fixing $t$, because of the internal elastic forces of the active contour which are along these curves. However, it is not necessarily smooth along the other family of isoparametric curves, the one obtained by fixing $s$, which are oriented along the direction of the inward motion. In order to obtain a smooth surface, $\mathbf{y}(s, t)$, from $\mathbf{x}(s, t)$ we solve the following regularization problem:

$$\text{Minimize} \iint \|\mathbf{y}(s, t) - \mathbf{x}(s, t)\|^2 \, ds \, dt + K \iint \left( \|\mathbf{y}_s(s, t)\|^2 + \|\mathbf{y}_t(s, t)\|^2 \right) ds \, dt, \tag{4}$$

where subscripts denote partial derivatives.

In (4), the surface $\mathbf{y}(s, t)$ is an elastic membrane which adapts to the shape of the sulcal surface $\mathbf{x}(s, t)$, while maintaining a certain degree of smoothness determined by the elasticity parameter $K$. Equation (4) is discretized and solved iteratively, resulting in a smoother surface parameterized by $\mathbf{y}(s,t)$, which is defined in the domain $\mathcal{D} = [0,1] \times [0,1]$. Fig. 4 illustrates the effect of this procedure on an original sulcus before smoothing. The resulting sulcus Fig. 4b is clearly smoother, but maintains the shape of the original sulcus.

## 2.5  Fixed-Point Algorithm

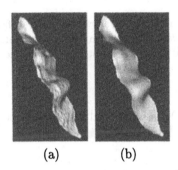

(a)          (b)

**Fig. 4.** A sulcus, (a) before, and (b) after the smoothing procedure.

The solution of (4) is a smooth parameterization of a sulcal ribbon. Although there is an infinite number of such parameterizations of a sulcus (or of any surface, as a matter of fact), any of them is adequate for visualization purposes, since the shape of a surface does not depend on the way that the surface is parameterized. However, for all the applications considered in the following section, it is at least desirable, if not necessary, to find a unique parameterization with specific properties. This is especially important in a procedure determining the average shape of a sulcus in which all the sulci whose average form is sought must be parameterized in a consistent way, so that corresponding points are averaged together. For example, Fig. 5 shows two surfaces, corresponding to two hypothetical sulci. The arrows show corresponding points, ie. points with the same $(s,t)$ parametric coordinates. The surfaces in (b) and (c) have identical shape, but clearly the parameterization in (b) is a much more reasonable match to that in (a).

One way to obtain a consistent, across subjects, surface parameterization, which is natural in the absence of landmarks along the sulcus, is to find a parameterization $\mathbf{x}(u,v)$ that has the following first fundamental form:

$$E = \lambda_s, \quad F = 0, \quad G = \lambda_t \tag{5}$$

where $\lambda_s$ and $\lambda_t$ are constants. Intuitively, such a parameterization can be obtained by stretching the parametric domain $\mathcal{D}$ by a factor of $\lambda_s$ horizontally, a factor $\lambda_t$ vertically, and folding it in 3D while preserving the angles between its isoparametric curves. If $\lambda_s = \lambda_t$, then the parameterization is homothetic, i.e. an isometry together with a uniform scaling factor.

Equation (5) implies that the surface with this first fundamental form must have isoparametric curves of constant speed (although the speeds of the u-curves and the v-curves differ if $\lambda_s \neq \lambda_t$). Moreover, the isoparametric curves intersect at right angles. In order to find such a parameterization, we apply a fixed point algorithm described in detail in [17], which iteratively reparameterizes the curves

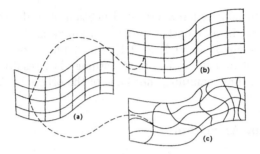

**Fig. 5.** Surfaces (a), and (b) have similar parameterizations. (c) shows the same surface as in (b) with a dramatically different parameterization. Points with similar parametric coordinates $(s, t)$ on the surfaces in (a) and (b) tend to fall in consistent locations along the two sulci; this is not true for (a) and (c).

$\mathbf{x}(s, j/N)$ and $\mathbf{x}(i/N, t)$ for each $i, j \in [0, 1, ..., N]$. This procedure typically converges in a few iterations.

# 3  Applications of Sulcal Mapping

## 3.1  Morphological Analysis of the Sulci

One of the fundamental problems in the emerging field of computational neuroanatomy is determining average shapes of brain structures and measuring the anatomical variability around them [2, 1, 18, 19, 8]. The parametric representation of the shape of the sulci presented in the previous section can form the basis for shape analysis of the sulcal structure and for determining average sulcal shapes. In order to obtain the average of a number of sulci, we apply the Procrustes fit, described in more detail in [2]. In this algorithm, the sulci are first translated to have a common centroid. Then, they are scaled so that the sum of the magnitudes of the vectors from the centroid of each sulcus to the points along the sulcus is equal to unity. Subsequently, the sulci are rotated iteratively until their distance from their average becomes minimal. This is a very fast algorithm, so typically a few iterations are sufficient for convergence.

If the resulting sulcal parameterizations of $N$ subjects in a group after the Procrustes fit are $\mathbf{p}_1(s, t)$, $\mathbf{p}_2(s, t)$, $\cdots, \mathbf{p}_N(s, t)$, $(s, t) \in \mathcal{D}$, then the average sulcus is

$$\overline{\mathbf{p}}(s, t) = \frac{1}{N} \sum_{i=1}^{N} \mathbf{p}_i(s, t). \qquad (6)$$

The covariance tensor around this mean can be readily obtained.

Obtaining a measure of the variance or the covariance tensor around the average shape inevitably depends on the specific parameterization scheme that was used. Although our parameterization is a sensible choice in the absence of specific landmarks along the sulcus, still it is one of many possible ones. In order to minimize the effects of the parameterization on the measurement of the variance around the average shape of a sulcus, in the experiments of Section 4 we measure the variance of the component of the residual vector $\mathbf{p}_i(s,t) - \overline{\mathbf{p}}(s,t)$ that is perpendicular to the tangent plane of the sulcus. This component depends primarily on the shape of the sulci and not on the way it is parameterized.

## 3.2 Spatial Normalization and Registration of 3D Images

Finding parametric representations of the sulcal ribbons also finds application in the spatial normalization and registration of brain images. We have previously reported a methodology [16, 13] that elastically warps one brain image to another, by mapping a number of surfaces in one brain to their homologous surfaces in the other brain. In [16, 13] the warping was based on the outer cortical and the ventricular surfaces, which can be extracted fairly easily from MR images. This method is extended in this paper to include the sulcal surfaces as additional features driving the 3D elastic warping. (A similar approach was described in [15], which used a different warping transformation as well as manually outlined sulci.)

Let $\mathbf{x}_1(s,t)$ and $\mathbf{x}_2(s,t)$ be the parameterizations of two homologous sulci. In our elastic warping algorithm we deform one sulcus to the other so that

$$\mathbf{x}_1(s,t) \longrightarrow \mathbf{x}_2(s,t) \forall (s,t) \in \mathcal{D}. \tag{7}$$

This effectively stretches one sulcus uniformly along each family of isoparametric curves so that it matches the other, while maintaining the angles at which the horizontal and vertical isoparametric curves intersect. The rest of the 3D image deforms following the equations of an elastic solid deformation.

**Non-Uniform Sulcal Stretching.** In the absence of either anatomical of functional landmarks, the directionally uniform stretching described above is the best guess for defining point-to-point correspondences between two sulci. However, often the structure of the sulci allows us to obtain a more accurate map from one sulcus to another. A notable example is the central sulcus, which has a fairly consistent folding pattern forming an S-like shape. This folding pattern is reflected by the principal curvatures along the sulcus, which can be therefore used for determining a nonuniform stretching of one sulcus to another that brings the curvatures of the stretched and the target sulci in best agreement.

In order to estimate the principal curvatures, $\kappa_1$ and $\kappa_2$, of the (discretized) surface $\mathbf{x}(s,t)$, we find a least-squares quadratic patch fit around each point of the sulcal ribbon and calculate the curvatures as described in [17].

Having defined the curvatures, we then find the 2D elastic transformation of $\mathcal{D}$ to itself, which is driven by a force field attempting to maximize the similarity of the curvatures along two sulci. This is essentially a *reparameterization* of one sulcus so that points of similar geometric structure in two homologous sulci have the same parametric coordinates $(s,t)$. The boundary conditions of this transformation fix the four corners of the sulcal ribbon, and allow the points along its four sides to slide freely under the influence of the external and the internal elastic forces. The details of this 2D elastic deformation are described in [20, 21].

# 4 Experiments

**Morphological Analysis.** Because of the functional importance of the central sulcus and the known distribution of function along it, mentioned previously as Penfield's homunculus, it is our primary interest to quantify its morphology. Therefore, we have focused our preliminary experiments on extracting and analyzing the central sulcus of five subjects. The sequence of steps, described in Section 2 were used initialize each active contour. A sulcal ribbon generated from the resultant trajectories is shown in Fig. 6. The parametric domain, sampled at regular intervals is superimposed on the sulcus in 3D, illustrating smooth uniform spacing along the $t$–isoparametric and $s$–isoparametric curves. Figure 8 shows that the ribbon obtained by the algorithm lies along the medial surface of the sulcus.

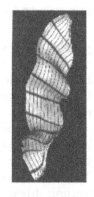

**Fig. 6.** A resulting sulcal surface.

After extracting the sulcal surfaces of the five subjects, we then applied the Procrustes fit algorithm as described in 3.1. The average sulcus, shown in 7, reveals two prominent folds, which further suggest a consistency in the folding pattern of the central sulcus in these five subjects.

Next, we applied our algorithm to three additional sulci: pre-central, superior frontal, and inferior frontal of the left hemisphere. The resulting sulci of two subjects are shown in Fig. 9 and a visual comparison suggests that sulci other than the central sulcus have fairly consistent gyrations. Most notably the superior frontal sulcus which appears to have one or two consistent folds, similar to the shape consistencies found in the central sulcus.

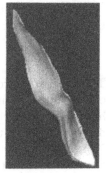

**Fig. 7.** The Procrustes average of the central sulcus from five subjects.

**Validation.** The performance of our algorithm was evaluated by quantitatively comparing the sulci obtained from our algorithm, for each of the five subjects, with a manual tracing of the same sulci. The central sulcus was traced on the axial slices; the outlines were then stacked to a 3D volume. Error measurements were obtained by recording the maximum distance in millimeters between the traced sulcus and the resulting sulcal representation from our algorithm. We obtained a maximum and average error for each central sulcus of the five subjects. The distance measure is calculated by growing a spherical neighborhood around each point in the parameterized surface until it intersects a manually traced point. The radius in *mm* of the resulting neighborhood is the error measure which we refer to as *Error 1*. This error measure, however, does not reflect deep parts of the actual sulcus which were not reached by the active contour. Specifically, each point in our parameterized surface $y(s, t)$ is close to some manually traced sulcal point. However, there might be parts of the traced sulci which are not reached by the active contour. In order to measure such errors and test the ability of our algorithm to cover a sulcus in its full extent, we also obtained a second error measure. This measure is similar to the one described above except that it measures the distance between each point in the *manually* traced sulcus and its nearest point in the parameterized sulcus. Ie. the neighborhood grows and is centered about each manually traced point rather than each point in the parameterized sulcus. At a deep region of the sulcus that is not reached by the active contour, this error measure is high. We refer to this error as *Error 2*.

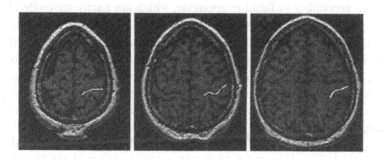

**Fig. 8.** Cross-sections of a resulting sulcal surface superimposed on the corresponding MR slices.

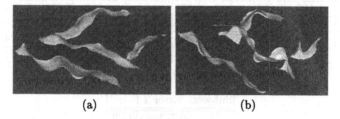

**Fig. 9.** (a) Four sulci(central, pre-central, superior frontal, and inferior frontal of the left hemisphere). (b) The same four sulci of another subject.

Each sulcus was manually outlined by two different raters; the errors are shown in Tables 10a and 10b. We also computed the differences between the two manual tracings by using the second error measure. The results show that the average errors fall roughly between .7mm and 1.6mm which are comparable to the average difference between the two raters which fall between .6mm and .9mm and have similar variance. We conclude that manual tracing would result in only a marginal improvement, at the expense of irreproducibility, subjectivity, and excessive human effort.

In considering the variability along the sulcus, it is necessary to correlate variability with error because variability measurements at regions of high error are dubious. The most meaningful variability information should be considered along the regions of the sulcus which correspond to low error. Interestingly, our results have shown that some of the most variable regions have low error. One fairly distinct region corresponds to a fold along the center of the sulcus, from which we have made two inferences. First, the low error indicates that our algorithm has been successful in following a seemingly difficult, high curvature region of the sulcus. Second, according to the homunculus, the facial regions of the body would somatotopically map to what we have found as a highly variable region of the central sulcus. One might expect such shape variability because of the high variability in facial expressions, which are partly controlled by that region of the primary motor cortex, as compared to the feet, hands, etc.

We note that the parameters in 3 and 4 were determined empirically. Detailed experiments validating the robustness of our method to them are reported in [22].

**3D Warping.** In this experiment we warped one volumetric MR image to another, using the outer cortical surface, the ventricular surface, and 4 sulci (central, pre-central, superior frontal, and inferior frontal, only of the left hemisphere) as features(see Fig. 9). A uniform stretching was applied to corresponding sulci to map them to each other. A cross-section from the warped image is shown in Fig. 11a, and in Fig. 11b overlayed on the cortical outline of the target image, which is shown in Fig. 11c.

| Subject | Error 1 | $\sigma$ | Error 2 | $\sigma$ | Subject | Error 1 | $\sigma$ | Error 2 | $\sigma$ |
|---------|---------|----------|---------|----------|---------|---------|----------|---------|----------|
| 1 | 0.969mm | 0.808 | 1.475mm | 1.322 | 1 | 1.168mm | 0.973 | 1.390mm | 1.302 |
| 2 | 1.156 | 0.892 | 1.150 | 1.101 | 2 | 0.952 | 0.818 | 0.954 | 1.040 |
| 3 | 0.825 | 0.724 | 1.589 | 2.467 | 3 | 0.722 | 0.697 | 1.550 | 2.278 |
| 4 | 1.168 | 0.816 | 1.114 | 0.940 | 4 | 1.103 | 0.760 | 0.874 | 0.736 |
| 5 | 0.691 | 0.729 | 0.720 | 0.718 | 5 | 0.677 | 0.642 | 0.887 | 0.826 |

(a)        (b)

| Subject | Error 2 | $\sigma$ |
|---------|---------|----------|
| 1 | 0.773mm | 0.720 |
| 2 | 0.684 | 0.636 |
| 3 | 0.637 | 0.644 |
| 4 | 0.830 | 0.848 |
| 5 | 0.673 | 0.596 |

(c)

**Fig. 10.** (a) Errors for first rater, (b) Errors for second rater, (c) Differences between first and second rater.

It is apparent from these images that a better registration was achieved at the left hemisphere (right side in the images, according to the radiology convention), which is the hemisphere of which the 4 sulci were used as features. Most notable is the registration around the central sulcus.

Experiments demonstrating the elastic reparameterization of the sulci, based on their principal curvatures are reported in [22].

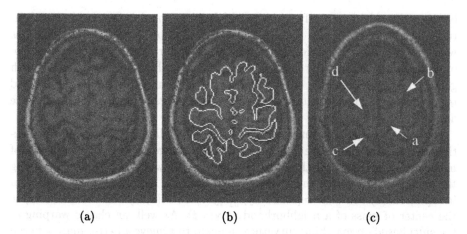

(a)　　　　　　　　　(b)　　　　　　　　　(c)

**Fig. 11.** 3D elastic warping using the outer cortical surface and 4 sulci of the left hemisphere (right side in the images) as landmarks. (a) A cross-section of the warped image. (b) The same cross-section overlayed on the cortical outline of the target image. (c) The corresponding cross-section of the target image. The arrows **a** and **b** highlight the sulci where a better registration was achieved. A poorer registration, in which the 4 sulci were not used as features, is seen along the analogous sulci, **c** and **d** on the other hemisphere.

## 5　Discussion

We have developed a quantitative methodology for describing the shape of the sulci, utilizing particular characteristics of the cortical folds. A force field guides a set of active contour points along the medial surfaces of sulci, thereby parameterizing the sulcal "ribbons". This technique was applied to five subjects, and its application was demonstrated in quantitative morphological analysis and spatial normalization and registration of brain images.

The advantage of our method is that a parameterized representation of the cortical folds is automatically obtained. The limitation of previous methods for medial axis finding is the difficulty in parameterization of the result. Traditional axis-width descriptors as described in [23, 6, 7] often generate noisy medial axes, or more importantly disconnected axes, making parameterization and subsequent shape analysis very difficult. Moreover, axes in the whole image are extracted, most of which do not correspond the sulci and therefore must be manually removed at a post-processing step.

Several extensions of this basic approach are possible. In particular, a current limitation of our algorithm is the requirement for the manual initialization of the active contour. The automation of this procedure is a very difficult task, primarily because of the complexity of the cortical structure. Specifically, although sulcal edges can be identified from the peaks of the absolute value of the minimum curvature of the outer cortical surface [24, 25, 26], the differentiation between the sulci eventually requires a higher level model. Our current and future work in this direction focuses on the use of prior probability distributions which reflect our expectation for finding a particular sulcal edge at a given coordinate $(u, v)$ of the outer cortical surface $\mathbf{b}(u, v)$. These priors, together with geometric properties of the outer cortex, such as curvatures, can potentially lead to the automatic identification of specific sulci, and the initial placement of the active contour along them.

Another extension of our algorithm is in the refinement procedure of Section 2.4. In particular, one could constrain the surface $\mathbf{y}(s, t)$ to the center of mass of the sulcus rather than $\mathbf{x}(s, t)$, therefore allowing it to freely slide along the medial surface rather than "being tied" to $\mathbf{x}(s, t)$. For example, the first term in equation (4) could be replaced by, $\iint \|\mathbf{y}(s, t) - \mathbf{c}(s, t)\|^2 ds dt$ where $\mathbf{c}(s, t)$ is the center of mass of a neighborhood at $\mathbf{y}(s, t)$. As well, an elastic warping of the sulci based on matching curvature can help to achieve a better map between subjects[21].

A current problem with the algorithm occurs when the active contour encounters an interruption, which frequently occurs in sulci such as the pre-central sulcus. If several active contour points exceed the threshold $\zeta$, as described in Section 2.3, the entire inward motion of the active contour terminates. In this case, the deepest edge of the sulcus will not be reached. If instead, the active contour continues, the fixed-point procedure of Section 2.5 will not parameterize the sulci consistently. We are currently pursuing a refinement of the algorithm which divides the active contour into two parts when an interruption is encountered. The parameterization will be applied separately to each section of the active contour.

## References

1. C. Davatzikos, M. Vaillant, S. Resnick, J.L. Prince, S. Letovsky, and R.N. Bryan. A computerized approach for morphological analysis of the corpus callosum. *J. of Comp. Assisted Tomography*, 20:88–97, Jan./Feb. 1996.
2. F.L. Bookstein. Biometrics, biomathematics, and the morphometric synthesis. *Bulletin of Mathematical Biology*, 58:313–365, 1996.
3. G. Szekely, A. Kelemen, C. Brechbuhler, and G. Gerig. Segmentation of 2-D and 3-D objects from MRI volume data using constrained deformations of flexible Fourier contour and surface models. *Medical Image Analysis*, 1:19–34, 1996.
4. M. Vaillant, C. Davatzikos, and R.N. Bryan. Finding 3D parametric representations of the deep cortical folds. *Proc. of the IEEE Workshop on Mathematical Methods in Biomedical Image Analysis*, pages 151–159, June 1996.
5. J.-F. Mangin, J. Regis, I. Bloch, V. Frouin, Y. Samson, and J. López-Krahe. A MRF based random graph modeling the human cortical topography. In *Proc. First Int. Conf., CVRMed*, pages 177–183, Nice, France, 1995.
6. S.M. Pizer, J.M. Coggins, C.A. Burbeck, B.S. Morse, and D. Fritsch. Object shape before boundary shape: Scale-space medial axes. *Journal of Mathematical Imaging and Vision*, 4:303–313, 1994.
7. B.S. Morse, S.M. Pizer, and A. Liu. Multiscale medial analysis of medical images. *Image and Vision Computing*, 12(6):327–338, July/August 1994.

8. P.M. Thompson, C. Schwartz, and A.W. Toga. High resolution random mesh algorithms for creating a probabilistic 3D surface atlas of the human brain. *Neuroimage*, 3:19–34, 1996.

9. G. Le Goualher, C. Barillot, L. Le Briquer, J.C. Gee, and Y. Bizais. 3D detection and representation of cortical sulci. *Proc. Computer Assisted Radiology, symposium on Computer and Communication Systems for Image Guided Diagnosis and Therapy*, pages 234–240, June 1995.

10. F. Kruggel. Automatical adaption of anatomical masks to the neocortex. *Proc. Int. Conf. on Computer Vision, Virtual Reality and Robotics in Medicine*, pages 231–236, April 1995.

11. M. Kass, A. Witkin, and D. Terzopoulos. Snakes: Active contour models. *International Journal of Computer Vision*, 1:321–331, 1988.

12. C.A. Davatzikos and J.L. Prince. An active contour model for mapping the cortex. *IEEE Trans. on Medical Imaging*, 14:65–80, 1995.

13. C. Davatzikos. Spatial normalization of 3D images using deformable models. *J. Comp. Assist. Tomogr.*, 20:656–665, July/August 1996.

14. S.R. Sandor. *Atlas-Guided Deformable Models for Automatic Labeling of Magnetic Resonance Brain Images*. PhD thesis, Un. of Southern California, 1994.

15. P. Thompson and A.W. Toga. A surface-based technique for warping three-dimensional images of the brain. *IEEE Trans. on Med. Imaging*, 15:402–417, 1996.

16. C. Davatzikos. Nonlinear registration of brain images using deformable models. *Proc. of the Workshop on Math. Meth. in Biom. Image Anal.*, pages 94–104, June 1996.

17. C. Davatzikos and R.N. Bryan. Using a deformable surface model to obtain a shape representation of the cortex. *IEEE Trans. on Med. Imaging*, 15:785–795, Dec. 1996.

18. M.I. Miller, G.E. Christensen, Y. Amit, and U. Grenander. Mathematical textbook of deformable neuroanatomies. *Proc. of the National Academy of Sciences*, 90:11944–11948, 1993.

19. A.C. Evans, D.L. Collins, S.R. Mills, E.D. Brown, R.L. Kelly, and T.M. Peters. 3D statistical neuroanatomical models from 305 MRI volumes. *Proc. of the IEEE Nucl. Sc. Symposium and Med. Imaging Conf.*, 3:1813–1817, 1993.

20. C. Davatzikos and J.L. Prince. Brain image registration based on curve mapping. *Proc. of the IEEE Workshop on Biomedical Image Analysis*, pages 245–254, 1994.

21. C. Davatzikos, J.L. Prince, and R.N. Bryan. Image registration based on boundary mapping. *IEEE Trans. on Med. Imaging*, 15(1):112–115, Feb. 1996.

22. M. Vaillant and C. Davatzikos. Finding parametric representations of the cortical sulci using an active contour model. *Medical Image Analysis*, 1997. accepted.

23. H. Blum and R.N. Nagel. Shape description using weighted symmetric axis features. *Patt. Recog.*, 10:167–180, 1978.

24. C. Davatzikos and R.N. Bryan. Using a deformable surface model to obtain a mathematical representation of the cortex. *Proc. of the IEEE Comp. Vision Symp.*, pages 212–217, Nov. 1995.

25. J.P. Thirion, O. Monga, S. Benayoun, A. Gueziec, and N. Ayache. Automatic registration of 3-D images using surface curvature. *SPIE Proc., Mathematical Methods in Medical Imaging*, 1768:206–216, 1992.

26. G. Subsol, J.P. Thirion, and N. Ayache. First steps towards automatic building of anatomical atlases. *INRIA, Technical Report N° 2216*, 1994.

# Bayesian Detection of Random Signals on Random Backgrounds

Harrison H. Barrett[1,2,3] and Craig K. Abbey[1,2]

1. Dept. of Radiology, University of Arizona, Tucson AZ 85724

2. Program in Applied Mathematics, University of Arizona, Tucson AZ, 85721

3. Optical Sciences Center, University of Arizona, Tucson AZ 85721

**Abstract.** This paper describes a general approach to signal detection with uncertainty in signal and/or background distributions. Attention is restricted to binary decision problems where the hypotheses can be expressed as signal-present vs signal-absent, but otherwise the treatment is general. Many familiar results come out as special cases.

## 1   Introduction

Bayesian signal detection plays two distinct roles in medical imaging. First, it is by definition the optimal way to detect tumors, stenoses or other signals whenever reliable prior information about the signal and its background is available. Second, the Bayesian detector, often referred to as the *ideal observer*, sets an upper limit to how well any observer can detect signals in images, and hence the performance of this observer is frequently used as a figure of merit for image quality.

When actually implementing Bayesian procedures, however, many practical difficulties arise. The essential information may not be available or may not accurately describe the imagery, and actual computation of the Bayesian discriminant may be difficult.

This paper focusses on the latter problem and summarizes methods to compute Bayesian discriminants for random signals in random backgrounds. Many of the results presented here are well known in the signal-detection literature but do not appear to be appreciated in medical imaging. The paper thus has a tutorial flavor, but it also presents practical recipes for computing the ideal discriminant for various kinds of signal and background uncertainty.

## 2   Hypothesis Testing with the Likelihood Ratio

Consider a binary decision problem where the task is to decide between two hypotheses, the null hypothesis $H_0$ and the alternative hypothesis $H_1$. In the context of signal detection, $H_0$ is signal-absent while $H_1$ is signal-present.

The decision is based on some data set, say $M$ data values $\{g_m, m = 1...M\}$ arranged as an $M \times 1$ column vector $\mathbf{g}$. We assume throughout this paper that each component of $\mathbf{g}$ is a continuous random variable. This model is not strictly justified with photon-counting systems, where a component of $\mathbf{g}$ represents the number of counts in some detector element. If the number of counts is reasonably large, however, the discrete nature of the data can often be ignored. For example, a Poisson probability law can be quite accurately approximated by a Gaussian if the mean number of counts is 10 or more [1]. We shall adopt the view that $\mathbf{g}$ takes on a continuous range of values and can thus be characterized by a probability density function. The probability density function of $\mathbf{g}$ if $H_i$ is true is denoted $p(\mathbf{g} | H_i)$. We shall not assume that components of $\mathbf{g}$ are uncorrelated or that the density function is independent of mean irradiance level, and no specific functional form for the densities will be assumed until we get to examples.

There are four possible outcomes of a binary decision process, two correct and two incorrect. If the decision is that $H_1$ is true when, in fact, it is true, then the decision is called a true positive or correct detection. If the decision is that $H_1$ is true when it is not, the decision is called a false positive or false alarm. True negatives and false negatives are defined analogously.

If the decision is non-randomized, in the sense that the same data vector will always result in the same decision, then any decision strategy on a binary task can be described as a two-step process: first compute some scalar test statistic from the data, then compare this scalar value to a threshold in order to make the decision. A plot of true-positive fraction vs false-positive fraction, obtained by varying the threshold, is called the *receiver operating characteristic* (ROC) curve.

A Bayesian approach to deciding between $H_0$ and $H_1$ is to assign costs to the four possible outcomes and to define the Bayes risk as the average cost. It is well known [2] [3] that the risk is minimized if the decision is based on the likelihood ratio, a random function of $\mathbf{g}$ defined by

$$\Lambda(\mathbf{g}) = \frac{p(\mathbf{g} | H_1)}{p(\mathbf{g} | H_0)}. \tag{1}$$

The Bayesian, armed with prior knowledge of $p(\mathbf{g} | H_0)$ and $p(\mathbf{g} | H_1)$, computes the likelihood ratio and compares it to a threshold that depends on the costs and prior probabilities of occurrence of the two hypotheses but not on the data. The decision is made in favor of $H_1$ if the test statistic exceeds the appropriate threshold. Since the costs and priors determine the threshold, they also determine the operating point on the ROC curve.

An observer who adopts this strategy and thus utilizes the available data in an optimal way with respect to Bayes risk is called an *ideal observer*. Stated differently, the ideal observer is one who uses the likelihood ratio as its test statistic. Equivalently, the ideal observer can compute the logarithm of $\Lambda$, called the log-likelihood ratio $\lambda$, and compare it to the logarithm of the threshold. Since the logarithm is a monotonic function, exactly the same decision is reached with either $\Lambda$ or $\lambda = \log \Lambda$, and the latter is frequently computationally easier.

The ideal observer is also optimal from several other viewpoints. In addition to minimizing the Bayes risk for any choice of costs and priors, it also maximizes the area under the ROC curve and leads to the maximum true-positive fraction at any specified false-positive fraction.

# 3  Task Specification

We now apply the general considerations of the last section to the problem of detecting a signal in an image [4] [5]. The $m$th component of the data vector $\mathbf{g}$ can be identified with the grey level in the $m$th pixel in the image.

Under the null hypothesis $\mathbf{H}_0$, the image $\mathbf{g}$ consists of a random background $\mathbf{b}$ plus a noise pattern $\mathbf{n}$. Both $\mathbf{b}$ and $\mathbf{n}$ are random $M \times 1$ vectors, and the distinction between them is somewhat arbitrary. The intuitive idea is that $\mathbf{b}$ is produced by imaging a scene through some imaging system, while $\mathbf{n}$ is associated with measurement noise. More importantly, the statistics of $\mathbf{n}$ for fixed $\mathbf{b}$ will be assumed to be determined fully by the basic physics of the measurement process. For example, the probability density function of $\mathbf{n}$ given $\mathbf{b}$, denoted $p_{\mathbf{n}}(\mathbf{n} \mid \mathbf{b})$, might be a zero-mean multivariate normal with a known (possibly $\mathbf{b}$-dependent) covariance matrix.

In addition to $p_{\mathbf{n}}(\mathbf{n} \mid \mathbf{b})$, we also need to know the probability density function of the background, denoted $p_{\mathbf{b}}(\mathbf{b})$, in order to fully determine $p_{\mathbf{n}}(\mathbf{n} \mid \mathbf{b})$. The background arises from imaging a scene through some imaging system, and the randomness in $\mathbf{b}$ comes from the ensemble of different scenes presented to the system. The density $p_{\mathbf{b}}(\mathbf{b})$ thus depends on both the ensemble of scenes and the characteristics of the imaging system, but we do not need to be very specific about these details at this point.

Under hypothesis $\mathbf{H}_1$, $\mathbf{g}$ consists of background, noise and an additional random vector $\mathbf{s}$ which we shall call the signal. In imaging terms, the signal is the image of some object that may or may not be present in the scene. As with the background, the statistics of the signal depend on both the ensemble of objects under consideration and on the details of the imaging system.

To be more precise about the statistics of the signal, we assume that it can be characterized by $K$ random parameters, which we can organize as a $K \times 1$ column vector $\boldsymbol{\alpha}$. For example, the random parameters may specify the location or orientation of the signal in the field, or they may index a family of shapes. In the extreme, we can assign one random parameter to each pixel in the image, so there is no loss of generality at all in writing the signal in parameterized form as $\mathbf{s}(\boldsymbol{\alpha})$. With this notation, the statistics of the signal are given by the probability density function $p_{\boldsymbol{\alpha}}(\boldsymbol{\alpha})$. We shall assume that $\boldsymbol{\alpha}$ is statistically independent of $\mathbf{b}$ and $\mathbf{n}$.

We also assume that the signal and background are additive. This assumption does entail some loss of generality since it rules out the common situation in optical imaging where the object of interest obscures the background (or is obscured by it). In medical imaging or other applications of penetrating radiation, however, it is reasonable to assume additive signal and background. Background due to scattered light or thermal emission can also often be treated as additive.

With these considerations, the two hypotheses are now specified as

$$H_0 : g = b + n, \qquad H_1 : g = b + n + s(\alpha). \qquad (2)$$

Under $H_0$, $g - b = n$, so the conditional density $p(g \mid b)$ is simply $p_n (g - b \mid b)$. The overall density $p(g \mid H_0)$ is then found by averaging over backgrounds:

$$p(g \mid H_0) = \int_\infty d^M b \, p_n (g - b \mid b) \, p_b (b) . \qquad (3)$$

If the noise statistics are independent of background, $p(g \mid H_0)$ is just the convolution of $p_n (n)$ and $p_b (b)$, but (3) is more general, allowing $p_n$ also to depend on $b$ (as it does with Poisson statistics).

The corresponding data density under $H_1$ is readily found. Since $n = g - b - s(\alpha)$ under this hypothesis, and we have assumed that $\alpha$ is statistically independent of $b$, we can write

$$p(g \mid H_1) = \int_\infty d^K \alpha \int_\infty d^M b \, p_n (g - b - s(\alpha) \mid b, \alpha) \, p_b (b) \, p_\alpha (\alpha) . \qquad (4)$$

This expression allows $p_n$ to depend on both $b$ and the signal parameters $\alpha$. If we considered only signal-independent noise, $p_n$ would be independent of both of these vectors, so this dependence is of interest only for noise mechanisms where the statistics depend on the mean irradiance level. Most notably, Poisson noise falls into this category. It is, however, a reasonable assumption that the signal is weak compared to the background; otherwise the detection task would be very easy. Thus, even for Poisson noise, we can assume that $p_n (n \mid b, \alpha) = p_n(n \mid b)$, so we have

$$p(g \mid H_1) = \int_\infty d^K \alpha \int_\infty d^M b \, p_n (g - b - s(\alpha) \mid b) \, p_b (b) \, p_\alpha (\alpha) . \qquad (5)$$

The likelihood ratio is the ratio of (5) to (3).

## 4 An Operator Formulation

With the version of $p(g \mid H_1)$ given in (5), the factor of $p_n (g - b - s(\alpha) \mid b)$ in the integrand is simply a shifted version of the corresponding factor in the integrand of $p(g \mid H_0)$ in (3). Since all noise densities of interest are analytic functions (and we are treating $g$ as a continuous variable), $p_n (g - b - s(\alpha) \mid b)$ can be expressed as a Taylor series in $s(\alpha)$.

To establish notation for this series, we first recall the familiar Taylor expansion for a scalar-valued function $\phi(x)$ of a single real variable x:

$$\phi(x + a) = \phi(x) + \frac{d\phi(x)}{dx} a + \frac{1}{2!} \frac{d^2\phi(x)}{dx^2} a^2 + \ldots = \sum_{k=0}^{\infty} \frac{\phi^{(k)}(x)}{k!} a^k, \qquad (6)$$

provided, of course, that all of the derivatives $\phi^{(k)}(x)$ exist. It is useful to rewrite (6) in operator form as

$$\phi(x+a) = \exp\left[a\frac{d}{dx}\right]\phi(x), \tag{7}$$

where the exponential differential operator is to be interpreted as

$$\exp\left[a\frac{d}{dx}\right] = \sum_{k=0}^{\infty}\frac{a^k}{k!}\frac{d^k}{dx^k}. \tag{8}$$

This operator is sometimes referred to as a *displacement operator* since it displaces the function $\phi(x)$ to $\phi(x+a)$.

One advantage of (8) is that it generalizes easily to the vector case. The multivariate Taylor expansion for a scalar-valued function of a real $M$-dimensional vector $\mathbf{x}$ is

$$\phi(\mathbf{x}+\mathbf{a}) = \exp(\mathbf{a}\cdot\boldsymbol{\nabla})\phi(\mathbf{x}), \tag{9}$$

where $\boldsymbol{\nabla}$ is the $M$-dimensional gradient operator and $\mathbf{a}\cdot\boldsymbol{\nabla}$ denotes a scalar product between $\mathbf{a}$ and this operator. In explicit component form, (9) means

$$\phi(\mathbf{x}+\mathbf{a}) = \phi(\mathbf{x}) + \sum_{i=1}^{N}a_i\frac{\partial}{\partial x_i}\phi(\mathbf{x}) + \frac{1}{2}\sum_{i=1}^{N}\sum_{j=1}^{N}a_ia_j\frac{\partial^2}{\partial x_i\partial x_j}\phi(\mathbf{x}) + \dots. \tag{10}$$

With this notation, we can write

$$p_{\mathbf{n}}(\mathbf{g}-\mathbf{b}-\mathbf{s}(\boldsymbol{\alpha})\,|\,\mathbf{b}) = \exp\left[-\mathbf{s}(\boldsymbol{\alpha})\cdot\boldsymbol{\nabla}_{\mathbf{g}}\right]p_{\mathbf{n}}(\mathbf{g}-\mathbf{b}\,|\,\mathbf{b}), \tag{11}$$

where $\boldsymbol{\nabla}_{\mathbf{g}}$ is the gradient with respect to $\mathbf{g}$.

Inserting (11) into (5) and shuffling the integrals, we find

$$p(\mathbf{g}\,|\,H_1) = \int_{\infty}d^K\alpha\,p_{\boldsymbol{\alpha}}(\boldsymbol{\alpha})\exp\left[-\mathbf{s}(\boldsymbol{\alpha})\cdot\boldsymbol{\nabla}_{\mathbf{g}}\right]\int_{\infty}d^M b\,p_{\mathbf{n}}(\mathbf{g}-\mathbf{b}\,|\,\mathbf{b})\,p_{\mathbf{b}}(\mathbf{b}). \tag{12}$$

From (3) we recognize that the integral over $\mathbf{b}$ is simply $p(\mathbf{g}\,|\,H_0)$, so we can write

$$p(\mathbf{g}\,|\,H_1) = \int_{\infty}d^K\alpha\,p_{\boldsymbol{\alpha}}(\boldsymbol{\alpha})\,p(\mathbf{g}-\mathbf{s}(\boldsymbol{\alpha})\,|\,H_0) \equiv \mathcal{D}p(\mathbf{g}\,|\,H_0), \tag{13}$$

where $\mathcal{D}$ is the operator defined by

$$\mathcal{D} = \int_{\infty}d^K\alpha\,p_{\boldsymbol{\alpha}}(\boldsymbol{\alpha})\exp\left[-\mathbf{s}(\boldsymbol{\alpha})\cdot\boldsymbol{\nabla}_{\mathbf{g}}\right]. \tag{14}$$

This simple operator form is possible only because we assumed that $p_{\mathbf{n}}(\mathbf{n}\,|\,\mathbf{b},\boldsymbol{\alpha}) = p_{\mathbf{n}}(\mathbf{n}\,|\,\mathbf{b})$.

From (14), we see that $\mathcal{D}$ is a weighted superposition of displacement operators in data space. The interpetation of an individual operator, $\exp\left[-\mathbf{s}(\boldsymbol{\alpha})\cdot\boldsymbol{\nabla}_{\mathbf{g}}\right]$ for fixed $\boldsymbol{\alpha}$, is straightforward; it displaces its operand by an amount $\mathbf{s}(\boldsymbol{\alpha})$. The effect of the overall operator $\mathcal{D}$ is determined by the density $p_\alpha(\alpha)$ of the signal parameters. If $p_\alpha$ were a delta function (non-random signals), the overall effect of $\mathcal{D}$ acting on $p(\mathbf{g} \,|\, H_0)$ would be a pure shift of that density, but since the averaging occurs after exponentiation, there can also be a distortion between $p(\mathbf{g} \,|\, H_0)$ and $p(\mathbf{g} \,|\, H_1)$.

On the other hand, the operator $\mathcal{D}$ does not change the normalization of its operand. It is easy to show that the integral over $\mathbf{g}$ of $\mathcal{D}p(\mathbf{g} \,|\, H_0)$ is unity, no matter what we choose for $\mathbf{s}(\alpha)$ or for $p_\alpha(\alpha)$ (so long as it is properly normalized).

Sometimes it is easiest to compute $\mathcal{D}p(\mathbf{g} \,|\, H_0)$ in the frequency domain. The $M$-dimensional Fourier transform of $p(\mathbf{g} \,|\, H_i)$, denoted $\Psi_i(\boldsymbol{\rho})$ and frequently referred to as the characteristic function, is given by

$$\Psi_i(\boldsymbol{\rho}) = \int_\infty d^M g \, p(\mathbf{g} \,|\, H_i) \exp\left(-2\pi i \boldsymbol{\rho}^t \mathbf{g}\right), \tag{15}$$

where $\boldsymbol{\rho}$ is an $M$-dimensional frequency vector. There is a simple relation between $\Psi_0(\boldsymbol{\rho})$ and $\Psi_1(\boldsymbol{\rho})$ for the case of signal detection with parameter uncertainty. Fourier-transforming (13), we find

$$\Psi_1(\boldsymbol{\rho}) = \Psi_0(\boldsymbol{\rho}) \int_\infty d^K \alpha \, p_\alpha(\alpha) \exp\left(-2\pi i \boldsymbol{\rho}^t \mathbf{s}(\alpha)\right) \equiv \Psi_0(\boldsymbol{\rho}) M(\boldsymbol{\rho}). \tag{16}$$

Thus the function $M(\boldsymbol{\rho})$ acts as a kind of MTF, transforming $\Psi_0(\boldsymbol{\rho})$ to $\Psi_1(\boldsymbol{\rho})$ (Note that $M(\mathbf{0}) = 1$).

With this operator notation, the likelihood ratio is now given by

$$\Lambda = \frac{\mathcal{D}p(\mathbf{g} \,|\, H_0)}{p(\mathbf{g} \,|\, H_0)}. \tag{17}$$

# 5   Examples

## 5.1  Signal known exactly, background known exactly, white Gaussian noise

We begin with a simple example having a well-known solution. We consider an exactly specified signal on a known background; this problem is frequently referred to as SKE/BKE (signal known exactly, background known exactly). We adopt a multivariate normal model for the only remaining random vector, the noise process $\mathbf{n}$. If we assume the noise is white, then the components of $\mathbf{n}$ are independent and identically distributed (iid) random variables, and we can write

$$p_n(\mathbf{n}) = N \exp\left[-\frac{1}{2\sigma^2} ||\mathbf{n}||^2\right] = N \exp\left[-\frac{1}{2\sigma^2} \sum_{m=1}^{M} n_m^2\right], \tag{18}$$

where $N$ is the normalizing constant. The density for $\mathbf{g}$ under $H_0$ is

$$p(\mathbf{g} \,|\, H_0) = N \exp\left[-\frac{1}{2\sigma^2} ||\mathbf{g} - \mathbf{b}||^2\right], \tag{19}$$

and under $\mathbf{H}_1$ it is

$$p\left(\mathbf{g}\,|\,\mathbf{H}_1\right) = \mathcal{D}p\left(\mathbf{g}\,|\,\mathbf{H}_0\right) = N\exp\left[-\frac{1}{2\sigma^2}\|\mathbf{g}-\mathbf{b}-\mathbf{s}\|^2\right]. \tag{20}$$

The likelihood ratio is easily found to be

$$\Lambda = \mathrm{const}\cdot\exp\left[\frac{1}{\sigma^2}\mathbf{s}^t(\mathbf{g}-\mathbf{b})\right] = \mathrm{const}\cdot\exp\left[\frac{1}{\sigma^2}\sum_{m=1}^{M}s_m(g_m-b_m)\right]. \tag{21}$$

The corresponding log-likelihood is

$$\lambda = \mathrm{const} + \mathrm{const}\cdot\mathbf{s}^t(\mathbf{g}-\mathbf{b}), \tag{22}$$

where

$$\mathbf{s}^t(\mathbf{g}-\mathbf{b}) = \sum_{m=1}^{M}s_m(g_m-b_m) \tag{23}$$

Thus the log-likelihood in this case is a matched filter applied to the difference between the observed image and the known background. The log-likelihood is a linear function of the data (*i.e.* a linear discriminant) and normally distributed, while the likelihood $\Lambda$ is nonlinear and log-normal.

## 5.2 SKE, white Gaussian noise, Gaussian background

Next we remove the restriction that the background be nonrandom. One useful model for $p_{\mathbf{b}}\left(\mathbf{b}\right)$ is a multivariate normal with mean $\overline{\mathbf{b}}$ and covariance matrix $\mathbf{K}_b$, both of which are presumed known *a priori*. With this model,

$$p\left(\mathbf{g}\,|\,\mathbf{H}_0\right) = N\exp\left[-\frac{1}{2}\left(\mathbf{g}-\overline{\mathbf{b}}\right)^t\mathbf{K}^{-1}\left(\mathbf{g}-\overline{\mathbf{b}}\right)\right], \tag{24}$$

where $N$ is another normalizing constant (not the same as in (18)) and $\mathbf{K}$ is the overall covariance matrix of the data. With the iid model for $\mathbf{n}$, $\mathbf{K}$ is given by

$$\mathbf{K} = \sigma^2\mathbf{I} + \mathbf{K}_b. \tag{25}$$

The signal-present density is

$$p\left(\mathbf{g}\,|\,\mathbf{H}_1\right) = \mathcal{D}p\left(\mathbf{g}\,|\,\mathbf{H}_0\right) = N\exp\left[-\frac{1}{2}\left(\mathbf{g}-\overline{\mathbf{b}}-\mathbf{s}\right)^t\mathbf{K}^{-1}\left(\mathbf{g}-\overline{\mathbf{b}}-\mathbf{s}\right)\right]. \tag{26}$$

The likelihood and log-likelihood are, respectively,

$$\begin{aligned}
\Lambda &= \mathrm{const}\cdot\exp\left[\mathbf{s}^t\mathbf{K}^{-1}\left(\mathbf{g}-\overline{\mathbf{b}}-\mathbf{s}\right)\right], \tag{27}\\
\lambda &= \mathrm{const}+\mathbf{s}^t\mathbf{K}^{-1}\left(\mathbf{g}-\overline{\mathbf{b}}-\mathbf{s}\right). \tag{28}
\end{aligned}$$

In this case $\lambda$ is a prewhitened matched filter applied to the image minus the mean background. It is still a linear discriminant and is still normally distributed.

## 5.3 Location uncertainty, iid Gaussian noise, nonrandom background

Next we consider the case where the background is nonrandom and the signal is known exactly except for its location in the image. For simplicity, we consider iid noise where $\mathbf{K}_n = \sigma^2\mathbf{I}$. If the background is nonrandom, that means that the data values $\{g_m\}$ are independent but not necessarily identically distributed since they can have different means. If we also take $b_m = $ constant, then the data values are iid under $\mathbf{H}_0$, but it is no difficulty to retain a general nonrandom background $\mathbf{b}$ in the equations. With these considerations, the probability density of the data under $\mathbf{H}_0$ is given by

$$p\left(\mathbf{g} \,|\, \mathbf{H}_0\right) = C \exp\left[-\frac{1}{2\sigma^2} \sum_{m=1}^{M} (g_m - b_m)^2\right]. \tag{29}$$

In a continuous notation, we can express a randomly shifted signal in a two-dimensional image as $s(\mathbf{r}) = h(\mathbf{r} - \Delta\mathbf{r})$, where $\mathbf{r}$ is a twodimensional position vector, $\Delta\mathbf{r}$ denotes the random shift, and $h(\mathbf{r})$ describes the signal shape. To make the transition to a discrete formulation, we take the $m$th component of the signal vector $\mathbf{s}$ to be $s(\mathbf{r})$ sampled at the points $\{\mathbf{r}_m, m = 1...M\}$, so $s_m = h(\mathbf{r}_m - \Delta\mathbf{r})$. The random parameter vector $\boldsymbol{\alpha}$ is $\Delta\mathbf{r}$, and the probability density of the data under $\mathbf{H}_1$ is

$$p\left(\mathbf{g} \,|\, \mathbf{H}_1\right) = C \int_{\infty} d^2\Delta r \, \mathrm{p}_{\Delta\mathbf{r}}\left(\Delta\mathbf{r}\right) \exp\left[-\frac{1}{2\sigma^2} \sum_{m=1}^{M} [g_m - b_m - h\left(\mathbf{r}_m - \Delta\mathbf{r}\right)]^2\right], \tag{30}$$

where the subscript $\infty$ on the integral sign indicates an integral over the infinite plane.

The likelihood ratio now takes a form derived by Nolte and Jaarsma [6],

$$\Lambda = \int_{\infty} d^2\Delta r \, \mathrm{p}_{\Delta\mathbf{r}}\left(\Delta\mathbf{r}\right)$$

$$\times \exp\left[-\frac{1}{2\sigma^2} \sum_{m=1}^{M} \left\{-2\left[g_m - b_m\right]\left[h\left(\mathbf{r}_m - \Delta\mathbf{r}\right)\right] + \left[h\left(\mathbf{r}_m - \Delta\mathbf{r}\right)\right]^2\right\}\right]$$

$$= \exp\left[-\frac{E_{\mathrm{sig}}}{2\sigma^2}\right] \int_{\infty} d^2\Delta r \, \mathrm{p}_{\Delta\mathbf{r}}\left(\Delta\mathbf{r}\right) \exp\left[\frac{1}{\sigma^2} \sum_{m=1}^{M} \left[g_m - b_m\right]\left[h\left(\mathbf{r}_m - \Delta\mathbf{r}\right)\right]\right], \tag{31}$$

where $E_{\mathrm{sig}}$ is the total signal energy, defined by

$$E_{\mathrm{sig}} = \sum_{m=1}^{M} \left[h\left(\mathbf{r}_m - \Delta\mathbf{r}\right)\right]^2. \tag{32}$$

Note that $E_{\mathrm{sig}}$ is approximately independent of $\Delta\mathbf{r}$ so long as the signal is constrained to lie within the borders of the image and the sampling is not too coarse compared to the scale of $s(\mathbf{r})$. Under these circumstances, $\exp[-E_{\text{sig}}/2\sigma^2]$ is just a constant factor in $\Lambda$. This nice feature would not have arisen had we not assumed a stationary noise model.

A suggestive way to rewrite (31) is to note that $\sum_m [g_m - b_m][h(\mathbf{r}_m - \Delta\mathbf{r})]$ can be interpreted as the output of a scanning matched filter operating on the data after subtracting the known background. We define this output as

$$t(\Delta\mathbf{r}) = \sum_{m=1}^{M} [g_m - b_m][h(\mathbf{r}_m - \Delta\mathbf{r})], \qquad (33)$$

so that

$$\Lambda = \text{const} \cdot \int_\infty d^2\Delta r\, p_{\Delta\mathbf{r}}(\Delta\mathbf{r}) \exp\left[t(\Delta\mathbf{r})/\sigma^2\right]. \qquad (34)$$

The optimal Bayesian test statistic in this problem is thus obtained by computing the output of a scanning matched filter for each shift $\Delta\mathbf{r}$, exponentiating it with weight $1/\sigma^2$, and then averaging the result with respect to the prior density on $\Delta\mathbf{r}$.

One obvious limit of (34) is when the signal location is fixed at the origin. Then $p_{\Delta\mathbf{r}}(\Delta\mathbf{r})$ is a Dirac delta function $\delta(\Delta\mathbf{r})$, and we again see that the log-likelihood is the output of a matched filter. In the opposite limit where $p_{\Delta\mathbf{r}}(\Delta\mathbf{r})$ is a constant over some finite field and zero outside it, $\Lambda$ is just the integral of $\exp\left[t(\Delta\mathbf{r})/\sigma^2\right]$ over this field. If $\sigma^2$ is small, this integral is dominated by the shifts $\Delta\mathbf{r}$ for which the filter output $t(\Delta\mathbf{r})$ is the largest.

This observation provides some justification for the common detection strategy of finding the peak value of the output of a scanning matched filter and comparing this value to a threshold in order to decide if the signal is present. Suppose that the peak occurs at $\Delta\mathbf{r} = \Delta\mathbf{r}_0$ and let $t(\Delta\mathbf{r}_0) = t_{\max}$. In the limit $\sigma^2 \to 0$, (34) can be written as

$$\Lambda \simeq \text{const} \cdot p_{\Delta\mathbf{r}}(\Delta\mathbf{r}_0) \exp\left[t_{\max}/\sigma^2\right] \int_\infty d^2\Delta r\, \exp\left\{[t(\Delta\mathbf{r}) - t_{max}]/\sigma^2\right\}. \qquad (35)$$

The corresponding log-likelihood ratio is

$$\lambda \simeq \text{const} + t_{\max}/\sigma^2 + \log\left[\int_\infty d^2\Delta r\, \exp\left\{[t(\Delta\mathbf{r}) - t_{max}]/\sigma^2\right\}\right]. \qquad (36)$$

The integral depends on the width of the function $\exp\{[t(\Delta\mathbf{r}) - t_{max}]/\sigma^2\}$, which in turn depends in a complicated way on the data and the bandwidth of the filter. As $\sigma^2 \to 0$, however, this function gets narrower and the integral gets smaller, while the term $t_{\max}/\sigma^2$ gets larger. Thus, for low noise levels, the log-likelihood ratio is simply $t_{\max}/\sigma^2$, justifying the common strategy.

Another interesting limit is threshold detection. For very weak signals, we can expand the exponential in (34) to obtain

$$\Lambda = \text{const} - \text{const} \cdot \sum_{m=1}^{M} [g_m - b_m]\langle h_m \rangle, \qquad (37)$$

where $\langle h_m \rangle$ is the location-averaged signal given by

$$\langle h_m \rangle = \int_\infty d^2\Delta r \, \mathrm{p}_{\Delta r}\left(\Delta r\right) h\left(r_m - \Delta r\right). \tag{38}$$

If all locations in the image are equally likely, then $\langle h_m \rangle$ is a constant independent of $m$, so $\Lambda$ is linearly related to the sum of the data values, $\sum_m g_m$. This sum is a useful test statistic in this problem only because we have assumed that the background is nonrandom. The presence of a signal increases the sum of the data values above the expected level it would have in the absence of a signal.

To summarize this section, the Bayesian strategy for detecting a signal with unknown location against a known background is:

(a) Subtract known background from image
(b) Apply matched filter at shift $\Delta r$
(c) Exponentiate it with weight $1/\sigma^2$
(d) Average with respect to the prior on $\Delta r$
(e) Compare to threshold

## 5.4 Random signal location, Gaussian background

We now combine the previous two examples and consider a signal with random location in a Gaussian random background. The likelihood ratio is this case is

$$\Lambda = \mathrm{const} \cdot \int_\infty d^2\Delta r \, \mathrm{p}_{\Delta r}\left(\Delta r\right) \exp\left\{ \left[ h\left(r_m - \Delta r\right) \right]^t \mathbf{K}^{-1} \left( \mathbf{g} - \bar{\mathbf{b}} \right) \right\}$$

$$= \mathrm{const} \cdot \int_\infty d^2\Delta r \, \mathrm{p}_{\Delta r}\left(\Delta r\right) \exp\left[ t\left(\Delta r\right) \right]. \tag{39}$$

where $t(\Delta r)$ is the output of a scanning prewhitening matched filter, viz.:

$$t(\Delta r) = \left[ h\left(r_m - \Delta r\right) \right]^t \mathbf{K}^{-1} \left( \mathbf{g} - \bar{\mathbf{b}} \right). \tag{40}$$

The recipe for signal detection in this problem is:

(a) Subtract mean background from image
(b) Prewhiten with total covariance matrix
(c) Matched filter at a particular shift
(d) Exponentiate
(e) Average over shifts
(f) Compare to threshold

## 5.5 Random signal location and scale, Gaussian background

Now suppose the signal is random both with respect to location and overall scale. One realization of the random signal in this case would be a vector $\mathbf{s}(\beta, \Delta r)$ for which the $m$th component is given by

$$s_m(\beta, \Delta r) = \frac{1}{\beta^2} h \left[ \frac{r_m - \Delta r}{\beta} \right]. \tag{41}$$

The factor $1/\beta^2$ ensures that all signals have the same integrated value regardless of the scale $\beta$. With these assumptions, the likelihod ratio is given by

$$\Lambda = \text{const} \cdot \int_\infty d^2 \Delta r \, p_{\Delta r} (\Delta r) \int_0^\infty d\beta \, p_\beta (\beta) \exp \left\{ \left[ \frac{1}{\beta^2} h \left[ \frac{\mathbf{r}_m - \Delta \mathbf{r}}{\beta} \right] \right]^t \mathbf{K}^{-1}(\mathbf{g} - \mathbf{b}) \right\}.$$

(42)

The detection recipe is now:

(a) Subtract mean background from image
(b) Prewhiten with total covariance matrix
(c) Compute the inner product with a scaled and shifted version of the signal
(d) Exponentiate
(e) Average over shifts and scales
(f) Compare to threshold

An interesting limit of this result is treated by Clarkson and Barrett elsewhere in this volume [7]. If it is valid to expand the exponential in (42) and retain only the term linear in $\mathbf{g}$, then the optimal discriminant can be realized as a wavelet transform.

## 5.6 Non-Gaussian background

All of the examples above have used a multivariate normal model for the background, but the general formalism allows other models as well. For example, many natural scenes are well described by a multivariate log-normal with a fractal autocorrelation function (one that varies as a non-integral power of the separation of two points).

To apply the Bayesian approach of this paper to detection on a general background, we must presume that we have some analytic model for $p(\mathbf{g} \,|\, H_0)$. From (13), the likelihood ratio can be written as

$$\Lambda(\mathbf{g}) = \frac{\int_\infty d^K \alpha \, p_\alpha(\alpha) p(\mathbf{g} - \mathbf{s}(\alpha) \,|\, H_0)}{p(\mathbf{g} \,|\, H_0)} = \int_\infty d^K \alpha \, p_\alpha(\alpha) \Lambda_\alpha(\mathbf{g}),$$

(43)

where $\Lambda_\alpha(\mathbf{g})$ is a conditional likelihood ratio defined by

$$\Lambda_\alpha(\mathbf{g}) = \frac{p(\mathbf{g} - \mathbf{s}(\alpha) \,|\, H_0)}{p(\mathbf{g} \,|\, H_0)}.$$

(44)

From (43) and (44), the detection recipe for a general background model is:

(a) Compute $p(\mathbf{g} \,|\, H_0)$ for specific background model
(b) Shift by $\mathbf{s}(\alpha)$ for fixed $\alpha$
(c) Compute conditional $\Lambda$ for fixed $\alpha$
(d) Average over $\alpha$
(e) Compare to threshold

# 6 Summary and conclusions

Bayesian methods are applicable to signal detection, and hence to the computation of detection-based figures of merit for image quality, whenever adequate information is available about the probability laws for the signal, background and measurement noise. Given this information, the Bayesian strategy is to compute the likelihood ratio $\Lambda$ and compare it to a threshold, calling the decision a detection if $\Lambda$ exceeds the threshold. This strategy is optimal by many criteria.

With signal randomness, the likelihood ratio is always a nonlinear function of the data; hence it cannot be realized by a linear filter. Nevertheless linear operations such as matched filters and wavelet transforms are useful stepping stones in signal detection; even though they are linear, the optimal nonlinear test statistic is a function of them.

# 7 Acknowledgements

The authors have benefitted greatly from discussions with Robert Wagner, Kyle Myers, Eric Clarkson and Jack Denny. This work was supported by the National Institutes of Health (NIH) through grant no. RO1 CA52643, but it does not represent the official position of NIH. In fact, so far as the authors know, NIH doesn't have any official positions.

# References

[1] H. H. Barrett and W. Swindell: Radiological Imaging: Theory of Image Formation, Detection and Processing, Revised edition. Academic Press, San Diego, 1006

[2] C. W. Helstrom: Elements of Signal Detection and Estimation. Prentice Hall, Englewood Cliffs NJ, 1995

[3] D. Middleton: An Introduction to Statistical Communication Theory. McGrawHill, New York, 1960.

[4] R.F. Wagner and H.H. Barrett: Quadratic tasks and the ideal observer. Proc. SPIE 727, 306-309 (1987).

[5] H. H. Barrett, K. J. Myers and R. F. Wagner: Beyond signal-detection theory. Proc. SPIE 626, 231-239 (1986).

[6] L. W. Nolte and D. Jaarsma: More on the detection of one of $M$ orthogonal signals. J. Acoust. Soc. Am. 41, 497-505 (1967).

[7] E. Clarkson and H. H. Barrett: Bayesian detection with amplitude, scale, orientation and position uncertainty. This volume.

# Approximate Distributions for Maximum Likelihood and Maximum *a posteriori* Estimates Under a Gaussian Noise Model

Craig K. Abbey[1,2], Eric Clarkson[1], Harrison H. Barrett[1,2,3],
Stefan P. Müller[4,5], and Frank J. Rybicki[5]

1. Dept of Radiology, University of Arizona, Tucson AZ, 85724

2. Program in Applied Mathematics, University of Arizona, Tucson AZ, 85721

3. Optical Sciences Center, University of Arizona, Tucson AZ, 85721

4. Dept. of Nuclear Medicine, Universitätsklinikum GH Essen, D-45122, Essen FRG

5. Brigham and Women's Hospital and Harvard Medical School, Boston MA 02115

**Abstract.** The performance of Maximum Likelihood (ML) and Maximum *a posteriori* (MAP) estimates in nonlinear problems at low data SNR is not well predicted by the Cramér-Rao or other lower bounds on variance. In order to better characterize the distribution of ML and MAP estimates under these conditions, we derive an approximate density for the conditional distribution of such estimates. In one example, this approximate distribution captures the essential features of the distribution of ML and MAP estimates in the presence of Gaussian-distributed noise.

## 1 Introduction

Quantitation tasks in medical imaging can be formulated as parameter estimation where the parameters of interest are derived from the image data [1][2]. Nonlinear tasks are those in which the parameters have a nonlinear relationship with the data. A nonlinear estimation task which has been used for optimization of medical imaging systems is the simultaneous estimation of amplitude and radius of a disk-shaped object which is blurred by the imaging system and corrupted by Gaussian-distributed noise [3][4]. Performance for this task has been evaluated using Maximum-Likelihood (ML) estimation; the present work analyzes ML estimates and Maximum *a posteriori* (MAP) estimates since they are commonly used to regularize ML estimates. As in the previous work, the analysis is restricted to nonsingular problems in which many pixel values are used to estimate a small number of identifiable parameters. A similar analysis to that presented here can be found in the work of Fessler *et al* for the high dimensional estimation task of image reconstruction [5][6].

Since the optimization of imaging systems requires evaluation of many system configurations, a convenient and computationally feasible method for predicting the distribution of ML and MAP estimates is desirable. A standard approach approximates the distribution of estimates using the unbiased form of the Cramér-Rao Bound (CRB) [7]. This approach is suitable for data that is linearly related to the image parameters, and it is generally quite good for parameters nonlinearly related to the data when the level of noise is low. However, as the signal-to-noise ratio (SNR) of the image data decreases, Monte-Carlo studies have shown the CRB inadequate for characterizing the distribution of parameter estimates [3].

This paper addresses the distribution of ML and MAP estimates at low SNR when the CRB is no longer valid. It is organized in three parts. First, the CRB is derived from an approximate Gaussian density in ML estimation by a linear approximation about the true parameter value. Second, we vary the point about which the linear expansion is performed. This step forms the basis of the proposed method and leads to an approximate density which is non-Gaussian for nonlinear estimation. Third, the method is demonstrated for a nonlinear estimation problem. In this particular problem, estimates are calculated for the amplitude and radius of a two-dimensional Gaussian feature embedded in white noise.

# 2 Derivation of approximate estimate density

This work focuses on the distribution of ML and MAP estimates $\hat{\boldsymbol{\theta}}$ of a $K$-dimensional parameter vector given the true parameter vector $\boldsymbol{\theta}^{\text{true}}$. We shall abuse standard notation slightly and denote the probability density function (pdf) for this distribution as $p\left(\hat{\boldsymbol{\theta}} = \boldsymbol{\theta}^{\text{ev}} \mid \boldsymbol{\theta}^{\text{true}}\right)$. With this notation we make explicit the difference between the random variable $\hat{\boldsymbol{\theta}}$ and the fixed (and presumed known) parameter vector at which we would like to evaluate the pdf, $\boldsymbol{\theta}^{\text{ev}}$.

The image data from which an estimate is computed are denoted by an $M$-dimensional vector $\mathbf{d}$ and are modeled as the sum of $\mathbf{s}\left(\boldsymbol{\theta}^{\text{true}}\right)$, a deterministic function of the true vector parameter and $\mathbf{n}$, a stochastic component. In the present example of nuclear medicine, the deterministic function $\mathbf{s}\left(\boldsymbol{\theta}\right)$ represents the profile of the feature of interest (the signal) after passing through the imaging system. The vector $\boldsymbol{\theta}$ represents the variable parameters in the signal function. The $M$-dimensional vector $\mathbf{n}$ represents the imaging system noise. Hence a component of the data is given by $d_i = s_i\left(\theta_1^{\text{true}}, \theta_2^{\text{true}}, \ldots, \theta_K^{\text{true}}\right) + n_i$, $i = 1, \ldots, M$. Unless otherwise noted, we use vector notation throughout this work, and in this format the model for describing the data is written

$$\mathbf{d} = \mathbf{s}\left(\boldsymbol{\theta}^{\text{true}}\right) + \mathbf{n}. \tag{1}$$

For ML estimation, Eqn (1) is sufficient to compute estimates. To compute MAP estimates, some prior knowledge of $\boldsymbol{\theta}^{\text{true}}$ must be specified in the form of a prior pdf $p(\boldsymbol{\theta}^{\text{true}})$. Since the logarithm of the prior is used exclusively throughout this work, it is convenient to define the pdf as

$$P\left(\boldsymbol{\theta}^{\text{true}}\right) = C \exp\left(-\mathbf{Q}\left(\boldsymbol{\theta}^{\text{true}}\right)\right), \tag{2}$$

where $C$ is a normalization constant independent of $\boldsymbol{\theta}^{\text{true}}$. The scalar function $\mathbf{Q}\left(\boldsymbol{\theta}^{\text{true}}\right)$ is often referred to as the Gibbs potential function [9] or as a penalty function [6] for its role in regularizing estimates. A common choice for this function is a quadratic function of $\boldsymbol{\theta}^{\text{true}}$, implying a Gaussian prior pdf.

We make the following assumptions about the estimation problem:

1. $\mathbf{s}\left(\boldsymbol{\theta}\right)$ is twice differentiable with respect to $\boldsymbol{\theta}$.

2. If used, the Gibbs potential function $\mathbf{Q}\left(\boldsymbol{\theta}\right)$ is also twice differentiable with respect to the variable $\boldsymbol{\theta}$.

3. The noise is independent of the signal.

4. The noise elements are normally distributed random variables with a known nonsingular covariance structure $\mathbf{K_d}$.

The first two assumptions are necessary to analyze the problem using standard results from multivariate calculus. For many imaging modalities, the image data follow Poisson counting statistics and thus appear to violate assumptions 3 and 4. However these assumptions often hold approximately. The Poisson is well approximated by a Gaussian at count levels typical of clinical imaging [8]. Furthermore, for low-contrast signals the dependence of the noise on the signal is negligible. Consequently the noise is well approximated by a signal-independent Gaussian pdf.

There are two reasons to consider an arbitrary known covariance $\mathbf{K_d}$ as opposed to the more usual assumption of independence in the noise vector. First, it allows us to analyze preprocessed data where the preprocessing has induced a correlation structure. Second, it provides a simple way to incorporate object variability [2] also known as "anatomical noise". Hence we will assume that the probability density function is an $M$-dimensional multivariate normal

$$\mathbf{n} \sim N_M\left(\mathbf{0}, \mathbf{K_d}\right). \tag{3}$$

Under the Gaussian noise model, an ML or MAP estimate $\widehat{\boldsymbol{\theta}}$ can be written as the vector $\boldsymbol{\theta}$ that maximizes the scalar equation

$$-\frac{1}{2}\left(\mathbf{d} - \mathbf{s}\left(\boldsymbol{\theta}\right)\right)^t \mathbf{K_d^{-1}}\left(\mathbf{d} - \mathbf{s}\left(\boldsymbol{\theta}\right)\right) - \mathbf{Q}\left(\boldsymbol{\theta}\right), \tag{4}$$

where the first term is derived from the log-likelihood function for the data under the noise model described above, and the Gibbs potential results from taking the logarithm of the prior in Eqn (2). For ML estimation, $\mathbf{Q}\left(\boldsymbol{\theta}\right)$ is absent.

With the constraints on differentiability described above, the estimator solves the nonlinear system of equations produced by taking the gradient with respect to $\boldsymbol{\theta}$ of the optimization function in Eqn (4),

$$G_{\widehat{\boldsymbol{\theta}}} K_d^{-1} \left[ d - s\left(\widehat{\boldsymbol{\theta}}\right) \right] - q_{\widehat{\boldsymbol{\theta}}} = 0. \tag{5}$$

The vector $q_{\widehat{\boldsymbol{\theta}}}$ is defined by $q_{\widehat{\boldsymbol{\theta}}} = \nabla Q\left(\widehat{\boldsymbol{\theta}}\right)$, and the matrix $G_{\widehat{\boldsymbol{\theta}}}$ is a $K \times M$ element matrix composed of first derivatives of $s\left(\boldsymbol{\theta}\right)$,

$$[G_{\boldsymbol{\theta}}]_{km} = \frac{\partial s_m\left(\boldsymbol{\theta}\right)}{\partial \theta_k},$$

evaluated at $\boldsymbol{\theta} = \widehat{\boldsymbol{\theta}}$. As stated in the introduction, we assume a low-dimensional $(K \ll M)$ and nonsingular $\left(\text{rank}\left(G_{\widehat{\boldsymbol{\theta}}}\right) = K\right)$ problem. This assumption ensures that the Observed Fisher Information Matrix [7][10], $F_{\boldsymbol{\theta}} = G_{\boldsymbol{\theta}} K_d^{-1} G_{\boldsymbol{\theta}}^t$ is invertible.

## 2.1 Derivation of the CRB from ML estimation of a linear system function

This section uses a linear approximation to $s\left(\boldsymbol{\theta}\right)$ to derive the CRB from ML estimation as described above. This analysis allows us to interpret the CRB beyond its usual role as a bound on variance [7][10], and it provides a theoretical platform for us to approximate the density $p\left(\widehat{\boldsymbol{\theta}} = \boldsymbol{\theta}^{\text{ev}} \,|\, \boldsymbol{\theta}^{\text{true}}\right)$ in the next section.

Consider the first-order Taylor-series approximation to $s\left(\boldsymbol{\theta}\right)$ expanded about $\boldsymbol{\theta}^{\text{true}}$,

$$s^{\text{lin}}\left(\boldsymbol{\theta}\right) = s\left(\boldsymbol{\theta}^{\text{true}}\right) + G_{\boldsymbol{\theta}^{\text{true}}}^t \left(\boldsymbol{\theta} - \boldsymbol{\theta}^{\text{true}}\right). \tag{6}$$

The vector function $s^{\text{lin}}\left(\boldsymbol{\theta}\right)$ is a linear approximation of the signal, which is assumed to be nonlinear with respect to the parameter $\boldsymbol{\theta}$. The resulting matrix of first derivatives is given by

$$\left[G_{\boldsymbol{\theta}}^{\text{lin}}\right]_{km} = \frac{\partial s_m^{\text{lin}}\left(\boldsymbol{\theta}\right)}{\partial \theta_k} = [G_{\boldsymbol{\theta}^{\text{true}}}]_{km}.$$

The density of ML estimates with $s^{\text{lin}}\left(\boldsymbol{\theta}\right)$ in place of $s\left(\boldsymbol{\theta}\right)$ will be used as the approximate density. We denote estimates under this "linearized" model by $\widehat{\boldsymbol{\theta}}^{\text{lin}}$.

Substituting Eqn (6) into Eqn (5) (with $q_{\widehat{\boldsymbol{\theta}}} = 0$ since we are considering ML estimation) yields

$$G_{\boldsymbol{\theta}^{\text{true}}} K_d^{-1} \left(d - s\left(\boldsymbol{\theta}^{\text{true}}\right) - G_{\boldsymbol{\theta}^{\text{true}}}^t \left(\widehat{\boldsymbol{\theta}}^{\text{lin}} - \boldsymbol{\theta}^{\text{true}}\right)\right) = 0.$$

If $F_{\boldsymbol{\theta}^{\text{true}}}^{-1}$ exists, the direct solution for the estimator is

$$\widehat{\boldsymbol{\theta}}^{\text{lin}} = \boldsymbol{\theta}^{\text{true}} + F_{\boldsymbol{\theta}^{\text{true}}}^{-1} G_{\boldsymbol{\theta}^{\text{true}}} K_d^{-1} \left(d - s\left(\boldsymbol{\theta}^{\text{true}}\right)\right).$$

Note that $\widehat{\boldsymbol{\theta}}^{\text{lin}}$ is a linear function of the data. Hence, the estimator is normally distributed with mean and variance following the laws of linear transformations

$$\widehat{\boldsymbol{\theta}}^{\text{lin}} \sim N_K \left( \boldsymbol{\theta}^{\text{true}}, \mathbf{F}_{\boldsymbol{\theta}^{\text{true}}}^{-1} \right).$$

Writing this multivariate pdf explicitly yields the following approximation to the desired pdf:

$$p \left( \widehat{\boldsymbol{\theta}} = \boldsymbol{\theta}^{\text{ev}} \mid \boldsymbol{\theta}^{\text{true}} \right) \simeq p \left( \widehat{\boldsymbol{\theta}}^{\text{lin}} = \boldsymbol{\theta}^{\text{ev}} \mid \boldsymbol{\theta}^{\text{true}} \right)$$

$$= \frac{\sqrt{\det \left( \mathbf{F}_{\boldsymbol{\theta}^{\text{true}}} \right)}}{(2\pi)^{K/2}} \exp \left( -\frac{1}{2} \left( \boldsymbol{\theta}^{\text{ev}} - \boldsymbol{\theta}^{\text{true}} \right)^t \mathbf{F}_{\boldsymbol{\theta}^{\text{true}}} \left( \boldsymbol{\theta}^{\text{ev}} - \boldsymbol{\theta}^{\text{true}} \right) \right). \qquad (7)$$

We refer to the density in Eqn (7) as the Cramér-Rao probability density function (CR-pdf). Under this first-order linear model, the estimator is unbiased and its covariance, $\mathbf{F}_{\boldsymbol{\theta}^{\text{true}}}^{-1}$ is the CRB on covariance for the nonlinear model of Eqn (1).

This derivation demonstrates two things. First, the CRB is recast as an approximate estimator covariance as opposed to its usual role as a lower bound on estimator performance. This difference does not represent an inconsistency in the use of the CRB since it is a lower bound only on the performance of unbiased estimators – a condition not usually met by ML and MAP estimators in nonlinear problems. Second, the limitations of this approach are related to the range of validity of the linear approximation and the magnitude of the noise in the data. For example, if $\mathbf{s}(\boldsymbol{\theta})$ were linear, the linear approximation in Eqn (6) would be valid everywhere, and consequently the CR-pdf would be exact. For weakly nonlinear problems with small levels of noise, the perturbations due to the noise will only rarely push estimates outside the range of validity of the linear approximation. In this case the CR-pdf is expected to be accurate as well. However, as the magnitude of the noise and the degree of nonlinearity increase, the noise will frequently push estimates far beyond the range of validity of the approximation, making the CR-pdf inaccurate.

## 2.2 The approximate density using a variable point of expansion

As discussed in the previous section, the CR-pdf is based on an approximation and thus has a limited range of validity about $\boldsymbol{\theta}^{\text{true}}$. One way to increase the range of validity is to expand $\mathbf{s}^{\text{lin}}(\boldsymbol{\theta})$ about the $\boldsymbol{\theta}^{\text{ev}}$ of interest. Applying this approach yields

$$\mathbf{s}^{\text{lin}}(\boldsymbol{\theta}) = \mathbf{s}(\boldsymbol{\theta}^{\text{ev}}) + \mathbf{G}_{\boldsymbol{\theta}^{\text{ev}}}^t (\boldsymbol{\theta} - \boldsymbol{\theta}^{\text{ev}}). \qquad (8)$$

In a fashion analogous to the derivation of the CDB-pdf, the matrix of first derivatives under this approximate model are given by

$$\left[ \mathbf{G}_{\boldsymbol{\theta}}^{\text{lin}} \right]_{km} = \frac{\partial s_m^{\text{lin}}(\boldsymbol{\theta})}{\partial \theta_k} = \left[ \mathbf{G}_{\boldsymbol{\theta}^{\text{ev}}} \right]_{km}.$$

In addition to the expansion of the signal about $\theta^{\mathrm{ev}}$, we now generalize the analysis to incorporate a second-order expansion of the prior term $\mathbf{Q}(\theta)$ about $\theta^{\mathrm{ev}}$.

$$\mathbf{Q}(\theta) \simeq \mathbf{Q}(\theta^{\mathrm{ev}}) + \mathbf{q}_{\theta^{\mathrm{ev}}}^t (\theta - \theta^{\mathrm{ev}}) + \frac{1}{2}(\theta - \theta^{\mathrm{ev}})^t \mathbf{D_Q}(\theta - \theta^{\mathrm{ev}}) \tag{9}$$

where $\mathbf{D_Q}$ is the matrix of second derivatives of the log prior defined by

$$[\mathbf{D_Q}]_{kk'} = \frac{\partial^2 \mathbf{Q}(\theta)}{\partial \theta_k \partial \theta_{k'}},$$

evaluated at $\theta = \theta^{\mathrm{ev}}$. In the case of a Gaussian prior, $\mathbf{D_Q}$ is the inverse-covariance matrix of the prior pdf and is independent of $\theta$. We again denote estimates under this linearized model by $\widehat{\theta}^{\mathrm{lin}}$.

Substituting Eqns (8) and (9) into Eqn (5) gives

$$\mathbf{G}_{\theta^{\mathrm{ev}}} \mathbf{K_d}^{-1}\left(\mathbf{d} - \mathbf{s}(\theta^{\mathrm{ev}}) - \mathbf{G}_{\theta^{\mathrm{ev}}}^t\left(\widehat{\theta}^{\mathrm{lin}} - \theta^{\mathrm{ev}}\right)\right) - \mathbf{q}_{\theta^{\mathrm{ev}}} - \mathbf{D_Q}\left(\widehat{\theta}^{\mathrm{lin}} - \theta^{\mathrm{ev}}\right) = 0,$$

which can be rewritten as

$$(\mathbf{F}_{\theta^{\mathrm{ev}}} + \mathbf{D_Q})\left(\widehat{\theta}^{\mathrm{lin}} - \theta^{\mathrm{ev}}\right) = \mathbf{G}_{\theta^{\mathrm{ev}}} \mathbf{K_d}^{-1}(\mathbf{d} - \mathbf{s}(\theta^{\mathrm{ev}})) - \mathbf{q}_{\theta^{\mathrm{ev}}}. \tag{10}$$

If $(\mathbf{F}_{\theta^{\mathrm{ev}}} + \mathbf{D_Q})$ is invertible, Eqn (10) can be solved for an explicit form of the parameter

$$\widehat{\theta}^{\mathrm{lin}} = \theta^{\mathrm{ev}} + (\mathbf{F}_{\theta^{\mathrm{ev}}} + \mathbf{D_Q})^{-1}\left(\mathbf{G}_{\theta^{\mathrm{ev}}} \mathbf{K_d}^{-1}(\mathbf{d} - \mathbf{s}(\theta^{\mathrm{ev}})) - \mathbf{q}_{\theta^{\mathrm{ev}}}\right).$$

As in section 2.2, $\widehat{\theta}^{\mathrm{lin}}$ is a linear function of the data and hence normally distributed with mean and covariance as follows

$$\left\langle \widehat{\theta}^{\mathrm{lin}} \right\rangle = \theta^{\mathrm{ev}} - (\mathbf{F}_{\theta^{\mathrm{ev}}} + \mathbf{D_Q})^{-1}\left(\mathbf{G}_{\theta^{\mathrm{ev}}} \mathbf{K_d}^{-1}\Delta\mathbf{s} + \mathbf{q}_{\theta^{\mathrm{ev}}}\right), \tag{11}$$

$$\mathrm{cov}\left(\widehat{\theta}^{\mathrm{lin}}\right) = (\mathbf{F}_{\theta^{\mathrm{ev}}} + \mathbf{D_Q})^{-1} \mathbf{F}_{\theta^{\mathrm{ev}}} (\mathbf{F}_{\theta^{\mathrm{ev}}} + \mathbf{D_Q})^{-1}, \tag{12}$$

where the vector $\Delta\mathbf{s}$ is defined as

$$\Delta\mathbf{s} = \mathbf{s}(\theta^{\mathrm{ev}}) - \mathbf{s}(\theta^{\mathrm{true}}).$$

The advantage of a variable point of expansion for the first-order approximation to $\mathbf{s}(\theta)$ is that the expansion can always be centered about $\theta^{\mathrm{ev}}$, the estimate of interest. As in section 2.2, $\mathrm{p}\left(\widehat{\theta}^{\mathrm{lin}} = \theta^{\mathrm{ev}} \mid \theta^{\mathrm{true}}\right)$ can be written with the explicit form of the multivariate normal density with the mean and covariance terms given in Eqns (11) and (12). The approximate density is then given by

$$\mathrm{p}\left(\widehat{\theta} = \theta^{\mathrm{ev}} \mid \theta^{\mathrm{true}}\right) \simeq \mathrm{p}\left(\widehat{\theta}^{\mathrm{lin}} = \theta^{\mathrm{ev}} \mid \theta^{\mathrm{true}}\right)$$

$$= \frac{\det(\mathbf{F}_{\theta^{\mathrm{ev}}} + \mathbf{D_Q})}{(2\pi)^{K/2}\sqrt{\det \mathbf{F}_{\theta^{\mathrm{ev}}}}}$$

$$\times \exp\left(-\frac{1}{2}\left(\mathbf{G}_{\theta^{\mathrm{ev}}} \mathbf{K_d}^{-1}\Delta\mathbf{s} + \mathbf{q}_{\theta^{\mathrm{ev}}}\right)^t \mathbf{F}_{\theta^{\mathrm{ev}}}^{-1}\left(\mathbf{G}_{\theta^{\mathrm{ev}}} \mathbf{K_d}^{-1}\Delta\mathbf{s} + \mathbf{q}_{\theta^{\mathrm{ev}}}\right)\right). \tag{13}$$

# 3 ML estimation of a simple "tumor" model

To test the approximate density of Eqn (13) in a low-dimensional nonlinear estimation problem, we consider ML estimation of amplitude $A$ and radius $R$ for a Gaussian signal in the presence of white noise. This example is intended as a simplification of the amplitude-radius problem considered in [3] where a more accurate model of the imaging system was used. Thus for this example

$$\boldsymbol{\theta} = \left[ \begin{array}{c} A \\ R \end{array} \right].$$

The nonlinear Cartesian model relating $\boldsymbol{\theta}$ to the data is

$$\mathbf{s}_m\left(\boldsymbol{\theta}\right) = A\exp\left(-\frac{1}{2}\frac{x_m^2 + y_m^2}{R^2 + \epsilon^2}\right).$$

The $x_m$ and $y_m$ specify the location of the $m$th pixel relative to the center of the tumor which is fixed at the center of the image. The model incorporates $32 \times 32$ pixel images; therefore $m$ runs from 1 to 1024. All distances are expressed in units of pixel length. The $\epsilon^2$ term, set to $\epsilon = \sqrt{2}$, is intended to provide a crude model of the blurring of the signal due to detector response and the system transfer function.

The method is illustrated by estimating $A$ and $R$ through Maximum Likelihood given that the true values of these parameters are $A^{\text{true}} = 10$ and $R^{\text{true}} = 4$. Three levels of noise are considered corresponding to pixel variances of $\sigma_{\text{d}}^2 = 50$, 100, and 200. 1000 Monte-Carlo (MC) samples for each pixel variance are compared to the two pdfs – the CR-pdf of Eqn. (7) and the approximate-density pdf of Eqn. (13) – by superimposing isocontours of each pdf onto sets of ML estimates in Figure 1. Thus, the accuracy of each pdf in describing the MC samples can be inspected visually. A more quantitative assessment of accuracy is the subject of future work.

Because the underlying distribution of the CR-pdf is Gaussian, its isocontours are constrained to be ellipses. At the lowest level of noise, i.e. $\sigma_{\text{d}}^2 = 50$, the isocontours of both pdfs are qualitatively similar and adequately enclose the MC sample estimates. In the case of the CR-pdf, this confirms that the CRB approximates the distribution of estimates. However, as the noise increases, i.e. $\sigma_{\text{d}}^2 = 200$, the non-Gaussian approximate pdf displays a curvature which better captures those ML estimates which fall relatively far from $\boldsymbol{\theta}^{\text{true}} = (10, 4)$. The elliptical isocontours of the CR-pdf are unable to enclose these points, showing graphically the inadequacy of the CRB in characterizing nonlinear estimates at high levels of noise.

# 4 Conclusions

This paper addresses the task of nonlinear estimation by developing an approximate probability distribution for ML and MAP estimates. Since ML and MAP

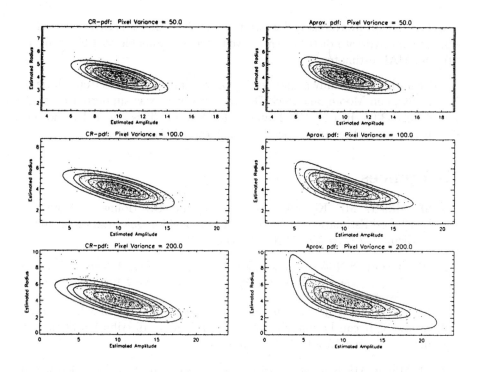

Figure 1: Plots of pdf contours of the CR-pdf in the left column and the approximate density of Eqn 13 in the right column. Plots are arranged vertically by the amount of noise (the variance) in the data. Plotted over the contours at each noise level are scatter plots from the Monte-Carlo samples of estimated amplitude and radius.

estimators are *implicitly* defined as the maximum of an objective functional based on the data likelihood, the challenge in this analysis is to find *explicit* distributions of the estimates.

Our approach begins by deriving the Gaussian CR-pdf from ML estimation where the signal is expressed as a first-order Taylor series approximation expanded about the true parameter vector $\theta^{true}$. We then vary the point about which the signal is expanded; the non-Gaussian approximate density is derived by setting the point of expansion to be $\theta^{ev}$, the vector at which the pdf is to be evaluated.

The CR-pdf and the approximate density are then evaluated for a simplified version of a previously studied nonlinear estimation problem [3] in which Monte-Carlo samples of ML estimates are produced from a signal embedded in white noise. Comparisons can be made by visually inspecting isocontours of the probability functions overlying the MC samples. When the data SNR is high, both densities are adequate for describing the estimates. Due to nonlinearity in the signal, at low SNR the scatter plots clearly depart from the elliptical isocontours of the Gaussian CR-pdf. However, isocontours of the non-Gaussian approximate density still capture the skewed distribution of the estimates. Hence, we believe that the approximate distribution derived here is a valuable tool for analyzing ML and MAP estimates.

The authors gratefully acknowledge many helpful comments from Marie Kijewski, Stephen Moore, and Jack Denny. This work was supported by grants R01-CA52643-05, R01-NS31902, and R01-CA55174. This paper does not necessarily represent the official views of the National Cancer Institute.

# References

[1] SP Müller, MF Kijewski, SC Moore, and BL Holman. "Maximum-Likelihood Estimation: A Mathematical Model for Quantitation in Nuclear Medicine," *J Nucl Med* 1990; 31:1693-1701.

[2] HH Barrett. "Objective assessment of image quality: Effects of quantum noise and object variability," *J Opt Soc Am A* 1990; 7:1266-1278.

[3] SP Müller, MF Kijewski, and SC Moore. "The efficiency of ML-estimation at low SNR can be inferred from the probability distribution of the estimates," *J Nucl Med* 1995; 36:119P.

[4] SP Müller, MF Kijewski, Christian Kappeler, and SC Moore. "Estimation performance at low SNR: Predictions of the Barankin Bound," in Medical Imaging 1995: Physics of Medical Imaging, Richard van Meter, Jacob Beutel, Editors. *Proc. SPIE* 2432:157-166.

[5] JA Fessler and AR Hero. "Cramér-Rao lower bounds for biased image reconstruction," in *Proc. Midwest Symposium on Circuits and Systems*, 1993, vol. 1, pp. 253-256.

[6] JA Fessler. "Mean and Variance of Implicitly defined Biased Estimators (such as Penalized Maximum Likelihood): Applications to Tomography," *IEEE Trans Image Proc*, EDICS 2.3, 1995.

[7] HL Van Trees. *Detection, Estimation and Modulation Theory*, (Wiley, New York, 1968).

[8] HH Barrett and W Swindell. *Radiological Imaging: Theory of Image Formation, Detection, and Processing* (Academic, New York, 1981), Vol. I.

[9] S Geman and D Geman. "Stochastic Relaxation, Gibbs Distributions and the Bayesian Restoration of Images," *IEEE Trans. on Pattern Analysis and Machine intelligence*, 1984 PAMI-6(6), pp 721-741.

[10] KV Mardia, JT Kent, and JM Bibby. *Multivariate analysis*, (Academic, San Diego, Calif., 1979).

# Continuous Gaussian Mixture Modeling

Stephen Aylward[1] and Stephen Pizer[2]

[1]Department of Radiology
[2]Department of Computer Science
Medical Image Display and Analysis Group
University of North Carolina
Chapel Hill, NC 27599

**Abstract.** When the projection of a collection of samples onto a subset of basis feature vectors has a Gaussian distribution, those samples have a generalized projective Gaussian distribution (GPGD). GPGDs arise in a variety of medical images as well as some speech recognition problems. We will demonstrate that GPGDs are better represented by continuous Gaussian mixture models (CGMMs) than finite Gaussian mixture models (FGMMs).

This paper introduces a novel technique for the automated specification of CGMMs, height ridges of goodness-of-fit. For GPGDs, Monte Carlo simulations and ROC analysis demonstrate that classifiers utilizing CGMMs defined via goodness-of-fit height ridges provide consistent labelings and compared to FGMMs provide better true-positive rates (TPRs) at low false-positive rates (FPRs). The CGMM-based classification of gray and white matter in an inhomogeneous magnetic resonance (MR) image of the brain is demonstrated.

## 1 Introduction

The crux of statistical pattern recognition and data analysis is the accurate modeling of the distributions of data. This paper presents a novel technique which is ideally suited for representing GPGDs. GPGDs arise in a variety of medical images such as MR images containing intensity inhomogeneities, X-ray CT images due to beam hardening, and SPECT images due to deficiencies in attenuation compensation. GPGDs also exist in some speech and handwriting recognition problems.

It has been demonstrated that within small regions of an MR image, a tissue's intensity will be Gaussian distributed, yet the parameters of those localized Gaussian distributions will vary as a result of an intensity inhomogeneity. Consider the proton density (PD) MR image in Fig. 1. It was acquired and converted to byte pixel values as described in [2]. It contains an intensity inhomogeneity which exists as a large scale dimming in the inferior cerebellum. The inhomogeneity can be quantified (Fig. 2) by Gaussian blurring the image at a scale of 15 pixels using only those pixel's having values between 100 and 200. More exact methods for measuring the inhomogeneity exist [4, 10, 16], but the stated approach is sufficient for our demonstration. The correlation between PD value and inhomogeneity

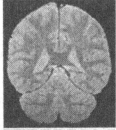

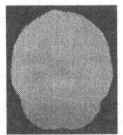

**Fig. 1.** Proton density MR image

**Fig. 2.** Estimated intensity inhomogeneity

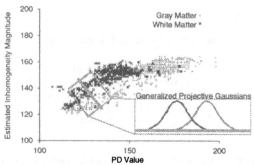

**Fig. 3.** Scatterplot of hand-labeled gray and white matter samples

magnitude is revealed by a scatterplot (Fig. 3) formed from 984 hand-labeled white matter and 788 gray matter samples from these images. In that scatterplot, every local collection of a tissue's samples has a Gaussian distribution, but a continuum of Gaussians is needed to represent each tissue's entire distribution; the distributions are GPGDs.

In speech recognition, it is commonly accepted that hidden Markov models using Gaussian distributions can represent certain aspects of the speech of a single person in a controlled situation, e.g., given a fixed level of stress. Smooth warpings can be applied to the parameters of those Gaussians to transition them to new situations and speakers [3]. To account for such variations in speaker and situation, multiple Gaussians are needed; the distributions resemble GPGDs.

When the correlations creating the GPGDs are well understood and easily measured, the most accurate models can be obtained by directly eliminating their effects and then using simple Gaussians [4, 10, 16]. When the correlations are not well understood or easily measured, Gaussian mixture models are appropriate.

Traditionally, FGMMs defined via maximum likelihood expectation maximization (MLEM) have been used to represent GPGDs. We will show that these distributions are more accurately and consistently represented by continua of means and variances. We call such continua "traces." We will show that the traces of a sampled GPGD can be extracted via height ridges of goodness-of-fit functions, and that these traces accurately and consistently define a CGMM of the underlying GPGD.

For this paper, the accuracy and consistency of the distribution models are quantified by the accuracy and consistency of the classifiers they define. That is, when a model $\Psi$ of a class i is used to provide class conditional probability estimates $P(\underline{x} \mid \Psi^{(i)})$ to a classifier, the accuracy and consistency of the labelings produced by that classifier determine the accuracy and consistency of the model. Assuming equal class priors $P(\Psi^{(i)})$ and maximum likelihood Bayes Rule classification, then

$$\text{label for } \underline{x} = \underset{i=1..\# \text{ of classes}}{\textbf{ARGMAX}} \left[ P\left(\Psi^i \middle| \underline{x}\right) = \frac{P\left(\Psi^i\right) P\left(\underline{x} \middle| \Psi^i\right)}{P(\underline{x})} = P\left(\underline{x} \middle| \Psi^i\right) \right] \quad [1]$$

A classifier's labeling accuracy is quantified by its TPRs and FPRs, and its labeling consistency is the standard error of those rates.

Section 2 introduces finite and continuous Gaussian mixture modeling. Section 3 presents our implementation of goodness-of-fit functions. These functions respond maximally when their parameters $\mu'$ and $\sigma'$ match those of the distribution from which the samples being tested originated. That section also discusses the how these functions are applied normal to the trace of a GPGD in order to extract that trace using a height ridge definition, and it ties the traces to the definition of a CGMM. Section 4 uses GPGDs, Monte Carlo simulations, and ROC analysis to compare FGMMs with CGMMs. Section 5 demonstrates the CGMM-based classification of tissues in an inhomogeneous MR image.

# 2  Gaussian Mixture Modeling

A mixture model is formed using multiple "component" distributions. In a Gaussian mixture model the component distributions are multivariate (N-dimensional) normal densities each of which is parameterized by $\phi$.

$$F(\underline{x};\Phi) = \frac{1}{(2\pi)^{N/2}|\underline{\underline{\Sigma}}|^{1/2}} e^{-\frac{1}{2}(\underline{x}-\underline{\mu})^t \underline{\underline{\Sigma}}^{-1}(\underline{x}-\underline{\mu})} \qquad \text{where} \qquad \Phi = \left\{\underline{\mu},\underline{\underline{\Sigma}}\right\} \qquad [2]$$

## 2.1  Finite Gaussian Mixture Modeling

If the number of components K is bounded, the Gaussian mixture model is a FGMM $\Psi$. It provides a probability for a sample $\underline{x}$ via

$$P(\underline{x} \mid \Psi) = \sum_{i=1}^{K} \omega^{(i)} F(\underline{x};\Phi^{(i)}) \text{ where } 1 = \sum_{i=1}^{K} \omega^{(i)} \text{ and } \Psi = \left\{\{\omega,\Phi\}^{(i)} \mid i = 1..K\right\} \qquad [3]$$

Most investigations involving mixture models use FGMMs trained via MLEM. While no FGMM training algorithm is best in all situations, MLEM is easy to implement and provides several desirable convergence properties such as monotonic convergence [5, 7, 8, 18]. MLEM, however, is an approximate gradient ascent algorithm, and it is subject to non-optimal local and global maxima. While MLEM is relatively robust to these non-optimal maxima [7, 15, 18], it will be shown that the FGMM component parameterizations produced via MLEM can vary greatly and be far from optimal given different sets of samples from the same distribution; FGMMs offer poor consistency. This inconsistency is aggravated by the reliance on the user to specify the number of components.

   While much research has focused on automatically determining an appropriate number of components for a given problem, a generally applicable approach has not be found [9, 18]. A FGMM's expected accuracy does not vary monotonically as a function of the number of components. Additionally, MLEM's non-optimal maxima can lead to poorly utilized components; the effective number of components in an FGMM may be less than the user specified number of components. GPGDs are comprised of an infinite number of components, so determining an appropriate finite number of components to approximate them with can be especially difficult.

## 2.2  Continuous Gaussian Mixture Modeling

A continuous mixture model consists of an uncountably infinite number of components whose parameters $\Psi$ span $N_t$ traces $T^{(j)}$ through the parameter space of its components, i.e., the domain of $\phi$. A CGMM provides a probability via

$$P(\underline{x} \mid \Psi) = \underset{\{\omega,\phi\}\in\Psi}{\text{MAX}} (\omega F(\underline{x};\phi)) \text{ where } \Psi = \left\{\{\omega,\Phi\} \,\middle|\, \begin{array}{l} \exists\, j \in 1..N_t \text{ s.t. } \Phi \in T^{(j)} \\ \text{and } \omega = P(\Phi) \end{array}\right\} \qquad [4]$$

This equation follows the simplifying assumptions made by Dempster, Laird, and Rubin [5] and states that since the underlying distribution is assumed to be a mixture, each sample is in fact generated by just one of the infinite number of components, the generating component is determined via maximum likelihood, and the generating component provides the best estimate of the sample's probability. The function $F(\underline{x};\phi)$ can be interpreted as providing a trace point conditional sample probability, and $\omega$ as providing a trace point *a priori* probability. Equation 3 can therefore be rewritten as

$$P\left(\underline{x} \mid \Psi\right) = \underset{\substack{\Phi \in T^{(j)} \in \Psi \mid j \in 1..N_t}}{\text{MAX}} \left(P(\Phi)P\left(\underline{x}|\Phi\right)\right) \tag{5}$$

The focus of this paper is the definition of the traces $T^{(j)}$ via height ridges of goodness-of-fit functions. A CGMM defined in this manner can accurately and consistently model the continua of means and variances which form a GPGD. For this paper, analysis is limited to GPGD's having one-dimensional traces.

# 3 Traces of Goodness-of-Fit

Each trace of a GPGD can be viewed as a continuum of central means (centers) with smoothly changing variances normal to that continuum (widths). A method has already been developed for representing the centers and widths of objects. That object representation method is known as the medialness core [12]. Medialness cores have been proven to be invariant to rotation, translation, intensity, and scale [12] and insensitive to a wide variety of image and boundary noise [11]. To apply medialness core methods to the representation of distributions, goodness-of-fit functions are used instead of medialness functions because goodness-of-fit functions are sensitive to sample density whereas medialness functions are sensitive to boundariness.

## 3.1. Univariate Gaussian Goodness-of-Fit

One class of goodness-of-fit functions is the univariate chi-squared measures. This class includes Pearson's statistic $\chi_P^2$, Read and Cressie's power divergent statistic $\chi_{R\&C}^2$, and the log likelihood ratio $\chi_{LLR}^2$ [14]. Since our goal is to develop mixture models using Gaussian components, the binned expected distribution $\underline{E}$ of these omnibus measures is derived from a univariate Gaussian. These functions are therefore referred to as Gaussian goodness-of-fit (GGoF) functions.

The parameters of these functions are $\mu'$ and $\sigma'$, the mean and standard deviation to be tested; $\mu'$ and $\sigma'$ define the expected distribution $\underline{E}$. This paper uses six bins B=6 centered at $\mu'$ and clipped so as to capture samples within $\pm 1.645\sigma'$ of $\mu'$. The GGoF functions are devised so as to be maximal when their parameters $\mu'$ and $\sigma'$ best match the $\mu$ and $\sigma$ of the population from which the samples originated. This is achieved by subtracting the standard goodness-of-fit functions from $\chi_{6-1}^2(\alpha = 0.99) = 15.09$ and then normalizing by that value (Equation 6). As a result of these modifications, a GGoF function's value is expected to be greater than zero for 99% of the sets of samples which originate from a Gaussian parameterized by $\mu'$ and $\sigma'$.

$$\chi_{LLR}^2\left(\mu',\sigma'\right) = \left(15.09 - 2\sum_{i=1}^{B} O_i \ln\left(\frac{O_i}{E_i}\right)\right)/15.09 \tag{6}$$

The accuracy and consistency of the local maxima of the $\chi_P^2$, $\chi_{R\&C}^2$, and $\chi_{LLR}^2$ GGoF functions were evaluated using 96 Monte Carlo simulations. Each simulation consisted of 5000 runs. The simulations considered four different training set sizes (20, 40, 80, 160 samples) from two distributions (a Gaussian with $\mu$=128 and $\sigma$=16 and a log-normal distribution using a log base of 1.6) and four different binning techniques (equirange, equiprobable, overlapped-equirange, overlapped-equiprobable) [1]. For each Monte Carlo run, the local maximum of the GGoF function was found via gradient ascent through ($\mu'$, $\sigma'$). The starting points for gradient ascent were selected from a 2D Gaussian distribution centered at each population's ideal parameter values ($\mu$, $\sigma$) having a standard deviation of 5% of those values. The accuracy of a local GGoF maximum was defined as the difference between the GGoF parameters ($\mu'$, $\sigma'$) of that maximum and the population's actual parameters ($\mu$, $\sigma$). Consistency was calculated as the standard error associated with each parameter $\mu'$ and $\sigma'$ of the maxima from each simulation.

Conclusions drawn include that 1) the binning method has more influence on accuracy and consistency than the GGoF function; 2) the accuracy and consistency of the estimates of $\mu$ do not vary significantly as a function of the number of samples, the GGoF function, or the binning technique; 3) $\chi^2_{LLR}$ with overlapped-equiprobable binning provides the most accurate and consistent estimates $\sigma$. As a result, $\chi^2_{LLR}$ with overlapped-equirange binning was used for all GGoF trace calculations.

## 3.2 Multivariate GGoF via Trace Tangents and Normals

To calculate multivariate GGoF values, the multivariate data about a given $\mu'$ are converted to multiple univariate distributions via projection onto a set of basis directions. The expected variance associated with each of those projections may differ. The multivariate GGoF value is the average $\chi^2_{LLR}$ value from each of those projections. We hypothesize that neighboring GGoF trace points capture a distribution's variance in the trace tangent direction, so each trace point needs only to capture variance normal to the trace.

To estimate a trace's normal (and tangent) directions as well as the expected variance of the distribution in each of those directions, our algorithm extends the geometric measures via statistics work conducted by Yoo [17]. Specifically, we suggest that eigenvectors of the local data's covariance matrix $\underline{\underline{\Sigma}}^{(L)}$ well approximate the normal (and tangent) directions of the GGoF trace, and the eigenvalues define expected variance ratios for each of the normal directions. Since $\underline{\underline{\Sigma}}^{(L)}$ is a function of only two variables, i.e., a mean $\mu'$ and a neighborhood size $s'$, its use in calculating multivariate GGoF functions allows those functions to be parameterized by just $\mu'$ and $s'$. $\underline{\underline{\Sigma}}^{(L)}$ approximation of the tangent allows a GGoF trace to be traversed without derivative calculations.

$\underline{\underline{\Sigma}}^{(L)}$ is measured using a Gaussian weighting $G(\bullet)$ of the samples $S$ about $\mu'$ so as to change smoothly given small changes in $\mu'$ or $s'$.

$$\underline{\underline{\Sigma}}^{(L)}_{ij}\left(\underline{\mu}',s'\right) = \sum_{\underline{z}\in S} G\left(\underline{z}|\underline{\mu}',3\sigma'\right)\left(\underline{z}_i - \underline{\mu}'_i\right)\left(\underline{z}_j - \underline{\mu}'_j\right) \Big/ \sum_{\underline{y}\in S} G\left(\underline{y}|\underline{\mu}',3s'\right) \qquad [7]$$

Define $\lambda_i$ for $i=1..N$ as the descending ordered eigenvalues of $\underline{\underline{\Sigma}}^{(L)}$ and $\underline{v}_i$ as their corresponding eigenvectors. If no additional information is available, it can be assumed that the maximum eigenvalued eigenvector $\underline{v}_1$ approximates the GGoF trace's tangent direction. The remaining eigenvectors specify the normal directions. Expected variances in each of the normal directions are specified by eigenvalue ratios; the expected variance in the eigen-direction, $\underline{v}_i | i=2..N$, is $(\sigma')^2 = (s')^2 \lambda_i/\lambda_2$.

To help understand the N+1 dimensional GGoF "space" ($\mu'$, $s'$) of an N dimensional distribution, slices through the 3D GGoF space of a 2D distribution in ($f_0, f_1$) can be calculated. Consider the scattergram shown in Fig. 4. Those 900 samples were generated from a simulated GPGD, Class A. Class A is defined by three approximating cubic B-splines and four isotropic control Gaussians (Table 1). Each spline governs one of the three parameters of the Gaussians, i.e., $f_0$, $f_1$, $\sigma$. To generate a sample, a parametric value $t$ is chosen from the uniform distribution U[0,1]. The three splines are evaluated at that $t$ value, an isotropic Gaussian distribution is thus defined, and from that distribution the sample is then generated. Figs. 5-7 are the GGoF values for fixed $s'$ and a range of $\mu'$ values using the samples in Fig. 4. 1D GGoF traces appear along the extent of the distribution.

| | Mean | | |
|---|---|---|---|
| | $f_0$ | $f_1$ | $\sigma$ |
| $G^{(0)}$ | 80 | 112 | 16 |
| $G^{(1)}$ | 112 | 56 | 1 |
| $G^{(2)}$ | 144 | 56 | 1 |
| $G^{(3)}$ | 192 | 112 | 16 |

**Table 1.** Control Gaussian of the GPGD, Class A

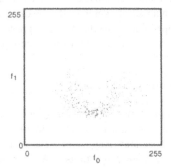

**Fig. 4.** Scattergram of 900 Class A samples

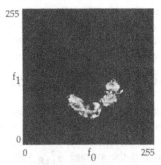

**Fig. 5.** Class A's GGoF space at s´=4

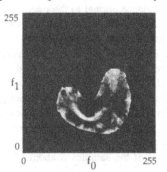

**Fig. 6.** Class A's GGoF space at s´=8

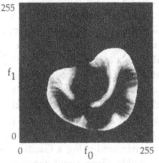

**Fig. 7.** Class A's GGoF space at s´=16

### 3.3 Gaussian Goodness-of-Fit Trace Extraction

As mentioned previously, GGoF traces are based on medialness cores. Techniques developed for medialness core extraction are used to extract GGoF traces. The three steps involved are trace stimulation, traversal, and traversal termination.

**Trace Stimulation.** A trace stimulation point has two components, $\mu^0$ and $s^0$. FGMM is used to specify $\mu^0$. Specifically, the user must select the number of FGMM components to use, the data are then modeled using FGMM, and the component mean which is nearest (measured via Euclidean distance) to two other component means is chosen as $\mu^0$. As a result, $\mu^0$ will generally be located within a dense region of a sampled GPGD. If multiple traces are requested, the remaining component means are used. The number of FGMM components used appears to be non-critical; for all CGMMs developed in this paper the stimulating FGMM used 7 components.

Specifying $s^0$ reduces to determining an initial neighborhood size for calculating $\underline{\underline{\Sigma}}^{(L)}$ at $\mu^0$. By assuming that the trace tangent at $\mu^0$ is well approximated by the maximum eigenvalued eigenvector of $\underline{\underline{\Sigma}}^{(L)}$, $s^0$ is the square root of the second largest eigenvalue. For this paper, the initial neighborhood size is set equal to the distance between $\mu^0$ and its closest neighboring FGMM mean. For the data in Fig. 4, $\mu^0$=(163.66, 80.08) and $s^0$=17.94.

**Trace Traversal.** The trace normals are approximated by the non-tangent eigenvectors of $\underline{\underline{\Sigma}}^{(L)}$ and a unit vector which points strictly in s. These directions define a hyperplane in GGoF space through which the local trace segment passes. When this normal plane is slightly shifted in the local trace tangent direction, a gradient ascent with respect to the GGoF values within that plane leads to a new trace point. For this paper, a step size of 0.1 feature space units is used to shift the normal plane, gradient ascent within that shifted plane is performed using Brent's line search method [13], and gradient ascent terminates when the gradient's projection onto the plane is less than 0.1% of its total magnitude. The point in the plane at which gradient ascent terminates is the new trace point. The new tangent direction is approximated by the eigenvector of local data's covariance matrix that has the maximum magnitude dot product with the previous trace point's tangent eigenvector. If the sign of the dot product is negative, the new tangent vector is negated to maintain the direction of traversal. This process is repeated until a traversal termination criterion is met.

**Trace Traversal Termination and Recovery.** Trace traversal terminates when a "well fitting" Gaussian cannot be found. Empirical evidence suggests that encountering a GGoF value of -10 or less is a reasonable stopping criterion. This criterion was used to terminate the traversal of every trace presented in this paper.

The rate of change of the trace is used to identify suspect trace points and halt their inclusion into the trace without causing termination of the traversal process. Such points are "stepped over" using the tangents of the previous valid trace point.

The $\underline{\mu}'$ component of a 1D GGoF trace of the data in Fig. 4 is shown in Fig. 8. The effect of recovery is visible as a break in the trace. To visualize the normal variance estimates provided by the trace, the 0, ±0.5, ±1, ±1.5, and ±2 $\sigma'$ points along the normal at each trace point can be plotted (Fig. 9). The next section details the conversion of a GGoF trace to a CGMM.

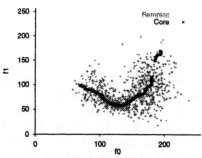

**Fig. 8.** $\underline{\mu}'$ of a GGoF trace of Fig. 4

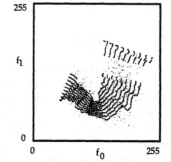

**Fig. 9.** Isocontours of the variance estimates

## 3.4 CGMMs via GGoF Traces

As defined in Equation 4, two values, $P(\underline{x}|\phi)$ and $P(\phi)$, are required at each trace point $\phi$ to define a CGMM $\Psi$. To calculate $P(\underline{x}|\phi)$, a trace point covariance matrix $\underline{\underline{\Sigma}}^{(\phi)}$ must be defined. The eigenvectors and eigenvalues of $\underline{\underline{\Sigma}}^{(\phi)}$ are defined by 1) the approximate normal directions and expected variances which were used to calculate $\phi$"s GGoF value (Section 3.2) and 2) the approximate tangent direction which is assigned a variance equal to the maximum expected variance in a normal direction.

A trace point's *a priori* probability $\mathbf{P}(\phi)$ is defined as the portion of samples it is expected to represent. The expected number of samples that will be represented by a trace point can be extrapolated based on the number of observed samples within a fixed standard deviation, i.e., s, of that point.

The CGMM defined via the GGoF trace depicted in Figs. 8 and 9 produces the probability density function depicted Fig. 10. Although the GGoF trace extended beyond the distribution, the low prior probabilities $\mathbf{P}(\phi)$ associated with those points reduce the negative effects of the over extension. The estimated density function should be compared with the population's actual density function which is shown in Fig. 11. There appears to be good correspondence. The next section focuses on quantifying that correspondence.

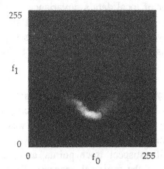

**Fig. 10.** CGMM estimated probability density function of Class A

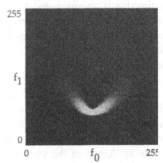

**Fig. 11.** Actual probability density function of Class A

# 4 CGMM's Accuracy and Consistency

To determine the accuracy and consistency of a classifier and thereby determine the accuracy and consistency of the distribution models it uses, Monte Carlo simulations and ROC analyses must be performed. This section begins by presenting an example classification result.

## 4.1 Example Results

The accuracy and consistency of a modeling technique is being determined by the accuracy and consistency of the labelings produced by classifiers that use the probability estimates provided by those models. Class A was defined in Section 3.2. A competing class, Class B, is defined as an isotropic Gaussian with $\mu=(128,128)$ and $\sigma=36$. Given the set of 900 training samples from Class B, the stimulation point $\mu^0=(160.37, 123.30)$ and $s^0=17.94$ is automatically chosen. The resulting trace point conditional isoprobability curves overlaid onto the training data scattergram are shown in Fig. 12. Using the Class A and Class B models developed thus far, every point in feature space can be assigned a label and an image can be developed which reflects those labelings with differing shades of gray. Fig. 13 is such an image with the optimal decision bounds between the classes overlaid in black.

The CGMMs of Classes A and B provide accurate labelings for the majority of feature space. To improve the CGMM's labelings, multiple traces can be used. While generally containing redundant information, additional traces do refine a CGMM. CGMMs using 7 traces per class (CGMM07) produce the labelings shown in Fig. 14. FGMMs using 7 components per class (FGMM07) produce the labelings shown in Fig. 15. Allocation to

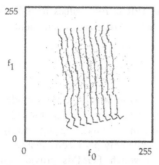

**Fig. 12.** Isoprobability curves of Class B's CGMM

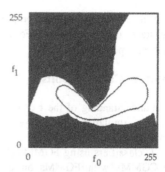

**Fig. 13.** Labeling of feature space produced by CGMMs with optimal decision bound overlaid

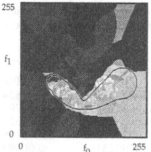

**Fig. 14.** Labelings by CGMM07

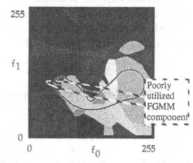

**Fig. 15.** Labelings produced by FGMM07

Different shades of gray correspond to allocation to different traces/components.
Light gray shades indicate assignment to Class A

each trace/component is indicated by different shades of gray; light grays indicate allocation to Class A. The presence of non-optimal FGMM maxima is clear; one Class A component is reduced to representing a sliver through feature space. That component is being poorly utilized, and its use does not correspond with the underlying distribution.

Given 2700 testing samples from each class, the Class A TPRs and FPRs in Table 2, Run1 are produced. Compared to FGMM07, CGMM07 offers an 718% decrease in the FPR with a less than 11% decrease in the TPR! To determine if these results were anomalous, new models were developed and tested using different samples from Classes A and B. Those results are summarized in Table 2, Run2. CGMM07 again produced the lowest FPR, but the differences are less dramatic.

While no conclusions should be drawn from these two runs, the results are quite encouraging. Not only does CGMM07 provide the lowest FPR values and competitive TPR

|  | Run1 | | Run2 | |
|---|---|---|---|---|
|  | **FPR** | **TPR** | **FPR** | **TPR** |
| **CGMM01** | 0.3233 | 0.8859 | 0.2281 | 0.6681 |
| **CGMM02** | 0.3215 | 0.8859 | 0.2178 | 0.7874 |
| **CGMM04** | 0.2604 | 0.8367 | 0.2200 | 0.8204 |
| **CGMM07** | **0.0385** | **0.8237** | 0.2318 | 0.8485 |
| **FGMM01** | 0.2933 | 0.8415 | 0.2878 | 0.8659 |
| **FGMM02** | 0.3259 | 0.9196 | 0.3185 | 0.9307 |
| **FGMM04** | 0.3315 | 0.9259 | 0.3218 | 0.9400 |
| **FGMM07** | 0.3152 | 0.9130 | 0.3067 | 0.9141 |

**Table 2.** Class B TPRs & FPRs from two different sets of training and testing data

values, but there is also an ordered progression in the TPR & FPR values for CGMM as the number of traces used is increased. For FGMM, the use of additional components does not always increase performance.

## 4.2 Monte Carlo Results

To gain an understanding of the expected consistency with which CGMMs model GPGDs, Monte Carlo simulations involving Class A and Class B were performed. Initial simulations revealed that even after 5000 repetitions of the modeling and testing task of Section 4.1, classifiers using FGMMs demonstrated extremely poor consistency. So as to compare CGMMs with FGMMs on a problem for which FGMMs provide consistent performance, the Monte Carlo experiments reported in this paper limited their analysis to the FGMMs and CGMMs of the GPGD, Class A. Each classifier was provided with an exact model of Class B. Given 100 Monte Carlo runs involving 900 Class A training samples and 2700 Class A and 2700 Class B testing samples yielded the average TPRs, FPRs, and standard error ranges shown in Table 4 (Fig. 16).

| | Average | | Standard Error | |
| | FPR | TPR | FPR | TPR |
|---|---|---|---|---|
| CGMM01 | 0.2002 | 0.7181 | 0.0057576 | 0.0165489 |
| CGMM02 | 0.2437 | 0.8192 | 0.0033732 | 0.0070245 |
| CGMM04 | 0.2702 | 0.8658 | 0.0025880 | 0.0032410 |
| CGMM07 | 0.2873 | 0.8862 | 0.0020565 | 0.0019929 |
| FGMM01 | 0.2779 | 0.8364 | 0.0009231 | 0.0009339 |
| FGMM02 | 0.2419 | 0.8660 | 0.0010374 | 0.0009371 |
| FGMM04 | 0.2216 | 0.8495 | 0.0011087 | 0.0014111 |
| FGMM07 | 0.1934 | 0.7990 | 0.0027022 | 0.0084882 |

**Table 3.** Average TPR/FPR values and their standard error ranges

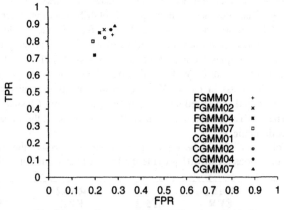

**Fig. 16.** Plot of average TPR & FPR values (Table 3)

Both modeling techniques demonstrate an ordered progression in consistency based on their hyperparameter, i.e., number of components or number of traces. FGMM's consistency, however, monotonically declines as additional components are used. CGMM's consistency monotonically improves as additional traces are used. CGMM07 is shown to offer very competitive consistency. ROC analysis is needed to compare the accuracy of these classifiers.

## 4.3 ROC Analysis

By changing the *a priori* probability (ROC observer bias) associated with Class B while keeping each class model and the testing data fixed, a continuum of FPR & TPR values are defined. These values form the ROC curves shown in Fig. 17.

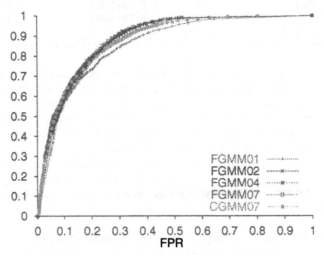

**Fig. 17.** ROC curves from fixed data, FGMMs and CGMMs

Using these curves, three measures can be made to quantitatively compare the classifiers' accuracy: the area under each curve; the maximum probability of generating a correct answer for each curve, i.e., Max-P(C) = MAX(TPR+(1-FPR)); and the TPR values of each curve at fixed FPR values [8]. Table 5 summarizes these measures.

|  | Area of ROC | Max-P(C) | TPR @ FPR=0.1 | TPR @ FPR=0.15 | TPR @ FPR=0.2 |
|---|---|---|---|---|---|
| CGMM07 | 0.8752 | 1.5893 | 0.6160 | 0.7068 | 0.7741 |
| FGMM01 | 0.8443 | 1.5530 | 0.5688 | 0.6704 | 0.7337 |
| FGMM02 | 0.8665 | 1.6048 | 0.5889 | 0.6961 | 0.7844 |
| FGMM04 | 0.8765 | 1.6126 | 0.6019 | 0.7166 | 0.7945 |
| FGMM07 | 0.8793 | 1.6159 | 0.6047 | 0.7155 | 0.7935 |

**Table 4.** Results of measures made on ROC curves in Fig. 19

The area under the CGMM07 curve is comparable to that of FGMM04 and only slightly less than FGMM07. CGMM07 provides performance similar to FGMM02, but well below FGMM04 and FGMM07. As demonstrated in both experiments of Section 4.1, CGMM07 provides the best TPR value for the smallest FPR tested, i.e., FPR=0.1. This ROC analysis, however, is based on a single instance of a model and does not reveal expected accuracy.

To determine the expected accuracy of CGMMs and FGMMs on the Class A / Class B problem, the Monte Carlo averaged TPR & FPR values reported in Section 4.2 are used. Specifically, the ROC curves passing through each classifier's Monte Carlo averaged TPR & FPR values can be explicitly calculated under the assumption that the class distributions are unit variance Gaussians. While that assumption is strictly incorrect for Class A, a Gaussian is a first order approximation to Class A's actual distribution. The significant measure produced from this ROC analysis is the probit measure d′, the spread of the means [6]. More accurate models have larger d′ values. Table 5 lists the relevant d′ values.

| | d′ | | d′ |
|---|---|---|---|
| CGMM01 | 1.418 | FGMM01 | 1.569 |
| CGMM02 | 1.607 | FGMM02 | **1.808** |
| CGMM04 | 1.719 | FGMM03 | 1.801 |
| CGMM07 | 1.768 | FGMM04 | 1.801 |
| CGMM14[1] | **1.810** | FGMM07 | 1.704 |

**Table 5.** Probit's d' value for ROC curves based on Monte Carlo averages (Table 3)

These values indicate that as additional cores are used, CGMMs can be expected to asymptotically outperform the best performing FGMM when representing Class A, a GPGD. That is, under first order assumptions for Classes A and B, the area under the CGMM14's ROC curve will be larger, the maximum probability of being correct for CGMM14 will be higher, and CGMM14 will provide a better TPR for every FPR value compared to the best performing FGMM, i.e., FGMM02.

Every one of the experiments performed suggests that for low FPRs, CGMMs composed of a sufficient number of GGoF traces can be expected to provide better TPRs than any FGMM via MLEM. The next sections presents some "real-world" results, the segmentation of an inhomogeneous medical image.

# 5 Inhomogeneous Magnetic Resonance Images

This section demonstrates the efficacy of CGMMs using GGoF traces for medical image data. Using the hand-labeled samples shown in Fig. 3, four GGoF traces can be automatically extracted to represent each class. Using these CGMMs, all of the points in the image can be labeled as either gray or white matter. While there will be errors since other tissues are present, the results are very promising; the gray matter mask formed is given in Fig. 18. The qualitative best FGMM was achieved using four components. FGMM04's gray matter mask is shown in Fig. 19.

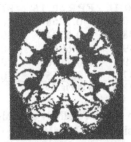
**Fig. 18.** CGMM04's gray matter mask

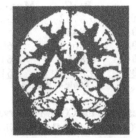
**Fig. 19.** FGMM04's gray matter mask

The differences between the CGMM and the FGMM masks are extremely small. The lack of a gold standard for this data prevents a quantitative comparison. These results are significant, however, in that they indicate that 1) CGMMs are a viable alternative for GPGDs given "real-world" data and 2) CGMMs do not require the user to specify a hyperparameter value, i.e., the number of components.

---

[1] Traces were stimulated using component means from FGMM14; See Section 3.3.

# 6  Conclusion

A CGMM of a GPGD can be defined using GGoF traces. When such models are used for classification, accurate labelings are produced. Initial experiments indicate that for small FPRs, this approach provides superior TPRs compared to FGMMs defined via MLEM. Given different collections of training data, the TPRs and FPRs associated with these labelings remain consistent relative to the consistency of the labelings produced by FGMMs. Furthermore, as additional GGoF traces are extracted, the accuracy and consistency of the CGMM improves asymptotically; defining CGMMs using GGoF traces avoids reliance on the user to specify critical hyperparameters such as the number of components, and it avoids the problems associated with local maxima in iterative parameter refinement processes, e.g., MLEM. The application of CGMMs using GGoF traces to medical image data and the existence of GPGDs in medical images is demonstrated via the classification of tissues in an inhomogeneous MR image. Current work is focusing on the extraction of higher dimensional (M>1) GGoF traces and the development of deformable distribution models using GGoF traces which adapt generic representations to form more optimal specific representations.

# 7  Acknowledgments

Special thanks goes to the members of Stephen Aylward's dissertation committee: James Coggins (advisor), Stephen Pizer (reader), Dan Fritsch, Steve Marron, Jonathan Marshall, and Keith Muller. This work was supported by the Medical Image Display and Analysis Group with partial funding from NIH grant P01 CA47982.

# References

1. Aylward, S.R., "Continuous Mixture Modeling via Goodness-of-Fit Cores," Dissertation, Department of Computer Science, University of North Carolina, Chapel Hill, 1997
2. Aylward, S.R. and Coggins, J.M., "Spatially Invariant Classification of Tissues in MR Images." *Visualization in Biomedical Computing,* Rochester, MN, 1994
3. Bellegarda, J.R. and Nahamoo, D., "Tied Mixture Continuous Parameter Modeling for Speech Recognition." *IEEE Transactions on Acoustics, Speech, and Signal Processing,* vol. 38, no. 12. 1990 p. 2033-2045
4. Dawant, B.M., Zijdenbos, A.P. and Margolin, R.A., "Correction of Intensity Variations in MR Images for Computer-Aided Tissue Classification." *IEEE Transactions on Medical Imaging,* vol. 12, no. 4. 1993 p. 770-781
5. Depmster, A., Laird, N., Rubin, D., "Maximum Likelihood for Incomplete Data via the EM Algorithm." *Royal Statistical Society,* vol. 1, no. 1. 1977
6. Egan, J.P., Signal detection theory and ROC analysis. Academic Press, Inc., New York, 1975
7. Jordan, M.I. and Xu, L., "Convergence Results for the EM Approach to Mixtures of Experts Architectures." *Technical Report,* Massachusetts Institute of Technology, Artificial Intelligence Laboratory, November 18, 1994
8. Liang, Z., Jaszezak, R.J. and Coleman, R.E., "Parameter Estimation of Finite Mixtures Using the EM Algorithm and Information Criteria with Application to Medical Image Processing." *IEEE Transactions on Nuclear Science,* vol. 39, no. 4. 1992 p. 1126-1133

9. McLachlan, G.J. and Basford, K.E., *Mixture Models.* Marcel Dekker, Inc., New York, vol. 84, 1988 p. 253

10. Meyer, C.R., Bland, P.H. and Pipe, J., "Retrospective Correction of Intensity Inhomogeneities in MRI." *IEEE Transactions on Medical Imaging*, vol. 14, no. 1. 1995 p. 36-41

11. Morse, B.S., Pizer, S.M., Puff, D.T. and Gu, C., "Zoom-Invariant Vision of Figural Shape: Effects on Cores of Image Disturbances." *Computer Vision and Image Understanding*, Accepted, 1997

12. Pizer, S.M., Eberly, D., Morse, B.S. and Fritsch, D.S., "Zoom-invariant Vision of Figural Shape: the Mathematics of Cores." *Computer Vision and Image Understanding*, Accepted, 1997

13. Press, W.H., Flannery, B.P., Teukolsky, S.A. and Vetterling, W.T., *Numerical Recipes in C.* Cambridge University Press, Cambridge, 1990

14. Read, T.R.C. and Cressie, N.A.C., *Goodness-of-fit statistics for discrete multivariate data.* Springer-Verlag, New York, 1988

15. Titterington, D.M., Smith, A.G.M. and Markov, U.E., *Statistical Analysis of Finite Mixture Distributions.* John Wiley and Sons, Chichester, 1985

16. Wells III, W.M., Grimson, W.E.L., Kikinis, R. and Jolesz, F.A., "Adaptive Segmentation of MRI Data." *IEEE Transactions on Medical Imaging*, vol. 15, no. 4. 1996 p. 429-442

17. Yoo, T. "Image Geometry Through Multiscale Statistics," Dissertation, Department of Computer Science, University of North Carolina, Chapel Hill, 1996

18. Zhuang, X., Huang, Y., Palaniappan, K. and Zhao, Y., "Gaussian Mixture Density Modeling, Decomposition, and Applications." *IEEE Transactions on Image Processing*, vol. 5, no. 9. 1996 p. 1293-1302

# New Statistical Models for Randoms-Precorrected PET Scans

Mehmet Yavuz and Jeffrey A. Fessler

Department of EECS, University of Michigan, Ann Arbor MI

**Abstract.** PET measurements are usually precorrected for accidental coincidence events by *real-time* subtraction of the delayed window
coincidences. Randoms subtraction compensates in mean for accidental
coincidences but destroys the Poisson statistics. We propose and analyze
two new approximations to the exact log-likelihood of the precorrected
measurements, one based on a "shifted Poisson" model, the other based
on saddle-point approximations to the measurement probability mass
function (pmf). The methods apply to both emission and transmission
tomography; however in this paper we focus on transmission tomography. We compare the new models to conventional data-weighted least
squares (WLS) and conventional maximum likelihood (based on the ordinary Poisson (OP) model) using simulations and analytic approximations. The results demonstrate that the proposed methods avoid the systematic bias of the WLS method, and lead to significantly lower variance
than the conventional OP method. The saddle-point method provides a
more accurate approximation to the exact log-likelihood than the WLS,
OP and shifted Poisson alternatives. However, the simpler shifted Poisson method yielded comparable bias-variance performance in the simulations. The new methods offer improved image reconstruction in PET
through more realistic statistical modeling, yet with negligible increase
in computation over the conventional OP method.

## 1  Introduction

In PET measurements, accidental coincidence (AC) events are a primary source
of background noise. AC events occur when photons that arise from separate
annihilations are mistakenly registered as having arisen from the same annihila-
tion. In transmission scans the photons that originate from different transmission
sources (rod or sector sources rotating around the patient) cause AC events. The
ratio of total AC events to "true" events is usually small in transmission scans
compared to emission scans. Nevertheless, the effect of AC events becomes severe for regions of high attenuation coefficients, because projections through
such regions result in low true coincidence rates. These low count rates can become comparable to AC rates. Thus estimates of the AC events are needed. One
can use the "singles" method [1] for this purpose, however this approach is not

This work was supported in part by NIH grants CA-60711 and CA-54362.

widely used because of the necessity for additional hardware and moreover usually singles rate vary during data acquisition [9]. Therefore, in most PET scans, the AC rates are estimated using delayed-window coincidences and the data are precorrected for AC events by real-time subtraction. Real-time subtraction of delayed window coincidences compensates in mean for AC events but destroys the Poisson statistics [7]. To avoid this problem, one needs to maintain the transmission and randoms measurements as two separate sinograms [8, 10]. However even if a PET system allows one to collect randoms (delayed coincidences) sinogram separately, this process would double the storage space for the acquired data. So in practice most PET centers collect and archive only the randoms precorrected data. We recommend separate acquisition and storage of delayed coincidences wherever feasible. The purpose of this paper is to provide accurate statistical methods for PET measurements with pre-subtracted delayed coincidences. Although our analysis and proposed models apply to both emission and transmission tomography, in this paper we focus on transmission tomography.

The exact log-likelihood for randoms precorrected data is intractable, so we describe and compare several approximations. For completeness, we first review the data-weighted least squares (WLS) method and the log-likelihood for the ordinary Poisson (OP) model for PET measurements. Then, we introduce a new "shifted" Poisson (SP) model [14] which matches both the first and second-order moments of the model to the underlying statistics of the precorrected data. We derive approximate analytic expressions for the variance of the different estimators and use the Cauchy-Schwarz inequality to show analytically that the proposed SP method yields lower variance than the OP method.

Secondly, we introduce a new saddle-point (SD) approximation for the pmf of precorrected measurements. The corresponding log-likelihood function is shown to have better agreement with the exact log-likelihood than the previous approximations. We apply the fast grouped-coordinate ascent algorithm [3] (with a few simple modifications) to maximize the proposed saddle-point objective function.

We also show results of 2D simulations showing that the WLS method leads to systematic bias and the OP method leads to higher variance than SP and SD methods. We also observe that SP and SD methods yield equivalent bias/variance performance whereas SP requires less computation. The contribution of this work lies in the fact that the proposed methods offer significant improvements in accuracy with minor computation increase.

## 2 Measurement Model

In conventional PET scans, the data are precorrected for AC events by *real-time* subtraction of the delayed-window coincidences [7]. The system detects coincidence events during two time windows: "prompt" window and "delayed" window. For each coincidence event in the prompt window, the corresponding sinogram bin is incremented. The statistics of these increments should be well approximated by a Poisson process. However, for coincidence events within the second delayed window, the corresponding sinogram bin is decremented, so the resultant "precorrected" measurements are *not* Poisson. Since prompt events and delayed events are independent Poisson processes, the precorrected measurements correspond to the difference of two independent Poisson random variables with variance equal to the sum of the means of the two random variables. In other words, randoms subtraction compensates in mean for AC events, but it also increases the variance of the measurement by an amount equal to the mean of AC events.

Let $\underline{Y} = [Y_1, \ldots, Y_N]'$ denote the vector of *precorrected* measurements. The precorrected measurement for the $n$th coincidence detector pair is:

$$Y_n = Y_n^{\text{prompt}} - Y_n^{\text{delay}}, \tag{1}$$

where $Y_n^{\text{prompt}}$ and $Y_n^{\text{delay}}$ are the number of coincidences within the prompt and delayed windows, respectively. Let $\mu = [\mu_1, \ldots, \mu_M]'$ denote the vector of unknown linear attenuation coefficients. For transmission scans, we assume that $Y_n^{\text{prompt}}$ and $Y_n^{\text{delay}}$ are statistically independent Poisson random variables with means $\bar{y}_n^{\text{p}}$ and $\bar{y}_n^{\text{d}}$ respectively as:

$$E\{Y_n^{\text{prompt}}\} = \bar{y}_n^{\text{p}}(\mu) = b_n e^{-l_n(\mu)} + r_n \tag{2}$$

$$E\{Y_n^{\text{delay}}\} = \bar{y}_n^{\text{d}} = r_n, \tag{3}$$

where $l_n(\mu) = \sum_{j=1}^{M} a_{nj} \mu_j$ is the total attenuation between $n$th detector pair. The $a_{nj} \geq 0$ factors have units of length and describe the tomographic system geometry. The $b_n > 0$ factors denote the blank scan counts and the $r_n \geq 0$ factors denote the mean of AC events.

Since $Y_n^{\text{prompt}}$ and $Y_n^{\text{delay}}$ are statistically independent and Poisson:

$$E\{Y_n\} = \bar{y}_n^{\text{p}}(\mu) - \bar{y}_n^{\text{d}} = b_n e^{-l_n(\mu)},$$

$$\text{Var}\{Y_n\} = \bar{y}_n^{\text{p}}(\mu) + \bar{y}_n^{\text{d}} = b_n e^{-l_n(\mu)} + 2r_n.$$

## 3 Exact Log-Likelihood

Let $\underline{y} = [y_1, \ldots, y_N]'$ be a realization of statistically independent random variables $\underline{Y}$ given in (1). Under the usual assumption of independence between different rays, one can express the exact distribution of $\underline{Y}$ using total probability:

$$P(\underline{Y} = \underline{y}; \mu) = \prod_{n=1}^{N} \sum_{m=0}^{\infty} P(Y_n^{\text{prompt}} = y_n + m; \mu) \, P(Y_n^{\text{delay}} = m)$$

$$= \prod_{n=1}^{N} \sum_{m=\lfloor -y_n \rfloor_+}^{\infty} \frac{[\bar{y}_n^{\text{p}}(\mu)]^{y_n+m} \, e^{-\bar{y}_n^{\text{p}}(\mu)}}{(y_n + m)!} \frac{r_n^m e^{-r_n}}{m!}, \tag{4}$$

where $\lfloor x \rfloor_+ = x$ if $x > 0$ and is 0 otherwise. The exact log-likelihood for $\mu$ becomes

$$L(\mu) = \log P(\underline{Y} = \underline{y}; \mu)$$

$$= \sum_{n=1}^{N} \log \left( \sum_{m=\lfloor -y_n \rfloor_+}^{\infty} \frac{[\bar{y}_n^{\text{p}}(\mu)]^{y_n+m}}{(y_n + m)!} \frac{r_n^m}{m!} \right) - (\bar{y}_n^{\text{p}}(\mu) + r_n). \tag{5}$$

Since image reconstruction is ill conditioned, usually one includes a roughness penalty $R(\mu)$ in the objective function. From the Bayesian point of view, this roughness penalty can be thought as a log-prior for $\mu$. Combining this penalty with the log-likelihood yields a penalized-likelihood objective function:

$$\Phi(\mu) = L(\mu) - R(\mu). \tag{6}$$

The goal is to estimate $\mu$ by maximizing $\Phi(\mu)$ over the nonnegative cone:

$$\hat{\mu} = \arg \max_{\mu \geq 0} \Phi(\mu). \tag{7}$$

Since the exact log-likelihood function (5) contains infinite summations, the above maximization is intractable. The following two sections develop tractable yet accurate approximations to $L(\mu)$.

# 4 Simple Approximations to the Exact Log-Likelihood

In this section, we first review the conventional approximations to $L(\mu)$: the WLS model and the conventional OP model. Then we introduce the SP model [14].

## 4.1 Quadratic Approximations

The quadratic approximation to the exact log-likelihood function results in the data-weighted least squares objective function $L_{WLS}(\mu)$ [12]:

$$L_{WLS}(\mu) = -\frac{1}{2} \sum_{n=1,\, y_n > 0}^{N} (l_n(\mu) - \hat{l}_n)^2 \frac{1}{\hat{\sigma}_n^2}, \tag{8}$$

where $\hat{l}_n = \log\left(\frac{b_n}{y_n}\right)$ is the method-of-moments estimate of the *line integral of the attenuation* $l_n(\mu)$ and $\hat{\sigma}_n^2 = \frac{y_n + 2r_n}{y_n^2}$. The $n$th weighting factor $\hat{\sigma}_n^2$ is an estimate of the variance of $\hat{l}_n(y_n)$ based on a second-order Taylor expansion around $\hat{l}_n(\bar{y}_n)$. This weighting is critical for the WLS method. The errors corresponding to projections with large values of $y_n$ are weighted more heavily. These projections pass through less dense objects and consequently have higher SNR values.

Alternatively, the choice of $\hat{\sigma}_n^2 = 1$ results in the unweighted least-squares (ULS) approach, which leads to much higher variance.

## 4.2 Ordinary Poisson (OP) Approximation

The conventional approach is to assume (approximate) that $\{Y_n\}_{n=1}^N$ are distributed as independent Poisson random variables with mean $\bar{y}_n = b_n e^{-l_n(\mu)}$, i.e.:

$$P(\underline{Y} = \underline{y}; \mu) \approx \prod_{n=1}^{N} \frac{[\bar{y}_n(\mu)]^{y_n} e^{-\bar{y}_n(\mu)}}{y_n!}. \tag{9}$$

The log-likelihood corresponding to this OP approximation is:

$$L_{OP}(\mu) = \sum_{n=1}^{N} y_n \log \bar{y}_n(\mu) - \bar{y}_n(\mu)$$

$$= \sum_{n=1}^{N} y_n \log(b_n e^{-l_n(\mu)}) - b_n e^{-l_n(\mu)}, \tag{10}$$

disregarding the constants independent of $\mu$.

## 4.3  Shifted Poisson (SP) Approximation

A better approach is to match both the first and second order moments by approximating the quantities $\{Y_n + 2r_n\}_{n=1}^{N}$ as having Poisson distributions with means $\{\bar{y}_n(\mu) + 2r_n\}$. This model leads to our proposed SP objective function:

$$L_{SP}(\mu) = \sum_{n=1}^{N} (y_n + 2r_n) \log(\bar{y}_n(\mu) + 2r_n) - (\bar{y}_n(\mu) + 2r_n),$$

$$= \sum_{n=1}^{N} (y_n + 2r_n) \log(b_n e^{-l_n(\mu)} + 2r_n) - (b_n e^{-l_n(\mu)} + 2r_n).$$

Note that although both $L_{WLS}$ and $L_{SP}$ match two moments, in WLS the second moment of $\hat{l}_n(y_n)$ is "fixed" independently of $\mu$, whereas in the SP model the moments vary with $\bar{y}_n(\mu)$ appropriately.

We have previously shown empirically that this model better agrees with the exact log-likelihood than either the WLS or OP model [14]. Next we provide an analytical result that corroborates those results.

## 4.4  Variance Analysis

To analyze the variance of each estimator, we applly the analytic approximations suggested in [2]. If $\bar{Y} = E\{\underline{Y}\}$, then using a first order Taylor expansion of $\hat{\mu}(\underline{Y})$ results in the following approximation to the covariance of $\hat{\mu}$ [2] :

$$\text{Cov}\{\hat{\mu}\} \approx P \,\text{Cov}\{\underline{Y}\} \, P^T \tag{11}$$

where $P = [-\nabla^{20}\Phi(\check{\mu}, \bar{Y})]^{-1} \nabla^{11}\Phi(\check{\mu}, \bar{Y})$ and $\check{\mu} = \arg\max_{\mu} \Phi(\mu, \bar{Y})$.

We apply (11) to find approximate expressions for the variance of the maximum likelihood estimators: $\hat{\mu}_{OP} = \arg\max_{\mu} L_{OP}(\mu)$ and $\hat{\mu}_{SP} = \arg\max_{\mu} L_{SP}(\mu)$. For this purpose we considered a highly simplified version of transmission tomography where the unknown is a scalar parameter, $i.e.$ $p = 1$. This simplified problem provides insight into the estimator bias and variance without the undue notation of the multi-parameter case. The objective functions used here can be expressed in the form:

$$\Phi(\mu, Y) = \sum_{n=1}^{N} h_n(\mu, Y).$$

Since the measurements are statistically independent, for the scalar problem the above approximation (11) reduces to:

$$\text{Var}\{\hat{\mu}\} \approx \left( \sum_{n=1}^{N} \frac{\partial^2 h_n(\check{\mu}, \bar{Y})}{\partial \mu^2} \right)^{-2} \sum_{n=1}^{N} \left[ \frac{\partial^2 h_n(\check{\mu}, \bar{Y})}{\partial \mu \, \partial Y_n} \right]^2 \text{Var}\{Y_n\}. \qquad (12)$$

With some tedious algebra, one can derive the following approximate expressions for variance of $\hat{\mu}_{OP}$ and $\hat{\mu}_{SP}$:

$$\text{Var}\{\hat{\mu}_{OP}\} \approx \frac{\sum_{n=1}^{N} a_n^2 (\bar{y}_n(\mu_t) + 2r_n)}{\left( \sum_{n=1}^{N} a_n^2 \bar{y}_n(\mu_t) \right)^2} \qquad (13)$$

$$\text{Var}\{\hat{\mu}_{SP}\} \approx \left[ \sum_{n=1}^{N} \frac{a_n^2 \bar{y}_n(\mu_t)^2}{\bar{y}_n(\mu_t) + 2r_n} \right]^{-1}, \qquad (14)$$

where $\mu_t$ denotes the true attenuation coefficient value and $\bar{y}_n(\mu) = b_n e^{-a_n \mu}$.

Letting $s_n = a_n^2 \bar{y}_n(\mu_t)$ and $t_n = a_n^2 (\bar{y}_n(\mu_t) + 2r_n)$, one can rewrite (13) and (14) as:

$$\frac{1}{\text{Var}\{\hat{\mu}_{OP}\}} \approx \frac{(\sum_n s_n)^2}{\sum_n t_n} \quad , \quad \frac{1}{\text{Var}\{\hat{\mu}_{SP}\}} \approx \sum_n \frac{s_n^2}{t_n}$$

Let $\underline{a}, \underline{b} \in \mathbb{R}^n$ such that $a_n = \dfrac{s_n}{\sqrt{t_n}}$, $b_n = \sqrt{t_n}$. Using Cauchy-Schwarz inequality: $|\underline{a}^T \underline{b}| \leq \|\underline{a}\|_2 \|\underline{b}\|_2$,

$$\sum_n s_n \leq \left( \sum_n \frac{s_n^2}{t_n} \right)^{\frac{1}{2}} \left( \sum_n t_n \right)^{\frac{1}{2}}$$

$$\left( \sum_n \frac{s_n^2}{t_n} \right)^{-1} \leq \frac{\sum_n t_n}{(\sum_n s_n)^2} \quad ,$$

so that within the accuracy of (11):

$$\text{Var}\{\hat{\mu}_{SP}\} \leq \text{Var}\{\hat{\mu}_{OP}\} , \qquad (15)$$

with equality if and only if $r_n/\bar{y}_n$ ratios are equal. For PET systems, these ratio terms are never constant, and in fact can be quite disparate. Thus we have shown the following result: the variance of the SP estimator will always be lower than the variance of the OP estimator.

# 5 Saddle-point (SD) Approximation

An alternative to the previous approximations for the exact pmf (4) of precorrected measurements is to make second order Taylor series approximations in the $z$-transform domain (i.e. on the probability generating function) and then to carry out the inverse transform. For this purpose, we have adopted the saddle-point method [5, 13].

Let $U \sim \text{Poisson}(\alpha)$, $V \sim \text{Poisson}(\beta)$ and $Y = U - V$ with pmf's $P_U(k)$, $P_V(k)$ and $P_Y(k)$ respectively. The generating function of $Y$ is:

$$G_Y(z) = \sum_k z^k P_Y(k) = G_U(z) \, G_V(z^{-1})$$

where $G_U(z) = \exp(\alpha(z - 1))$ and $G_V(z) = \exp(\beta(z - 1))$. In terms of the generating function, $P_Y(k)$ is given by the contour integral

$$P_Y(k) = \frac{1}{2\pi j} \oint_{C+} z^{-k-1} G_Y(z) \, dz = \frac{1}{2\pi j} \oint_{C+} e^{\Phi_k(z)} \, dz, \qquad (16)$$

where $j = \sqrt{-1}$ and the contour $C^+$ must lie in the region of convergence of $G_Y(z)$ and enclose the origin, and

$$\Phi_k(z) = -(k+1)\log(z) + \alpha(z-1) + \beta(z^{-1} - 1)$$

$$\frac{d\Phi_k(z)}{dz} = \Phi_k^{(1)}(z) = -\frac{(k+1)}{z} + \alpha - \frac{\beta}{z^2}$$

$$\frac{d^2\Phi_k(z)}{dz^2} = \Phi_k^{(2)}(z) = \frac{(k+1)}{z^2} + \frac{2\beta}{z^3}.$$

We observe that $\Phi_k(z)$ (and hence the integrand $e^{\Phi_k(z)}$) is convex for $z \in \mathbb{R}$, $z > 0$ and $k \geq 0$. The integrand has a minimum at $x_o \in \mathbb{R}$, $x_o > 0$ which is called the saddle point, i.e.:

$$\Phi_k^{(1)}(x_o) = -\frac{(k+1)}{x_o} + \alpha - \frac{\beta}{x_o^2} = 0 \quad \text{and} \quad x_o > 0$$

which yields

$$x_o = \frac{(k+1) + v_k}{2\alpha} = \frac{2\beta}{-(k+1) + v_k}, \qquad (17)$$

where $v_k = x_o^2 \Phi_k^{(2)}(x_o) = \sqrt{(|k| + 1)^2 + 4\alpha\beta}$.

Following [5], we deform the contour $C^+$ in (16) into a vertical line through saddle point $x_o$, as $z = x_o + jy$, $-\infty < y < \infty$ and a semicircle around the left half plane at infinity. This contour is permissible for $k \geq 0$, since the only singularities of the integrand are at $z = 0$ and $z = \infty + j0$. If $|z| \to \infty$ for $\Re[z] < x_o$ then $e^{\Phi_k(z)} \to 0$. Hence the contribution of the semicircle around the left half plane at infinity vanishes and (16) reduces to

$$P_Y(k) = \frac{1}{2\pi} \int_{-\infty}^{\infty} e^{\Phi_k(x_o + jy)} \, dy. \qquad (18)$$

Expanding $\Phi_k(z)$ in Taylor's series around $z = x_o$, one obtains:

$$\exp\left[\Phi_k(z)\right] = \exp\left[\Phi_k(x_o) + \frac{1}{2}\Phi_k^{(2)}(x_o)(z - x_o)^2 + \sum_{l=3}^{\infty}\frac{1}{l!}\Phi_k^{(l)}(x_o)(z - x_o)^l\right]$$

$$= \exp\left[\Phi_k(x_o) + \frac{1}{2}\Phi_k^{(2)}(x_o)(z - x_o)^2\right]\left[1 + \frac{\Phi_k^{(3)}(x_o)}{6}(z - x_o)^3 + \ldots\right],$$

since $\Phi_k^{(1)}(x_o) = 0$. The integral (18) becomes

$$P_Y(k) = \frac{e^{\Phi_k(x_o)}}{2\pi}\int_{-\infty}^{\infty}e^{\frac{1}{2}\Phi_k^{(2)}(x_o)(jy)^2}\left[1 + \frac{\Phi_k^{(3)}(x_o)}{6}(jy)^3 + \ldots\right]dy$$

$$= \frac{e^{\Phi_k(x_o)}}{\sqrt{2\pi\Phi_k^{(2)}(x_o)}}[1 + R] = \frac{x_o^{-k}e^{v_k - \alpha - \beta}}{\sqrt{2\pi v_k}}[1 + R] \qquad (19)$$

where

$$R = \frac{\Phi_k^{(4)}(x_o)}{8\left[\Phi_k^{(2)}(x_o)\right]^2} + \ldots$$

Using the algorithm by Rice [11], the residuum R can be written as:

$$R = \frac{1}{24(k+1)}\left[\frac{-5 + 12\sqrt{1+\eta} - 9(1+\eta)}{(1+\eta)^{3/2}}\right] + O\left[\left(\frac{1}{k+1}\right)^2\right]$$

where $\eta = \frac{4\alpha\beta}{(k+1)^2}$. The residuum asymptotically goes to zero as $k \to \infty$ and more importantly we have observed empirically that the approximation error is negligibly small even for very small values of $k$. Neglecting R in (19) results in our saddle-point approximation for the pmf $P_Y(k)$ as:

$$P_Y(k) \simeq P_Y^s(k) = \frac{x_o^{-k}e^{v_k - \alpha - \beta}}{\sqrt{2\pi v_k}}, \quad k \geq 0. \qquad (20)$$

For $k < 0$ the integrand in (16) is not guaranteed to be convex for $z > 0$. Moreover, the integrand does not vanish along the semicircle around the left half plane at infinity. Thus we use the change of variables $w = 1/z$ in (16), so that:

$$P_Y(k) = \frac{1}{2\pi j}\oint_{C+}w^{k-1}G_Y(w^{-1})\,dw = \frac{1}{2\pi j}\oint_{C+}e^{\check{\Phi}_k(w)}\,dw \qquad (21)$$

where

$$\check{\Phi}_k(w) = (k - 1)\log(w) + \alpha(w^{-1} - 1) + \beta(w - 1).$$

Following similar steps as the case for $k \geq 0$, the saddle point approximation for $k < 0$ can be shown to be :

$$P_Y(k) \simeq P_Y^s(k) = \frac{w_o^k e^{v_k - \alpha - \beta}}{\sqrt{2\pi v_k}}, \quad k < 0 \qquad (22)$$

where

$$w_o = \frac{-(k-1)+v_k}{2\beta} = \frac{2\alpha}{(k-1)+v_k}.$$

Thus, combining (20) and (22) the saddle-point (SD) approximation for the log-likelihood (5) is:

$$L_{SD}(\mu) = \sum_{n=1}^{N} \log P_Y^s(y_n; \bar{y}_n(\mu))$$

$$= \sum_{n=1}^{N} h_n^s(\mu) \tag{23}$$

where

$$h_n^s(\mu) = \begin{cases} y_n \log\left(\dfrac{\bar{y}_n(\mu)+r_n}{y_n+1+u_n(\mu)}\right) - \bar{y}_n(\mu) + u_n(\mu) - \dfrac{1}{2}\log u_n(\mu) \,, \ y_n \geq 0 \\[4mm] y_n \log\left(\dfrac{\bar{y}_n(\mu)+r_n}{y_n-1+u_n(\mu)}\right) - \bar{y}_n(\mu) + u_n(\mu) - \dfrac{1}{2}\log u_n(\mu) \,, \ y_n < 0 \end{cases} \tag{24}$$

with $u_n(\mu) = \sqrt{(|y_n|+1)^2 + 4(\bar{y}_n(\mu)+r_n)r_n}$ and disregarding constants independent of $\mu$.

Note that this approximation is considerably simpler than the exact log-likelihood (5), since no infinite sums or factorials are needed. Nevertheless, it is remarkably accurate as shown below. Also, one can observe that as $r_n \to 0$, $h_n^s(\mu) \to [y_n \log \bar{y}_n(\mu) - \bar{y}_n(\mu)] = L_{OP}(\mu)$ (to within constants independent of $\mu$), which is expected because for $r_n = 0$ the ordinary Poisson model is appropriate.

Fig. 4 shows a representative comparison of the exact log likelihood function and the approximations for noiseless data as a function of $\mu$. Although $L_{SP}(\mu)$ fits the exact log-likelihood better than $L_{WLS}(\mu)$ and $L_{OP}(\mu)$, clearly $L_{SD}(\mu)$ has the best agreement with the exact log-likelihood $L(\mu)$. In a large number of additional comparisons not shown due to space considerations, we have observed that $L_{SD}(\mu)$ agrees remarkably well with the exact log-likelihood $L(\mu)$ and clearly better than the other models.

## 6   2D Simulations

To study bias and variance properties of the estimators based on the above approximations, we performed 2D simulations. For $\mu$ we used the synthetic attenuation map shown in Fig. 1, which represents a human *abdomen* with linear attenuation coefficient 0.0096/mm. The image was a 128 by 64 array of 4.5 mm pixels. We simulated a PET transmission scan with 192 radial bins and 256 angles uniformly spaced over 180 degrees. The $a_{nj}$ factors correspond to 6 mm wide strip integrals on 3 mm center-to-center spacing. The $b_n$ factors were generated using pseudo-random log-normal variates with standard deviation of 0.3 to account for detector efficiency variations, and scaled so that $\sum_n \bar{y}_n$ was one million counts. The $r_n$ factors corresponded to a uniform field of 5% random coincidences. Pseudo-random transmission measurements were generated according to (2) and (3). For regularization, we used the modified quadratic penalty [4], which matches the spatial resolution of different estimators.

We generated 100 independent realizations of the transmission measurements. For each measurement realization, an estimate of the attenuation map was reconstructed using 20 iterations of the grouped-coordinate ascent algorithms [3] applied to the objective functions (8), (10), (11) and (23). We computed both the sample mean and sample standard deviation images for all methods.

Fig. 2 shows horizontal profiles through the sample mean images. These profiles show that WLS is *systematically* negatively biased, whereas the OP, SP and SD models are free of systematic bias. (The overshoot at the edges is due to the quadratic penalty used in the reconstruction. Even with noiseless data, this blurring effect will still be present.)

To study the variance, we computed the *ratio* of sample standard deviation images of different estimators, over all interior pixels. Fig. 3 shows the histogram of the standard deviation ratios. The OP model yields, on the average, 20% higher standard deviation than the both SP and SD models. In other words, to achieve the same noise level, the OP method would require about 40% greater scan time.

Although the standard deviation values could be decreased by using higher count rates, the ratio of standard deviations of different estimators will remain approximately same for higher count rates [2].

We performed additional simulations using the thorax phantom with nonuniform attenuation [14]. The results were comparable.

# 7   Estimates of the AC rates  $(\hat{r}_n)$

One needs to know the mean of the AC events $(r_n)$ in order to compute $L_{SP}(\mu)$ and $L_{SD}(\mu)$. Since the $r_n$ terms are not readily available from the real (precorrected) data, some estimates of the randoms must be used.

Fig. 5 displays the scatter plot of real delayed coincidence sinograms for blank scan and transmission scan data. Each point in the plot corresponds to a specific detector pair. The similarity of both delayed coincidence measurements suggests that one can acquire the delayed coincidence events during the blank scan and use them (after properly normalizing for different scan durations) as an estimate of the AC rates for transmission scans performed on the same PET system. We performed additional simulations (not shown) in which we substituted a simple constant for $r_n$ rather than the true values into the SP and SD objective functions. This approximation resulted in only a slight increase in the standard deviation (around 2%) of the SP and SD estimates without any systematic bias. These results demonstrate that both the SP and SD approximations are robust to errors in the $r_n$ estimates.

# 8 Discussion

AC events are a primary source of background noise in positron emission tomography. After the AC events are precorrected, the measurement statistics are no longer Poisson. For transmission scans, WLS method and ML method based on ordinary Poisson (OP) model lead to systematic bias and higher variance, respectively, compared to our proposed shifted Poisson (SP) model for measurement statistics which matches both the first and second-order moments.

We proposed a new approximation for the exact log-likelihood which is derived using saddle-point approximation to the pmf of precorrected measurements. Both the analysis of the error term and the log-likelihood plots and 1D simulations (not shown due to space considerations) show that the new approximation agrees very closely with the exact log-likelihood compared to previous approximations.

2D simulations show that both SP and SD models perform very closely. They are both free of systematic bias and yield reduced standard deviation (about 20%) compared to OP model. As we observed very close agreement between exact log-likelihood and SD approximation both from the log-likelihood plots and 1D simulations, we were expecting SD method to perform better than SP method. However, for the 2D simulations reported here, the SP method performed as well as SD method. Thus the SP method is particularly attractive since it requires comparable computation to OP method but has reduced variance. We plan to compare the SD and SP methods to the uniform Cramer-Rao bounds [6].

The high correlation between delayed coincidence events of blank and transmission scans suggest that one can use AC rates estimated from blank scans. We have seen that even using constant AC rates in 2D simulations resulted in only a slight increase in the standard deviation without any systematic bias. Thus the proposed SP and SD methods are robust enough for practical use.

We plan to apply the proposed method to emission tomography, where even higher AC rates than the transmission tomography are common, particularly in 3D PET. Moreover, in 3D PET, very large data sets are likely to preclude separate acquisition of random coincidences, so the real-time subtraction methods are usually used for emission scans. So the potential benefit of the proposed models should be even greater.

# References

1. M E Casey and E J Hoffman. Quantitation in positron emission computed tomography: 7 A technique to reduce noise in accidental coincidence measurements and coincidence efficiency calibration. *J. Comp. Assisted Tomo.*, 10(5):845–850, 1986.
2. J A Fessler. Mean and variance of implicitly defined biased estimators (such as penalized maximum likelihood): Applications to tomography. *IEEE Tr. Im. Proc.*, 5(3):493–506, March 1996.
3. J A Fessler, E P Ficaro, N H Clinthorne, and K Lange. Grouped-coordinate ascent algorithms for penalized-likelihood transmission image reconstruction. *IEEE Tr. Med. Im.*, 16, April 1997. To appear.

4. J A Fessler and W L Rogers. Spatial resolution properties of penalized-likelihood image reconstruction methods: Space-invariant tomographs. *IEEE Tr. Im. Proc.*, 5(9):1346–58, September 1996.

5. C Helstrom. Approximate evaluation of detection probabilities in radar and optical communications. *IEEE Tr. Aero. Elec. Sys.*, 14(4):630–40, 1978.

6. A O Hero, J A Fessler, and M Usman. Exploring estimator bias-variance tradeoffs using the uniform CR bound. *IEEE Tr. Sig. Proc.*, 44(8):2026–41, August 1996.

7. E J Hoffman, S C Huang, M E Phelps, and D E Kuhl. Quantitation in positron emission computed tomography: 4 Effect of accidental coincidences. *J. Comp. Assisted Tomo.*, 5(3):391–400, 1981.

8. E Ü Mumcuoğlu, R M Leahy, and S R Cherry. Bayesian reconstruction of PET images: methodology and performance analysis. *Phys. Med. Biol.*, 41:1777–1807, 1996.

9. J M Ollinger and J A Fessler. Positron emission tomography. *IEEE Signal Proc. Mag.*, 14(1):43–55, January 1997.

10. D G Politte and D L Snyder. Corrections for accidental coincidences and attenuation in maximum-likelihood image reconstruction for positron-emission tomography. *IEEE Tr. Med. Im.*, 10(1):82–89, March 1991.

11. S O Rice. Uniform asymptotic expansions for saddle point integrals-application to a probability distribution occuring in noise theory. *Bell Syst. Tech J.*, 47:1971–2013, November 1968.

12. K Sauer and C Bouman. A local update strategy for iterative reconstruction from projections. *IEEE Tr. Sig. Proc.*, 41(2):534–548, February 1993.

13. D L Snyder, C W Helstrom, A D Lanterman, M Faisal, and R L White. Compensation for readout noise in CCD images. *J. Opt. Soc. Amer. Ser. A*, 12(2):272–83, February 1995.

14. M Yavuz and J A Fessler. Objective functions for tomographic reconstruction from randoms-precorrected PET scans. In *Proc. IEEE Nuc. Sci. Symp. Med. Im. Conf.*, 1996. To appear.

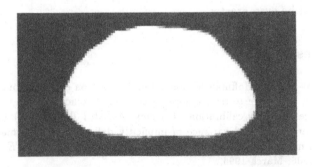

**Fig. 1.** Simulated abdomen attenuation map.

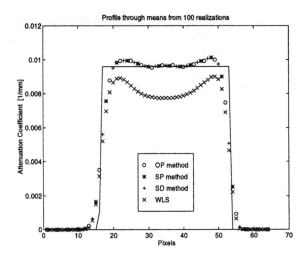

**Fig. 2.** Horizontal profile through the sample mean images for abdomen phantom. The WLS method has a systematic negative bias. The ordinary Poisson (OP), shifted Poisson (SP) and saddle-point (SD) methods are free of this systematic negative bias.

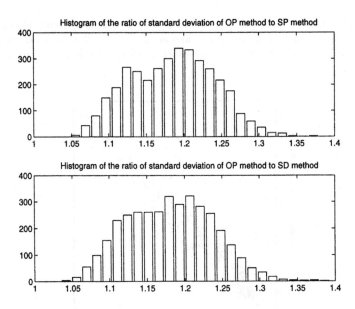

**Fig. 3.** Histogram of the ratio of standard deviations in reconstructions of the abdomen phantom. The ordinary Poisson (OP) method yields, on the average, 20% higher standard deviation than the proposed shifted Poisson (SP) and saddle-point (SD) methods.

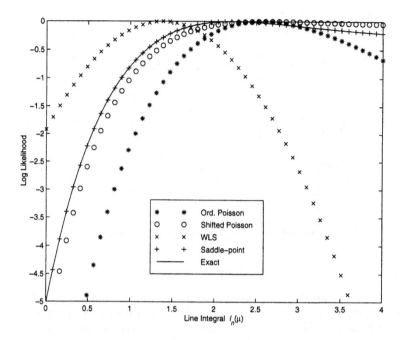

**Fig. 4.** Representative comparison of exact log-likelihood function with objective functions of different models as a function of line integral $l_n(\mu)$. Randoms rate is 5%. The proposed saddle-point approximation agrees with exact log-likelihood significantly better than the other models.

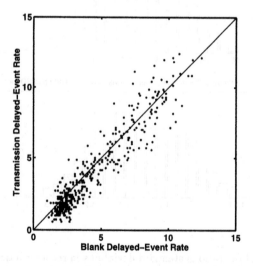

**Fig. 5.** Scatter plot of delayed coincidence event of blank and transmission scans.

# Registration of 3D Medical Images Using Simple Morphological Tools

J.B. Antoine Maintz, Petra A. van den Elsen, and Max A. Viergever

Image Sciences Institute, PO Box 85500, AZU-E.01.334, NL-3508 GA Utrecht, the Netherlands. Email: Twan.Maintz@cv.ruu.nl

**Abstract.** Multimodal medical images are often of too different a nature to be registered on the basis of the image grey values only. It is the purpose of this paper to construct operators that extract similar structures from these images that will enable registration by simple grey value based methods, such as maximization of cross-correlation. These operators can be constructed using only basic morphological tools such as erosion and dilation. Simple versions of these operators are easily implemented on any computer system. We will show that accurate registration of images of various modalities (MR, CT, SPECT and PET) can be obtained using this approach.

## 1 Introduction

Registration and hybrid visualization of 3D medical images has received ample attention from researchers in the past few years. The reasons for this may be clear: there are numerous applications in diagnostic as well as treatment settings, benefitting from integrating the complementary character of multimodal images. Notable application fields include neurosurgery and radiation therapy planning (Taylor, Lavallée, Burdea & Mösges 1996). For example, in the latter field, dose calculation is done best using a CT image, while often the target area can best be identified in an MR image. A second important reason is the recent availibility of computing power and computer architecture that can handle the entire bulk of 3D data –even though the size of clinical images has also grown considerably– while older methods often required data reduction of the images to, *e.g.*, a limited point set, surface, or abstract representation. Such computing power gives access to a class of so-called *voxel based* methods, which are preferable to previous methods in most cases.

Existing 3D rigid –*i.e.*, restricted to translational and rotational transformations– registration methods can be divided into extrinsic (external attachment based) and intrinsic (patient related) approaches (van den Elsen, Pol & Viergever 1993). Examples of extrinsic registration methods include methods based on fiducial markers (van den Elsen & Viergever 1994), a facial mould (Schad, Boesecke, Schlegel, Hartmann, Sturm, Strauss & Lorenz 1987) or a stereotactic frame (Vandermeulen 1991). Compared to these methods, voxel based methods (Woods, Maziotta & Cherry 1993, Hill, Studholme & Hawkes 1994, Maintz, van den Elsen & Viergever 1994, Maintz, van den Elsen & Viergever 1995, Studholme, Hill & Hawkes 1995, Viola & Wells III 1995, van den Elsen, Maintz, Pol & Viergever 1995, Maintz, van den Elsen & Viergever 1996, Maes, Collignon, Vandermeulen, Marchal & Suetens 1996*a*, Maes, Collignon, Vandermeulen, Marchal & Suetens 1996*b*) are more patient friendly, and show higher reproducibility. Moreover, retrospective registration is now possible, as are extensions to non-rigid registration. Examples of intrinsic registration approaches other than voxel based methods are landmark registration (Evans, Marrett, Collins & Peters 1989, Hill, Hawkes, Crossman, Gleeson, Cox, Bracey, Strong & Graves 1991), surface based registration (Levin, Pelizzari, Chen, Chen & Cooper 1988, Pelizzari, Chen, Spelbring, Weichselbaum & Chen 1989), and hybrids of these techniques. Compared to these methods, voxel based methods are better reproducible and less labour intensive. Voxel based methods are considered extremely promising with respect to accuracy (Viergever, Maintz, Stokking, van den Elsen & Zuiderveld 1995).

In this paper, we investigate the use of morphological operators for voxel based registration. Multimodal medical images are often of too different a nature to be registered directly on the basis of the image grey values only. It is the purpose of this paper to construct operators that extract similar structures from these images that will enable registration by maximization of the cross-correlation or a similar measure. The methods constructed are related to conventional surface based methods. However, instead of binary-valued surfaces we employ real-valued 'surfaceness' images obtained from the original images, thus employing more of the available image content. The operators involved can be constructed using only concatenations of basic image operations such as computing the maximum or minimum of a small region. We will show that accurate registration of images from various different modalities (MR, CT, SPECT and PET) can be obtained using this approach.

## 2 Methods

In the following section we will define the morphological operators featuring in our registration approach. The features extracted from the images by these operators can be used for registration by optimizing the cross-correlation value. Section 2.2 details the cross-correlation maximization algorithm. The next sections describe the morphological operator compounds that can be employed in three specific applications: CT-MR registration (2.3), MR-SPECT registration (2.4), and MR-PET registration (2.5). The final section (2.6) describes verification methods for the registrations obtained. Registration results of the developed methods will be shown in section 3.

### 2.1 Morphological operations

The operators used in this paper stem from the field of mathematical morphology (Serra 1982, Haralick, Sternberg & Zhuang 1987, Serra 1988); all are well known and frequently used there. They are simple in the sense that they usually have an intuitive geometrical interpretation, and that they allow straightforward implementations on a computer platform, although fast and elegant approaches require quite some sophistication.

The *erosion* $\varepsilon$ of a function $f(x)$ by a symmetrical planar structuring element $B$ is defined as $\varepsilon(f)(x) = \inf_{b \in B}(f(x - b))$. The dual operation of erosion is called *dilation* ($\delta$), which is defined by $\delta(f)(x) = \sup_{b \in B}(f(x - b))$. The effects of the erosion and dilation operations are usually intuitively clear: erosion will "eat away", abrade the boundary of objects, whereas dilation will expand objects at the boundary.

Erosion and dilation are dual operations, *i.e.*, erosion of $f(x)$ equals dilation of the complement of $f(x)$. They are not inverses, owing to the non-linear character of the operations; there are multiple input images that produce the same result when eroded. The smallest pseudo-inverse, *i.e.*, the composition of erosion and dilation, has some interesting properties. The morphological *opening* $\gamma$ is defined as the composition of erosion and dilation, the morphological *closing* $\varphi$ is defined as the composition of dilation and erosion: $\gamma = \delta\varepsilon$ and $\varphi = \varepsilon\delta$. Their effects are again intuitively clear: a closing removes holes and thin cavities, and an opening opens up holes that are near (with respect to the size of the structuring element) a boundary, and removes small object protuberances. An example is given in figure 1.

Since the erosion and dilation operations act most prominently on object boundaries, the *differences* between the eroded, the dilated and the original images bring out edge information of the original. The *morphological gradient* $g$ is defined as the difference between a dilated and an eroded image: $g(f) = \delta(f) - \varepsilon(f)$. This 'thick' gradient

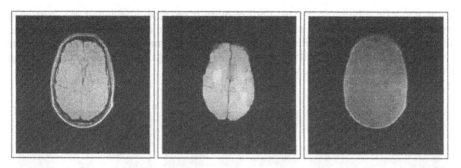

**Fig. 1.** Example of opening (middle) and closing (right) by a square structuring element on a grey valued MR image (left).

can be decomposed into two 'half' gradients: an 'inner' gradient $g^- = f - \varepsilon(f)$ adhering to the inside of objects, *i.e.*, to the bright side of the edge, and an outer gradient $g^+ = \delta(f) - f$.

The ideas of erosion and dilation can also be employed for contrast enhancement and deblurring of grey valued images. The contrast can be enhanced by replacing each pixel value by either the dilated or eroded value, whichever one was closer to the original value:

$$f_{\text{enh}} = \begin{cases} \delta(f) & \delta(f) - f \le f - \varepsilon(f) \\ \varepsilon(f) & \text{otherwise.} \end{cases}$$

This technique can be shown to exactly reconstruct a convex homogeneous object that has been blurred by Gaussian convolution. This result does not hold in the general case, but nonetheless pleasing results can be obtained, as figure 2 shows. Upon iterating the deblurring operation, it always converges to a stable result (Kramer & Bruckner 1975).

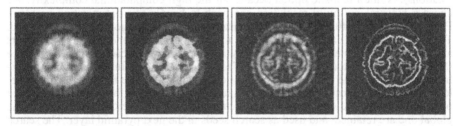

**Fig. 2.** Example of deblurring applied to a SPECT image. From left to right: the original $128 \times 128$ SPECT image, the image after a single step of deblurring with a $3 \times 3$ square, the inner gradient of the original, and the inner gradient of the deblurred version.

It is often desirable to remove small objects from images, while keeping larger objects completely intact. The standard opening does not have the right properties to do this, because the shape of objects is not completely preserved. An approach to remedy this is to use *opening by reconstruction*. Before defining this, we need the concept of *geodesic dilation* $\delta_g = \min(\delta(f), g)$, where $g$ is a 'control' image: $f$ is dilated in the usual way, but constrained so as to never grow 'outside' of the control image $g$.

If the geodesic dilation is iterated until stability is reached, it is called *reconstruction by dilation*. The opening by reconstruction, finally, is the composition of erosion, and reconstruction by dilation. Here, the erosion removes small and thin objects, and the following reconstruction by dilation brings the remaining objects back to their original form. An example can be seen in figure 3.

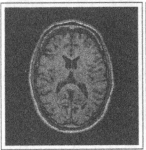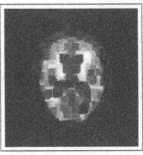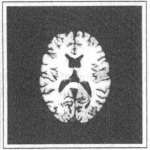

**Fig. 3.** Example of opening by reconstruction of an MR image. Left: original image. Middle: eroded image. Right: final image, after reconstruction and subsequent thresholding. The original image is used as the control image in the reconstruction.

## 2.2 Registration method

Our aim is to use the morphological operators described in the previous section to extract feature images from multimodal images that show enough similarity as to allow for rigid registration by maximizing the cross-correlation value.

An exhaustive search of the 6-dimensional parameter space (three translations, three rotations), is not a realistic option because of the high computational complexity. We chose a *hierarchical* multi-resolution approach to handle this optimization problem. From each of the feature images to be registered a multi-resolution pyramid is created. The bottom layer of each pyramid equals the original image, and a number of layers are created by repeated downsampling by a factor of two in each dimension. Three (SPECT/PET) to five (high resolution CT) layers are created. In the top layer an exhaustive search of the parameter space is now feasible. We use the term 'exhaustive' loosely here, as we restrict the parameter space to realistic transformations. The global optimum found in the search, as well as local optima within a certain percentage of the global one are retained, and used as search seeds in the next pyramid layer. The search spaces in adjacent layers are narrowly tuned lest to miss a local optimum.

## 2.3 Application: CT and MR registration

Direct use of the morphological (inner) gradient often causes misregistration when the cross-correlation is optimized in the above described way, especially where images with a large slice thickness are concerned. The reason for this is that various edges, notably the skull and skin edges, are frequently very close together, which causes the wrong edges to be aligned by the registration algorithm. We therefore extended the method to only use the skin edge. To detect this edge using a morphological inner gradient, we first need to remove all internal structures in the images, so the inner gradient acts upon an image containing only the skin edge. These internal structures can be removed by applying a closing for the removal of dark structures followed by an opening for the removal of bright structures. In the case of MRI, the nature of the images is such that the opening is not even necessary. The only parameters that need to be established are the sizes of the structuring elements used, which should be large enough to obtain the desired effect, while kept sufficiently small to minimize distortion effects. The operations actually used can be found in table 1. As the table shows, a different approach is used for MR T1 and T2 weighted images, which is necessitated by the completely different nature of the images. With poor quality initial images, both the CT and MR final edgeness images can still be improved (*i.e.* made more homogeneous) by applying a threshold. The actual threshold value does not appear to be critical, and we fixed it to 20% of the image maximum after processing. Figure 4 shows examples of the final feature images.

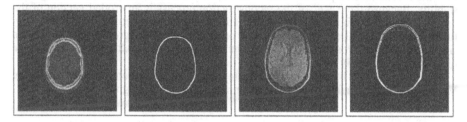

**Fig. 4.** Examples of the original and edgeness feature images used in CT (left two images) to MR (right two images) registration.

It may seem –when looking at the final feature images– that the method reduces to surface based registration. The feature images, however, are not nearly binary, but have an extensive grey range, nor are the depicted structures thin. These very properties ensure proper convergence of the registration method.

### 2.4 Application: SPECT to MR-T1 registration

With SPECT[1] to MR-T1 registration, we use the same approach as with CT to MR registration: to avoid the risk of misregistration, *i.e.*, the alignment of anatomically non-corresponding edges upon using simple edgeness images, we use a morphological operator to select the skin edge from the MR. The edgeness is then computed both from MR and SPECT by applying a morphological inner gradient. The SPECT edgeness image can be improved upon by using morphological deblurring as a preprocessing step. Examples of the SPECT feature images can be seen in figure 2 and of the MR feature image in figure 4.

### 2.5 Application: PET to MR registration

Registration of PET[2] to MR-T1 images based on the skin edge is not feasible, since the skin edge cannot be seen in a PET image like in a SPECT image. Our PET/MR registration is therefore based on the cortex edge, rather than the skin edge as with SPECT/MR registration.

---

[1] In this application we use $^{99m}$Tc-HMPAO perfusion SPECT images.

[2] In this application we use FDG (fluorodeoxyglucose) or ethyl 8-fluoro-5,6-dihydro-5-methyl-6-oxo- H-imidazo [1,5-$\alpha$]-[1,4] benzodiazepine-3-carboxylate (Flumazenil) PET images.

The extraction of the cortex edge from the PET image is relatively easy, since it is the dominant edge of the image. We improve the inner gradient image in much the same way as before (cf. CT to MR registration) by removing internal structures with a closing and an opening. In addition, since PET images are somewhat more blurry than MR images, we sharpen the image by a deblurring operation.

In the MR image, we suppress the skin edge, and endeavor to 'select' only the cortex edge. We can achieve this by removing all structure outside of the cortex in the MR image, by applying an opening to it. This can either be a plain opening or an opening by reconstruction. While the latter produces less artefacts, it is also more time consuming to perform. The disadvantage of using an opening is that the cortex and the structures outside of it need to be well separated in order for the opening to create the desired result. Although this condition is met for transverse image slices above the eyes, it breaks down for slices near the base of the brain. A solution to this is to simply stop the reconstruction process after a number of iterations, instead of iterating until stability. Because the 'seed' of the reconstruction process is an eroded version of the original image (see figure 3), the first iterations will reconstruct the cortex, and only further iterations will allow the skin and other structures to 'grow back'. Since the size of the applied erosion is known, the number of iterations after which to stop the reconstruction is easily estimated.

The proposed PET feature images for registration can be seen in figure 5, and the MR feature images before computing the inner gradient in the figures 1 and 3.

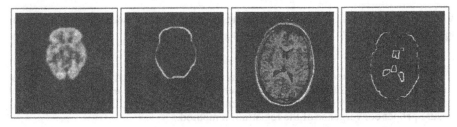

**Fig. 5.** Example of PET and MR feature images as used in PET to MR registration. The left two images show an original PET slice and the corresponding slice from the feature volume, and the right two images show an original and feature MR slice.

For PET to MR-T2 registration, the above described method for PET to MR-T1 registration can be used. However, since the cortex edge is much brighter in T2 weighted images than in T1 weighted MR images, we can suffice with a simpler feature extracting scheme for the MR image: an opening followed by a threshold and an inner gradient.

## 2.6 Accuracy verification of the registration

In this paper, we use the methods of visual inspection and comparison to registration based on fiducial skin markers in all of the applications. The visual inspection was performed by segmenting meaningful contours from a slice of one image, and overlaying them onto a corresponding slice from a registered image. This procedure is carried out using around four transversal slices, as well as the midsagittal and midcoronal slice from the MR image involved. The 'fit' of the contours is then assessed visually. In the case of CT to MR registration, we additionally used a cadaver study for validation, and also compared the registration results to those obtained by an earlier method: $L_w$ *correlation*, a method which is based on optimizing the cross-correlation of edgeness images extracted from the original images involved by means of convolution with

| From \ To | MR-T1 | MR-T2 |
|---|---|---|
| CT | CT: close(4), open(8), inner grad.<br>MR: close(4), inner grad. | CT: close(4), open(8), inner grad.<br>MR: open(1), threshold(low), close(2), inner grad. |
| SPECT | SPECT: deblur, inner grad.<br>MR: close(4), inner grad. | |
| PET | PET: deblur, close(3), open(3), inner grad.<br>MR: open by reconstruction, inner grad. | PET: deblur, close(3), open(3), inner grad.<br>MR: open(4), threshold(low), inner grad. |

**Table 1.** Summary of morphological registration methods. Bracketed numbers indicate the structuring element half size used (in millimeters). Only square structuring elements were used.

Gaussian derivatives, see (Maintz, van den Elsen & Viergever 1997). Since this method was designed specifically for CT to MR registration, it could not be used to verify the registrations involving SPECT or PET. Finally, with PET to MR registration and CT to MR registration, 9 patients were implanted with four fixed markers, which were used to establish a comparative registration (West et al. 1996). The verification methods used are summarized in table 2.

| | visual inspection | skin markers | fixed markers | comparison to $L_w$ correlation | cadaver study |
|---|---|---|---|---|---|
| CT/MR | ✓ | ✓ | ✓ | ✓ | ✓ |
| PET/MR | ✓ | ✓ | ✓ | np | np |
| SPECT/MR | ✓ | ✓ | – | np | np |

**Table 2.** Summary of verification methods used. Legend: ✓: method used, –: method not used, **np**: use of the method is not possible.

# 3 Results

## 3.1 Application: CT to MR registration

**Studies validated by fiducial skin markers and $L_w$ correlation** The patients involved in these studies were supplied with three markers glued to the skin just before image acquisition (van den Elsen, Viergever, van Huffelen, van der Meij & Wieneke 1991, van den Elsen & Viergever 1994). The markers are attached near the temporomandibular joints and at the nasion. The marked points can be located with subslice accuracy using near-automatic —two user-identified seed points are required for each marker— methods in each of the images involved. The marker based registration is then performed by aligning (in the least squares sense) the three points located in each of the images involved.

In previous work (Maintz et al. 1995, Maintz et al. 1997), we examined the use of edgeness images –as generated from CT and MR volumes by means of computing a scaled gradient magnitude– for registration purposes. The edgeness computing operator, called $L_w$, appeared well suited for the task of CT to MR registration.

The two studies involved[3] were registered by means of the new morphologically based method, as well the above mentioned skin marker and $L_w$ based methods. As a measure for the difference between the various registration results, we use the *maximum* and *mean* distance between two corresponding voxels as transformed by the different registration results. We compute these distances taking into account all voxels within a sphere containing the entire head, so these measures are in fact overstimates of the 'true' error, *i.e.* the error based only on patient related voxels. Table 3 shows the maximum and mean distances between all of the registrations. Please note that these distances are not error measures, as the registration used for reference will also contain a certain error. The results of the visual inspection was that shifting the registered contours did not improve the morphologically based registration, and that in a number of image areas there is a clear preference for the morphologically based match over the marker based registration.

|  | | Study 1 | | | Study 2 | |
|---|---|---|---|---|---|---|
|  | | Morph. | $L_w$ | | Morph. | $L_w$ |
| Maximum distance | Marker | 6.8 | 3.3 | Marker | 4.2 | 6.0 |
|  | Morph. | | 4.3 | Morph. | | 5.8 |
|  | | Morph. | $L_w$ | | Morph. | $L_w$ |
| Mean distance | Marker | 3.9 | 1.9 | Marker | 2.8 | 3.4 |
|  | Morph. | | 2.6 | Morph. | | 3.3 |

**Table 3.** Maximum and mean distances (in millimeters) between CT to MR registrations as obtained by marker based, $L_w$ based, and morphologically based registrations.

**Studies validated by fixed fiducial markers** The patient group involved here comprises seven patients, each implanted with four fixed fiducial markers, any trace of which was removed from the images before feature detection was applied. The reference registration was computed based on the fiducials. The validation of our morphologically based registration was done in a more elaborate way than in the previous study, namely by computing the maximum and median distance between the two registrations in ten small anatomically relevant volumes of interest, which were located in the MR image by clinical experts[4]. Per patient, six registrations were performed: the CT was registered to a proton density (PD) weighted MR image, a T1 weighted MR image, a T2 weighted MR image, and geometrically rectified (Chang & Fitzpatrick 1992) ver-

---

[3] Study I contained a 256 matrix, 200-slice transversal T1-weighted FFE sequence MR image, with voxel dimensions of $0.98 \times 0.98 \times 1.0mm$, obtained on a 1.5 T Philips Gyroscan S15, and a 256 matrix, 100-slice transversal CT image, with voxel dimensions $0.94 \times 0.94 \times 1.55mm$, obtained on a Philips Tomoscan 350. Study II contained a 256 matrix, 100-slice transversal T1-weighted FFE sequence MR image, with voxel dimensions $0.9 \times 0.9 \times 1.55mm$, obtained on a Philips Gyroscan T5, and a 256 matrix, 128-slice transversal CT image, with voxel dimensions $0.7 \times 0.7 \times 1.5mm$, obtained on a philips Tomoscan LX. These images are –in terms of image quality– at the high end of current clinical practice.

[4] The method of computing the maximum distance differs from the one used in the previous study, since this particular validation study was part of an off-site blinded registration validation protocol. This is also the reason why median distances are used in this validation study instead of mean distances.

sions[5] of all of the MR images[6]. An advantage of this patient group is that the fixed markers are most likely more reliable than the skin markers used in the previous section. The image quality in this group is considerably poorer, but not unrealistically so with respect to today's clinical practice. The results can be viewed in table 4. Note that, in this particular study, the geometrical rectification of the MR sets did not significantly alter the registration results.

The results of the visual inspection were less good than in the previous section. Although the actual inspection is made more difficult by the relatively poor quality of the images and the thicker slices, it is obvious that, at least for a number of patients, the morphologically based registrations could be improved.

| Study # | Maximum distances | | | | | | | Median distances | | | | | | |
|---|---|---|---|---|---|---|---|---|---|---|---|---|---|---|
| | 1 | 2 | 3 | 4 | 5 | 6 | 7 | 1 | 2 | 3 | 4 | 5 | 6 | 7 |
| CT-MR(PD) | 4.7 | 11.0 | 19.0 | 6.8 | 8.2 | 9.9 | 4.7 | 4.0 | 5.5 | 8.9 | 2.7 | 4.0 | 4.5 | 3.7 |
| CT-MR(T1) | 7.4 | 12.8 | 8.4 | 9.1 | 9.1 | 10.5 | 4.0 | 5.6 | 7.0 | 7.6 | 8.4 | 4.7 | 4.8 | 3.6 |
| CT-MR(T2) | 4.2 | 3.4 | 6.1 | 5.1 | 6.0 | 6.3 | 5.0 | 3.4 | 3.2 | 5.3 | 4.8 | 4.6 | 4.0 | 4.4 |
| CT-MR(PD rect) | 1.4 | 9.9 | 7.3 | 9.0 | 7.4 | 6.4 | 1.4 | 1.2 | 6.7 | 6.9 | 7.2 | 3.0 | 3.2 | 0.8 |
| CT-MR(T1 rect) | 5.2 | 10.5 | 7.5 | 14.2 | 8.6 | - | 1.7 | 4.6 | 6.7 | 6.9 | 11.7 | 4.2 | - | 1.1 |
| CT-MR(T2 rect) | 4.9 | 6.5 | 5.4 | 3.4 | 3.7 | 6.2 | 4.4 | 4.5 | 5.3 | 4.6 | 3.2 | 3.0 | 5.1 | 3.8 |

**Table 4.** Maximum and median distances (in millimeters) computed over 10 anatomically relevant volumes of interest, between our morphologically based registrations and a reference registration based on fixed fiducials. The dash indicates the rectified MR volume was not available.

**Study validated by a cadaver study** One cadaver study[7] was included in the validation experiments. Cadaver based validation has several attractive properties: The images are free of motion artefacts, there is no need to pay heed to radiation dose with the CT acquisition, i.e., the field-of-view can be chosen arbitrarily large, and external and internal markers can be attached and inserted without paying much attention to possible tissue damage. On the other hand, post-mortem changes in the anatomy could possibly make the data unrealistic.

The reference registration (Hemler, van den Elsen, Sumanaweera, Napel, Drace & Adler 1995) was obtained by inserting four glass hollow rods ($1.5/3.0mm$ inside/outside diameter) into the head of a human cadaver at different angles. These tubes were filled with a contrast agent, and detected in each of the modalities. The center lines of the detected tubes were used to compute the maximum and mean distances. Before applying the morphologically based registration method, the tube structures were eliminated from the images.

Since the contained (scanned) volume of the head in the CT image is of a size seldom encountered in clinical practice, these data provide us with an opportunity to simulate more clinically relevant registration cases by selecting an appropriate volume from the CT image, while keeping the reference registration based on the entire scanned

---

[5] Except for patient 6, MR T1.

[6] The CT images were 512 matrix, approximately 30 tranversal slices, with voxel dimensions $0.65 \times 0.65 \times 4.0mm$, obtained on a Siemens Dr-H. The MR (PD, T1 and T2-weighted) images were 256 matrix, approximately 23 transversal slices, SE sequence, with voxel dimension $1.25 \times 1.25 \times 4.0mm$, obtained on a 1.5T Siemens SP.

[7] The CT image was a 512 matrix, 180-slice transversal image, with voxel dimensions of $0.67 \times 0.67 \times 1.0mm$, obtained on a GE HiSpeed Advantage Helical CT. The MR image was a 256 matrix, 124-slice transversal 3D GRASS sequence image, with voxel dimensions $1.09 \times 1.09 \times 1mm$, obtained on a GE Signa 1.5T.

volume. Also, from the original volumes images with thicker slices were simulated. The morphologically based registration was applied to all of the original and simulated volumes separately, and the registration results were compared to the reference registration based on the entire high-resolution volumes. The maximum and mean distances are given in table 5. The visual inspection showed that the registrations were accurate, with the exception of the registration using only the lower part of the CT volume. In the latter case an error in the order of a few pixels could be observed in some image areas.

| Images used | Maximum distance | Mean distance |
|---|---|---|
| original volumes | 1.1 | 0.4 |
| 3mm slices | 2.5 | 1.0 |
| 5mm slices | 3.7 | 2.1 |
| lower CT volume only | 4.6 | 2.2 |
| upper CT volume only | 2.1 | 0.7 |

**Table 5.** The maximum and mean distances (in millimeters) between the morphologically based registrations and the reference registration of a cadaver study.

## 3.2 Application: SPECT and MR registration

In this application, $^{99m}$Tc-HMPAO SPECT images were registered to T1-weighted MR images[8]. The patient group comprised five patients, and the reference registration was provided by means of fiducial skin markers. Initially, the patient group was much larger, but, owing to the cumbersome nature in terms of image acquisition –the group consisted of children with tics and concentrative disorders– only in five cases could the markers be used successfully. This in itself is already an argument in favor of retrospective registration techniques. The maximum and mean distances between the marker based (reference) registration and the morphologically based registration of the five remaining patients are listed and table 6. The visual inspection gives the impression of imprecise

| | Study # | | | | |
|---|---|---|---|---|---|
| | 1 | 2 | 3 | 4 | 5 |
| Maximum distance | 15.6 | 7.8 | 6.2 | 12.6 | 10.9 |
| Mean distance | 8.3 | 3.9 | 3.0 | 6.5 | 8.5 |

**Table 6.** The maximum and mean distances (in millimeters) between the marker based (reference) registration and the morphologically based registrations of five SPECT to MR registrations.

results when viewing most of the marker based registrations. Two of the morphologically based registrations could also be improved upon. The inaccuracy is also reflected in the relatively large errors in the table. We suspect the sometimes severe motion artefacts in the images to hamper proper registrations.

We can as yet not draw definite conclusions regarding the quality of the morphologically based registration, because of the poor quality of the images used, and the lack of precision in the marker based reference registation. More images need to be acquired for proper tuning and verification of the morphologically based registration method.

---

[8] The MR images were 256 matrix, 127 slice, FFE sequence T1-weighted transversal images, with voxel dimensions $0.78 \times 0.78 \times 1.25mm$, obtained on a Philips Gyroscan T5. The SPECT images were 64 matrix, with approximately 50 slices, $^{99m}$Tc-HMPAO transversal images, with voxel dimensions $3.91 \times 3.91 \times 3.56mm$, obtained on a Picker PRISM 3000.

## 3.3  Application: PET to MR registration

Within this application, we used two types of validation: fixed implanted fiducial markers, and skin fiducial markers. In both cases visual inspection was also applied. The verification is the same as in the case of the CT to MR registration application: with the fixed markers, the median and maximum distances in ten anatomically relevant volumes of interest are computed, whereas with the skin markers the maximum and mean distances in a sphere containing the entire head are computed.

**Studies validated by fixed fiducial markers** Seven patient studies were used in these experiments (of which five concern patients also used in the CT to MR registration as validated by fixed fiducials). Of each patient, three MR studies and a PET study were acquired[9]. Of five patients the MR studies were also geometrically corrected (Chang & Fitzpatrick 1992). The registration results can be seen in table 7. Visual inspection is hard compared to CT to MR inspection, owing to the relatively poor image quality. The accuracy as assessed from visual inspection correlates well in a qualitative sense with the differences listed in table 7.

| Study # | Maximum distances | | | | | | | Median distances | | | | | | |
|---|---|---|---|---|---|---|---|---|---|---|---|---|---|---|
| | 1 | 2 | 3 | 4 | 5 | 6 | 7 | 1 | 2 | 3 | 4 | 5 | 6 | 7 |
| PET-MR(PD) | 8.0 | 7.7 | 8.1 | 5.6 | 7.6 | 9.8 | 7.5 | 3.6 | 4.9 | 3.6 | 3.4 | 4.9 | 6.4 | 5.8 |
| PET-MR(T1) | 5.5 | 10.6 | 3.8 | 3.9 | 5.9 | 5.1 | 4.0 | 2.6 | 8.6 | 2.3 | 2.5 | 4.8 | 3.7 | 3.3 |
| PET-MR(T2) | 7.2 | 12.7 | 6.4 | 15.0 | 4.0 | 13.1 | 8.8 | 3.7 | 6.3 | 3.2 | 11.6 | 2.3 | 8.1 | 5.4 |
| PET-MR(PD rect) | 5.4 | 6.9 | 5.2 | 6.6 | 9.2 | - | - | 3.6 | 6.6 | 3.6 | 4.3 | 5.9 | - | - |
| PET-MR(T1 rect) | 6.2 | 4.4 | 4.5 | - | 7.7 | - | - | 4.5 | 3.2 | 3.7 | - | 5.1 | - | - |
| PET-MR(T2 rect) | 5.4 | 9.0 | 4.1 | 10.9 | 3.6 | - | - | 3.9 | 7.7 | 3.4 | 10.6 | 2.2 | - | - |

**Table 7.** Maximum and Median distances (in millimeters) computed over 10 anatomically relevant volumes of interest, between our morphologically based registrations and a reference registration based on fixed fiducials. If there is a dash in the table, the rectified MR volume was not available.

**Studies validated by skin fiducial markers** Four patient studies were involved in these experiments. Of three patients MR T1 weighted, MR T2 weighted, PET FDG, and PET Flumazenil images[10] were made. Of the fourth patient only an MR T1 weighted and a PET FDG study was made. For various logistic reasons, notably the short half life of the [11]C based Flumazenil, no markers were used in the Flumazenil studies. The markers in one of the FDG studies could not be detected properly because the used (clinically defined) field-of-view did not allow for proper inclusion of one of the markers. The remaining maximum and mean distances between the marker based registrations and the morphologically based registrations are listed in table 8. The visual inspection

---

[9] The MR images were respectively PD, T1 and T2-weighted transversal SE sequence images, with a 256 matrix, containing approximately 23 slices, with voxel dimension $1.25 \times 1.25 \times 4.0mm$, obtained on a 1.5T Siemens SP. The PET image was a 128 matrix, 15 slice transversal FDG ([18]F-fluorodeoxyglucose) image with voxel dimensions $2.59 \times 2.59 \times 8.0mm$, obtained on a Siemens/CTI ECAT 933/08-16.

[10] The T1 weighted MR images were 256 matrix, 127 slice FFE sequence images, with voxel dimensions $0.98 \times 0.98 \times 1.2mm$. The T2 weighted images were 256 matrix, 130 slice TSE sequence images, with voxel dimensions equal to the T1 weighted image. Both MR images were obtained on a Philips Gyroscan T5. The PET images, both Flumazenil and FDG studies, were 128 matrix, 31 slice images with voxel dimensions $2.35 \times 2.35 \times 3.38mm$, obtained on a Siemens/CTI ECAT 951/31R.

| | Maximum distances | | | | Minimum distances | | | |
|---|---|---|---|---|---|---|---|---|
| Study # | 1 | 2 | 3 | 4 | 1 | 2 | 3 | 4 |
| FDG-T1 | - | 7.5 | 4.6 | 8.8 | - | 5.1 | 2.4 | 6.6 |
| FDG-T2 | - | 11.7 | 13.8 | - | - | 8.9 | 11.0 | - |

**Table 8.** The maximum and mean distances (in millimeters) between the marker based and morphologically based registrations of the FDG and MR studies involved.

reveals that accurate marker detection is limited by the blurry nature of the PET images. Marker based alignment is therefore not the best of standards for PET to MR registration. The morphologically based registrations appear accurate in most cases, but in some cases a visible mismatch can be perceived when viewing the midsagittal plane. There seems to be no difference between the quality of registrations involving FDG PET images and the ones using Flumazenil PET images. The registrations involving T1 weighted MR images appear more accurate than the ones using T2 weighted MR images.

# 4 Discussion

We have applied the morphologically based registration techniques on many more image pairs than addressed in this paper. The ones reported here are those pairs that come with a reference registration that can be used for at least some validative measure. The methods perform satisfactorily in all cases of CT to MR registration with images of regular clinical protocols (although results are better when high resolution data is used), but –as the above sections showed– mismatches may still occur when functional images are involved. Generally, significant misregistrations can easily be perceived when inspecting the registration visually. It is not difficult to adapt the feature extraction procedure in these cases such that a satisfactory match is obtained. However, such interventions destroy the automatic nature of the whole registration process. As can be learned from West *et al.* (1996), our MR to PET registration accuracy measurements are comparable to most other registration algorithms, even though many methods in this study use manual intervention to optimize the registration.

In conclusion, simple morphological tools are capable of registering CT and MR images accurately and robustly, and provide acceptable PET to MR and SPECT to MR registrations in most cases. We have not found a simple procedure that adequately registers SPECT or PET with MRI in all cases considered; the variability in the data is too large to enable a fully robust registration paradigm.

A point we want to emphasize is that the reference registrations should not be regarded as a gold standard, *i.e.*, the distances in the tables should not be interpreted as errors. Such distances are at best *indicative* of the quality of the morphological registrations. In a number of cases, especially in the CT to MR application, it was clear from visual inspection that the morphologically based registration was of superior quality. Moreover, even with high resolution volumes (voxel volume $1mm^3$), experts sometimes could not distinguish between the quality of two matches, although the maximum distance between them exceeded $3mm$. This can have a number of causes, amongst which are local image distortion, the fact that the distance overestimates the 'true' error, the *rigid* transformation paradigm, the fact that a registration algorithm will perform better in those image areas dominant in the feature images (*i.e.*, at the edges used in the registration), *etc.*

In the opinion of these authors, voxel based registration methods will eventually outperform others. We are currently experimenting with mutual information based methods as developed by Collignon and co-workers (Collignon, Maes, Delaere, Vandermeulen,

Suetens & Marchal 1995), which produces visually attractive results on *almost all* of the image pairs used in this paper. However, these methods are as yet unsuitable for registration tasks that are severely time-constrained (such as intra-operative registration) or tasks that do not allow registration by means of a rigid transformation only (*e.g.* involving abdominal scans). Speed of the registration method is heavily dependant on the information content of the images involved. In this paper, by applying morphological operators, we have dramatically reduced the total information content of images, while simultaneously extracting feature information of corresponding anatomical structures. Also, we have shown that multi-resolution approaches can be used in the maximization procedure. Preliminary experiments corroborate that both the multi-resolution approach and the information reduction could be incorporated into mutual information based registration.

## 5 Acknowledgments

*This research was supported in part by the industrial companies Philips Medical Systems, KEMA, Shell Industrial Exploration and Production, and ADAC Europe, as well as by the Netherlands ministries of Education & Science and Economic Affairs through a SPIN grant, and by the Netherlands Organization for Scientific Research (NWO), through a travel grant. Dr Paul Hemler and Dr Thilaka Sumanaweera are kindly acknowledged for their work on the cadaver study. Dr Jan Buitelaar and Alice van Dongen, MA are greatfully acknowledged for their assistance with the SPECT images. The images with implanted fixed markers used in the validation of the CT/MR and PET/MR registrations were acquired as part of the project "Evaluation of Retrospective Image Registration", NIH R01MS/CA 3392 6-01, coordinated by Dr Michael Fitzpatrick, Vanderbilt University. We are indebted to Jay West and Dr Michoel Fitzpatrick for their help regarding these images. We also wish to thank Dr René Debets, Dr B. Sadzot and Christian Degueldre for their assistance in acquiring the PET images, and Dr Linda Meiners for helping out with the related MR protocol.*

## References

Chang, H. & Fitzpatrick, J. M. (1992), 'A technique for accurate magnetic resonance imaging in the presence of field inhomogeneities', *IEEE Transactions on medical imaging* **11**, 319–329.

Collignon, A., Maes, F., Delaere, D., Vandermeulen, D., Suetens, P. & Marchal, G. (1995), Automated multimodality image registration using information theory, *in* Y. Bizais & C. Barillot, eds, 'Information Processing in Medical Imaging', Kluwer Academic Publishers, Dordrecht, pp. 263–274.

Evans, A. C., Marrett, S., Collins, L. & Peters, T. M. (1989), Anatomical-functional correlative analysis of the human brain using three dimensional imaging systems, *in* R. Schneider, S. Dwyer III & R. Jost, eds, 'Medical imaging: image processing', Vol. 1092, SPIE press, Bellingham, WA, pp. 264–274.

Haralick, R. M., Sternberg, S. R. & Zhuang, X. (1987), 'Image analysis using mathematical morphology', *IEEE transactions on pattern analysis and machine intelligence* **9**(4), 532–550.

Hemler, P. F., van den Elsen, P. A., Sumanaweera, T. S., Napel, S., Drace, J. & Adler, J. R. (1995), A quantitative comparison of residual error for three different multimodality registration techniques, *in* Y. Bizais, C. Barillot & R. di Paola, eds, 'Information processing in medical imaging', Kluwer, pp. 389–390.

Hill, D. L. G., Hawkes, D. J., Crossman, J. E., Gleeson, M. J., Cox, T. C. S., Bracey, E. C. M. L., Strong, A. J. & Graves, P. (1991), 'Registration of MR and CT images for skull base surgery using pointlike anatomical features', *British journal of radiology* **64**(767), 1030–1035.

Hill, D. L. G., Studholme, C. & Hawkes, D. J. (1994), Voxel similarity measures for automated image registration, *in* R. Robb, ed., 'Visualization in biomedical computing', Vol. 2359, SPIE Press, Bellingham, WA, pp. 205–216.

Kramer, H. P. & Bruckner, J. B. (1975), 'Iterations of a non-linear transformation for enhancement of digital images', *Pattern recognition* **7**, 53–58.

Levin, D. N., Pelizzari, C. A., Chen, G. T. Y., Chen, C. & Cooper, M. D. (1988), 'Retrospective geometric correlation of MR, CT, and PET images', *Radiology* **169**(3), 817–823.

Maes, F., Collignon, A., Vandermeulen, D., Marchal, G. & Suetens, P. (1996a), Multi-modality image registration by maximization of mutual information, *in* 'Mathematical methods in biomedical image analysis', IEEE computer society press, Los Alamitos, CA, pp. 14–22.

Maes, F., Collignon, A., Vandermeulen, D., Marchal, G. & Suetens, P. (1996b), 'Multi-modality image registration by maximization of mutual information', *IEEE Transactions on medical imaging* . In press.

Maintz, J. B. A., van den Elsen, P. A. & Viergever, M. A. (1994), Using geometrical features to match CT and MR brain images, *in* L. Beolchi & M. Kuhn, eds, 'Medical imaging, analysis of multimodality 2D/3D images', Vol. 19 of *Studies in Health, Technology and Informatics*, IOS Press, Amsterdam, pp. 43–52.

Maintz, J. B. A., van den Elsen, P. A. & Viergever, M. A. (1995), Comparison of feature-based matching of CT and MR brain images, *in* N. Ayache, ed., 'Computer vision, virtual reality, and robotics in medicine', Vol. 905 of *Lecture notes in computer science*, Springer-Verlag, Berlin, pp. 219–228.

Maintz, J. B. A., van den Elsen, P. A. & Viergever, M. A. (1996), 'Evaluation of ridge seeking operators for multimodality medical image matching', *IEEE Transactions on pattern analysis and machine intelligence* 18(4), 353–365.

Maintz, J. B. A., van den Elsen, P. A. & Viergever, M. A. (1997), 'Comparison of edge-based and ridge-based registration of CT and MR brain images', *Medical image analysis* 1(2), 151–161. in press.

Pelizzari, C. A., Chen, G. T. Y., Spelbring, D. R., Weichselbaum, R. R. & Chen, C. T. (1989), 'Accurate three-dimensional registration of CT, PET, and/or MR images of the brain', *Computer assisted tomography* 13(1), 20–26.

Schad, L. R., Boesecke, R., Schlegel, W., Hartmann, G. H., Sturm, G. H., Strauss, L. G. & Lorenz, W. (1987), 'Three dimensional image correlation of CT, MR, and PET studies in radiotherapy treatment of brain tumors', *Computer assisted tomography* 11, 948–954.

Serra, J. (1982), *Image analysis and mathematical morphology*, Academic press.

Serra, J. (1988), *Image analysis and mathematical morphology, volume 2: theoretical advances*, Academic press.

Studholme, C., Hill, D. L. G. & Hawkes, D. J. (1995), Multi resolution voxel similarity measures for MR-PET registration, *in* Y. Bizais & C. Barillot, eds, 'Information Processing in Medical Imaging', Kluwer Academic Publishers, Dordrecht, pp. 287–298.

Taylor, R. H., Lavallée, S., Burdea, G. C. & Mösges, R. (1996), *Computer-integrated surgery*, Technology and clinical applications, MIT Press, Cambridge, MA.

van den Elsen, P. A., Maintz, J. B. A., Pol, E. & Viergever, M. A. (1995), 'Automatic registration of CT and MR brain images using correlation of geometrical features', *IEEE Transactions on medical images* 14(2), 384–398.

van den Elsen, P. A., Pol, E. J. D. & Viergever, M. A. (1993), 'Medical image matching– a review with classification', *IEEE Engineering in medicine and biology* 12(1), 26–39.

van den Elsen, P. A. & Viergever, M. A. (1994), 'Marker guided multimodality matching of the brain', *European radiology* 4, 45–51.

van den Elsen, P. A., Viergever, M. A., van Huffelen, A. C., van der Meij, W. & Wieneke, G. H. (1991), 'Accurate matching of electromagnetic dipole data with CT and MR images', *Brain topography* 3(4), 425–432.

Vandermeulen, D. (1991), Methods for registration, interpolation and interpretation of three-dimensional medical image data for use in 3-D display, 3-D modelling and therapy planning, PhD thesis, University of Leuven, Belgium.

Viergever, M. A., Maintz, J. B. A., Stokking, R., van den Elsen, P. A. & Zuiderveld, K. J. (1995), Matching and integrated display of brain images from multiple modalities, *in* 'Medical Imaging', Vol. 2434, SPIE Press, Bellingham, WA, pp. 2–13.

Viola, P. & Wells III, W. (1995), Alignment by maximization of mutual information, *in* 'International conference on computer vision', IEEE computer society press, Los Alamitos, CA, pp. 16–23.

West et al., J. (1996), Comparison and evaluation of retrospective intermodality image registration techniques, *in* M. H. Loew & K. M. Hanson, eds, 'SPIE proc MI', Vol. 2710, pp. 332–347.

Woods, R., Maziotta, J. & Cherry, S. (1993), 'MRI-PET registration with automated algorithm', *journal of computer assisted tomography* 17(4), 536–546.

# Deformation for Image Guided Interventions Using a Three Component Tissue Model

P. J. Edwards, D. L. G. Hill, J. A. Little, D. J. Hawkes

Radiological Sciences
UMDS, Guys Hospital
London SE1 9RT, U.K.
p.edwards@umds.ac.uk

**Abstract.** In image guided neurosurgery it is necessary to align pre-operative image data with the patient. The rigid body approximation is usually applied, but is often not valid due to tissue deformation. Most non-rigid registration algorithms, such as those used for atlas matching, provide a smooth deformation, which does not model the characteristics of different tissues accurately since, for example, bone will appear to deform. We suggest that a physically based model of tissue could provide a powerful tool for tracking tissue movement. Since the algorithm must ultimately run in real time, we have developed a simplified model of tissue deformation based on a three component system. Regions are labelled as either rigid, deformable or fluid. A novel strategy to avoid folding in the transformation is described. Our model was applied to MRI and CT data from a neurosurgery patient with epilepsy. The test data is limited and the current implementation is in 2D, but initial results are promising.

## 1 Introduction

Image guided surgery requires that data from pre-operative images be registered to the patient on the operating table. Most commercial systems assume the rigid body approximation, i.e the image data is aligned with the patient by translation and rotation only. In certain cases, such as surgery in the skull base where soft tissue is close to bone, rigid body transformations give a good approximation. Often, however, this is not the case.

The problem we are addressing can be summarised as follows. Prior to a surgical or other interventional procedure, high quality 3D images (usually MRI or CT) are obtained. During the procedure some spatial information might be available from, perhaps, a surgical localiser, intra-operative video, intra-operative ultrasound, X-ray fluoroscopy, or interventional MRI or CT. This information is less complete and often less detailed than the pre-operative representation. The spatial information provided may be more accurate, however, as tissue deformation might have occurred since the pre-operative scan. Given this more accurate yet incomplete data we wish to estimate the location, size and shape of certain structures visible in the pre-operative images yet invisible to the surgeon.

The particular example we will be studying is neurosurgery of a patient with epilepsy. The procedure itself and explanations for the resulting deformation will be discussed in section 2. Significant deformation of the brain is apparent. The aim of this work is to make use of knowledge about the physical properties of tissue to make the best approximation of the positions of structures from the intra-operative data we are given.

Much effort has been applied to the related 'atlas problem' in which images from different individuals are registered to a common coordinate system [1, 2]. The most widely used algorithms register brain images into a bi-commisural co-ordinate system, as used by the Talaraich atlas [3]. Various deformation algorithms have been proposed for the atlas problem, including elastic or viscous matching [4, 5] thin plate splines [6] and multi-rigid correlation warps [7].

There is much less published work which incorporates deformations into registration of images of an individual taken at different times to account for tissue movement. Exceptions to this include matching of x-ray projections to nuclear medicine bone scans using kriging [8] and elastic matching of MRI and CT of the thorax [9].

All the above techniques provide a smooth deformation between landmark, contour or volume data. The physical properties of tissues are not considered. Waters [10, 11] created a physical model of facial tissue. The application is very different to that described here, the object being production of realistic facial expressions. Unlike ours, their model did not include fluid regions.

We previously presented a crude method involving separate transformation of individual structures [12] which produced unwanted discontinuities. Recent work by our own group has incorporated rigid regions into a smoothly interpolated medium and produced successful results on deformed neck MRI images [13].

The algorithm presented here uses a fundamentally different approach. A simple physical model allowing rigid, deformable and fluid tissues is created. Rigid regions are constrained and fluid regions have no energy associated with deformation. The deformable region can have a number of energy characteristics. Tension, spring, stiffness and area constraints have been examined and compared and a novel fold avoidance strategy implemented. The current implementation is 2D though the method can be extended to 3D.

This paper presents, to the best of our knowledge, the first application of deformable models to image guided interventions in which tissue deformation would invalidate the rigid body assumption.

## 2 Clinical Application

The algorithm we have developed may well have many applications in image guided surgery, both inside and outside the head. As a first step we will consider the applicability of the technique to neurosurgery of a patient with epilepsy.

Some patients who present with recurrent grand mal epilepsy and have not responded to drug therapy are considered suitable candidates for neurosurgery. The aim of the procedure is to remove any lesion associated with the pathology and specifically the epileptic focus, whilst avoiding critical functioning cortex. At King's College Hospital, London, a large craniotomy is performed and electrode mats are placed in the subdural space (see fig. 1). For a few days postoperatively, stimulation studies are performed to establish which areas show critical function and any seizures are monitored to identify the epileptic focus.

A second procedure is then undertaken to remove the pathological tissue. In general, the electrode mats are simply removed and either a diagram of their position or a photograph from the first operation is used to relate stimulation data to the patient in-theatre. There are inherent inaccuracies in such a process which make epilepsy surgery a good candidate for image guidance.

A problem for conventional rigid body guidance, however, is that there is often considerable brain shift during these procedures. For this paper we will be examining one particular case, though brain shift has been identified as a common feature of such operations [14].

The trend is for the brain to undergo a reduction in volume. This may be partly due to measures taken intra-operatively to lower intracranial pressure.

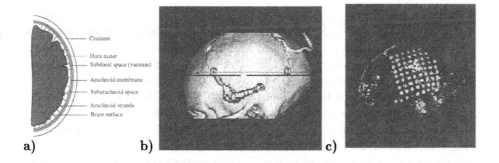

**Fig. 1.** Electrode mat placement - (a) schematic of the cranium , (b) skull surface from CT showing craniotomy and (c) the electrodes from CT.

## 3   Method

The technique we use is based on the opposition of forces between the pre-operative model and intra-operative sample data. The model is created from a segmentation of the pre-operative scans and is specific to the individual patient. A sample energy function is constructed which increases with the discrepancy between the current position and the data. The total energy, which we minimise, is the sum of the sample and model components.

$$E_{total} = E_{model} + E_{sample} \qquad (1)$$

This is similar to the method used for active contour models, where $E_{sample}$ is usually an edge strength measure and $E_{model}$ could be a contour model or generic anatomical model [15]. In our case $E_{model}$ is specific to the individual patient and is extracted from the pre-operative scans. The sample data are landmarks that in practice would be obtained during the operation.

Initially, the model energy will be zero and the sample energy large (assuming a substantial deformation has occurred). As we minimise the total energy the model will deform and approach a good match with the sample data. It is clear that the balance between the model and sample energies is important in achieving the desired result. We will return to this question in section 3.1.

## 3.1 Sample Energy

The sample data for the current example are landmark positions. The associated energy function is

$$E_{sample} = \alpha \sum_{i=1}^{m} \frac{(\mathbf{L}_i - \mathbf{L}'_i)^2}{\sigma_i^2}, \tag{2}$$

where $m$ is the number of landmarks, $\mathbf{L}_i$ is destination position of landmark $i$, $\mathbf{L}'_i$ is its position given the current model parameters and $\sigma_i$ is the standard deviation of the measurement. In this way we are providing a least-squares fit of the data subject to our model. The factor $\alpha$ is a weighting which relates the sample energy to that of the model and allows the required dimensionality. The value chosen depends on the desired weighting given to the model compared to the landmarks. As $\alpha \to \infty$ the landmarks are interpolated exactly.

One could argue, since the selection of the landmarks will not be exact, that it is reasonable to allow the model to alter the landmark positions. This does not represent the statistics of landmark measurement correctly, however. It is wrong to suggest that all landmarks should move in the direction of lower model energy, since the model is not based on knowledge of landmark measurement.

For our purposes, we suggest that the best estimation for the updated model position is where the landmarks are moved exactly to their new locations. It may be possible to constrain the landmarks exactly in later versions of the algorithm. In the current implementation we set $\sigma_i$ to be small (1 pixel) for each landmark and increase the value $\alpha$ at each stage of grid subsampling (by a factor equivalent to the number of nodes). This ensures close adherence to the landmark data.

It is worth noting that higher dimensional sample data could be incorporated simply by using an appropriate $E_{sample}$. Such an energy term could be created for contours, surfaces and voxel data (see section 5).

## 3.2 Model Energy

To construct the model, we split the image region into a grid of $n$ nodes which are related by elements connecting them. These elements are either simple connections between two nodes or a triangle with a node at each corner. We have $n$ nodes with positions $\mathbf{N}_i$. Let $\delta_i$ be a subset of the neighbourhood of nodes connected to $\mathbf{N}_i$, chosen so as to avoid elements being counted twice. The total energy is the sum over all elements and can be written as

$$E_{model}(\mathbf{N}_1, \mathbf{N}_2 \cdots \mathbf{N}_n) = \sum_{i=1}^{n} \sum_{\mathbf{N}_j \in \delta_i} E_{element}(\mathbf{N}_i, \mathbf{N}_j), \tag{3}$$

The energy, $E_{element}$, of a connection will be a function of the node positions at either end.

Each node is labelled according to its physical properties. It has been proposed that rigid regions could be simply assigned a higher stiffness than deformable areas [16]. This means, however, that time is spent computing the deformations of an area that does not deform.

We adopt a different approach. It is assumed for the purposes of neurosurgery that there is only one rigid body, the skull, and that it is rigidly registered. In surgical practice this rigid registration could be provided by pins or markers inserted into bone. This means that the rigid node positions can be fixed and are not adjusted during the energy minimisation.

Fluid node connections are assigned zero energy, i.e. there is no cost associated with their deformation, allowing them to move almost freely. The exception to this is that an energy associated with very small area is applied to avoid folding. This will be discussed in more detail in section 3.2. The assignation of zero energy to fluid regions is analogous to a zero continuity weighting in inverse visual problems as proposed by Terzopoulos [17].

Deformable elements should have an energy which attempts to describe the physical properties of the tissue. Work has been published on mechanical properties of the cranial cavity [18], so such a model may seem reasonable. It is mathematically difficult, however, to build such a model. There is also an efficiency consideration. If the algorithm is expected to be useful during surgery it must provide results within a reasonable time. We have compared a number of simple energy terms that are based on intuitional physical characteristics rather than real measurements of tissue properties. These are outlined in the following sections.

### Tension

$$E_{tension}(\mathbf{N}_i, \mathbf{N}_j) = |\mathbf{N}_j - \mathbf{N}_i - \mathbf{N}^0{}_{i,j}|^2 \tag{4}$$

Here, $\mathbf{N}^0{}_{i,j}$ is the relaxed vector between the two nodes. This is equivalent to having 1D spring elements along each of the axes which attempt to keep the X and Y distances between the nodes constant. This can be compared to a thin membrane [17]. This energy is computationally simple. There is a cost associated with any movement other than pure translation of all nodes.

### Stiffness

$$E_{stiffness}(\mathbf{N}_i, \mathbf{N}_j, \mathbf{N}_k) = |\mathbf{N}_j + \mathbf{N}_k - 2\mathbf{N}_i|^2 \tag{5}$$

The stiffness energy is a curvature term, so requires three points. In this case, $\mathbf{N}_j$ and $\mathbf{N}_k$ are two nodes which are connected to $\mathbf{N}_i$, of equal size and opposite direction when relaxed. This minimises the same energy as the thin plate spline. This term is computationally simple. There is an energy associated with any movement other than affine transformations.

## Spring

$$E_{spring}(\mathbf{N}_i, \mathbf{N}_j) = (|\mathbf{N}_j - \mathbf{N}_i| - l_{i,j})^2 \tag{6}$$

This energy term is a 2D spring, where the distance between the nodes is calculated and subtracted from the relaxed distance, $l_{i,j}$. The whole grid is then a simple network of springs. The modulus term requires calculation of a square root, which is comparatively expensive. An energy is associated with movement other than rigid body transformations.

## Area

$$E_{area}(\mathbf{N}_i, \mathbf{N}_j, \mathbf{N}_k) = \frac{|(\mathbf{N}_j - \mathbf{N}_i) \times (\mathbf{N}_k - \mathbf{N}_i)|^2}{A_{i,j,k}^2} + \frac{A_{i,j,k}^2}{|(\mathbf{N}_j - \mathbf{N}_i) \times (\mathbf{N}_k - \mathbf{N}_i)|^2} \tag{7}$$

The area term requires three nodes which form a triangle. The cross product is twice the area of the triangle with corners $\mathbf{N}_i$, $\mathbf{N}_j$ and $\mathbf{N}_k$. $A_{i,j,k}$ is its relaxed value, i.e the initial area of that element. The function has a minimum value of 2 when $|(\mathbf{N}_j - \mathbf{N}_i) \times (\mathbf{N}_k - \mathbf{N}_i)| = A_{i,j,k}$, and tends to infinity as the area tends to zero. This has the effect of trying to minimise any change in the total area and is similar to the incompressibility term used by Waters [11]. Rigid body transformations, shears and area preserving scalings have no cost. A 3D implementation of this energy term would attempt to preserve volume.

**Folding** A problem that occurs with many deformation algorithms, both iterative and non-iterative, is that the transformation collapses or folds over in some regions. This can be described mathematically as the Jacobian of the transformation becoming negative, or the mapping no longer being one-to-one.

Some methods to overcome this have been devised. For example, Christensen et al [5] check the Jacobian on every iteration of their viscous fluid model and perform regridding when it falls below a fixed value. For our purposes we wish to stop any of our triangular elements from collapsing. To achieve this a further energy term is added to both fluid and deformable regions.

$$E_{fold}(\mathbf{N}_i, \mathbf{N}_j, \mathbf{N}_k) = \begin{cases} \frac{F^2}{\gamma^2} + \frac{\gamma^2}{F^2}, & \text{if } F \leq \gamma; \\ 2 & \text{Otherwise.} \end{cases} \tag{8}$$

where,

$$F(\mathbf{N}_i, \mathbf{N}_j, \mathbf{N}_k) = \frac{|(\mathbf{N}_j - \mathbf{N}_i) \times (\mathbf{N}_k - \mathbf{N}_i)|}{A_{i,j,k}}, \tag{9}$$

This is similar to the area energy term given by (7), but $\gamma$ represents a fraction of the area above which the energy is constant. The equation is chosen so as to be continuous and differentiable, to be constant for all but small areas

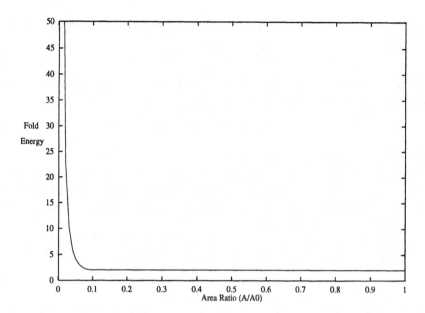

**Fig. 2.** The fold energy function, which stops the area collapsing to zero.

and asymptotically large as the area tends to zero. A graph of the function for $\gamma = 0.1$ is shown in figure 2. Simply adding this energy does not rule out folding. An iterative minimisation algorithm may well jump over one of the infinities in $E_{fold}$. A sensible minimum bracketing scheme is clearly required. This will be discussed in the next section.

## 3.3 Minimisation

We need to decide on an algorithm for minimising our energy function. Since all of the energies described in the previous sections have derivatives which are calculable with similar effort to the energy, a scheme which uses derivatives would seem sensible. The algorithm we have chosen to use is conjugate gradient descent.

We have re-implemented the Numerical Recipes routine [19], improving some of the memory overheads and porting to C++. The initial bracketing routine is also significantly different and is discussed in more detail.

The basis of the algorithm is that an initial vector is chosen (down the path of maximum gradient) and 1D minimisation is performed in that direction. Subsequent directions are conjugate to the previous vector and this process is iterated until an adequate solution is found.

The 1D minimisation can be described as follows. Starting at a point $\mathbf{P}$, where

$$\mathbf{P}^T = (\mathbf{N^o}_1^T, \cdots, \mathbf{N^o}_n^T) \tag{10}$$

and $\mathbf{N^0}_i$ is the current position of the $i^{\text{th}}$ node, and given a direction $\mathbf{D}$, where

$$\mathbf{D}^T = (\mathbf{D}_1^T, \cdots, \mathbf{D}_n^T) \tag{11}$$

and $\mathbf{D}_i$ is the vector for the $i^{\text{th}}$ node in the direction in which we wish to minimise, construct an energy function,

$$E(\lambda) = E_{total}(\mathbf{P} + \lambda \mathbf{D}), \tag{12}$$

then perform 1D minimisation over $\lambda$.

Before 1D minimisation begins a solution must be bracketed. Usually this is done by taking larger and larger steps in a downhill direction until the energy increases. Such a strategy is extremely likely to jump over one of the infinities associated with the fold energy.

Instead we calculate the nearest fold in direction $\mathbf{D}$. For a given triangular element with corners $\mathbf{N}_i$, $\mathbf{N}_j$ and $\mathbf{N}_k$ folding occurs when

$$|(\mathbf{N}_j - \mathbf{N}_i) \times (\mathbf{N}_k - \mathbf{N}_i)| = 0 \tag{13}$$

i.e. the area is zero and $\mathbf{N}_i$, $\mathbf{N}_j$ and $\mathbf{N}_k$ are collinear. Substituting current positions $\mathbf{N^0}_i$ and directions $\mathbf{D}_i$, for each element we get:

$$|((\mathbf{N^0}_j + \lambda \mathbf{D}_j) - (\mathbf{N^0}_i + \lambda \mathbf{D}_i)) \times ((\mathbf{N^0}_k + \lambda \mathbf{D}_k) - (\mathbf{N^0}_i + \lambda \mathbf{D}_i))| = 0 \tag{14}$$

This produces a quadratic in $\lambda$ which is easily solvable. The calculation is performed for all triangles in the model and the lowest value is taken as the limit of our search space. The bracketing process then consists of moving downhill towards this limit until the fold energy forces the function upwards. This ensures that the solution that we bracket is a non-folding one.

To aid efficiency, minimisation is performed in a multigrid fashion, starting with a very coarse grid and interpolating to finer grids until the desired accuracy is achieved. At each subsampling of the grid a new node is placed at the mid-point of each pair of adjacent nodes (including diagonals). The initial and destination positions of the new nodes are calculated as the mid-point in the same way.

The final and initial positions of the grid give a transformation in either direction. For our purposes we wish to distort the pre-operative model to match the data points, so interpolation is carried out in the forward direction using a perspective transformation on all rectangles in the initial configuration.

## 4 Results

To examine the workings of our model let us first look at a small scale grid and see how the different compartments interact. Fig. 3 shows an arrangement of elements with rigid (dark), deformable (light) and fluid (blank) regions. Under stretching, a large proportion of the deformation is taken up by the fluid region. When compressing, the fluid region collapses but does not pass through the rigid region because of the non-folding constraint.

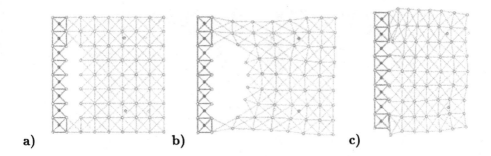

a)            b)             c)

**Fig. 3.** A model grid (a) relaxed, (b) stretched and (c) compressed.

The epilepsy data that we will apply the algorithm to is shown in fig. 4. These are corresponding 2D slices taken from registered pre-operative MRI and post-operative CT. These images were automatically registered using an information theory approach [20]. Considerable reduction of the brain volume is apparent. The only data given to the algorithm are seven landmarks on the brain surface and a segmented image showing the rigid, deformable and fluid regions. This is intended to mimic the kind of data that may be available during the procedure, i.e. a rigid registration of the skull using marker pins and sparse surface points on the brain. The segmentation is based on the brain extracted from MRI and the skull from CT, which are the images likely to form the pre-operative model. Fig. 5 shows the segmented image and an example set of model elements.

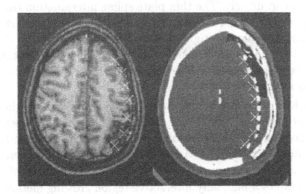

**Fig. 4.** Corresponding slices from pre-operative MRI (left) and postoperative CT (right) showing brain volume reduction. The landmarks used are marked with crosses.

The results of minimisation for our different energy functions and some combinations thereof are shown in fig. 6. In these figures the CT is thresholded at a

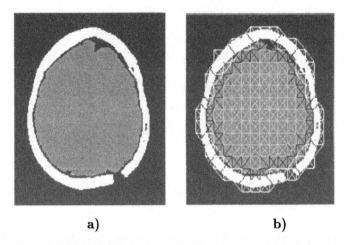

a)                                    b)

**Fig. 5.** Model construction, (a) the pre-operative segmentation and (b) the corresponding model elements.

high level so as to show only the bone and electrodes. The warped MRI dataset is overlaid so as to show the relative position of the electrodes, skull and brain. Since no depth landmarks were used to define the warp the two electrodes placed in the inter-hemispheric fissure serve as an independent check. It should also be noted that the mid-line as seen in the postoperative CT is not significantly distorted.

Obviously, the rigid registration (fig. 6(a)) maps neither the brain surface nor depth features accurately. The thin plate spline interpolation (fig. 6(b)) was performed using radial basis function methods with extra landmarks to mimic the knowledge that the skull is rigid. The mid-line is significantly deformed by this transformation and its movement is too great. The spring energy function (fig. 6(c)) gives a much better result, though the central electrodes show that the mid-line has again moved too far.

All the solutions provided by our model show wispy lines in the discontinuous region where there is a fluid gap. This is due to imperfect segmentation. Some small regions of soft tissue, probably dura, which are close to the skull have been identified as rigid. Such tissue is then seen to be 'dragged' across the discontinuity. The segmentation process itself is not the subject of this paper, but for these examples a manually interactive region growing method was used. One would not necessarily expect perfect results from such a method.

The area term on its own produces a poor result. The surface of the brain is seen to 'leak' out in-between the landmarks. This is visible as a curved wave-like brain surface inside the fluid region. The internal deformation is also contorted, as can be seen by following the mid-line. This is not surprising since the area of the brain has clearly decreased and area conservation is the only constraint on each element. In combination with other energies a better result can be achieved. It may be relevant to have such an energy term if some model which predicts

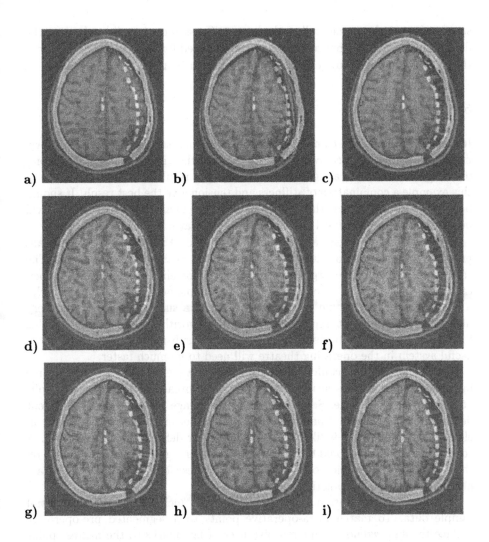

**Fig. 6.** The resulting deformation for (a) rigid registration, (b) interpolated thin plate spline, and (c) spring, (d) area, (e) area+membrane, (f) area+spring, (g) tension, (h) stiffness, and (i) tension+stiffness energy functions.

grey and white matter volume from anaesthesia data can be established.

The tension energy term also overestimates the motion of the mid-line, whereas the stiffness term falls short. A direct addition of the tension and stiffness terms gives a good result.

It is interesting to note that the thin plate spline interpolation result is very different to that obtained using the stiffness energy function. Since both attempt to minimise curvature one might expect a similar result. A likely reason for the difference is that the thin plate spline minimises curvature over the whole of 2D space, whereas the numerically calculated stiffness term is valid only over the deformable region and hence curvature is minimised for this area. The fact that this region is bounded by a discontinuity will greatly affect the deformation.

## 5 Discussion

It is clear that the three component strategy has successfully captured the movement of the brain surface away from the skull in the given example. The choice of energy function has a significant effect on the resulting deformation and in this example a combination of stiffness and tension give the best result. It should be stressed, however, that this is an isolated example and further validation will be required before any hard conclusions can be drawn.

The strategy for fold avoidance is successful. Folding was a significant problem without this addition, especially in or near the fluid regions. The calculation of the fold energy adds to the inherent efficiency problems associated with such models. Though the multigrid implementation is of some help, a 128×128 grid takes some 2-3 hours to relax on a sun sparc 20/66. It is very likely that more efficient implementation of the algorithm could improve on this figure, for example by better interpolation when subsampling the grids, but a useful system in the operating theatre will need to be much faster.

One solution that could substantially improve efficiency is a quad tree implementation. In the current coarse-to-fine approach all elements are split at every change of scale. Some regions of the image do not exhibit sufficient deformation to warrant fine scale elements. A better strategy is to split an element only when this is likely to provide further deformation information. A condition for splitting could be a threshold on the energy gradients (or forces) on the interpolated finer grid nodes. Calculation of these forces would also facilitate a more intelligent interpolation scheme.

Further implementation developments would include higher dimensional sample data. To match intra-operative points to a segmented pre-operative surface the sum would be squared distances of landmarks to the nearest point on the surface. Where two full surfaces are to be registered the volume enclosed by the gap between them may be a useful measure. Where two sets of images are available a voxel similarity measure such as correlation or mutual information could be used.

The algorithm will need to be extended to 3D. All the energy equations can easily be extended to represent a 3D grid. The area terms will then become volume terms so calculation of the folding criteria will require solution of cubic equations. This is a small overhead in comparison to the increase in the number of nodes. It is also likely that gravity will play a part in the true deformation of the brain and should be incorporated into the model. Further components to the model, such as white and grey matter delineation, may also be appropriate.

Validation of algorithms such as the one presented here will remain an issue of critical importance. What is clear is that our model gives reasonable prediction of the position of deep structures given only a few sparse surface points. This is representative of the data that could be available during neurosurgery on an epilepsy patient. It is very likely that such a model will be useful for this and other neurosurgery applications.

# 6 Acknowledgements

The work in this paper was funded by the UK EPSRC (grant no. GR/J90183). J. Little is funded by Philips Medical Systems (EasyVision/EasyGuide Advanced Development). We are grateful to our clinical collaborators Prof. Charles Polkey, Dr. Tim Cox, Prof. Michael Gleeson, and Mr. Anthony Strong for their ongoing support, and to the radiography staff at the Guy's and St Thomas' NHS Trust, and the Maudsley Imaging Centre.

# References

1. A. C. Evans, S. Marrett, J. Torrescorzo, S. Ku, and L. Collins. MRI-PET correlation in three dimensions using a volume-of-interest (VOI) atlas. *J. Cereb. Blood Flow Metab.*, 11:A69–A78, 1991.
2. K. J. Friston, C. D. Frith, P. F. Liddle, and R. S. J. Frackowiak. Plastic transformation of PET images. *J. Comput. Assist. Tomogr.*, 15:635–639, 1991.
3. J. Talairach and P. Tournoux. *A coplanar stereotaxic atlas of a human brain.* Thieme, Stuttgart, 1988.
4. R. Bajcy and S. Kovacic. Multiresolution elastic matching. *CVGIP: Graphical Models and Image Processing*, 46:1–21, 1989.
5. C. A. Christensen, R. D. Rabbitt, M. I. Miller, S. C. Joshi, U. Grenader, A. Coogan, and D. C. Van Essen. Topological properties of smooth anatomic maps. In Y. Bizais, C. Barillot, and R. Di Paola, editors, *Information Processing in Medical Imaging*, pages 101–112. Kluwer Academic Publishers, 1995.
6. F. L. Bookstein. Thin-plate splines and the atlas problem for biomedical images. In A. C. F. Colchester and D. J. Hawkes, editors, *Information Processing in Medical Imaging*, 1991.
7. D. L. Collins, A. C. Evans, C. Holmes, and T. M. Peters. Automatic 3d segmentation of neuro-anatomical structures. In Y. Bizais, C. Barillot, and R. Di Paola, editors, *Information Processing in Medical Imaging*, pages 139–152. Kluwer Academic Publishers, 1995.
8. K. V. Mardia and J. A. Little. Image warping using derivative information. In F. L. Bookstein, J. S. Duncan, N. Lange, and D. C. Wilson, editors, *Mathematical Methods in Medical Imaging III*, pages 16–31. SPIE Proceedings 2099, July 1994.
9. M. Moshfeghi. Elastic matching of multimodality medical images. *CVGIP: Graphical Models and Image Processing*, 53(3):271–282, 1991.
10. K. Waters. A physical model of facial tissue and muscle articulation derived from computer tomography data. In *SPIE 1808 Visualization in Biomedical Computing*, pages 574–583, 1992.
11. D Terzopoulos and K. Waters. Analysis and synthesis of facial image sequences using physical and anatomical models. *IEEE Trans. PAMI*, 15(6):569–579, 1993.
12. P. J. Edwards, D. L. G. Hill, J. Little, V. A. S. Sahni, and D. J. Hawkes. Medical image registration incorporating deformations. In D. Pycock, editor, *Proc. 6th Brit. Machine Vision Conf.*, volume 2, pages 691–699, 1995.

13. J. Little, D. L. G. Hill, and D. J. Hawkes. Deformations incorporating rigid structures. In *Proc. Mathematical Methods in Biomedical Image Analysis*, pages 104–113. IEEE Computer Society Press, 1995.

14. D. L. G. Hill, C. R. Maurer, M. Y. Wang, R. J. Maciunas, and J. M. Barwise, J. A. Fitzpatrick. Estimation of intraoperative brain surface movement. In *Proc. MRCAS/CVRMed, in press*, 1997.

15. M. Kass, A. Witkin, and D. Terzopoulos. Regularization of inverse visual problems involving discontinuities. *Int. J. Computer Vision*, 8(4):321331, 1986.

16. A. K. F. Lui and D. J. Bone. Integrating graphical editing into sparse data interpolation using non-uniform thin plate splines. In *Proc. 1st Int. Conf. on Visual Information Systems*, pages 541–550. Melbourne, Australia, 1995.

17. D. Terzopoulos. Regularization of inverse visual problems involving discontinuities. *IEEE trans. Pattern Analysis and Machine Intelligence*, 8(4):413–424, 1986.

18. S. Hakim, J. G. Venegas, and J.D. Burton. The phisics of the cranial cavity, hydrocephalus and normal pressure hydrocephalus. *Surgical Neurology*, 5:187–210, 1976.

19. W.H. Press, S.A. Teukolsky, W.T. Vetterling, and B.P. Flannery. *Numerical Recipes in C, 2nd Edition*. Cambridge University Press, 1992.

20. C Studholme, D.L.G. Hill, and D.J. Hawkes. Automated 3-D registration of MR and CT images of the head. *Medical Image Analysis*, 1(2), 1996.

# Registration of Abdominal CT and SPECT Images Using Compton Scatter Data

Katarina Sjögreen, Michael Ljungberg, Kjell Erlandsson, Lars Floreby[1] and
Sven-Erik Strand
Department of Radiation Physics, The Jubileum Institute
[1] Department of Applied Electronics
Lund University
Sweden

**Abstract.** The present study investigates the possibility to utilize Compton scatter data for registration of abdominal SPECT images. A method for registration to CT is presented, based on principal component analysis and cross-correlation of binary images representing the interior of the patient. Segmentation of scatter images is performed with two methods, thresholding and a deformable contour method. To achieve similarity of organ positions between scans, a positioning device is applied to the patient. Evaluation of the registration accuracy is performed with *a)* a [131]I phantom study, *b)* a Monte Carlo simulation study of an anthropomorphic phantom, and *c)* a [123]I patient trial. For *a)* r.m.s. distances between positions that should be equal in CT and SPECT are obtained to $1.0\pm 0.7$ mm, which thus for a rigid object is at sub pixel level. From *b)* results show that r.m.s. distances depend on the slice activity distribution. With a symmetrical distribution deviations are in the order of 5 mm. In *c)* distances between markers on the patient boundary are at the maximum 16 mm and on an average 10 mm. It is concluded that by utilizing the available Compton scatter data, valuable positioning information is achieved, that can be used for registration of SPECT images.

## 1 Introduction

Registration of tomographic nuclear medicine images to intra and inter-modality data has several beneficial applications, such as co-alignment of serial scans for temporal analysis, or for mapping of tracer uptake onto anatomical images from X-ray CT and MRI. Several techniques have been developed and employed [1,2], most commonly for matching of brain images, see e.g. [3,4] by use of global rigid transformations [5]. Registration has also an important application in the field of quantitative measurements for absorbed dose determinations in radionuclide therapy (RNT) [2,6-10]. For the present study, the primary purpose is to obtain information on the density distribution required as input for attenuation and scatter corrections for SPECT, and for dose calculations for RNT. For patients with disseminated malignant disease in abdominal regions CT is often performed as a standard routine, and the intention is to utilize the density information carried by CT data. Registration of abdominal and thoracic data is a somewhat different problem from registering images of the head, due to the elasticity of abdominal structures and a considerable organ movement during acquisition because of respiration, heartbeats, etc. Common features that can be correlated with certainty may be problematic to find; external markers must be positioned at exactly the same positions in relation to abdominal organs, and internal landmarks must be possible to outline for both imaging modalities. Another problem for registration with SPECT is the lack of information on the patient contour. To overcome these problems, Erdi et al used a patient specific cast with fiducial markers [7]. Scott et al attached a fiducial band to the patient [9] and have also been using anatomical landmarks. Point markers were used by Koral et al [8] while Kramer et al [6,10] used a combination of anatomical and external landmarks or fiducial markers. Transmission scanning has also been used for outlining and registration of the thorax, see e.g. [11].

The present study explores the possibility of utilizing information acquired with a broad energy window in the Compton region to estimate the contour of the patient. The main objective is to investigate whether it is feasible to use this information [12], normally rejected at acquisition, for registration of SPECT and CT. Compton scatter projections can for most modern gamma camera systems be acquired simultaneously with photopeak data. Hence, no co-alignment procedure is required, as may be the case for sequential emission and transmission studies e.g. Problems with positioning of markers for contour estimation may also be avoided. The registration is performed by principal component analysis and cross-correlation. Filled contour images with uniform distribution are used, to overcome problems imposed by differing spatial resolution and intensity distribution of the images. As with any contour based method, an approximation is that the positions of organs in relation to the body boundaries are equal. A positioning device has been developed which is employed according to a standardized protocol at every occasion. Several factors have influence on the accuracy, such as the activity distribution and the method used for contour delineation in the scatter images. Two segmentation methods have been applied, and evaluation has been performed by 1) Monte Carlo simulated $^{131}$I data by use of an anthropomorphic computer phantom, 2) a $^{131}$I phantom study and 3) a patient examination performed with a $^{123}$I-labelled monoclonal antibody.

## 2 Material and Method

### 2.1 Model

For the present application, quantitative information of SPECT images is to be improved by use of CT data that are acquired for diagnostic purposes other than dose planning alone. A prerequisite has therefore been to perform registration without degrading the quality of either SPECT or CT data. Several assumptions have been adopted in the model and the intention is here to state them clearly. The trunk is viewed as being constituted of three principal regions; the rather stabile thorax and pelvis, and the intermediate elastic abdomen that may be stretched and twisted extensively. For the thoracic region, positions of structures are assumed to be determined mainly by the alignment of the rib cage. The pelvic girdle similarly constitutes a base for the caudal organs of the abdomen. Positioning of these two regions is set in focus by thorough alignment of the head, arms, thorax, pelvis and legs according to a standardized protocol. Provided that alignment is performed equally, positions of intermediate abdominal organs are assumed to be

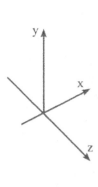

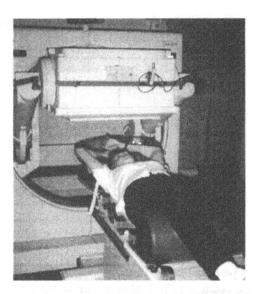

**Fig. 1.** The patient position at acquisition. Arms and head are resting in a plastic shell, a sail cloth is put underneath the patient. The laser for alignment in the x direction is attached to the gamma camera head.

similar. Then, in this position, post acquisition rotations around the z axis (Fig.1) combined with translations in the x and y directions are supposed to suffice to make data fit. Z coordinates are obtained by a marker system and are assumed to properly represent the axial position of the entire slice. Image data are thus treated as sets of parallel rigid planes. Warping or stretching have not been implemented at this stage, neither rotations that would involve reslicing the 3D image sets.

## 2.2 Patient Position

In order to achieve an equal position for both CT and SPECT, a conform positioning system has been developed (see Fig.1 and 2). At both facilities the patient is lying with the arms raised above the head. Arms and head rest in a plastic shell that has been designed to combine comfort and position consistency. A specially designed pillow is placed under the knees. The patient couch is flat and covered by a hard plastic marker board in which an N-shaped line has been milled. For SPECT studies a 1 m long 3 mm diameter [57]Co source is inserted to the N-shape, while for CT scans the empty line is used as marker. The patient is positioned in relation to the marker by use of laser beams that define reference axes in the x and z directions relative to the camera field-of-view (FOV). In order to facilitate fine adjustment of the position, two sheets of sail cloth are placed between the patient and the marker plate; cloth to cloth slide easily against each other. Adjustment is made until ink marks on stabile structures such as jugulum, sternum and also the umbilicus, coincide with the laser beams. A girdle is wrapped around the waist and couch to help the patient stay immobile.

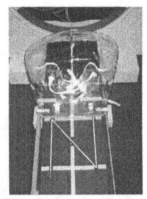

**Fig. 2.** The shell for positioning of arms and head, and the N marker board which is placed underneath the patient at acquisition.

## 2.3 Compton Scatter Data

As the count-rate distribution in the scatter images depends on the selection of the Compton energy window, the spectral distribution has been analyzed with Monte Carlo simulation studies [13]. Simulations were performed for [131]I and [123]I, with photon spectra according to tabulated data [14], in the geometry described in 2.7. The spectral distribution of the registered photons in the gamma camera was separated into contributions from photons having passed through the patient unscattered, having been scattered once, twice or three times or more, as shown in Fig.3 for [131]I. The width and location of the Compton window were selected with respect to the intensity of multiply scattered photons, which were considered likely to represent peripheral parts of the patient. Another requirement was that photons from the [57]Co marker of 122 keV should be detected in the scatter window but not interfere with photopeak counts.

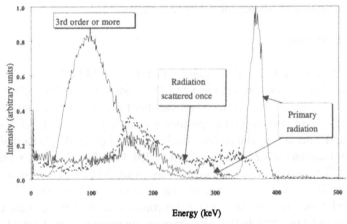

**Fig. 3.** Registered photon energies in the gamma camera, separated into contributions from primary radiation, radiation scattered once, or three times or more. Second order scatter was similar to the first order component and has been omitted to make the figure clearer. The simulation included all major photon energies and the above spectrum displays an average of four opposite projections of the Zubal phantom.

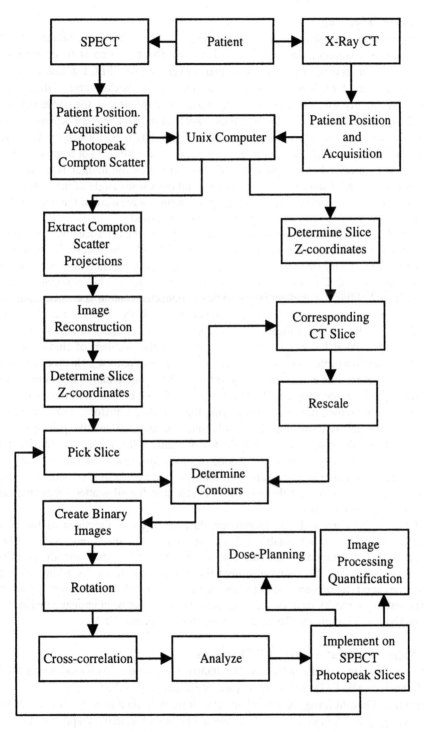

**Fig. 4.** Flow chart illustating the registration procedure

## 2.4 Image Processing

The registration procedure is illustrated in Fig.4. After acquisition, image sets are transferred to a common DEC alpha workstation. The first step is to determine z coordinates. In transversal slices, the N-shaped marker used for SPECT appears as three intense points, and for CT as three "holes" in a homogeneous background. If the marker plate is accurately aligned, the two outer points are situated at the same position throughout the image set, while the lateral coordinate of the middle point depends on the slice axial position. Semiautomatic detection of the points is performed by assigning three subregions in which the coordinate of the maximum (SPECT) or minimum (CT) intensity is determined. Axial positions of slices in which the marker is present are determined from the distances between markers and the known angle of the N-vertices. A linear fit of the z coordinates to the slice number returns a measure of the overall slice thickness, and positions of remaining slices are extrapolated.

A SPECT scatter slice is then selected interactively and the CT slice with the closest z position is chosen. Both images are resampled to 128 or 256 matrices and rescaled to equal pixel size. Binary filled contour images are created, representing the interior of the body exclusively. For CT images this is achieved by applying a Sobel gradient operator [15] and thresholding the gradient image so that a connected contour is created. Spurious edges inside the patient boundary are removed interactively. Every pixel inside the boundary is then assigned a logical unit number by use of a recursive region growing algorithm; recursion has been found useful because the problem of finding a stop condition is circumvented. For scatter data, noise and low contrast influence the shape of the boundaries, thus enhancing the need for a robust segmentation algorithm. Two different techniques have been applied, as further described below. Both binary images are rotationally aligned in the x-y plane using the Hotelling transform [15,4] which is based on principal component analysis and rotates the image so that the principal axes are aligned with the image axes. Either the CT or scatter SPECT image is translated in the x and y directions by an amount obtained by cross-correlation analysis, executed in the frequency domain. Obtained values on rotations and translations are stored. A new SPECT slice is selected and the procedure is repeated for all scatter slices that can produce adequate contours.

Obtained rotations and translations are then analyzed as functions of the axial location. Translations are established as the average in the x and y directions respectively. For rotations, a moving average is estimated so that smooth interslice differences regarding the rotation around the z axis may occur. Resulting scaling, translations and rotations are applied to image sets and for SPECT the same operations are applied to photopeak data. Image processing routines have been implemented in IDL (Interactive Data Language, Research Systems Inc, Colorado, USA).

## 2.5 Segmentation of Scatter SPECT Images

Scatter slices are reconstructed by an iterative maximum likelihood expectation maximization (ML-EM) algorithm [16] and are slightly smoothed.

**Interactive Thresholding.** A logarithmic transform is applied in order to enhance the low intensity parts. A global threshold is selected giving a boundary shape that at visual inspection is considered representative of the unthresholded image. For some slices of the experimental and clinical studies, unrealistically abrupt edges are generated, due to scattered radiation from the couch and also noise. Contours have then been smoothed manually by guidance from the unthresholded images.

**Deformable Contours or Snakes.** One robust approach to the segmentation problem is provided by the concept of deformable contours, or "snakes" [17]. Generally, it relies on the idea to minimize a cost function (Eq.1) including terms for "internal energy" and "external forces." For the present application, the first term approximates the arc length of the contour while the second term includes each contour point's deviation from a particular gray level. By introducing polar coordinates, the outline of the scatter contour is represented by a scalar function $r(k)$ which denotes the radial distance from the center at the angle $k$. Polar coordinates are obtained by bilinear interpolation of pixel values in slightly smoothed images. For each of the $N$ snake points $m$ candidates are defined and the actual optimization is performed by use of dynamic programming [18]. The cost function

$$E = \sum_{k=0}^{N-1} \sqrt{ ( r(k)\cdot\cos\frac{2\pi k}{N} - r(k-1)\cdot\cos\frac{2\pi(k-1)}{N} )^2 + ( r(k)\cdot\sin\frac{2\pi k}{N} - r(k-1)\cdot\sin\frac{2\pi(k-1)}{N} )^2 }$$
$$+ w \cdot | I_p( r(k) , \frac{2\pi k}{N} ) - I_{ref} | \quad (1)$$

is thus minimized with respect to $r(k)$, which for each $k$ can take one of $m$ discrete values. $I_p$ is the gray level of the polar image representation and $I_{ref}$ is a reference gray level to which the contour is attracted. The parameter $w$ weights the influence of the external force term. For the present study, the parameters were set to $N=36$, $m=21$ and $w= 0.1$. Trials were performed with $I_{ref}$ set to 5, 10, 15 and 18 % of maximum intensity of each image slice.

## 2.6 Acquisitions

For SPECT acquisitions, a scintillation camera (DIACAM, Siemens Gammasonic Inc., IL,USA) connected to a Nuclear Mac computer (Scientific Imaging Inc) was used. SPECT projections in 120 angles were acquired in a 128×128 matrix and 360° rotation mode. Transversal images of 128×128 pixels were reconstructed by an iterative ML-EM algorithm [16] with 30 iterations per transversal slice. Images were slightly smoothed using a median 3×3 and a 3 ×3 boxcar average kernel.

A phantom study was performed using a Lucite DeLuxe elliptical phantom (Data Spectrum Inc, NC, USA) filled with water and four spheres containing $^{131}$I. The largest sphere was situated in the phantom center and the remaining three, positioned around the center with radii between 7 and 8 cm. A high energy collimator was employed and the pixel size was 3.8 mm. The phantom was aligned in relation to the marker plate by use of the laser beams. Acquisition was made in two energy windows, one of ±15% centered over the photopeak of 364 keV and a second of 50 - 150 keV over the Compton scatter region.

The patient trial was performed for a clinical evaluation study of a monoclonal antibody directed towards colon cancer, labelled with $^{123}$I. An activity of 146 MBq was injected and imaging performed 8 hours after injection. SPECT and whole body images then mainly showed uptake in the superior part of the abdomen and the bladder.

Acquisition was performed in a photopeak energy window of ±20% centered at 164 keV (to detect the primary photons of 159 keV), and a scatter window of 90 keV ±66%. A LEAP collimator was used and the pixel size was 3.8 mm.

CT scanning was performed with a Philips Tomoscan LX. For all studies the program for abdominal scanning was used. The transaxial FOV was 350 mm, the matrix size 512×512 and the axial sampling made with a slice thickness of 10 mm and no interslice gaps. Scanning of the phantom was performed in the geometry described above, with iodine contrast medium inserted to the spheres.

## 2.7 Monte Carlo Simulation

A Monte Carlo study for [131]I was performed with the SIMIND code [13] for the DIACAM camera configuration and a high energy collimator. A patient like source distribution was obtained by utilizing the anthropomorphic computer Zubal-phantom [19]. The distribution of [131]I was chosen to resemble an actual patient study and is given in Table 1. An amount of 768 million photons were simulated for 64 projections. Data were stored in 64×64 matrices with a pixel size of 6.25 mm. The spectral distribution of the primary photons included all major photon energies [14]. Septal penetration was not included in the simulation.

## 2.8 Evaluation

To evaluate the intrinsic accuracy of the computer algorithm, binary images were registered to themselves with a changed pixel size and randomly introduced translations and rotations between ±5 pixels and ±10 degrees. Binary images of human shape were obtained from the Zubal-phantom by setting all pixels representing the body equal to a constant value. Two measures of registration accuracy were used. The sum of absolute differences (SAD) was calculated and expressed as a fraction of the total number of pixels representing the patient for the actual slice. In order to get a length measure of the accuracy, differences between induced and obtained rotations and translations were evaluated and expressed as residual distances between pixels that should be identical. For this measure, the value of the rotational inaccuracy is dependent on the radial position. A radius of one fourth of the image dimensions was chosen since often, organs of interest are not situated at the very edges of the FOV. The accuracy was evaluated as

| Source organ | Relative number of emitted photons | Situated between Zubal-phantom slices |
|---|---|---|
| Urine | 12 | 127 -- 211 |
| Spleen | 15 | 112 -- 136 |
| Liver | 15 | 112 -- 149 |
| Liver tumor | 30 | 120 -- 131 |
| Bladder | 12 | 185 -- 211 |
| Heart | 7 | 80 -- 111 |
| Thyroid | 12 | 62 -- 66 * |

**Table 1.** Activity distribution for the [131]I Monte Carlo simulation study of the anthropomorphic Zubal-phantom.

a function of axial position, giving an estimate of the influence of the slice shape.

The extent and accuracy to which contours generated from Compton scatter data can be used for registration was then investigated. CT and [131]I SPECT scatter images known to represent identical anatomical regions, with well defined slice thickness, were obtained from the Zubal-phantom. Images representing the density distribution and here used for CT data were produced by converting the codes for the different organs to density values from Schneider et al [20]. [131]I SPECT slices were obtained by Monte Carlo simulation. Segmentation of scatter images was performed with both described methods. Prior to segmentation scatter images were rotated and translated at random within $\pm 7$ pixels and $\pm 10$ degrees. Registration was performed and rotational and translational residuals evaluated for several slices, giving an estimate of the influence of the activity distribution.

A phantom study was performed to evaluate the influence of scattered radiation from the patient couch and the accuracy of the axial fit. As obtained rotations and translations differed slightly in the axial direction, averages were calculated and applied to SPECT photopeak and CT image sets respectively. As measure of accuracy the 3D coordinate of the center-of-mass for each sphere was determined. Sphere boundaries were outlined in consecutive images by interactively choosing a threshold value for photopeak SPECT images and by use of the technique previously described for contour determination for CT.

Patient trials provide the most relevant accuracy measure. At this stage, the method has been evaluated for one [123]I SPECT patient only. Three point markers, [57]Co for SPECT and lead for CT, were fastened to the patient at the relatively stable structures sternum and the left and right side of the rib cage. Obtained rotations and translations were analyzed as a function of axial position and divided into three groups, one for each marker, over which the average was calculated. Obtained values were implemented on image data and the accuracy evaluated by determining the r.m.s. distance between markers. Because of limited spatial resolution for SPECT, markers appeared in several slices and so mean coordinates in the x, y and z directions were determined.

## 3 Results

A summary of the results is presented in Table 2.

| Intrinsic Accuracy | SAD: $6.2 \pm 0.4$ % | Rms distance: | $0.6 \pm 0.2$ | pixels |
|---|---|---|---|---|
| Phantom Experiment | x: $1.9 \pm 0.2$ | y: $0.3 \pm 0.1$ | z: $1.0 \pm 0.3$ | |
| Monte Carlo | slice numbers | 70 -- 110 | 110 -- 150 | 150 -- 230 |
| Simulation | Interactive Threshold | $4.7 \pm 1.9$ | $8.9 \pm 1.9$ | $4.1 \pm 2.3$ |
| | Snakes, 10% | $8.5 \pm 2.9$ | $10.6 \pm 3.3$ | $5.2 \pm 2.3$ |
| | Snakes, 5% | $10.8 \pm 4.0$ | $7.8 \pm 2.5$ | $7.3 \pm 3.2$ |
| Patient | Averages: x: 7 | y: 11 | z: 12 | |

**Table 2.** Summary of results in mm, except where stated otherwise

The intrinsic accuracy for the registration algorithm as evaluated by SAD, was on an average obtained to $6.2\pm0.4\%$ and was less than 7.5 % for all slice shapes. Expressed as residuals, intrinsic deviations were at maximum 1.2 pixels, and at average $0.6\pm0.2$ pixels. A maximum rotational deviation of 0.9 degrees was obtained, corresponding to 0.5 pixels at the half radius, i.e. 32 pixels from the rotation center.

For the simulated $^{131}$I study and segmentation performed with the thresholding method, accuracies of 0.5 to 13.3 mm were obtained, corresponding to 0.2 and 5.3 pixels respectively. A maximum rotational deviation of 4 degrees was obtained and for translations 7.6 mm. The larger deviations, ranging from 6 to 13.3 mm with an average of approximately 9 mm, occurred in density slices between 110 and 150. Lower deviations, 0.5-9 mm, were obtained for slices 70 - 110, and 150 - 230, with averages of about 5 and 4 mm for each region respectively. A similar pattern was seen when segmentation was performed with the deformable contour model; accuracies here depended on the choice of $I_{ref}$ and the axial position, i.e. the slice number of the Zubal-phantom. When $I_{ref}$ was set to 10%, an average deviation of 8.5 mm was obtained for density slices 70 - 110 and for slices 150 - 230, 5.2 mm. For slices in between, numbers 110 to 150, this result was 10.6 mm. With $I_{ref}$ set to 5%, deviations were on the average larger, however for slices 110-150 a result of 7.8 mm was obtained. For 15% and 18%, obtained results were similar to that of 10% except for some 20 slices in the inferior abdomen for which deviations were large. Fig.5 shows corresponding photopeak and scatter SPECT images and also density slices representing CT data. For the slices through the heart and bladder the activity is focused in the center giving a rather symmetrical scatter count rate distribution. For a slice through the liver, the activity concentration is prominent in the right side of the patient giving a tilted scatter distribution. In between the major organs, scatter distributions are fairly homogeneous,

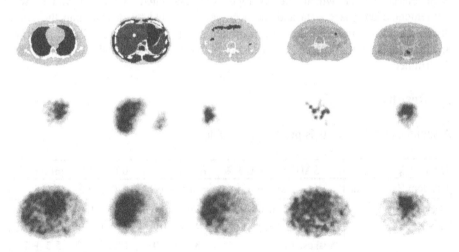

**Fig. 5.** Transversal images obtained by Monte Carlo simulation of the 3D anthropomorphic Zubal-phantom, with activity distribution according to Table 1. Top row: Density slices, middle row: photopeak $^{131}$I SPECT images, bottom row: scatter images. Shown images correspond to density slices 92, 120, 145, 170 and 195 and represent slices through the heart, superior liver, inferior liver, intestines and the bladder respectively.

and to some extent reflecting the activity distribution of neighboring slices.

Deviations for the phantom study were obtained to less than 2.9 mm for all directions and were on average 1.9, 0.3 and 1 mm in the x, y, z directions respectively.For the patient evaluation trial, obtained r.m.s. distances between markers in the CT and SPECT images were at maximum 16 mm. In the z direction, values depended slightly on the number of slices included at determination of the SPECT marker position. Obtained deviations in the x, y and z directions were on an average 7, 11 and 12 mm, between 6 and 9 mm, 9 and 12 mm, 4 and 16 mm, respectively.

## 4 Discussion

Several aspects need to be considered for registration of abdominal tomographic images. Inherent limitations to both the resolution and the determination of tissue positions are imposed by the continuous movements of organs and the temporal variation of stomach, bowel, bladder content etc. The liver e.g. has been reported to move as much as 3-8 cm between inhalation and expiration [2]. A related problem is achievement of a conform and reproducible patient position, and for systems employing fiducial markers, the accuracy to which the patient may be positioned in relation to the markers (or vice versa). Erdi et al [7] arrived at accuracies of 1-2 cm by use of a cradle with external markers. For the present positioning system several patient examinations have been performed, although only one has been used for evaluation of accuracy. Generally the hard couch has been well tolerated. Rather, patients have been bothered by lying with their arms raised during the 30 minutes SPECT acquisition. The sail cloth has been found useful for positioning of the patient in relation to the laser beams. In the evaluation trial, the activity retention in the abdomen was low and thus images were noisy. Obtained deviations are at the maximum 16 mm, indicating that acceptable alignment may be achieved although further evaluation is required.

An approximation in the present model is that images have been considered as parallel and rigid slices. CT images acquired through the swayback have shown that the patient may be slightly twisted in the axial direction, so that the angle around the z axis vary throughout the abdomen. The relation between all slices has therefore not been fixed as is done in a 3D rigid body model. By allowing smooth variations for the rotation around the z axis in the intermediate abdomen, some elasticity has been incorporated. As images are considered parallel, uncertainties regarding the rotation around the x and y axes are introduced. Positions of the pelvis, thorax and the intermediate part respectively have been difficult to obtain and eventual rotations have been assumed to be accounted for by the positioning device. The possibility to determine the axial location of abdominal slices by use of only scatter slices is believed to be limited. In the present study a marker plate was applied which also provided a conform couch shape at the different facilities.

Results from the phantom study show that the axial location may be accurately determined from the positioning device and that the registration accuracy for a rigid object is at sub pixel level. By results from the simulated study, deviations in the order of 5 mm are obtained for images in which the events are symmetrically distributed. In density slices where the liver is present, which for scatter data correspond to additional slices because of the spatial distribution of the scattered radiation, deviations are higher. Accuracies thus depend on the intensity homogeneity which in turn depends on the activity distribution and also, as seen in the experimental studies, on scattered radiation from the patient couch. For boundary determination, this imposes difficulties because the appropriate threshold value varies with the lateral position. The deformable contour model initially tested here, may provide a robust tool for automated contour determination. Deviations are somewhat larger as compared to the manual thresholding method, however has the advantage of being automatic and thus less time consuming. Further optimization need to be performed in order to optimize the reference threshold value or some other criterion to be used for contour search.

Another factor that has shown to have influence on the scatter images is the method for reconstruction. Initially slices were reconstructed by filtered back projection, but iterative reconstruction later showed to be favorable due to the streak artefacts produced by filtered back projection, that for peripheral parts of the abdomen were not negligible. Other factors influencing the overall accuracy are thought to be the axial sampling density i.e. the slice thickness and the presence of interslice gaps for CT, the spatial resolution for different imaging modalities and the width and location of the Compton scatter energy window.

Achievement of a representative and independent system for evaluation of registration accuracy requires special attention, see e.g. [21]. As the objective is to register positions of organs and lesions, evaluation should focus on the positions of internal structures. However, the SPECT tracers used in this study were not homogeneously distributed in certain organs, making this approach less feasible. Special markers for evaluation of accuracy were applied, providing an independent measure of the accuracy on the patient boundary.

The concept of using Compton scatter data for guidance of contour determination to be used for registration has shown promising results. Future work will include development of the registration method to improve the use of data in three dimensions and further investigation of the segmentation problem.

## Acknowledgements

The authors would like to thank Karin Wingårdh, B.Sc, and Magnus Tagesson, M.Sc, for support during the patient studies. This work has been supported by grants from the Swedish Cancer Foundation grant 2353-B96-10XBB, the Gunnar, Arvid and Elisabeth Nilsson Foundation, the Mrs Berta Kamprad Foundation, the John and Augusta Persson Foundation and the Lund University Hospital Funds.
This research was supported by Swedish Radiation Protection Institute, grant SSI P 893.95.

## References

1.  D.A. Weber, M. Ivanovic: Correlative Image Registration. Seminars in Nucl Med XXIV, 311-323 (1994)
2.  G Flux: Multimodality image registration and its application to the dosimetry of intralesional radionuclide therapy. Doctoral Thesis (1995)
3.  C.A. Pelizzari et al: Accurate Three-Dimensional Registration of CT, PET, and/or MR Images of the Brain. J Comput Assist Tomogr 13, 20-26 (1989)

4. N.M. Alpert et al: The Principal Axes Tranformation - A Method for Image Registration. J Nucl Med 31, 1717-1722 (1990)
5. P.A. van den Elsen et al: Medical Image Matching - A Review with Classification. IEEE Eng Med Biol 12, 26-39 (1993)
6. E.L. Kramer et al: CT-SPECT Fusion to Correlate Radiolabeled Monoclonal Antibody Uptake with Abdominal CT Findings. Radiology 172, 861-865 (1989)
7. Y.E. Erdi et al: A new fiducial alignment system to overlay abdominal computed tomography or magnetic resonance anatomical images with radiolabeled antibody Single-Photon Emission Computed Tomographic scans. Cancer 73, 923-931 (1994)
8. K.F. Koral et al: CT-SPECT fusion plus conjugate views for determining dosimetry in iodine-131-monoclonal antibody therapy of lymphoma patients. J Nucl Med 35, 1714-1720 (1994)
9. A.M. Scott et al: Image registration of SPECT and CT images using an external fiduciary band and three-dimensional surface fitting in metastatic thyroid cancer. J Nucl Med 36, 100-103 (1995)
10. E.L. Kramer, M.E. Noz: CT-SPECT Fusion for Analysis of Radiolabeled Antibodies: Applications in Gastrointestinal and Lung Carcinoma. Nucl Med Biol 18, 27-42 (1991)
11. S. Eberl et al: Automated interstudy image registration technique for SPECT and PET. J Nucl Med 37, 137-145 (1996)
12. T. Pan et al: Segmentation of the Body and Lungs from Compton Scatter and Photopeak Window Data in SPECT: A Monte Carlo Investigation. IEEE Trans Biomed Eng 3, 1657-1661 (1993)
13. M. Ljungberg, S-E. Strand: A Monte Carlo Program Simulating Gamma Camera Imaging. Computer Methods and Programs in Biomedicine 29, 257-272 (1989)
14. D.A. Weber et al: MIRD: Radionuclide Data and Decay Schemes. The Society of Nuclear Medicine Inc (1989)
15. R.C. Gonzalez, R.E. Woods: Digital Image Processing. Addison-Wesley Publishing Company Inc (1992)
16. T.S. Pan et al: Design of an efficient 3D projector and backprojector for SPECT. Proceedings of the International Meeting on Fully 3D Image Reconstruction in Radiology and Nuclear Medicine 181-185 (1995)
17. M. Kass et al: Snakes: Active Contour Models. International Journal of Computer Vision 321-331 (1988)
18. A.A. Amini et al: Using Dynamic Programming for Solving Variational Problems in Vision. IEEE Transactions on pattern analysis and machine intelligence 12, 855-867 (1990)
19. G. Zubal et al: Computerized three-dimensional segmented human anatomy. Med Phys 21, 299-302 (1994)
20. U. Schneider et al: The calibration of CT Hounsfield units for radiotherapy treatment planning. Phys Med Biol 41, 111-124 (1995)
21. P.F. Hemler et al: Registration error quantification of a surface based multimodality image fusion system. J Nucl Med 22, 1049-1056 (1995)

# Definition of Volume Transformations for Volume Interaction

Thomas Schiemann and Karl Heinz Höhne

Institute of Mathematics and Computer Science in Medicine (IMDM),
University Hospital Hamburg-Eppendorf, Germany
e-mail: schiemann@uke.uni-hamburg.de

**Abstract.** Volume transformations of medical images play an important role for many applications such as registration of different modalities, mapping atlases onto clinical data, or simulation of surgical procedures. While registration and atlas mapping can for the major number of applications be performed without tight time constraints, it is essential for simulation systems that they allow real-time interaction. As any computational method in volumes is usually very time consuming, current approaches do mainly concentrate on surface manipulations instead of transforming the entire volume. This paper describes an approach, which overcomes this problem by first defining the volume manipulation on basis of surface models, which ensure real time performance, and in a second step the transformation is applied to the entire volume by interpolating the mapping parameters using scattered data interpolation methods.

## 1 Introduction

Geometric volume transformations often are a matter of interest when handling tomographic images in medicine. Currently, registration procedures are the main area of application and have already entered clinical routine. For the purpose of multi-modal registration, a global affine transformation of one of the volumes is usually sufficient [5, 15] if we assume that image distortions introduced by the scanning devices have been corrected in advance. The situation gets much more complex if we enter the field of atlas registration, which requires non-linear transformations for compensation of morphological differences between the atlas and the subject under consideration.

Simulation procedures build another large field where volume transformations can be used and cover a variety of medical applications:

- Simulation of classical surgical procedures: Open the operation field and shift, remove, replace, or sculpture structures.
- Simulation of endoscopic procedures: Blow up the area of investigation and deform the esophagus, the stomach, or the intestine as the endoscope is pushed through them.
- Simulation of growing morphological structures: Select a seed-area and let the included structures grow (for study of genesis), or insert a seed point for a lesion and see the effects of its growth.

– Assessment of inter-individual variation: Select corresponding structures of different individuals and map them onto each other or onto a common reference.

It is obvious that non-linear volume transformations are again required for all such procedures. These transformations usually lead to expensive computations, while for simulation of surgery or endoscopy real-time execution is required for enabling realistic feedback. Therefore current systems [1, 3, 8, 13] concentrate on transformation of surfaces only, which introduces a number of drawbacks, because all structures are hollow and can hence not represent reality.

In this paper we describe a method, which offers true volume transformations at any stage of a simulation procedure. While the definition of the transformation is still based on surface models in order to provide real-time interaction, the volume transformation is computed in the entire volume by interpolating the mapping parameters using scattered data interpolation methods.

## 2    Method

This section covers three different topics, which are necessary to apply volume transformations within an volume interaction environment [6], which is suitable for different applications. The volume interaction environment allows segmentation [11] of volume objects from different tomographic sources (CT, MRI, histological slices) and exploration of these objects via comprehensive 3D visualization techniques [9, 14].

The first subsection describes, how to introduce surface models into the volume context, for example models of medical devices like the tip of an endoscope, or surface representations of morphological structures, which are contained in the volume. The different ways of interaction with the surface model within the volume context are described in second subsection, and the third subsection shows how to extend the definition of the volume transformation from the surface models to the entire volume.

### 2.1    Surface model

The first objective is to set up a surface model for real-time interaction in the context of the volume. The design of the model shall have several degrees of freedom such that it can be adapted to different applications. We are therefore using a model $M$ with two layers of parameters. It can be formalized as

$$M(P_0, n_1, n_2, n_3; \Sigma, \alpha).$$

The first layer describes an orthogonal coordinate system with origin at $P_0$ and directions $n_i$. This coordinate system spans a hull with shape parameters $\Sigma$ and $\alpha$. The parameter $\Sigma$ can take discrete values from a limited set, where each element corresponds to a fixed basic shape of the model (tab. 1). There are three classes of shapes corresponding to elemental solids $\mathcal{E}$ (e.g. ellipsoid or cone), compositions $\mathcal{C}$ of solids, which are usually approximations of medical devices, and triangular meshes $\mathcal{T}$ for keeping surface representations of volume objects.

The parameter $\alpha$ is a tuple of variable length with boolean, integer, or float elements. Their number and type is depending on the value of $\Sigma$. Typical parameters, which are determined by $\alpha$ are extent, mesh width, number of elements composed (for class $\mathcal{C}$), or whether the solids are closed or open. The possible values for $\Sigma$, which have been realized so far are listed in table 1, and figure 1 shows the model's appearance for different values of $\Sigma$ and $\alpha$.

The parameter value $\Sigma = \mathcal{T}$ differs from all other parameters in the way, that the corresponding model is not determined by a closed analytical description, but instead uses a pure enumeration of surface elements. This option is necessary for storing arbitrary surface models, which are usually obtained from volume objects by triangulation. For this purpose we are using the marching cubes technique [7] extended by a method for reducing the number of triangles [16].

| $\Sigma$ | Shape | $\Sigma$ | Shape | $\Sigma$ | Shape | $\Sigma$ | Shape |
|---|---|---|---|---|---|---|---|
| $\mathcal{E}_1$ | Plane | $\mathcal{E}_5$ | Star | $\mathcal{C}_1$ | Arrow | $\mathcal{T}$ | Triangular mesh |
| $\mathcal{E}_2$ | Ellipsoid | $\mathcal{E}_6$ | Torus | $\mathcal{C}_2$ | Dumbbell | | |
| $\mathcal{E}_3$ | Cone | $\mathcal{E}_7$ | Cylinder | $\mathcal{C}_3$ | Ultrasound-sensor | | |
| $\mathcal{E}_4$ | Cube | | | $\mathcal{C}_4$ | Head of endoscope | | |

**Table 1.** Values for the basic shape parameter $\Sigma$ and corresponding appearances of the model. The values $\mathcal{E}_i$ represent elemental solids, $\mathcal{C}_i$ represent compositions of solids, and $\mathcal{T}$ stands for triangular meshes of arbitrary shape.

For later use of the model it is essential that it can be displayed very fast. Therefore the model is also represented in the typical fashion of computer graphics as three lists of points $\{P_i\}$, lines $\{L_i\}$, and triangles $\{T_i\}$.

$\{P_i\}$ $(i = 1, \ldots, n_P, \quad P_i \in I\!\!R^3)$ includes the hull-points after discretization of the model according to $\Sigma$ and $\alpha$.

$\{L_i\}$ $(i = 1, \ldots, n_L, \quad L_i \in \{1, \ldots, n_P\}^2)$ is a list of line-elements and determines, which two points from $\{P_i\}$ shall each be linked by a line, if the model is displayed as a wire-frame.

$\{T_i\}$ $(i = 1, \ldots, n_T, \quad T_i \in \{1, \ldots, n_P\}^3)$ is a list of triangle-elements and determines, which three points from $\{P_i\}$ shall each build a triangular patch, if the model is displayed with shaded surfaces.

In figure 1 the different appearances of the model are shown as wire-frames without any further context in order to enhance the method of construction. But as the model shall serve as an aid for definition of volume transformations, it is essential that it can be displayed in a natural way within the context of the

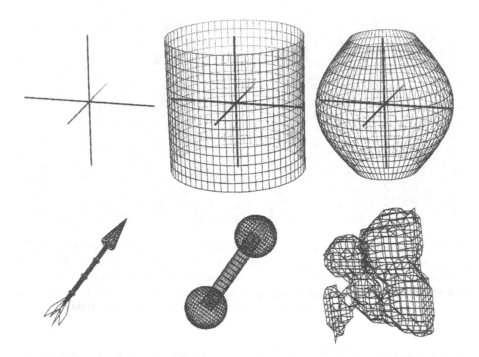

**Fig. 1.** Different appearances of the surface model. Top row: Coordinate system without hull and with two different cylindrically shaped hulls shaped hulls ($\Sigma = \mathcal{E}_7$) corresponding to two different settings for the parameter-vector $\alpha$, which in this case determines the curvature. Bottom row: Two compositions of elemental solids (arrow $\Sigma = \mathcal{C}_1$, and dumbbell $\Sigma = \mathcal{C}_2$), and a surface representation of a part of the intestine ($\Sigma = \mathcal{T}$).

volume. The rendering routines for the model are hence considering all geometric mapping parameters, which are used for any image (2D or 3D) obtained from the volume. The surface rendering uses the z-buffer of 3D images in order to be consistent regarding hidden surfaces. If the model is visualized with shaded surfaces, the illumination parameters are also equivalent to those of the volume based image (fig. 2 left). When the model is to be displayed on 2D slices of the volume, this can be performed by orthogonal 3D visualization (fig. 2 middle), or the list of triangles $\{T_i\}$ can be used to compute the intersection of the model with the slice for showing the outline of the intersection (fig. 2 right).

## 2.2 Interaction

The last subsection described the static construction of the surface model and how to adapt it to different circumstances. For its primary use of defining volume transformations, the second important question is how to modify the surface model intuitively and quickly. As we want to use the method on a common work-

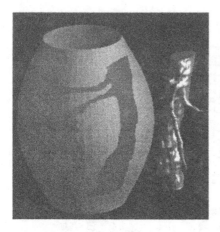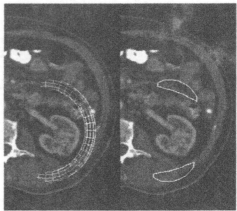

**Fig. 2.** Visualization of the surface model on images obtained from the volume. Left: Perspective 3D rendering within the context of volume objects. Hidden surfaces and illumination are computed on common parameters in order to achieve a consistent appearance of the model. Right: Display of the model on planes of the volume either by orthogonal 3D rendering (left) or outlining of the intersection area (right).

station, the only input device we can use is a standard mouse. Any interaction with the model must therefore be performed in the following way:

1. User action (= movement of mouse)
2. Derivation of a 3D modification of the model from the 2D movement
3. Computation of the transformation of the whole model
4. Output of the transformed model (on the screen)

Steps 1 and 4 do not need much discussion, as step 1 is a natural method for any interaction with standard computers, and step 4 means the 3D rendering procedures, which are based on well known computer graphics techniques [4]. Steps 2 and 3 are however critical for the goal of an intuitive and fast method.

**Interaction with the surface model** For transformation of the model according to the user action with the mouse there is a large set of modes, which can be grouped into three different classes (fig. 3):

- Global functions of different sub-classes are used for an overall general modification of the model: Polynomial functions up to second order are used to perform global movements (first order) or simple distortions (second order). More general mappings are used to model elastic deformations (e.g. via thin-plate-splines or warping schemes).
- Local displacements of the model's hull are expressed by displacements of the mesh points. Any mesh point can be selected for interactive displacement, and several points can be grouped for common modifications.

- <u>Parameter modifications</u> of the parameter vector $\alpha$. For these modes mouse movement will result in modification of one or several elements of $\alpha$, e.g. for changing the geometry of a model for a surgical device.

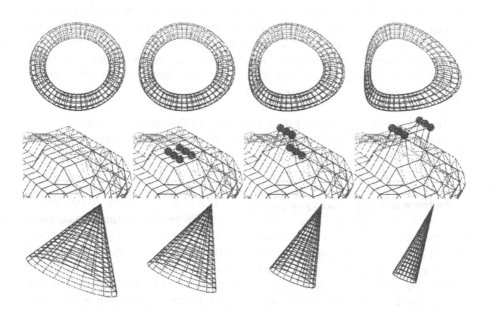

**Fig. 3.** Different classes of interaction, where each image represents a state during a continuous interaction. The model can be transformed via global functions (top), local modifications of the mesh points (middle), or changes of the parameter vector $\alpha$ (bottom).

The main problem, when having only a 2D mouse for definition of a 3D transformation is the lack of a third dimension. The common way to solve this problem is to use the keyboard for switching to the missing dimension. For example, a free 3D rotation could in this way be defined by assigning the X-rotation to the up-down movement, the Y-rotation to the left-right movement, and the Z-rotation to the left-right movement, while a certain key is pressed. This is of course not intuitive and causes major difficulties for many users. Hence we prefer to use one of the following two methods for definition of 3D actions:

- The number of degrees of freedom for the model's transformation can be reduced. In this way every dimension of the transformation can be assigned to one of the mouse directions. A 3D translation could e.g. be restricted to a plane or to the direction perpendicular to an object surface. The restricting elements can usually be determined from the context of the application.
- The 3D transformation could be defined indirectly by definition of an auxiliary item, which can be defined more easily. For example, a free rotation

could be defined by selection of a point, towards which a certain axis of the model shall be rotated.

**Computation of the transformation of the model**  The method described above ensures, that the interaction with the model can be performed as intuitive as possible with a 2D mouse. For real-time execution it is now critical, that the transformation can be applied with as little computational expense as possible. The detailed way of computing the transformation of the model depends on the actually selected transformation mode. In principle, there are the following two main steps, which have to be performed:

1. Transformation of all hull points according to the transformation.
2. Transformation of all hull points from object space into the space of the image, in which the model is to be displayed. This means multiplication of every point with a homogeneous $(4 \times 4)$-matrix.

As there is a large variety of possible volume transformations to be defined, it is impossible to make a clear general statement on the computational costs. For affine transformations, the computation is very cheap, because for the transformation itself it is sufficient to transform the coordinate system of the model only, resulting in a new matrix, which can be combined with the image matrix of the second step. For general non-linear transformations, the expense depends directly on the complexity of the active transformation mode: While displacing groups of mesh points is cheap, because only a local small portion of the model needs to be transformed, polynomial mappings require by far more computation time, and parameter modifications may be expensive if the model's geometry is complex.

One possible way of saving time, which can be taken under any circumstances, is to keep the complexity regarding the model's number of surface elements as low as possible. Especially during the initial state of an application it is usually acceptable to work with models in lower resolution.

## 2.3  Volume interpolation

The model described in the previous two subsections offers the functionality of interactively defining volume transformations in a very general fashion. As our main intention is to obtain true volume transformations, the transformation has to be spread from the surfaces of the model to every single voxel in the volume in order to assign a displacement vector to every discrete point. Techniques, which could be used for this are known as scattered data interpolation methods, because the given data points are not well ordered for parameter-guided standard interpolation. In general, we have to deal with the following interpolation problem:

We have a set of source points $\{A_i\}$, which are taken from the surface model in the original state, and a set of target point $\{Z_i\}$, which are taken from the transformed surface model. The problem is to find an at least steady function

$$f(P) : \mathbb{R}^3 \to \mathbb{R}^3 \qquad \text{with } f(A_i) = Z_i \text{ for all } i.$$

We have investigated two different interpolation schemes for this problem:

**Interpolation with weighted local interpolators** The most obvious approach is to construct $f$ as a weighted sum of locally interpolating functions $f_i$:

$$f(P) = \sum_{i=1}^{n} \omega_i(P) \, f_i(P),$$

where

$$f_i : \mathbb{R}^3 \to \mathbb{R}^3, \qquad f_i(A_i) = Z_i \text{ for all } i,$$

and

$$\omega_i : \mathbb{R}^3 \to \mathbb{R}$$

are normalized weight functions with

$$\omega_i(A_i) = 1 \text{ for all } i, \qquad \omega_i(A_j) = 0 \text{ for all } i \neq j,$$

$$\omega_i(P) \geq 0 \text{ and } \sum_{i=1}^{n} \omega_i(P) = 1 \text{ for all } P \in \mathbb{R}^3.$$

This approach has originally been proposed in [12]. For our method we followed a choice for $f_i$ and $\omega_i$, which is described in [10]:

$$f_i(P) = Z_i + L(P - A_i),$$

where $L : \mathbb{R}^3 \to \mathbb{R}^3$ is a linear functional, which minimizes a global error function. The weights are chosen as

$$\omega_i(P) = \frac{\sigma_i(P)}{\sum_{j=1}^{n} \sigma_j(P)}$$

with

$$\sigma_i(P) = \frac{1}{\|P - A_i\|^2}$$

The construction of this interpolation scheme follows basically geometric ideas. It is therefore not surprising, that artifacts are occurring, if the range of displacements is increasing. This problem does not occur with the second approach:

**Interpolation with thin-plate splines** Interpolation with thin-plate splines has successfully been introduced to 2D image processing [2] and can directly be generalized for 3D applications. The construction of thin-plate splines origins from mechanics, which results in much better behavior for even strong displacements compared to interpolation with linear local interpolators. The interpolating function $f$ is constructed as a linear combination of functions of the form

$$U(r) = r^2 \log r^2 \qquad (r \in I\!\!R, \ r > 0),$$

and an affine correction term:

$$f(P) = \sum_{i=1}^{n} \Omega_i U(\|P - A_i\|) + L(P) + Q_0,$$

where $\Omega_i, Q_0 \in I\!\!R^3$, and $L : I\!\!R^3 \to I\!\!R^3$ is again a linear functional. The function $U$ is a fundamental solution of the biharmonic equation $\Delta^2 U = 0$. The Vectors $\Omega_i$ and $Q_0$ and the coefficients of $L$ are determined by solving the following system of linear vector equations, which formalize the interpolation condition and normalization:

$$\sum_{i=1}^{n} \Omega_i U(\|A_j - A_i\|) + L(A_j) + Q_0 = Z_j \quad j = 1, \ldots, n$$

$$\sum_{i=1}^{n} \Omega_i = 0$$

$$\sum_{i=1}^{n} \Omega_i x_i = 0$$

$$\sum_{i=1}^{n} \Omega_i y_i = 0$$

$$\sum_{i=1}^{n} \Omega_i z_i = 0, \quad \text{where } A_i = (x_i, y_i, z_i)^T$$

**Volume resampling** The remaining task is now, to actually perform the volume transformation by resampling the new volume. As the integer-coordinates of the input volume are mapped onto float-coordinates in the output-volume, a single input voxel will usually be spread on several output voxels, or several input voxels will share one output voxel (for shrinking transformations). Different resampling solutions have been published for this problem [17]. In the current phase of this project we are using a straight-forward approach, which transforms the 6 neighbors of every voxel and fills the volume spanned by these neighbors in the output volume with the value of the central voxel. This filling is weighted according to the percentage, which is covered in the respective output voxel.

# 3 Results

The proposed methods have been implemented in ANSI-C on standard UNIX-workstations (e.g. DEC alpha). They have been embedded in a comprehensive medical volume interaction system (VOXEL-MAN) and can thus be invoked in conjunction with many different applications. The following subsections describe two different areas, in which the method can be applied.

## 3.1 Normalization of Shape

For comparison of different individuals it is useful to transform different volumes into a common general shape. Such procedures are frequently proposed for brain studies, especially in the field of computerized atlases.

If the brain is assumed to be roughly ball shaped, different brains can be transformed to spheres and can hence be compared in their new normalized shape. For this purpose we are using the described model in star-shape ($\Sigma = \mathcal{E}_5$). The center of the star is located in the center of the brain, and every ray gets the length, which makes it touch the outer surface. The rays have a certain width, which ensures that they are long enough to leave the sulci. Figure 4 shows a 3D image of a brain with the corresponding ray ends each marked by small balls. The ray end points form the set $\{A_i\}$ of source points.

We then take a star with equal number of rays but uniform length of 100 voxels and take their end points as the set of target points $\{Z_i\}$. After computation of the thin-plate spline the volume is transformed and we end up with a ball shaped brain as shown in figure 5.

While this application does in general not require real-time definition of the mapping, our approach has the advantage, that corrections on the set of source points $\{A_i\}$ can easily and quickly be performed. Such corrections might e.g. be necessary when pathological changes in morphology are present.

## 3.2 Simulation of surgical procedures

For simulation of surgical procedures the described method offers the choice of two different ways of interaction depending on the question, whether the surface model represents the surgical device or the examined structure. We illustrate this application with the example of a needle examination of a kidney.

The first principle is to use the surface model as a representative for the needle by using the cylindrical shape ($\Sigma = \mathcal{E}_7$) with the interaction modes of free rotation and translation along a fixed direction (determined by the rotation). Hence the needle can be rotated and shifted along the specified axis within the context of the volume objects (fig. 6 left). The mesh points around the tip of the needle are "sensitive" and recognize, when they hit volume structures. Hence two sets of points can be obtained after having shifted the needle into the kidney: Those points on the boundary of the kidney, which were hit by the sensitive grid points when the tip of the needle penetrated the kidney, form the source points $\{A_i\}$ for the coming volume transformation. The current positions of

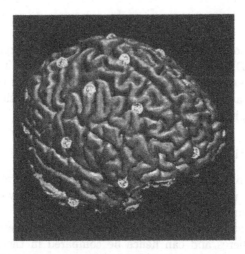

**Fig. 4.** 3D image of a brain obtained from MRI. The markers show the end points of the rays corresponding to the star shaped model.

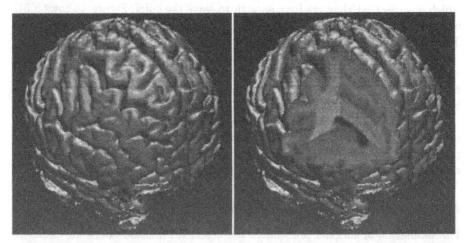

**Fig. 5.** Brain after volume transformation into a uniform shape. On the right a portion of the brain has been removed for showing the effect of true volume instead of surface transformation.

the sensitive needle points form the target points $\{Z_i\}$. After computation of the volume transformation we obtain images like in figure 7, which show the deformed kidney.

The second principle is to fill the surface model with a triangular description of the considered kidney ($\Sigma = \mathcal{T}$, fig. 6 right). The interaction mode is set to translation perpendicular to the last hit surface element. When now moving the mouse, we immediately see a feedback of the deformed kidney surface, because for the surface model the transformation can be computed very fast. Again the

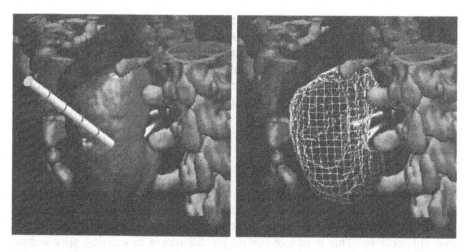

**Fig. 6.** View of the left kidney and surrounding structures (bone, intestine) obtained from a spiral CT dataset of an upper abdomen. The surface model mimics a needle and can be moved within the volume scene (left). When the needle touches the kidney, the deformation can not be visualized immediately, because the kidney is present in its volume representation. This situation changes, if the kidney is replaced with the corresponding surface model (right) in order to allow real-time manipulations. (The kidney is displayed as a wire-frame only instead of shaded surfaces in order to enhance its different representation compared to the volume objects).

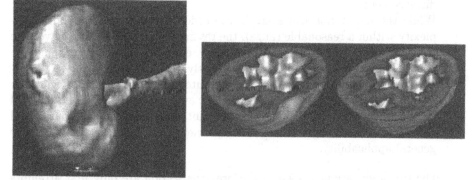

**Fig. 7.** Volume based renderings of the kidney after computation of the true volume transformation defined in figure 6. The imprint of the needle is clearly visible in the lower section of the organ. The cuts through the kidney show the treatment's effects on internal structures. For comparison the very right image shows the corresponding structure without deformation.

computation of the true volume transformation can be released at any time of the procedure, e.g. in order to assess internal structures (fig. 7).

While both principles have the advantage of real-time interactivity, they both also have the disadvantage of showing only one aspect of the procedure at a time - either the surgical instrument or the considered structure. This problem can be handled by switching from one principle to the other, which can be done at any stage of the procedure.

# 4 Conclusion

We have described a framework for interactive definition and execution of volume transformations. As it is not based on any conditions on the type of the considered volumes or their contents, the method has a very large range of possible applications. This is one of the major differences to existing approaches, which are usually suited to single questions. Another difference is the fact, that our approach results in true volume transformations, which are important for a comprehensive assessment of the structures contained in the volume.

It is clear that such a complex system has many points, which are going to be subject for improvement:

- The set of interaction modes has to be expanded towards algorithms for mechanical simulations like finite element methods. This will improve the realism of the local deformations, which are currently based on mesh point displacements.
- While the interaction times are in the order of real-time (for model complexity within a reasonable range), the resampling procedure for the volume transformation has to be performed more efficiently in order to apply the true volume transformation more frequently during the procedure.
- The surface model will be subject for automatic procedures for adaption to different applicational contexts, e.g. for automatically finding an optimal laparoscopic path. While there is no doubt that many applications would benefit from such algorithms, this also means to leave the scope of very general applicability.

The two applications shown in the previous section are only first attempts in showing the practicability of the method. Other possible applications could only briefly be mentioned and will - as the two others - be subject of further developments.

# 5 Acknowledgments

We are grateful to all members of our department, who have supported this work. The described methods have been realized within the VOXEL-MAN framework, which is the main project of our research group: Bernhard Pflesser, Andreas Pommert, Kay Priesmeyer, Martin Riemer, Rainer Schubert, and Ulf Tiede.

# References

1. Ayache, N.: Medical computer vision, virtual reality and robotics. *Image and Vision Computing 13*, 4 (1995), 295–313.
2. Bookstein, F. L.: *Morphometric tools for landmark data.* Cambridge University Press, Cambridge, 1991. (ISBN 0-521-38385-4).
3. Cotin, S., Delingette, H., Ayache, N.: Real Time Volumetric Deformable Models for Surgery Simulation. In Höhne, K. H., Kikinis, R. (Eds.): *Visualization in Biomedical Computing 1996.* Lecture Notes in Computer Science 1131, Springer-Verlag, Heidelberg, 1996, 535–540.
4. Glaeser, G.: *Fast Algorithms for 3D-Graphics.* Springer-Verlag, Heidelberg, 1995. (ISBN 3-540-94288-2).
5. Hill, D. L., Studholme, C., Hawkes, D. J.: Voxel Similarity Measures for Automated Image Registration. In Robb, R. A. (Ed.): *Visualization in Biomedical Computing 1994, Proc. SPIE 2359.* Rochester, MN, 1994, 205–216.
6. Höhne, K. H., Pflesser, B., Pommert, A., Riemer, M., Schiemann, T., Schubert, R., Tiede, U.: A new representation of knowledge concerning human anatomy and function. *Nature Med. 1*, 6 (1995), 506–511.
7. Lorensen, W. E., Cline, H. E.: Marching cubes: A high resolution 3D surface construction algorithm. *Comput. Graphics 21*, 4 (1987), 163–169.
8. MacDonald, D., Avis, D., Evans, A. C.: Multiple Surface Identification and Matching in Magnetic Resonance Images. In Robb, R. A. (Ed.): *Visualization in Biomedical Computing 1994, Proc. SPIE 2359.* Rochester, MN, 1994, 160–169.
9. Pommert, A., Bomans, M., Höhne, K. H.: Volume visualization in magnetic resonance angiography. *IEEE Comput. Graphics Appl. 12*, 5 (1992), 12–13.
10. Ruprecht, D., Müller, H.: Free form deformations with scattered data interpolation methods. In Farin, G. et al. (Eds.): *Geometric Modelling (Computing Suppl. 8).* Springer-Verlag, 1993, 267–281.
11. Schiemann, T., Bomans, M., Tiede, U., Höhne, K. H.: Interactive 3D-segmentation. In Robb, R. A. (Ed.): *Visualization in Biomedical Computing II, Proc. SPIE 1808.* Chapel Hill, NC, 1992, 376–383.
12. Shepard, D.: A two-dimensional interpolation function for irregularly spaced data. In *Proc. of the 23rd National Conference of the ACM.* ACM-Press, New York, 1968, 517–524.
13. Thompson, P., Toga, A. W.: A Surface-Based Technique for Warping Three-Dimensional Images of the Brain. *IEEE Trans. Med. Imaging 15*, 4 (1996), 402–417.
14. Tiede, U., Schiemann, T., Höhne, K. H.: Visualizing the Visible Human. *IEEE Comput. Graphics Appl. 16*, 1 (1996), 7–9.
15. van den Elsen, P. A., Pol, E.-J. D., Viergever, M. A.: Medical image matching — A review with classification. *IEEE Engng. Med. Biol. 12*, 1 (1993), 26–39.
16. Wilmer, F., Tiede, U., Höhne, K. H.: Reduktion der Oberflächenbeschreibung triangulierter Oberflächen durch Anpassung an die Objektform. In Fuchs, S., Hoffmann, R. (Eds.): *Mustererkennung 1992, Proc. 14. DAGM-Symposium*, Springer-Verlag, Berlin, 1992, 430–436.
17. Wolberg, G.: *Digital Image Warping.* IEEE Computer Society Press, Los Alamitos, CA, 1990.

# Nonlinear versus Linear Models in Functional Neuroimaging: Learning Curves and Generalization Crossover

Niels Mørch[1,2], Lars K. Hansen[2], Stephen C. Strother[3], Claus Svarer[1]
David A. Rottenberg[3], Benny Lautrup[4], Robert Savoy[5], Olaf B. Paulson[1]

[1] Neurobiology Research Unit
Copenhagen University Hospital, Rigshospitalet
DK-2100 Copenhagen Ø, Denmark

[2] Department for Mathematical Modelling
Technical University of Denmark
DK-2800 Lyngby, Denmark

[3] Radiology and Neurology Departments
University of Minnesota
and
PET Imaging Service
Minneapolis VA Medical Center
Minnesota, 55417, USA

[4] Niels Bohr Institute
University of Copenhagen
DK-2100 Copenhagen Ø

[5] Massachusetts General Hospital
Boston, Massachusetts, USA

**Abstract.** We introduce the concept of generalization for models of functional neuroactivation, and show how it is affected by the number, $N$, of neuroimaging scans available. By plotting generalization as a function of $N$ (i.e. a "learning curve") we demonstrate that while simple, linear models may generalize better for small $N$'s, more flexible, low-biased nonlinear models, based on artificial neural networks (ANN's), generalize better for larger $N$'s. We demonstrate that for sets of scans of two simple motor tasks—one set acquired with $[O^{15}]$water using PET, and the other using fMRI—practical $N$'s exist for which "generalization crossover" occurs. This observation supports the application of highly flexible, ANN models to sufficiently large functional activation datasets.
**Keywords**: Multivariate brain modeling, ill-posed learning, generalization, learning curves.

## 1  Introduction

Datasets that result from functional activation studies of the living, human brain typically consist of two corresponding sets of observables, the *microscopic* and the *macroscopic* [26]. The brains haemodynamic response, reflecting the microscopic neuronal firing pattern, is measured by modern three-dimensional (3D) imaging techniques such as positron emission tomography (PET) and functional magnetic resonance imaging (fMRI) by integrating in space and time [21]. Along with the resulting set of 3D image volumes (scans) a corresponding set of macroscopic descriptors governs the overall conditions of the experiment. This set can include experimentally controlled factors, such as paradigm labels and variables, and physiological and demographic measures, such as age and heart-rate. The micro- and macroscopic observables are generally both sets of multivariate, stochastic variables. Arranging the microscopic variables (the 3D image volumes) in vectors $\mathbf{x}$ and the macroscopic variables in vectors $\mathbf{g}$ a functional activation dataset $\mathcal{D}$ consisting of $N$ observations can be written as

$$\mathcal{D} = \{(\mathbf{x}_j, \mathbf{g}_j) \mid j = 1, \ldots, N\} \ . \tag{1}$$

Generally, we will assume the observations to be random, independent samples of an underlying stationary process with distribution $P(\mathbf{x}, \mathbf{g})$. As we shall see this distribution plays a central role in the analysis of functional activation datasets [18].

In the following we discuss the so-called "curse of dimensionality" that results from the extremely ill-posed nature of typical functional activation datasets [6,23]. The problem is discussed in terms of probability density estimation and we briefly mention ways to remedy the inevitable over-parameterization that otherwise occurs in modeling procedures based on such datasets [12]. The main point we hope to convey is how model generalization—as studied intensively in other fields dealing with probability density estimation and multivariate modeling [8,13,17,20]—applies to functional neuroimaging [18], and specifically how it is affected by the number, $N$, of available observations.

## 2 Models of Functional Activation Datasets

In terms of $\mathbf{x}$ and $\mathbf{g}$ the analysis of functional activation datasets can be phrased as the estimation (of properties) of $P(\mathbf{x}, \mathbf{g})$. For instance, we can estimate the conditional mean, $E\{\mathbf{x}|\mathbf{g}\}$, using multivariate linear models as in [7], thus effectively modeling the expected scan from a set of macroscopic variables. Or, we can estimate the alternative conditional mean $E\{\mathbf{g}|\mathbf{x}\}$, using multivariate linear models as in [18], effectively modeling the expected value of a set of macroscopic variables from the scan[1].

In general, we employ parameterized models of the properties we wish to estimate. In this work we focus on models that estimate $E\{\mathbf{g}|\mathbf{x}\}$. Being a function of $\mathbf{x}$ we denote these models $f_\theta(\mathbf{x})$, explicitly indicating the dependency on the set of parameters $\theta$. Parameter values are estimated using some or all of the available data. We call such a set of data used for parameter estimation the *training set*,

$$\mathcal{D}_{train} = \{(\mathbf{x}_j, \mathbf{g}_j) \mid j = 1, \ldots, N_{train}\} \ . \tag{2}$$

---

[1] In fact, it can be shown that the two linear models are analogous and simple relations between the parameters exist.

For a given set of parameters model performance is quantified using the *cost function*, $c(\mathbf{x}, \mathbf{g}, \theta)$, which is often derived from maximum likelihood (ML) arguments [4,10,14]. Parameter values are estimated by optimizing the cost function based on the observations in the training set (we say that the model is trained, hence the name). Averaged over the training set this evaluates to

$$C(\mathcal{D}_{train}, \theta) = \iint c(\mathbf{x}, \mathbf{g}, \theta) P_{train}(\mathbf{x}, \mathbf{g}) \, d\mathbf{x} \, d\mathbf{g} \; . \tag{3}$$

By using the empirical density estimate $P_{train}(\mathbf{x}, \mathbf{g}) = \frac{1}{N_{train}} \sum_{j=1}^{N_{train}} \delta(\mathbf{x} - \mathbf{x}_j, \mathbf{g} - \mathbf{g}_j)$ we get the so-called *training error*

$$C(\mathcal{D}_{train}, \theta) = \frac{1}{N_{train}} \sum_{j=1}^{N_{train}} c(\mathbf{x}_j, \mathbf{g}_j, \theta), \quad (\mathbf{x}_j, \mathbf{g}_j) \in \mathcal{D}_{train} \; . \tag{4}$$

The choice of cost function will depend on the noise model and potential constraints we impose on the model outputs (e.g. to make them interpretable as probabilities). For more details on these issues see [3,10,14].

Equipped with a training set, a model, and a cost function we are ready to gain knowledge about $P(\mathbf{x}, \mathbf{g})$ and, hopefully, underlying information processing relationships in the human brain. However, several important additional issues must be considered before attempting to build practical models. Rather than using (4) to model $E\{\mathbf{g}|\mathbf{x}\}$ from the observations directly we can reduce the computational burden dramatically by taking the extremely ill-posed nature of typical functional activation datasets into account.

## 2.1 Ill-posed Datasets

While we often include only a few descriptors in the macroscopic variables $\mathbf{g}$ making them low-dimensional, the microscopic variables $\mathbf{x}$ that represent the scans are often high-dimensional. Despite preprocessing that, among other things, mask out voxels outside the brain more than 40000 voxels often remain. Using $\mathcal{I}$ to denote the space in which all possible observations fall (i.e., the *input space*) we have $\dim(\mathcal{I}) \sim 10^4$. The space spanned by the actual observations in the dataset is called *signal space* and denoted $\mathcal{S}$. Often no more than a few hundred observations are available, so $\dim(\mathcal{S}) \sim 10^2$.

Typically $\dim(\mathcal{S}) \ll \dim(\mathcal{I})$, making $\mathcal{S}$ a small subspace of $\mathcal{I}$. This is exactly what characterizes extremely ill-posed datasets. In Fig. 1 an ill-posed situation is illustrated. Input space is 3D Euclidean space indicated by the dashed vectors. With only two observations in the dataset represented by the solid vectors, signal space is a 2D subspace, i.e. a plane. The dataset does not contain information about the parts of $\mathcal{I}$ that are orthogonal to $\mathcal{S}$.

Because the dimension of $\mathcal{S}$ is low we have a correspondingly low number of degrees of freedom available in any subsequent modeling, and naive estimation based directly on the observation pairs $(\mathbf{x}, \mathbf{g})$ will result in strong linear relations between the estimated parameters; the original basis in which observations in

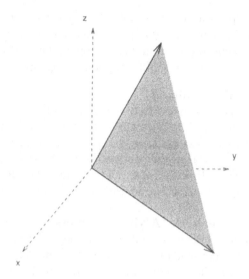

**Fig. 1.** Illustration of an ill-posed dataset. With input space, $\mathcal{I}$, being three-dimensional (represented by the dashed vectors) the signal space, $\mathcal{S}$, which is the space spanned by the two observations in the dataset (represented by the solid vectors), is the plane indicated in gray. The dataset contains no information about the parts of input space that are orthogonal to signal space because $\dim(\mathcal{S}) < \dim(\mathcal{I})$.

input space are represented is a poor choice when it comes to representing observations efficiently in signal space. We can easily construct other, more efficient bases, however, that reduce the dimensionality of the *representation* without loss of information [12,19]. The only requirement is that the basis chosen spans signal space. One particularly choice of basis is to use the observations in the dataset themselves. Even-though efficient in reducing an extremely ill-posed problem to an only marginally ill-posed one bases that reveal more about the signal structure are available. In particular, a singular value decomposition (SVD) basis [11,15,16] has been shown to reveal an interesting subspace structure [12,22,23]. In the following $\mathbf{v}$ will denote the projection of a scan $\mathbf{x}$ onto an efficient basis that spans signal space; for more details see [18].

## 2.2 Model Flexibility and Bias

Having reduced the extremely ill-posed dataset to a marginally ill-posed one where the dimension of each observation, $\mathbf{v}$, equals the number of observations, it is now part of the modeling task to impose further constraints in order to avoid over-fitting. Different model families approach this in various ways, by limiting model flexibility and thus the effective dimensionality of the parameterization to match the available degrees of freedom.

In the following we focus on models for classification. Assuming the macroscopic variables to be univariate labels we seek to build models that optimally classify the microscopic variables[2], $\mathbf{x}$, into the correct classes. In other words, we seek a *decision boundary* in signal space that allows the observations to be correctly classified according to their macroscopic labels. More specifically we will apply two model families that differ in model flexibility:

- **Fishers Linear Discriminant**
  Fishers Linear Discriminant (FLD) is a family of linear classifier that are based on a cost function that measures the difference between class means relative to the within class variance [4,14]. The term linear refers to the fact that the models are linear in the parameters which makes parameter estimation straight forward. However, this relatively high *bias* limits the flexibility of the relationships (decision boundaries) that the models can implement.

- **Artificial neural network (ANN) classifiers**
  Artificial neural networks is a family of parameter efficient models that deal with the curse of dimensionality by employing nonlinearities [2,9]. The models are nonlinear in the parameters in contrast to FLD. This complicates parameter estimation but makes the models less biased and allow them to implement a much more flexible and wider range of relationships (decision boundaries) [10,24].

## 3   Generalization

Although cost functions allow us to quantify model performance the training error in (3) is the average over the *specific* and *limited* training set only. If the distribution of observations in this set, $P_{train}(\mathbf{x}, \mathbf{g})$, does not match the true distribution, $P(\mathbf{x}, \mathbf{g})$, sufficiently well the cost function value will not reflect model performance correctly. Rather, as training sets are often small we should use *generalization error*,

$$G(\theta_{train}) = \iint c(\mathbf{x}, \mathbf{g}, \theta_{train}) P(\mathbf{x}, \mathbf{g}) \, d\mathbf{x} \, d\mathbf{g} \ . \tag{5}$$

as our measure of model quality. Unfortunately this requires complete knowledge of $P(\mathbf{x}, \mathbf{g})$ which, of course, we do not have. Instead we can estimate generalization either analytically [1,20] or empirically [24]. The latter is often called *test error*

$$\widehat{G}(\theta_{train}) = C(\mathcal{D}_{test}, \theta_{train}) \tag{6}$$

$$= \frac{1}{N_{test}} \sum_{j=1}^{N_{test}} c(\mathbf{x}_j, \mathbf{g}_j, \theta_{train}), \quad (\mathbf{x}_j, \mathbf{g}_j) \in \mathcal{D}_{test} \tag{7}$$

and evaluated using an independent set of observations organized in a *test set*

$$\mathcal{D}_{test} = \{(\mathbf{x}_j, \mathbf{g}_j) \mid j = 1, \ldots, N_{test}\} \ . \tag{8}$$

---

[2] In practice we use $\mathbf{v}$ of course, thus efficiently representing the scans using a basis that spans signal space.

In (5) we have indicated how generalization error depends on the training set via the estimated parameters $\theta_{train}$. To eliminate this dependency we average over training sets of size $N_{train}$ to yield the *expected generalization error*

$$E_{N_{train}}(G) = \int G(\theta_{train})P(\mathcal{D}_{N_{train}})\, d\mathcal{D}_{N_{train}} \ , \tag{9}$$

which can be estimated empirically by using the test error in (7) to estimate $G(\theta_{train})$. Clearly, using a set of the available observations to independently estimate generalization reduces the number of observations left for training. The optimal split of the available data into training- and test sets constitutes a non-trivial problem that has been studied in the context of ANN's and statistical re-sampling techniques [5]. In the remainder of this paper we will fix the size of the test set as well as the observations therein to allow measures of model performance that are unbiased—or at least comparable between different model families.

### 3.1 Learning Curves and Generalization Crossover

Using generalization we are now ready to investigate how the number of observations in the training set, $N_{train}$, affects model performance. We hypothesize that, as $N_{train}$ increases, generalization error will decrease. This downwards slope of the so-called *learning curve* is caused by the improved estimates of $P(\mathbf{x}, \mathbf{g})$ (on which the models are based) that increasingly larger training sets provide.

For a given model family the learning curve will eventually flatten out as additional observations no longer improve model performance due to limitations in the models themselves. This naturally leads to the further hypothesis that learning curves look different for different model families. Models that are very flexible typically need many examples to obtain stable parameter estimates. These models will in return generalize very well. In contrast, the implicit constraints in highly biased models enable them to obtain stable parameter estimates from fewer observations. However, they may not generalize as well as their more flexible counterparts. Thus, while generalization error is highest for very flexible models for small training sets, it decreases to a lower level than for highly biased, less flexible models as $N_{train}$ increases. This means that a *generalization crossover* occurs at which point the data support the use of the more flexible models. The situation is illustrated in Fig. 2.

## 4 Methods

To estimate learning curves data from two functional activation studies, both involving simple motor tasks, was used.

### 4.1 [O$^{15}$]Water PET Scanning

A set of 30 subjects were each scanned 8 times using a Siemens-ECAT 953B PET scanner while alternately resting and performing a simple finger opposition

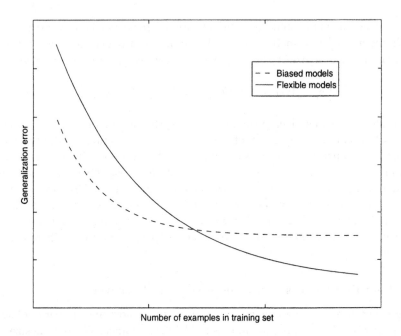

**Fig. 2.** Model generalization as a function of number of observations, $N_{train}$, used to estimate model parameters. Generalization error decreases with increasing $N_{train}$ for both highly flexible and more biased models. The decrease is more rapid for the latter, whereas the former reaches a lower level for large values of $N_{train}$. At the point of generalization crossover enough data is available to support the use of more flexible, low-biased models.

task with their left hand [22]. For each subject four scans were acquired in each of the two states yielding a total of 240 scans.

Before scanning [$O^{15}$]water was automatically injected in the subjects right arm leaving the left arm free to perform the task. With the eyes covered by a patch an auditory timing signal was delivered by insert earphones.

For baseline (rest) scans, subjects were instructed to lie still and remain awake; they received no stimulation. For motor activation scans, the subjects left arm was positioned perpendicular to the scanning couch. At the start of the injection, the timing signal was initiated and the finger-thumb opposition task continued for 60 s. The finger-thumb opposition task consisted of sequential opposition of the thumb and successive digits, and back again $(2, 3, 4, 5, 4, 3, 2, 3, 4, \ldots)$ at a rate of 1 Hz.

PET scanning commenced when the radioactive material reached the brain, typically 10–20 s after injection, and data acquisition continued for 90 s. Each scanning session consisted of eight 90 s PET scans separated by 10 min rest periods to allow for $O^{15}$ decay, for a total experimental time of approximately 90 min. The first, third, fifth, and seventh scans were acquired in the baseline state, and the second, fourth, sixth, and eighth scans were acquired in the activated state. Scans corrected for randoms, dead-time, and attenuation, but not for scatter, were reconstructed using 3D filtered back-projection.

## 4.2 fMRI Scanning

A single subject performing a left-handed finger-to-thumb opposition task was scanned during eight 180 s runs. In each run 24 baseline, 24 activation, and 24 baseline whole brain echo planar scans were acquired (2.5s/scan) with an interslice distance of 8 mm and an in plane voxel resolution of $3.1 \times 3.1$ mm$^2$. This yielded a total of 576 scans. During activation the task was timed with an auditory signal at a rate of 1 Hz.

## 4.3 Scan Alignment and Preprocessing

The PET and fMRI scans were intra-subject aligned using AIR (Automated Image Registration) [27] and only the PET scans were then stereo-tactically normalized to a simulated PET reference volume in Talairach space [25] using the 12 parameter linear transformation described in [28] (see [22] for more details). This yielded scans with 48 slices, inter-slice distance of 3.4 mm and in plane voxel resolution of $3.1 \times 3.1$ mm$^2$. After masking out voxels outside the brain an SVD basis was computed based on the entire[3] set of scans.

## 4.4 Modeling

After normalizing the singular vectors, $\mathbf{v}$, to zero mean and a standard deviation of one, a fixed test set was randomly selected (100 for the PET data and 200 for the fMRI data). The remaining observations were utilized to yield training sets of increasing size. A number of training sets of each size (25 for the PET data and 20 for the fMRI data) were randomly sampled with replacement[4] from the singular vectors. For each of the resulting training sets a linear (FLD) and a nonlinear (ANN) classifier were estimated. Model performance was then assessed using the fixed test set. The linear and nonlinear classifiers are based on different cost functions, so to allow a quantitative comparison generalization was measured as the mean misclassification on the independent test set.

# 5 Results

Figure 3 depicts the learning curves for the linear and nonlinear classifiers on the PET data. The two curves are slightly offset horizontally to better show the

---

[3] Basing models on an SVD of the entire set of observation limits results from generalization measures to the specific set of subjects in the PET case, and the specific subject in the fMRI case. Thus, generalization error does not implicate the extent to which models generalize to subjects other than those included in the datasets.

[4] Estimators based on sampling with replacement (also known as bootstrapping), where the same observation may appear more than once in the same sample, are asymptotically central [5]—however counter-intuitive this may seem.

error-bars that indicate one standard deviation of the mean for each training set size. As hypothesized both learning curves decrease. The nonlinear classifier

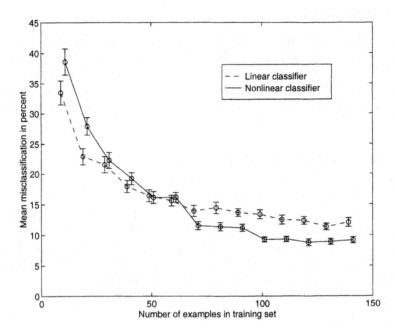

**Fig. 3.** For an $[O^{15}]$water PET study of a simple finger opposition task model generalization (measured as the mean misclassification on an independent test set) is plotted as a function of number of observations, $N_{train}$, used to estimate model parameters. Generalization error decreases with increasing $N_{train}$ for the linear as well as the nonlinear classifiers. However, generalization error decreases more rapidly and settles at a higher level for the linear classifier than for its nonlinear counterpart. Thus, for this task linear classifiers seem optimal for small datasets. As more observations become available we are better off using the more flexible nonlinear classifiers.

seems to generalize worse for small training sets but perform relatively better as $N_{train}$ increases. Indeed, a generalization crossover occurs for training sets with around 60 examples, and as $N_{train}$ increases further generalization error for the nonlinear classifier settles at a lower level than that of its linear counterpart.

For the fMRI dataset Fig. 4 shows a similar picture. Again the learning curves for the linear and nonlinear classifiers cross as the number of observations in the training set is increased. Thus, for small training sets we can not reject the linear model.

## 6 Discussion

We have introduced a general framework for the analysis of functional activation datasets. In this framework the extremely ill-posed nature of typical datasets

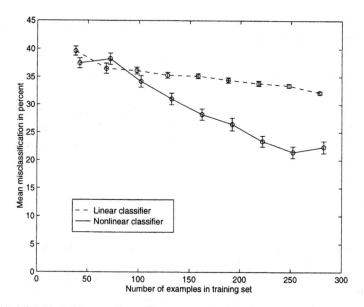

**Fig. 4.** For an fMRI study of a left-handed finger-to-thumb opposition task model generalization (measured as the mean misclassification on an independent test set) is plotted as a function of number of observations, $N_{train}$, used to estimate model parameters. Generalization error decreases with increasing $N_{train}$ for the linear as well as the nonlinear classifiers. However, generalization error decreases more rapidly and settles at a higher level for the linear classifier than for its nonlinear counterpart. Again, the linear classifiers can not be rejected for small datasets. As more observations become available we are better off using the more flexible nonlinear classifiers.

imposes an immense computational burden on any modeling procedures. We have shown how a simple coordinate transform reduces data representation without loss of information, thus minimizing the computational load.

The importance of not measuring model performance on the same set of data used to estimate the model parameters has been stressed, and we have sketched how independent test sets provide empirical estimates of generalization. We have hypothesized how generalization error decreases as more observations become available for parameter estimation. Decreasing learning curves satisfying our hypothesis have been demonstrated on two functional activation datasets of PET and fMRI scans of subjects performing simple motor tasks.

By employing model families that differ in flexibility we have further shown the effect of model flexibility on the slope of the learning curves. For the studied tasks we have identified generalization crossovers, at which point enough observations are available to support the use of a more flexible, nonlinear model. We believe this to have implications for the future of modeling in functional neuroimaging; as more and more data become available the support for more sophisticated and flexible models increase. While introducing problems of their own (by e.g. not being linear in their parameters), these models can potentially lead to increased knowledge of the systems that govern information processing in the living, human brain.

# 7 Acknowledgments

This work has been funded in part by the Human Brain Project grant P20 MH57180, the Danish Research Councils for the Natural and Technical Sciences through the Danish Computational Neural Network Center, CONNECT, the Danish Research Council for Medical Science, and the Danish Research Academy.

# References

1. H. Akaike. Fitting autoregressive models for prediction. *Annals of the Institute of Statistical Mathematics*, 21:243–247, 1969.
2. C. M. Bishop. *Neural Networks for Pattern Recognition*. Clarendon Press, Oxford, 1995.
3. J. S. Bridle. Training stochastic model recognition algorithms as networks can lead to maximum mutual information estimation of parameters. *Advances in Neural Information Processing Systems*, 2:211–217, 1990.
4. R. O. Duda and P. E. Hart. *Pattern Classification and Scene Analysis*. John Wiley & Sons, 1973.
5. B. Efron and R. J. Tibshirani. *An Introduction to the Bootstrap*. Monographs on Statistics and Applied Probability. Chapman & Hall, 1993.
6. J. H. Friedman. On bias, variance, 0/1-loss, and the curse-of-dimensionality. *Journal of Knowledge Discovery and Data Mining*, 1996. In press.
7. K. J. Friston, J.-P. Poline, A. P. Holmes, C. D. Frith, and R. S. J. Frackowiak. A multivariate analysis of PET activation studies. *Human Brain Mapping*, 4:140–151, 1996.
8. B. Hassibi and D. G. Stork. Optimal brain surgeon. *Advances in Neural Information Processing Systems*, 5:164–174, 1992.
9. J. Hertz, A. Krogh, and R. G. Palmer. *Introduction to the Theory of Neural Computation*. Addison-Wesley, 1994.
10. M. Hintz-Madsen, M. W. Pederson, L. K. Hansen, and J. Larsen. Design and evaluation of neural skin classifiers. In Y. Tohkura, S. Katagiri, and E. Wilson, editors, *Proceedings of 1996 IEEE Workshop on Neural Networks for Signal Processing*, pages 223–230, 1996.
11. J. E. Jackson. *A User's Guide to Principal Components*. Wiley Series on Probability and Statistics, John Wiley and Sons, 1991.
12. B. Lautrup, L. K. Hansen, I. Law, N. Mørch, C. Svarer, and S. C. Strother. Massive weight sharing: A cure for extremely ill-posed problems. In H. J. Hermann, D. E. Wolf, and E. P. Pöppel, editors, *Proceedings of Workshop on Supercomputing in Brain Research: From Tomography to Neural Networks, HLRZ, KFA Jülich, Germany*, pages 137–148, 1994.
13. Le Cun, Y., J. S. Denker, and S. Solla. Optimal brain damage. *Advances in Neural Information Processing Systems*, 2:598–605, 1990.
14. K. V. Mardia, J. T. Kent, and J. M. Bibby. *Multivariate Analysis*. Academic Press, 1979.

15. J. R. Moeller and S. C. Strother. A regional covariance approach to the analysis of functional patterns in positron emission tomographic data. *Journal of Cerebral Blood Flow and Metabolism*, 11:A121–A135, 1991.

16. J. R. Moeller, S. C. Strother, J. J. Sidtis, and D. A. Rottenberg. Scaled subprofile model: A statistical approach to the analysis of functional patterns in positron emission tomographic data. *Journal of Cerebral Blood Flow and Metabolism*, 7:649–658, 1987.

17. J. Moody. Prediction risk and architecture selection for neural networks. In V. Cherkassky, J. H. F. H., and H. Wechsler, editors, *From Statistics to Neural Networks, Theory and Pattern Recognition Applications*, pages 147–165. Springer Verlag, 1992.

18. N. Mørch, L. K. Hansen, I. Law, S. C. Strother, C. Svarer, B. Lautrup, U. Kjems, N. Lange, and O. B. Paulson. Generalization and the bias-variance trade-off in models of functional activation. *IEEE Transactions on Medical Imaging*, 1996. Submitted.

19. N. Mørch, U. Kjems, L. K. Hansen, C. Svarer, I. Law, B. Lautrup, S. Strother, and K. Rehm. Visualization of neural networks using saliency maps. In *Proceedings of 1995 IEEE International Conference on Neural Networks*, volume 4, pages 2085–2090, 1995.

20. N. Murata, S. Yoshizawa, and S.-I. Amari. Network information criterion—determining the number of hidden units for an artificial neural network model. *IEEE Transactions on Neural Networks*, 5:865–872, 1994.

21. M. I. Posner and M. E. Raichle. *Images of Mind*. W. H. Freeman, 1994.

22. S. C. Strother, J. R. Anderson, K. A. Schaper, J. J. Sidtis, J. S. Liow, R. P. Woods, and D. A. Rottenberg. Principal component analysis and the scaled subprofile model compared to intersubject averaging and statistical parametric mapping: I. "Functional connectivity" of the human motor system studied with [$^{15}$O]water PET. *Journal of Cerebral Blood Flow and Metabolism*, 15:738–753, 1995.

23. S. C. Strother, J. R. Anderson, K. A. Schaper, J. J. Sidtis, and D. A. Rottenberg. Linear models of orthogonal subspaces & networks from functional activation PET studies of the human brain. In Y. Bizais, C. Barillot, and R. D. Paola, editors, *Proceedings of the 14th International Conference on Information Processing in Medical Imaging*, pages 299–310. Kluwer Academic Publishers, 1995.

24. C. Svarer, L. K. Hansen, and J. Larsen. On design and evaluation of tapped-delay neural network architectures. In H. R. Berenji et al., editors, *Proceedings of 1993 IEEE International Conference on Neural Networks*, pages 45–51, 1993.

25. J. Talairach and P. Tournoux. *Co-planar stereotaxic atlas of the human brain*. Thieme Medical Publishers Inc., New York, 1988.

26. A. W. Toga and J. C. Mazziotta. *Brain Mapping*. Academic Press, 1996.

27. R. P. Woods, S. R. Cherry, and J. C. Mazziotta. A rapid automated algorithm for accurately aligning and reslicing positron emission tomography images. *Journal of Computer Assisted Tomography*, 16:620–633, 1992.

28. R. P. Woods, J. C. Mazziotta, and S. R. Cherry. Automated image registration. In K. Uemura et al., editors, *Quantification of Brain Function. Tracer Kinetics and Image Analysis in Brain PET*, pages 391–400. Elsevier Science Publishers B. V., 1993.

# Synthetic Resampling Methods for Variance Estimation in Parametric Images

Ranjan Maitra

Statistics and Data Mining Research Group
Bellcore, Morristown NJ 07960, USA *

**Abstract.** Parametric imaging procedures offer the possibility of comprehensive assessment of tissue metabolic activity. Estimating variances of these images is important for the development of inference procedures in a diagnostic setting. Unfortunately, the complexity of the radio-tracer models used in the generation of a parametric image makes analytic variance expressions intractable. A natural extension of the usual resampling approach is infeasible because of the computational effort. This paper suggests a computationally practical approximate simulation strategy to variance estimation. Results of experiments done to evaluate the approach in a simplified model one-dimensional problem are very encouraging. The suggested methodology is evaluated here in the context of parametric images extracted by mixture analysis; however, the approach is general enough to extend to other parametric imaging methods.

## 1 Introduction

The ability to assess quantitatively the biologic status of tissue from a sequence of dynamic Positron Emission Tomography (PET) scans is one of the most powerful features of this radiologic tool. The most common approach in this regard is a technique called ROI analysis. Here, the reconstructed pixel values in each scan are averaged over a given region (ROI) to yield a time series, called the *time-activity curve* (TAC), and then the regional biologic parameter values are estimated by fitting non-linear models to the time series. There are concerns regarding image registration while drawing these regions with the help of other imaging modalities such as X-ray Computed Tomography (CT) or Magnetic Resonance Imaging (MRI), as well as the potential for inaccurate metabolic parameter estimation because of the possible selection of inhomogeneous regions [22]. From a practical standpoint however, the most important concern is that outside the selected regions, the reconstructed PET data are only interpreted qualitatively, thus compromising the quantitative potential of this expensive technology.

Parametric imaging attempts to offer comprehensive pixel-wise assessments of tissue metabolic activity. The technique builds on fitting radio-tracer models to the time-course reconstructed PET data at each pixel. However, the presence of noise and heterogeneity between the reconstructed pixel values makes

* Research supported in part by the National Institutes of Health grant CA-57903 at the University of Washington, Seattle, USA.

direct fitting of models inappropriate [12, 24], and underlines the need for more refined approaches (Blomqvist [1], Cunningham and Jones [4], Gjedde [9, 10], Herholz [13], Patlak, et al. [23], O'Sullivan [20, 22]).

The full quantitative potential of PET can be realized if it is possible to draw scientific inferences from these parametric images. To this end, in recent years, there has been considerable attention directed to the analysis of multi-subject cerebral activation studies using [O-15]-water [8, 26]. Such studies are interesting in determining, for instance, how the brain processes different cognitive tasks and functions. However, in a clinical setting, there is a practical need for inference tools to guide diagnostic decisions from single-patient studies [14, 15]. In this context, Blomqvist et al. [2] noted the desirability of developing methodology to estimate variances in parametric images. Such mechanisms will permit the evaluation of hypotheses related not only to the mean parameter over regions but also regional heterogeneity measures. The statistical significance of any hypothesis test is based on the assumption that under the null hypothesis, the behavior of the test statistic can be explained in terms of purely random variation. In setting up such a test, estimates of dispersion are needed. Unfortunately however, the nonlinear formulations used in the construction of parametric images make analytic variance formulae intractable. The simulation approach of Haynor and Woods [11] could theoretically be extended to develop a variation of the bootstrap method of Efron [6]. This would involve simulating inhomogeneous Poisson processes, independent over time, in the observation (sinogram) domain with (time-dependent) mean intensities estimated by the count data, applying image reconstruction and parametric image generation to obtain an ensemble of simulated functional images. The resampled parametric images could then be used to estimate the dispersions. Unfortunately, the cumulative computational burden of the number of reconstruction steps needed in the simulation makes such an approach impractical.

This paper suggests a synthetic simulation approach via the parametric bootstrap [6] executed in the imaging domain. Under idealized projection conditions, each reconstructed PET scan is well approximated by a multivariate Gaussian distribution. The mean of this distribution is estimated by the reconstructed image. Computationally feasible and accurate dispersion estimates developed in Maitra and O'Sullivan [16, 19] and Maitra [17, 18] are exploited and the result validated for a realistic range of total expected counts. This model is used to simulate dynamic PET sequences, from each of which biologic parameters are extracted. This yields a bootstrap sample of the functional images, which can be used to assess variability. The advantage of this approach over the one that extends the strategy in [11] is that it eliminates the computationally expensive reconstruction step when simulating from the observation process.

The main contributions of this paper are presented in two sections. Section 2 develops the methodology used in the simulation of dispersion estimates. Section 3 reports on the experiments done to validate the approximate Gaussian distributional assumption of reconstructed PET scans, as well as those done to assess the performance of the suggested methodology. Since the latter is not possible to evaluate in a two-dimensional PET setup, the suggestions are evaluated on experiments performed on a model one-dimensional problem with reconstruction characteristics similar to PET. Finally, Section 4 summarizes the contributions of this paper and poses questions for future research.

## 2 Theory and Methods

### 2.1 Distribution of a Time-course Reconstructed PET Sequence

The reconstruction algorithm in PET for the distribution of radio-tracer in tissue at a fixed time-point is the filtered backprojection algorithm:

$$\hat{\lambda}_i^h = \sum_{\theta=1}^{n_\theta} \sum_{d=1}^{n_d} e_h(u_i \cos\theta + v_i \sin\theta - d) y_{d,\theta}. \tag{1}$$

Here $y = \{y_{d,\theta}; d = 1, 2, \ldots, n_d; \theta = 1, 2, \ldots, n_\theta\}$ is the corrected sinogram data, $e_h(\cdot)$ is the reconstruction filter with resolution size (FWHM) $h$, $\lambda = \{\lambda_i; i = 1, 2, \ldots, I\}$ is the source distribution and $\hat{\lambda}^h$ the corresponding reconstruction.

Theoretically, it can be shown that the asymptotic distribution of the reconstructed PET scan at a fixed time-point under idealized projection conditions is multi-Gaussian [17, 18]. The mean of this distribution is estimated by the reconstructed image and unbiased estimates of the variances can be obtained accurately by applying the methods outlined in [16, 19]. The Fourier reduction detailed in [17, 19] that combines the assumption of relative uniformity of the variances in the observed bins with the properties of the Radon transform is used to assess the correlations. This technique is a computationally elegant implementation of the spatially invariant correlation structure of Carson et al. [3].

The above results can be used to suggest an approximate distribution for a dynamic sequence of reconstructed PET scans. The data recorded by the detector over time are independent. Further, the reconstruction of the radio-tracer uptake at any one time-point, does not involve the observations at any other; hence, the reconstructions are themselves independent over time. This gives

**Result 1** *The asymptotic distribution of the time-course reconstructed PET sequence $\{\hat{\lambda}^h(t); t = 1, 2, \ldots, T\}$ is a Gaussian random field.*

### 2.2 Synthetic Simulation Approach to Estimating Dispersions

Result 1 implies that for high expected total emissions, the distribution of the time-course reconstructed PET sequence can be approximated by a Gaussian random field. This is used to construct a practical modification to the resampling scheme outlined earlier. The exact implementation is as follows:

1. Obtain a time-course reconstructed image sequence of radio-tracer uptake from the PET study. Also, obtain the variance estimates of the reconstructed pixel values for each of these scans. Approximate the correlations between

the reconstructed pixel values in each scan by the spatially invariant correlation structure developed in [17, 18, 19]. From this reconstructed PET sequence, obtain a functional image of the estimated pixel-wise tissue biologic parameters.

2. Simulate from a Gaussian random field with mean estimated by the above reconstructed time-course sequence. The spatially invariant correlation structure means that Fourier methods can be used in the simulation of correlated multivariate Gaussian realizations (see appendix for details). From each simulated PET sequence, obtain pixel-wise simulated images of the desired biologic parameters.

3. Estimate dispersion of the estimated functional image from this bootstrap sample.

This approach is practical because it eliminates the cumulative computational overhead of performing many reconstruction steps while obtaining resampling estimates of variability.

# 3 Evaluation of Suggested Strategy

## 3.1 Diagnostic Checks

Diagnostic checks were performed to evaluate the approximation of the distribution of a reconstructed PET scan by the multivariate Gaussian distribution and a spatially invariant correlation structure at realistic total expected emissions rates. There are two levels of approximation here: (1) appropriateness of the asymptotic Gaussian distributional assumption in a typical PET scan, and (2) assumption of a spatially invariant Fourier correlation structure. Both of these need to be tested. To this end, experiments were performed on a set of simulation PET experiments.

**Experiments** The model chosen in the diagnostic checks was a version of the Shepp-Vardi-Kaufmann phantom [25] digitized on a $128 \times 128$ grid (Figure 3.1a). The sinogram domain had $128 \times 320$ distance-angle bins. A sample realization is shown in Figure 3.1b. Evaluations were done over a range of realistic total expected emissions. These were allowed to vary over 9 distinct values (equispaced on a $\log_2$ scale) between $10^4$ and $10^6$. This range is comparable to that seen in individual scans in a typical dynamic PET study using the radio-tracer [F-18]-deoxyglucose. For each of these total expected counts, 1000 realizations were generated in the observation domain and reconstructions obtained. The resolution size (FWHM) of the filter for each reconstruction was set so as to provide optimal reconstructions at the corresponding total expected counts. The reconstructions were standardized to have zero mean and unit variance. The reference distribution was the sum of squares of these standardized reconstructed pixel values, where the summation index was over all those pixels that were not

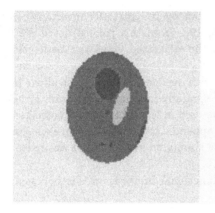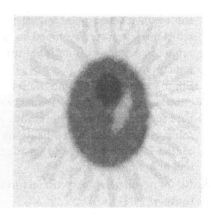

**Fig. 1.** (a) The Vardi-Shepp phantom used in the simulations. (b) Sample reconstruction.

in the background of the imaging region. The statistic used was

$$W_2 = \sum_{i=1, i \notin \mathcal{B}}^{I} \frac{\left[\hat{\lambda}_i^h - \mathrm{E}(\hat{\lambda}_i^h)\right]^2}{\mathrm{Var}(\hat{\lambda}_i^h)} \tag{2}$$

where $\mathcal{B}$ represents the pixels in the background of the image. The diagnostic checks were performed by comparing the distribution of this statistic $W_2$ with that obtained by summing up the corresponding squared coordinates of sample realizations generated from a multivariate Gaussian distribution with zero mean and unit variance and the appropriate spatially invariant correlation structure.

**Results** This section reports the results of our diagnostic checks. The goodness-of-fit for the distribution of $W_2$ was evaluated both in terms of descriptive plots and analytically. For descriptive analyses, quantile-quantile plots of the test sample were compared with those generated using the reference sample. Linearity in the plots implies agreement with the asymptotic multi-Gaussian distribution.

Figure 2 plots the quantiles of the empirical distribution of $W_2$ against those obtained from the sample drawn from the reference distribution for the range of counts. The plots are by and large linear and, as expected, the quality of the linear fit improves with increasing count. However, the slope is lower than unity with increasing count rate. This can be explained by the fact that for higher total expected emissions, the optimal bandwidth required in smoothing the reconstructions for consistency is lower and as seen in several studies [3, 17, 19], the dispersions are under-approximated at lower smoothing levels.

To further our understanding of the performance of the diagnostic evaluations, the two-dimensional PET experiments were repeated by fixing the total

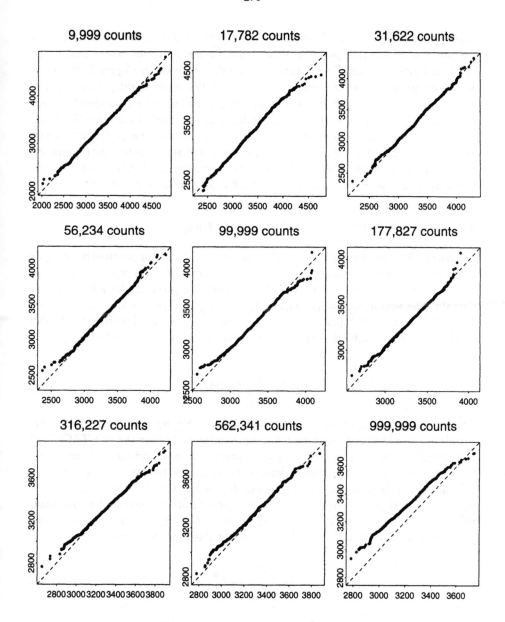

**Fig. 2.** Quantile-quantile plots of the empirical distribution of $W_2$ generated from the reference distribution against those obtained from simulations obtained from the model. The asymptotic fit is tested by looking at a range of counts.

expected emissions at the highest level $(10^6)$ and varying the bandwidth over the range of nine corresponding values used in the previous experiments. The plots (not reported here) were generally similar to those in Figure 2. However, at higher bandwidths, the upper quantiles of $W_2$ were slightly heavier. The slope of the plot went down, away from unity with decreasing bandwidth, thus strengthening our view that it is the under-approximated dispersions for lower bandwidths that made the diagnostic suspect in the previous experiments. These experiments again underline the need for improved schemes for approximating dispersions in reconstructed PET scans; however, the multi-Gaussian distributional approximation to a reconstructed PET scan seems reasonable.

## 3.2 Variance Estimation in Parametric Images

**Mixture Models** The mixture analysis approach [20, 22] to parametric imaging is one of many methods suggested in the literature. Let $\lambda_i(t)$ represent the true source distribution in the $t$'th time-bin at the $i$'th pixel in the PET imaging domain. The vector $\lambda_i(\cdot) = \{\lambda_i(t); t = 1, 2, \ldots, T\}$ is called the true *time-activity curve* (TAC) at the $i$'th pixel. A $K$-component mixture model represents the $i$'th pixel TAC as a weighted average of $K$ underlying curves (sub-TACs) $\xi_k, k = 1, 2, \ldots, K$.

$$\lambda_i(t) = \sum_{k=1}^{K} \pi_{ik} \xi_k(t) \tag{3}$$

where the mixing proportions $\{\pi_{ik}; k = 1, 2, \ldots, K\}$ lie in the $K$-dimensional simplex. The physical basis for such a representation is that the sub-TACs ($\xi$'s) correspond to the different tissue types represented in the image and the underlying $\pi_i$.'s indicate the anatomic tissue composition of the underlying pixel.

Parametric imaging maps the metabolic parameter of interest, $\vartheta$, at each pixel in the image. The mixture analysis approach fits the metabolic parameter $\vartheta^{(k)}$ to each tissue sub-TAC $\xi_k(\cdot)$ and following (3) regards each pixel biologic parameter as a composition of the component tissue parameters,

$$\vartheta_i = \sum_{k=1}^{K} \pi_{ik} \vartheta^{(k)} \tag{4}$$

*Estimation Algorithms* For functional imaging, the data are a time-course sequence of reconstructed PET scans $\hat{\lambda}^h = \{\hat{\lambda}^h(t); t = 1, 2, \ldots, T\}$. The number of tissue types, $K$, the sub-TACs $\xi_k(\cdot)$, and the mixing proportions $\pi_{ik}$'s have to be determined. $K$ is obtained from anatomic considerations or through clustering or other sophisticated algorithms [20, 22]. Estimation of $\xi$'s and $\pi$'s is usually done alternately to fit the model,

$$\hat{\lambda}_i^h(t) \sim \sum_{k=1}^{K} \pi_{ik} \xi_k(t); \quad t = 1, 2, \ldots, T. \tag{5}$$

The problem of estimating $\xi$'s, given the $\pi$'s, is a low-dimensional problem and usually robust to the choice of the estimation method. On the other hand, the dimensionality of the $\pi_{ik}$'s is high and so the estimation problem is delicate. Many methods have been proposed: among them is a quadratic (weighted) least-squares algorithm which constrains $\pi_{ik}$'s to belong to the $K$-dimensional simplex.

The tissue metabolic parameters $\vartheta^{(k)}$'s are estimated from the $\xi_k(\cdot)$'s and the pixel metabolic parameters are estimated following (4):

$$\hat{\vartheta}_i = \sum_{k=1}^{K} \hat{\pi}_{ik} \hat{\vartheta}^{(k)} \qquad (6)$$

**Experiments** Experiments were conducted to assess the performance of the suggested approach for estimating the pixel-wise variances of the functional parameters, $\vartheta$'s. Since it is not possible, with existing computational power, to estimate/compute the true variances in a two-dimensional PET setup needed for purposes of comparison, evaluations were done in a simplified one-dimensional deconvolution setting with projection characteristics as described in [21]. A 6-component mixture model was specified. Since as explained earlier, most of the variability is in the estimation of the mixing proportions, the component sub-time activity curves $\xi$'s (and hence $\vartheta^{(k)}$'s) were known. The relationship between

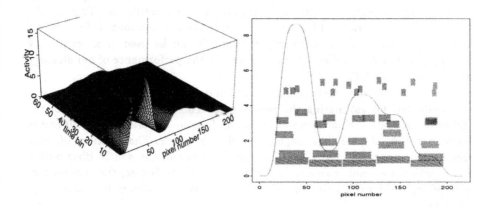

**Fig. 3.** (a) Perspective plot of the source distribution $\lambda(\cdot)$ used in the experiments. (b) The selected regions (ROI) (shaded bars) and the true source distribution at the fifth time-point (broken line). Size of the shaded bars is proportional to the ROI size.

$\xi_k$'s and $\vartheta^{(k)}$'s was specified by the equation

$$\xi_k(t) = \vartheta^{(k)} \exp\{-h_k t\}; \qquad k = 1, 2, \ldots, 6. \qquad (7)$$

This implies that $\vartheta^{(k)} = \xi_k(0)$. This is called the "amplitude parameter". $h_k$ is another functional parameter (the "half-life") but this parameter was not of interest in this experiment. The source distribution $\lambda(\cdot)$ (Figure 3a) was specified using (3) with mixing proportions ($\pi_{ik}$'s) that were blurred step functions [5]. The target functional parameter was defined using the $\pi$'s and the $\vartheta^{(k)}$'s in (4).

Time activity curves over 60 time-points were reconstructed at 216 bins (pixels) from realizations of an inhomogeneous Poisson process in the observation domain [5]. The reconstructions were smoothed by a Gaussian kernel with bandwidth preset to correspond to smoothing parameters that are reasonable for the given total expected emissions. The $\pi_{ik}$'s were estimated from $\hat{\lambda}^h(\cdot)$ and used to obtain $\hat{\vartheta}$'s.

1000 simulated reconstructions of the TAC were obtained by simulating the observed process and $\hat{\vartheta}$'s were extracted from each $\hat{\lambda}^h(\cdot)$. Sample pixel-wise standard deviations of these $\hat{\vartheta}_i$'s were assumed to be the "ground truth" in our performance evaluations.

Realizations were simulated from the approximate multi-Gaussian model for the estimated TACs $\hat{\lambda}^h(\cdot)$. Bootstrap samples of $\hat{\vartheta}$'s were obtained as outlined in Section 2.2 and standard deviations calculated. The experiment was done with bootstrap sample sizes $m=10$, 30 and different total expected emissions and replicated 500 times in order to study the distributional properties of these bootstrapped standard deviations.

The above experiment was performed using an extension of the simulation approach in [11]. Sample data sets were simulated in the observation domain followed by reconstruction and mixture analysis to obtain sample parametric data sets from where variances of the parameters were estimated. This simulation strategy is impractical to implement in the two-dimensional PET context; however, in the one-dimensional experiments, it can be used as a benchmark for our synthetic resampling scheme, indicating the performance of our strategy when applied to PET.

The suggested modified simulation method for estimating dispersions was also evaluated for estimating the covariances. This was done in terms of the ability to estimate the variances of the mean functional parameter in 40 homogeneous regions of sizes that ranged from 6 to 36 pixels. The locations of these regions are shown in Figure 3b. The true intensity of the source distribution at the fifth time-point is shown in the background. As before, the experiments were performed for different ranges of counts as well as different bootstrap sample sizes.

**Results** The results of the experiments conducted to evaluate the modified bootstrap approach are presented here. Figure 4a is a plot of the functional parameter — the "amplitude" — along with a sample estimate obtained using mixture analysis. The suggested method was evaluated in terms of its ability to assess the variance of this estimate. The percent relative absolute bias, averaged over pixels ranged from around 4–5% for all count rates and bootstrap sample sizes. Figure 4b shows a set of pixel-wise bootstrapped standard deviation estimates (points). Here the bootstrap sample size, $m=10$. The "true" standard deviation is shown by means of the broken line in Figure 4b. This was estimated from replicating the experiment 1000 times. The standard deviations were high in regions where the value of the parameter was high. The bootstrapped standard deviation estimates were post-processed by smoothing with the variable-span smoother of Friedman [7] which uses a local cross-validation scheme to adaptively estimate the resolution size of the smoothing filter. The smoothed estimate (Figure 4b, bold line) gave a better fit. Variability of the estimates was measured by the average, over pixels, of the mean percent absolute error in estimated standard deviation. Table 1 summarizes the bias and the variability

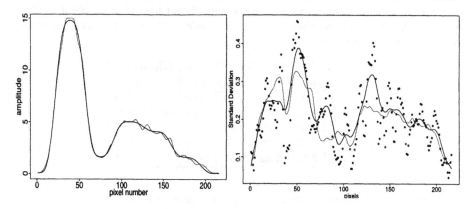

**Fig. 4.** (a) true amplitude (broken line) and a sample estimate (bold line); (b) true pixel-wise standard deviation (broken line) of the estimated amplitude and its unsmoothed (points) and smoothed (bold line) estimates (10 bootstrap replications).

measures of the estimated bootstrap standard deviations for both the synthetic

**Table 1.** Bias and variability measures for smoothed bootstrap standard deviation estimates over different total expected counts and bootstrap sample sizes. The bias measure is the percent relative bias averaged over pixels and the variability measure is the mean relative percent absolute error in estimating standard deviations averaged over pixels. Corresponding measures for unsmoothed estimates are in parenthesis. The measures in the left block were obtained using the synthetic resampling approach while those in the right block were obtained using the usual resampling strategy.

| Counts | Bias | | Variability | | Bias | | Variability | |
|---|---|---|---|---|---|---|---|---|
| $(\times 10^5)$ | *10 rep* | *30 rep* | *10 rep* | *30 rep* | *10 rep* | *30 rep* | *10 rep* | *30 rep* |
| **1.02** | 4.6 | 4.8 | 17.3 | 14.0 | 4.8 | 4.9 | 17.4 | 13.9 |
| | (5.6) | (3.7) | (27.7) | (21.6) | (5.2) | (3.8) | (27.7) | (21.4) |
| **2.05** | 5.1 | 5.1 | 16.1 | 12.9 | 5.0 | 5.0 | 16.2 | 12.9 |
| | (3.8) | (5.4) | (27.6) | (21.3) | (5.2) | (4.1) | (27.5) | (21.4) |
| **4.10** | 5.1 | 4.9 | 15.5 | 12.3 | 4.8 | 5.1 | 15.4 | 12.3 |
| | (5.3) | (3.7) | (27.3) | (21.0) | (5.1) | (3.7) | (27.4) | (20.9) |

resampling approach (left block) as well as the usual resampling strategy (right block). There is virtually no difference between either method, suggesting good performance of our approximate resampling scheme for variance estimation of parametric images. Further, the percent relative absolute biases are not altered appreciably as a result of the smoothing; however, the variability measures are considerably improved. The bias and variability rates do not differ appreciably

**Table 2.** Bias and variability measures for estimated standard deviations of mean estimated functional parameters over regions and different bootstrap sample sizes. Bias and variability measures are similar to those in Table 1. The reported percentages are averaged over regions of the same size.

| ROI size | Bias | | | Variability | | |
|---|---|---|---|---|---|---|
| (pixels) | *10 rep* | *20 rep* | *30 rep* | *10 rep* | *20 rep* | *30 rep* |
| 6 | 4.5 | 2.69 | 3.09 | 25.88 | 21.61 | 19.91 |
| 14 | 3.64 | 2.54 | 2.40 | 21.54 | 16.51 | 14.56 |
| 20 | 3.91 | 2.68 | 2.52 | 20.34 | 14.69 | 13.11 |
| 28 | 3.55 | 2.19 | 1.66 | 19.92 | 13.79 | 11.48 |
| 36 | 3.18 | 2.02 | 2.00 | 19.52 | 13.79 | 11.66 |

for different total expected counts, for the unsmoothed estimates. This points suggests that the unsmoothed estimators. As expected, the error rates decrease with increasing bootstrap sample size.

The errors in estimating standard deviations of the estimated mean functional parameter over the 40 homogeneous regions are presented in Table 2. The variability measures decreased with increasing size of region; a corresponding, albeit slight, phenomenon was also reported for the bias measures. Since summing over larger regions tends to have a smoothing effect, this is expected. However, since the variability measures are still high, this suggests the need for post-processing the estimates.

# 4  Discussion

The main contribution of this paper is a practical approach to variability assessment in parametric images obtained from dynamic sequences of reconstructed Positron Emission Tomography (PET) scans. The approach hinges on the approximation of the distribution of the reconstructed PET sequence by a Gaussian random field. The dispersions are specified by the Fourier methods outlined in Maitra [17]. Diagnostic checks were performed to test the validity of our suggestion, in the context of simulation PET experiments. Further, a one-dimensional analogue of the PET reconstruction problem was used to evaluate the performance of the approach in estimating the variances of the estimated parameters, with encouraging results. Though the focus has been the estimation of pixel-wise variances of parametric images using the mixture analysis of O'Sullivan [20, 22], the technique is general enough to be applied to variance assessment in parametric images obtained by approaches other than mixture analysis.

A number of issues remain to be addressed. As seen in the experiments, the estimation process can be improved by post-processing the estimated variances. The crude smoothing algorithm we have used does not perform well in the presence of correlated coordinates, which is very likely in our case. Hence, the obtained error rates may potentially be decreased by a more sophisticated choice of smoothing parameter. Another question of interest is determining the number of bootstrap samples. Further, the diagnostic tests indicate that there is need for better dispersion estimation procedures, especially at lower bandwidths. An attraction of the Fourier method of estimating correlations is the computational efficiency in generating correlated data — such an approach is not necessarily possible even in the one-dimensional model where we have accurate correlation computation procedures [16, 17]. Hence, there is need for developing better dispersion estimation procedures, and also efficient simulation procedures that can generate data with similar correlation structures. Another issue is the incorporation of correction factors that are routinely applied to the PET reconstructions in order to account for detector geometry and other effects. Since the ultimate goal of this exercise is to develop practical inference tools to guide diagnostic decisions, these issues will have to be addressed. With the increasing use of three-dimensional scanners, modest moves are beginning to be made in the direction of using these reconstructions for quantitative purposes. Extending the suggested technique to such settings would be invaluable for diagnosis. Thus, while this seems a promising new technique towards variability estimation in functional images, a number of questions remain to be investigated. To this end, a promising beginning with great potential can be said to have been made.

## APPENDIX: FOURIER SIMULATION METHODS

In matrix notation, the reconstruction equation can be expressed as

$$\hat{\lambda}^h = S_h (K'K)^{-1} K' y \tag{8}$$

where $y$ is the corrected projection data, $K$ is the discretized version of the Radon transform, and $S_h$ represents the smoothing operation of resolution size (FWHM) $h$ that is applied to the raw reconstructions in order to obtain acceptable solutions [21]. Under the assumption of relative uniformity of variances of the observed $y$'s, it can be shown [17, 18, 19] that the reconstruction $\hat{\lambda}^h$ has a spatially invariant correlation structure given by

$$\mathrm{Corr}(\hat{\lambda}_i^h, \hat{\lambda}_i^h) = \frac{C_h(|\,i - j\,|)}{C_h(0)}, \tag{9}$$

where $\Upsilon = \{C_h(0), C_h(1), \dots, C_h(I)\}$ is the first row of the approximately Fourier matrix $S_h(K'K)^{-1}S_h$.

Let $Z = \{Z_1, Z_2, \dots, Z_I\}$ be independent standard Gaussian random variables. Denote $\check{Z}$ and $\check{\Upsilon}$ as the corresponding Fast Fourier transforms of $Z$ and $\Upsilon$, respectively. $\check{\Upsilon}$ is real-valued and positive, and so is $\check{\Psi} = \sqrt{\check{\Upsilon}}$. Defining $B_h$ as the

the matrix formed by the rows obtained by permuting the inverse Fourier transform of $\check{\Psi}$, we get $B_h B_h' = S_h (K'K)^{-1} S_h$. Let $X = \{X_1, X_2, \ldots, X_I\} = B_h Z$. Then $X$ can be readily obtained from $Z$ by discrete convolution with $\Psi$. This step can be achieved via Fast Fourier transforms. Further, $X$ forms a set of correlated zero-mean, unit-variance Gaussian variables with the desired correlation structure. Let $R_i = \hat{\lambda}_i^h + \hat{\tau}_i X_i$, where $\hat{\tau}_i^2$ is the variance estimate of $\hat{\lambda}_i^h$ detailed in [17, 18, 19]. Then $R = \{R_1, R_2, \ldots, R_I\}$ is a realization from the asymptotic distribution of $\hat{\lambda}$. The realizations are readily simulated because of the Fast Fourier Transforms used in obtaining correlated realizations.

## Acknowledgements

I would like to thank Professor Finbarr O'Sullivan, my dissertation advisor in the Department of Statistics at the University of Washington, for introducing me to this problem and for the many hours of helpful advice and invaluable insights that I have received from him. Some of the routines used in the one-dimensional experimental evaluations were written by Kingshuk RoyChoudhury of the Department of Statistics at the University of Washington: his help is gratefully acknowledged.

## References

1. Blomqvist, G., "On the Construction of Functional Maps in Positron Emission Tomography", *J. Cereb. Blood Flow and Metab.*, 4:629-32, 1984.
2. Blomqvist, G., Eriksson L., and Rosenqvist G., "The Effect of Spatial Correlation on Quantification in Positron Emission Tomography" *Neuroimage*, 2:2, 1995.
3. Carson, R. E., Yan, Y., Daube-Witherspoon, M. E., Freedman, N., Bacharach, S. L. and Herscovitch, P., "An Approximation Formula for the Variance of PET Region-of-Interest Values", *IEEE Trans. Med. Imag.*, 12:240-50, 1993.
4. Cunningham, V. J., and Jones, T., "Spectral Analysis of Dynamic PET Studies", *J. Cereb. Blood Flow and Metab.*, 13:15-23, 1993.
5. Choudhury, K. R. and O'Sullivan, F., "A Statistical Examination of FBP and ML for Estimating Mixture Models from Dynamic PET Data", *1995 IEEE Nucl. Sci. Symp. and Med. Imag. Conf. Record*, 3:1237-1241, 1995.
6. Efron, B., "The Jackknife, the Bootstrap and Other Resampling Plans", SIAM, 1982.
7. Friedman, J. H., "A Variable Span Smoother", *Tech. Rep. No. 5, Lab. for Comp. Stat., Dept. of Stat., Stanford Univ., Stanford, CA*, 1984.
8. Friston, K. J., Frith, C. D., Liddle, P. F., and Frackowiak R. S., "Comparing Functional (PET) Images: The Assessment of Significant Change", *J. Cereb. Blood Flow Metab.*, 11:690-99, 1991.
9. Gjedde, A., "High- and Low-affinity Transport of Glucose from Blood to Brain", *J. Neurochem.*, 36:1463-71, 1981.
10. Gjedde, A., "Calculation of Cerebral Glucose Phosphorylation from Brain Uptake of glucose analogs in vivo: a re-examination", *Brain Res. Rev.*, 4:237-74, 1982.
11. Haynor, D. R. and Woods, S. D., "Resampling Estimates of Precision in Emission Tomography", *IEEE Trans. Med. Imag.*, 8:337-43, 1989.

12. Herholz, K. and Patlak, C. S., "The Influence of Tissue Heterogeneity on Results of Fitting Nonlinear Model Equations to Regional Tracer Uptake Curves. With an Application to Compartmental Models used in Positron Emission Tomography", *J. Cereb. Blood Flow Metab.* 11:10-24, 1991.

13. Herholz, K., "Non-stationary Spatial Filtering and Accelerated Curve-fitting for Parametric Imaging with Dynamic PET", *Eur. J. Nucl. Med.*, 14:477-84, 1988.

14. Heiss, W. D., Kessler, J., Karbe, H., Fink, G. R., and Pawlik, G., "Cerebral Glucose Metabolism as a Predictor of Recovery from Aphasia in Ischemic Stroke", *Arch. Neurol.*, 50:958-64, 1993.

15. Heiss, W. D., Kessler, J., Slansky, I., Mielke, R., Szelies, B., and Herholz, K., "Activation PET as an Instrument to Determine Theraupetic Efficacy in Alzheimer's Disease", *Ann. N. Y. Acad. Sci.*, 695:327-31, 1993.

16. Maitra, R. and O'Sullivan, F., "Estimating the Variability of Reconstructed PET Data : A Technique Based on Approximating the Reconstruction Filter by a sum of Gaussian kernels", *1995 IEEE Nucl. Sci. Symp. and Med. Imag. Conf. Record*, 3:1411-14, 1995.

17. Maitra, R., "Variability Estimation in Linear Inverse Problems", *Ph. D. dissertation*, Department of Statistics, University of Washington, 1996.

18. Maitra, R., "Estimating Precision in Functional Images", *J. Comp. Graph. and Stat.*, 6:1:1-11, 1997.

19. Maitra, R. amd O'Sullivan, F., "Variability Assessment in PET and Related Generalized Deconvolution Models", *J. Amer. Stat. Assoc.*, submitted, 1997.

20. O'Sullivan, F., "Imaging Radiotracer Model Parameters in PET : A Mixture Analysis Approach", *IEEE Trans. Med. Imag.*, 12:399-412, 1993.

21. O'Sullivan, F., Pawitan, Y. and Haynor, D., "Reducing Negativity Artifacts in Emission Tomography: Post-Processing Filtered Backprojection Solutions", *IEEE Trans. Med. Imag.*, 12:653-663, 1993.

22. O'Sullivan, F., "Metabolic Images from Dynamic Positron Emission Tomography studies", *Stat. Meth. in Med. Res.*, 3:87-101, 1994.

23. Patlak, C. S., Blasberg, R. G., and Fenstenmacher, J. D., "Graphical Evaluations of Blood-to-brain Transfer Constants from Multiple-time Uptake Data", *J. Cereb. Blood Flow Metab.* 3:1-7, 1983.

24. Schmidt, K., Miles, G. and Sokoloff, L., "Model of Kinetic Behavior of Deoxyglucose in Heterogeneous Tissues in Brain: a Reinterpretation of the Significance of Parameters fitted to Homogeneous Tissue Models", *J. Cereb. Blood Flow Metab.* 11:10-24, 1991.

25. Vardi, Y., Shepp, L. A. and Kaufman, L. A., "Statistical model for Positron Emission Tomography", *J. Amer. Statis. Assoc.*, 80:8-37, 1985.

26. Worsley, K. J., Evans, A. C., Marrett, S. and Neelin, P., "A Three-dimensional Statistical Analysis for CBF Activation Atudies in Human Brain", *J. Cereb. Blood Flow Metab.*, 12:900-18, 1992.

# Space-Time Statistical Model for Functional MRI Image Sequences

H. Benali [1], I. Buvat [1], J.L. Anton [2], M. Pélégrini [1], M. Di Paola [1], J.Bittoun [3], Y. Burnod [2] and R. Di Paola [1]

[1] U66 INSERM, CHU Pitié Salpêtrière, 75634 Paris
[2] CJF 93-03, CREARE, 9 quai Saint Bernard, 75005 Paris
[3] U2R2M-CIERM, 78 rue du Général Leclerc, 94275 Le Kremlin-Bicêtre

**Abstract**: Changes in cerebral blood oxygenation and flow during activation of human brain can be measured using functional magnetic resonance imaging (fMRI) data acquired during periodic sensory stimulation. Ideally, spatial and temporal correlations in the acquired data should all be taken into account to derive statistical parametric maps (SPM) and to identify significant changes in fMRI signal. This paper proposes a multivariate statistical model for brain activation detection accounting for both the spatial and temporal correlations. This model considers a space-time variant error and a spatial Markov random field process is used to yield an unbiased estimate of the SPM. As the number of pixels is large enough, the asymptotic theory is used to derive a threshold allowing the identification of activated areas in the SPM. The method is illustrated on sensorimotor experiments performed on normal subjects using 1.5T gradient-echo MRI.

## 1 Introduction

Non-invasive detection of blood oxygenation dependent contrast (BOLD) in human brain by fMRI provides a powerful tool for neurophysiological and cognitive research [1-3]. The fMRI technique is particularly attractive because of its spatial and temporal resolution. Because BOLD contrast is fairly small, with activation inducing signal increase ranging from 5 to 10% [4, 5], a sensitive method is needed to detect the activation sites. Moreover, changes in fMRI brain images are not only due to activation, but also to other variables, such as pulsatile blood flow, imaging artifacts or patient motion. Despite these problems, two objectives are currently pursued using fMRI: 1) Mapping the response to a stimulus onto an anatomical image, i.e., identifying regions for which there is a specific correlation between a time-dependent sensorimotor task and a measured change in physiology; 2) Characterizing the transfer function of the brain. This paper addresses only the first objective.

The most common methods used to detect activation sites are the subtraction-based methods. More sophisticated techniques have also been described and can be divided up into two main categories: 1) Pixel-based techniques which process the time series corresponding to each pixel and test the hypothesis that there are no differences between the signal measured during the control and the stimulation periods [6-8]. These methods deal with one pixel at a time to derive the SPM pixel by pixel and ignore the spatial correlation between neighboring pixels, although some of these methods take spatial correlation into account for a further analysis of the SPM [4, 9, 10]; 2) More recently, multivariate statistical methods have been proposed to process simultaneously all the time series corresponding to the different pixels [11-15]. To our knowledge, no methods deal with both spatial and time correlation to estimate the SPM. In this paper, we propose an original approach which takes into account the spatial and time correlation in the detected signal using a multivariate statistical space-time model. The asymptotic theory is used to determine the parameters involved in the model. Solving the model yields an SPM theoretically free of space-time correlated noise. The method is illustrated using sensorimotor experiments performed on normal volunteers with 1.5T gradient-echo MRI.

## 2 Removing the intrinsic brain signal

In fMRI, it has been reported that the delay associated with the hemodynamic response in the signal change is 5 to 8 s from stimulus onset to 90% maximum, and 5 to 9 s from stimulus cessation to 10% above baseline signal [16]. Therefore, "equilibrium processes" (i.e. processes that are stable in time) can be studied by acquiring the images after an equilibrium state has been reached, e.g., either 20 s after the stimulus onset (activation equilibrium), or 20 s after the subject has stopped any task (baseline equilibrium). Under these conditions, it is reasonable to assume that the fMRI signal is constant within a state and that the time correlation caused by the hemodynamic response to the sensory input can be ignored. In this paper, only brain states observed at equilibrium were considered. Our purpose was to develop a method for detecting areas in which significant changes occurred between baseline equilibrium (corresponding to periods of time during which the subject was not performing any particular sensorimotor task) and activation states (during which the subject performed a given sensorimotor task).

Let $a_i(t)$ be the signal observed in a pixel $i$ during the activation equilibrium $A$, and $b_i(t)$ be the intrinsic brain signal observed during the baseline equilibrium $B$. For each pixel $i$, the time course observed during the activation equilibrium $A$ will be referred to as the T-component vector $a_i$, while the time course observed during the baseline equilibrium $B$ will be referred to as the T-component vector $b_i$. Both $a_i$ and $b_i$ consist of R repeated "trials" of K consecutive time points acquired during $A$ and $B$ respectively ($RxK=T$). Although $a_i$ is observed during the activation task, it may still include a component $r_i$ representing intrinsic brain activity and/or venous signal which are not related to the stimulus, in addition to the signal $s_i$ induced by the stimulus:

$$a_i = r_i + s_i. \tag{1}$$

To detect only the signal $s_i$ induced by the stimulus, it is helpful to discount the brain signal $r_i$ which is not directly related to the stimulus. For that purpose, we proposed a multivariate conditioning method [13] accounting for the correlation which may exist between the time courses observed in different pixels. If **B** denotes the NxK matrix of the signals observed in N pixels at K equally sampled time points during a baseline trial, and **A** is the NxK matrix of signals observed at K equally sampled time points during the activation trial which immediately followed the baseline trial, the conditioned signal $\mathbf{Y}$ (NxK matrix of $y_i(t)$) is obtained by [17]:

$$\mathbf{Y} = \mathbf{A} - \mathbf{B}(\mathbf{B}^t\mathbf{B})^{-1}\mathbf{B}^t\mathbf{A} = \mathbf{PA}, \tag{2}$$

where

$$\mathbf{P} = \mathbf{Id_N} - \mathbf{B}(\mathbf{B}^t\mathbf{B})^{-1}\mathbf{B}^t \tag{3}$$

is the orthogonal projector onto the space orthogonal to the space spanned by $\{b_i\}_{i=1,...,N}$ and $\mathbf{Id_N}$ is the (NxN) identity matrix. The conditioned signal $\mathbf{Y}$ represents the part of the signal in $\mathbf{A}$ which is not correlated with the intrinsic brain signal $\mathbf{B}$. Conditioning is performed independently for each trial including K baseline and K activation images, leading to R matrices $\mathbf{Y}$. These matrices are then appended to yield a new Nx(KxR) matrix, i.e. an NxT matrix $\mathbf{Y}$, describing the conditioned signals for all trials.

# 3 Space-time statistical model

## 3.1 The fixed effect model

The sequence $\mathbf{Y}$ of the T conditioned images, each having N pixels, can be considered as N time series $y_i$ (i=1...N) of T components $y_{ij}$ (j=1...T). $y_i$ represents the time course of the signal in pixel i. Due to the conditioning process, $y_i$ does not depend on the intrinsic brain signal $\mathbf{B}$. The fixed effect model is defined as follows [18, 19]:

a) The activation signal $\mathbf{Y}$ can be separated into the unknown component $\mathbf{Z}$ which is the "true" part of the activation signal and an unknown random error $\mathbf{E}$ (representing noise):

$$\mathbf{Y} = \mathbf{Z} + \mathbf{E}. \tag{4}$$

The errors $\mathbf{E}$ are orthogonal to $\mathbf{Z}$. It is the true (fixed effect) component $\mathbf{Z}$ which is of real interest and which has to be estimated.

b) The expectation of $\mathbf{Y}$ is the fixed effect part:

$$E(\mathbf{Y}) = \mathbf{Z}, \tag{5}$$

i.e., the random errors $\mathbf{E}$ have a zero mean.

c) The error variance is separable in space and in time as follows:

$$var(\mathbf{E}) = \mathbf{W} \otimes \Gamma, \tag{6}$$

where $\mathbf{W}$ is the NxN symmetric positive matrix of spatial covariance of the errors $e_i$, $\Gamma$ is the TxT symmetric positive matrix of temporal covariance of the errors $e_i$ and $\otimes$ represents the outer product. Both $\mathbf{W}$ and $\Gamma$ are assumed to be known.

d) There is a Q (Q<K) dimensional linear space $\mathcal{C}$ such that $\mathbf{Z}$ belongs to $\mathcal{C}$.

This last hypothesis implies that the unknown part $Z$ of the activation signal could be estimated by projecting $Y$ onto the subspace $S$.

## 3.2 Least-square fitting with space-time correlated errors

The least-square estimate of $Z$ is obtained by minimizing the residuals between the acquired data $Y$ and the unknown fixed part $Z$ given a space-time correlation model, by means of a matrix $T$ for time correlation and a matrix $N$ for space correlation, i.e. by minimizing:

$$\mathcal{E}(|Y-Z|^2_{T\otimes N}). \qquad (7)$$

The minimum of equation 7 is reached for $S$ spanned by the $Q$ eigenvectors $u_k$ associated with the largest $Q$ eigenvalues $\lambda_k$ (in matrix $\Lambda$) of the matrix [18]:

$$Y^t N Y T. \qquad (8)$$

The optimal estimation of the fixed part $Z$ is therefore obtained by projecting the conditioned data $Y$ onto the subspace $S$. To perform the eigendecomposition of the matrix $Y^t N Y T$, the appropriate matrices $N$ and $T$ must be determined. The choice of these matrices is closely related to the spatial and temporal statistical properties of the data. If the number $N$ of pixels is large enough, the asymptotic theory can be used to estimate these matrices. Asymptotically, the optimal estimate of $S$ is obtained when $N$ is equal to $W^{-1}$ and $T$ is equal to $\Gamma^{-1}$ [20-22]. As a result, $Z$ is estimated by projecting $Y$ onto the basis of the $Q$ eigenvectors $u_k$ (represented by the matrix $U$) using the matrices $W^{-1}$ and $\Gamma^{-1}$:

$$Z = Y\,\Gamma^{-1}\,U^t\,(U\,\Gamma^{-1}\,U^t)^{-1}\,U = V\,\Lambda\,U, \qquad (9)$$

with:

$$V = Y\,\Gamma^{-1}\,U^t\,\Lambda^{-1}. \qquad (10)$$

## 3.3 Space-time correlation model

The fixed effect model is attractive since it can take into account the spatial and temporal correlations of the signal. However, the covariance matrices $W$ and $\Gamma$ are not known a priori and have to be estimated. This requires the introduction of a time correlation model and of a space correlation model.

**Time correlation model.** For equilibrium studies, the hemodynamic response to the sensory input, which describes the time dispersion of the observed activation after the stimulus onset, can be ignored. Indeed, it is reasonable to assume that the fMRI signal is constant for a brain state at equilibrium. In this particular case, the statistical study of MRI noise showed that the noise $e_i$ is not correlated in time ($\Gamma = Id_T$) and presents an identical normal distribution [23, 24].

**Spatial correlation model.** To model the spatial correlation of the errors $e_i$, the spatial relationships between pixels must be introduced by means of the covariance matrix $W$. The process $Y$ is considered as a second-order spatially stationary process defined at pixels i (i=1,...,N). The covariance matrix $W$ of elements $w_{ik}$ can then be written as follows:

$$w_{ii} = \sigma^2,$$

and

$$w_{ik} = cov(i - k), \tag{11}$$

where cov(i-k) is the covariance function, depending on the relative locations of the pixels i and k. The variogram $\gamma$ is conventionally used to determine the type of stationary dependence in the data and to deduce an appropriate spatial model. The variogram is defined as follows:

$$\gamma(i - k) = \sigma^2 - cov(i - k). \tag{12}$$

For a second-order spatially stationary process, an estimator of the variogram based on the method-of-moments [25] is:

$$2\gamma(h) = \frac{1}{n_h} \sum_{(i,k)\in N(h)} (y_i - y_k)^2 \tag{13}$$

where N(h) is the set of pixels (i,k) at lag (i-k)=h, and $n_h$ is the number of pairs of pixels in N(h).

Various parametric variogram models are presented in [26]. If the variogram model adequately describes the spatial dependencies of the data, then the estimated covariance matrix $W$ used to estimate the fixed part $Z$ should be optimal. Experiments showed that the exponential variogram model closely fitted the measured variograms. This model is given by:

$$2\gamma(h) = 0 \qquad \text{if h=0,}$$
$$2\gamma(h) = \tau_0 + \tau_1 (1- \exp (- \tau_2 h)) \text{ otherwise.} \tag{14}$$

The choice of this model will be justified further in the result section.
Using equations 12 and 14, the covariance function cov can be derived:

$$2\sigma^2 = \tau_1,$$
$$cov(i - k) = \sigma^2 \exp (- \tau_2 (i - k)). \tag{15}$$

Because the covariance function is exponential, the process $y_i$ can be interpreted as a realization of a first-order autoregressive Gaussian process, also called a Gaussian Markov process [25]. When defining $\rho = \exp(-\tau_2)$, which represents the first order spatial correlation, it can be shown that [27]:

$$\mathbf{W} = \sigma^2 \begin{pmatrix} 1 & \rho & \rho^2 & \cdots & \rho^{N-1} \\ \rho & 1 & \rho & \cdots & \rho^{N-2} \\ \rho^2 & \rho & 1 & \cdots & \rho^{N-3} \\ & & \cdots & & \\ \rho^{N-1} & & & \cdots & 1 \end{pmatrix} \qquad (16)$$

i.e.,

$$\mathbf{W}^{-1} = \frac{1}{(1-\rho^2)\sigma^2} \begin{pmatrix} 1 & -\rho & 0 & \cdots & 0 \\ -\rho & 1+\rho^2 & -\rho & \cdots & 0 \\ 0 & -\rho & 1+\rho^2 & \cdots & 0 \\ & & \cdots & & \\ 0 & & & \cdots & 1 \end{pmatrix}. \qquad (17)$$

In summary, the solution of the fixed effect model using the matrices $\Gamma^{-1}$ and $\mathbf{W}^{-1}$ as estimated above yields an estimate of $\mathbf{Z}$, the fixed component of the model, which is assumed to represent the noise-free signal related to the stimulus. $\mathbf{Z}$ is expressed in terms of the eigenimages $v_k$ (in matrix $\mathbf{V}$) obtained from the eigendecomposition (equation 10). The eigenimages $v_k$ are the maps of the greatest signal variations which are not due to the error $\mathbf{E}$ or to the intrinsic brain signal. These maps will be used to calculate the SPM. This requires the study of the statistical distributions of each eigenimage $v_k$, to locate areas of statistically significant signal variations in the SPM. In this work, only $v_1$ will be considered, since it corresponds to the greatest signal variations.

## 3.4 Statistical distribution of the SPM

General null hypotheses and demonstrations of the asymptotic Gaussian distributions of $u_k$ and $\lambda_k$ can be found in [21]. Using these results, the asymptotic distributions of the eigenimages $v_k$ can be derived [13]. If $\lambda^*_k$ and $v^*_k(i)$ denote the asymptotic random variables $\lambda_k$ and $v_k(i)$ when $N$ tends to infinity, the statistics $\sqrt{\lambda_k}\, v_k(i)$ follows a Gaussian distribution with mean $\sqrt{\lambda^*_k}\, v^*_k(i)$ and with a variance equal to:

$$\xi_k^2 = \sum_{j \neq k}^{K} \left[ \frac{\sigma^2}{\lambda^*_j - \sigma^2} + \left( \frac{\sigma^2}{\lambda^*_j - \sigma^2} \right)^2 \right] \lambda^*_j v^*_j(i)^2. \qquad (18)$$

The statistical parametric map ($SPM_k$) associated to the eigenimage $v_k$ defined by:

$$SPM_k(i) = \frac{\sqrt{\lambda_k}\, v_k(i)}{\xi_k} \qquad (19)$$

is therefore asymptotically normal with mean $\sqrt{\lambda^*_k}\, v^*_k(i)$ and with a variance equal to 1.

To detect the activation sites, the null hypothesis $H_0$ is that the fixed component $z_i$ is zero, which implies that $v^*_k(i)=0$ [13]. For each pixel i, $H_0$ can therefore be tested using SPM(i) which, if $H_0$, is true, should asymptotically follow a standardized normal distribution with mean 0.

To summarize the previous sections: a single parameter $\rho$ can be estimated from the variogram of the conditioned signal $Y$ (Eq. 13). Then, the eigenimages $v_k$ can be calculated from the eigendecomposition of the matrix $Y^t W^{-1} Y \Gamma^{-1}$. These eigenimages can be used to derive the statistical parametric map for activation (Eq. 19).

# 4 Materials and methods

## 4.1 Sensorimotor task

Twenty right-handed volunteers were studied. All subjects were healthy, had no known neurological problems and gave their informed consent following the guidelines of the Human Studies Committee of "Hôpital du Kremlin-Bicêtre". The subjects performed a sensorimotor discrimination task, consisting of right hand fingers to thumb opposition movements.

## 4.2 Functional MR image acquisition

MR images were acquired using a 1.5T Signa MR imaging system (General Electric Medical Systems) with a standard head coil. A sagittal medial anatomical image was first used to find the intercommissural line in order to detect the somatomotor hand area. Frontal MR images were then acquired around the central sulcus. The FOV was 24 cm, the pixel dimension was 1.88 mm x 0.94 mm and the slice thickness was 5 mm. For display, the images were interpolated to .94 mm x .94 mm pixel size. At each of the three contiguous frontal sections selected, the following images were acquired: 1) a frontal anatomical image (spin echo T1-weighted, TR = 500 ms, TE = 11 ms), 2) functional images (gradient echo sequence, TR = 80 ms, TE = 60 ms, flip angle = 20°). Three sets of 5 functional images were acquired for each state (sensorimotor task and baseline), yielding 30 images in total, corresponding to 15 baseline and 15 activation images. The first image of a 5 image trial was always acquired 20 s after the subject had started the task (activation trial) or had stopped the task (baseline trial). Each image acquisition time was 20.5 s. In addition, 30 more baseline images were acquired, after the subject had stopped any task for 20 s.

## 4.3 Data pre-processing

**Image registration**. Subject motion during the experiment may introduce artifacts in any analysis method which assumes the spatial stability of pixels in the set of images. Even a motion with an amplitude less than the pixel size can produce artifacts [28]. To reduce this potential source of errors, an inter-frame motion was automatically compensated for. Because of the relatively large thickness of the slices

(5 mm) and the small amplitude of expected motion, the approximation of an "in plane" rigid displacement was considered to be valid. Three parameters describing planar translation and rotation between a reference image (usually the first image in the series) and each image in the series were estimated by maximizing the correlation coefficient between the reference image and the image to be aligned [29]. Fractional pixel displacements were taken into account using a cubic interpolation [30].

**Segmentation of the brain.** After compensating for head motion artifacts, a binary mask including the brain was obtained by an automatic thresholding procedure. All activation and baseline images of the analyzed series were added together and the resulting image was smoothed using a 5x5 Gaussian kernel. The histogram of this smoothed image presented 2 peaks, one corresponding to pixels included in the brain, another corresponding to pixels outside the brain. The Otsu procedure [31] was used to determine the intensity threshold between these two peaks and to segment the brain. Only those pixels inside the brain region were considered further in the analysis.

## 4.4 Results

To illustrate the accuracy of the space-time model, one typical study is presented. Two time series, with and without activation, corresponding to the same subject are considered.

**Variogram model.** From the conditioned data $Y$, the spatial correlation parameters $\tau_0$, $\tau_1$ and $\tau_2$ (Eq. 13 and 15) were estimated in the 4 nearest neighbors at distance h in the vertical and horizontal directions using the weighted-least-square estimates. Fig. 1 shows the agreement between the estimated variogram and the exponential variogram model. The weighted-least-square estimates ($\tau_0$, $\tau_1$, $\tau_2$) were (38.37, 24.91, 1.15). These parameters corresponded to a spatial variance $2\sigma^2 = 24.91$ and to a first order spatial correlation $\rho = \exp(-1.15)=.315$.

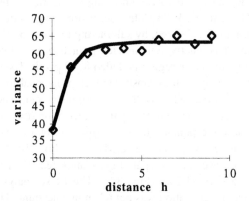

**Fig. 1.** Estimated variogram of the residuals in the 4-nearest neighbors (diamonds). The solid line is the weighted-least-squares fit using an exponential model $2\gamma(h) = 38.37 + 24.91\ (1-\exp(-1.15h))$.

This result shows that the exponential variogram model matches the spatial variance structure of the data, i.e. that the first autoregressive Gaussian process accurately describes the spatial correlation in the data.

**SPM analysis without activation signal**. The characteristics of the SPM obtained by the proposed multivariate approach were first illustrated using data with no activation signal, i.e., by taking the series of 30 baseline images, arranging them as 6 trials of 5 images as if 3 trials had in fact been acquired during an activation task, and processing the resulting "fake" baseline/activation image series. The SPM corresponding to the normalized first eigenimage was derived. Since there was no activation, the distribution of the SPM calculated according to equation 19 should follow a standardized normal distribution. The histogram of the calculated SPM is shown in Fig. 2. The SPM distribution is indistinguishable from that predicted by the asymptotic theory.

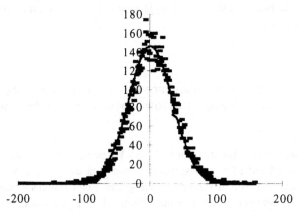

**Fig. 2.** Histogram of the calculated SPM (bars) compared to the predicted standardized normal distribution (solid line). x-axis values have been multiplied by 100.

The final stage of the analysis involves choosing a statistical threshold to identify the activated areas. Using the "fake" baseline/activation image series described above, a conventional t-test map was derived, by subtracting the sum of 15 baseline images from the sum of 15 "fake" activation images (which were actually also baseline images). For this study, the brain region included 8800 pixels. Using a 5% threshold on the t-test map, the number of false-positive pixels was equal to 759 (8.6%) (Fig. 3a). Two SPM were then derived from the space-time model. The first SPM was calculated without taking into account the spatial correlation ($\rho=0$, i.e. **W=Id**). When using a 1.96 threshold corresponding to a .05 type I error to detect the activation regions, 491 false-positive pixels were detected (5.6%) (Fig. 3b). A second SPM was calculated by taking into account the spatial correlation (eq. 17, $\rho=.315$). 109 false-positive pixels were detected (1.2%) (Fig. 3c.). The t-test analysis was much too conservative since spatial correlation was not taken into account. These results show that accounting for the multivariate nature of the data, and especially for the spatial correlation, could significantly reduce the number of false-positive pixels.

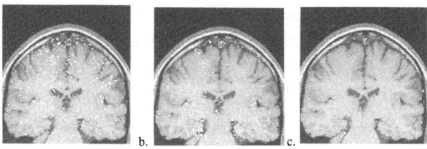

a.　　　　　　　　b.　　　　　　　　c.

**Fig. 3.** Maps of the false-positive pixels superimposed on the anatomical image, when using a 5% statistical threshold. t-test map (a), space-time model with $\rho=0$ (b) and space-time model with $\rho=.315$ (c).

**SPM analysis for activation studies.** For the same subject, the baseline/activation time series of 30 images was analyzed as previously described. The SPM obtained from the activation study was calculated using equation 19 with $\rho=0$ (i.e., ignoring spatial correlation) and $\rho=.315$. A threshold of 1.96 corresponding to a .05 type I error was then used to detect pixels with activation signal. The thresholded SPM with activation regions consisting of at least 6 pixels are shown in Fig. 4. The SPM obtained using the proposed method can be compared to the conventional t-test image derived from the subtraction of the sum of the 15 baseline images from the 15 activation images (Fig. 4a). The number of activation regions detected using the t-test was too large since no correction was made for the large number of multiple comparisons. The proposed approach reduced the number of falsely activated pixels and might yield to a more accurate detection of the activated areas (Fig. 4c). These areas were well correlated to the spatial form of the gray matter [2]. The activation curve corresponding to the average signal intensity for the pixels inside the detected regions using the space-time model ($\rho=.315$) is shown in Fig. 5. As expected, the average signal intensity inside the detected regions followed the activation time course used in the experiment.

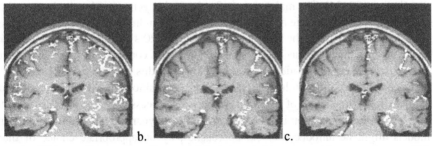

a.　　　　　　　　b.　　　　　　　　c.

**Fig. 4.** SPM superimposed on the anatomical image. t-test map (a), space-time model with $\rho=0$ (b), space-time model with $\rho=.315$ (c). A 5% statistical threshold was used and only regions of at least 6 connected pixels were represented.

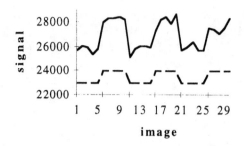

**Fig. 5**. Activation curve (solid line) corresponding to the average signal intensity of the pixels inside the detected regions in Fig. 4c. The on-off cycle matches the task-control paradigm (dashed line).

## 5 Discussion

Multivariate data analysis is an appealing approach to deal with brain fMRI data. Unlike methods analyzing the time series observed for each pixel independently, the multivariate approach permits a simultaneous processing of the time series observed in all pixels of interest, taking advantage of the complementary information provided by the set of pixels. Moreover, it makes it possible to introduce a priori knowledge about the spatial and temporal covariance properties of the data, potentially improving the sensitivity and the specificity of the analysis. In this paper, we proposed a space-time statistical model leading to the determination of the significant activation map. This model first focuses on the signal changes specific to the activation state using a previously described conditioning procedure [13]. The noise-free part of the conditioned signal is then estimated using the fixed effect model, and an SPM is deduced. Its statistical distribution is derived using the asymptotic theory.

The fixed effect model requires the covariance matrix of the error **E** to be separable in space (**W**) and in time (**Γ**). It further assumes that these matrices are known or can be estimated. This requires the statistical properties of the acquired data to be studied. In MRI, it has been shown that the time errors have an identical independent normal distribution [23, 24]. The main source of noise is that generated by the body and the receiver coil. As the image acquisition time for our studies was 20.5 s, and as images were acquired only after the subject had been at least 20 s in the same state (baseline or activation), the noise has been considered to be not correlated in time. The matrix **Γ** was then taken as the identity matrix. However, this hypothesis will have to be revisited when dealing with echo planar data acquisition or with non equilibrium studies. In [6], the theory of a stationary Gaussian process was used and addressed the problem of autocorrelation in time, due to the hemodynamic response function. Such models might be introduced in our approaches, by an appropriate choice of the **Γ** matrix.

Regarding the spatial correlation of the data, it is well known that the adjacent pixels error are highly correlated by the initial acquisition process. Our results showed that for our studies, the exponential variogram model was well adapted to the acquired data. The spatial covariance function of the errors was then an exponential function.

In that particular case, the errors $e_i$ can be interpreted as a realization of a first-order autoregressive Gaussian process, i.e. a Gaussian Markov random field. Given this model, the matrix $W$ depends on a single parameter $\rho$ which can be estimated using a weighted-least-square optimization algorithm [25]. A related approach based on Euler characteristic was used in [4, 10] to derive an appropriate threshold for SPM. By contrast, our method takes the spatial correlation into account *when calculating* the SPM, not only for determining an appropriate threshold.

Given the space and time covariance of the signal described by the matrices $W^{-1}$ and $\Gamma^{-1}$, solving the model gives an estimate of the noise-free part of the conditioned data, using the eigendecomposition of the matrix given in equation 8. This eigendecomposition leads to eigenimages which represent the main signal variability, supposedly due to the activation paradigm. The normalized eigenimages are defined as statistical parametric maps.

To estimate the significant activation areas in the SPM, the statistical properties of the eigenimages must be determined. Based on theoretical results regarding the asymptotic distribution of principal components [21, 22] we showed that, given the large number of pixels involved, the normalized eigenimages (i.e. the SPM) present a standardized Gaussian distribution under the null hypothesis (no activation signal). When processing data with no activation signal (i.e. "fake" baseline/activation image series), the distribution of the SPM calculated according to equation 19 followed the expected standardized normal distribution. When thresholding this SPM using a value of 1.96 corresponding to a .05 type I error probability, 5.6% false-positive pixels were detected using the proposed multivariate model, and the number of false-positive pixels was further reduced (1.2%) when accounting for the spatial correlation in the model. These preliminary results suggest that the space-time model might increase the specificity for the detection of activation areas compared to the more conventional t-test method and to the method we previously described [13]. Indeed, in these approaches, the spatial correlation is not taken into account. For activation studies too, our preliminary results suggest that the proposed multivariate spatio-temporal model might improve the sensitivity and the specificity of the detection of activated areas. This remains to be proven however.

# 6 Conclusion

We described a space-time multivariate model for fMRI brain activation detection. This statistical approach takes into account both the spatial and temporal correlations to estimate an unbiased statistical parametric map (SPM). A Gaussian Markov random process was considered to model the spatial correlation of the noise into the multivariate statistical model. As the number of pixels was large enough, the asymptotic theory could be used to derive the SPM statistical distribution and determine a threshold for the detection of significant activation areas. Preliminary results showed that taking into account the spatio-temporal correlations reduced the number of false-positive pixels. Further studies will be necessary to assess the practical value of the proposed method. As the model permits the introduction of various forms of time correlation by means of the time covariance matrix, a study of the time correlation induced by the hemodynamic response function will also be performed to take full advantage of the potentialities of the model when this function cannot be ignored.

# 7 References

1. J.W. Belliveau, D.N. Kennedy, R.C. McKinsky, B.R. Buchbinder, R.M. Weisskoff, M.S. Cohen, J.M. Vivea, T.J. Brady and B.R. Rosen: Functional mapping of the human cortex by resonance imaging. Science 254, 621-768 (1991)
2. P.E. Roland: Brain activation. New York: Wiley-Liss 1992
3. R.G. Shulman, A.M. Blamire, D.L. Rothman and G. McCarthy: NMRI and spectroscopy of humain brain function. Proc. Natl. Acad. Sci. USA 89, 1837-1841 (1993)
4. K.J. Worsley, A.C. Evans, S. Marrett and P. Neelin: A three-dimensional statistical analysis for CBF activation studies in human brain. J. Cereb. Blood Flow Metab. 12, 900-918 (1992)
5. W. Schneider, B.J. Casey and D. Noll: Functional MRI mapping of stimulus rate effects across visual processing stages. Human Brain Mapping 1, 117-133 (1994)
6. K.J. Friston, P. Jezzard and R. Turner: Analysis of functional MRI time-series. Human Brain Mapping 1, 153-171 (1994)
7. E. Bullmore, M. Brammer, S.C.R. Williams, S. Rabe-Hesketh, N. Janot, A. David, J. Mellers, R. Howard and P. Sham: Statistical methods of estimation and inference for functional MR image analysis. Magn. Reson. Med. 35, 261-277 (1996)
8. K. Sekihara and H. Koizumi: Detecting cortical activities from fMRI time-course data using the MUSIC algorithm with forward and backward covariance averaging. Magn. Reson. Med. 35, 807-813 (1996)
9. K.J. Friston, C.D. Frith, P.F. Liddle and R.S.J. Frackowiak: Comparing functional (PET) images: the assessment of significant change. J. Cereb. Blood Flow Metab. 11, 690-699 (1991)
10. K.J. Worsley, S. Marrett, P. Neelin, A.C. Vandal, K.J. Friston and A.C. Evans: A unified statistical approach for determining significant signals in images of cerebral activation. Human Brain Mapping 4, 58-73 (1996)
11. K.J. Friston, C.D. Frith, R.S.J. Frackowiak and R. Turner: Characterizing dynamic brain responses with fMRI: a multivariate approach. NeuroImage 2, 157-167 (1995)
12. S.C. Strother, J.R. Anderson, K.A. Schaper, J.S. Sidtis and D.A. Rottenberg: Linear models of orthogonal subspaces and networks from functional activation PET studies of the human brain. In: Y. Bizais, C. Barillot and R. Di Paola (eds): Information Processing in Medical Imaging. Dordrecht: Kluwer Academic Publishers 1995, pp. 299-310
13. H. Benali, J.L. Anton, M. Di Paola, F. Frouin, O. Jolivet, R. Carlier, J. Bittoun, Y. Burnod and R. Di Paola: Conditioned statistical model for functional MRI studies of the human brain. In: Y. Bizais, C. Barillot and R. Di Paola (eds): Information Processing in Medical Imaging. Dordrecht: Kluwer Academic Publishers 1995, pp. 311-322

14. J.L. Anton, H. Benali, E. Guigon, M. Di Paola, J. Bittoun, O. Jolivet and Y. Burnod: Functional MR imaging of the human sensorimotor cortex during haptic discrimination. NeuroReport 7, 2849-2852 (1996)

15. W. Backfrieder, R. Baumgartner, M. Samal, E. Moser and H. Bergmann: Quantification of intensity variations in functional MR images using rotated principal components. Phys. Med. Biol. 41, 1425-1438 (1996)

16. P.A. Bandettini, A. Jesmanowicz, E.C. Wong and J.S. Hyde: Processing strategies for time-course data sets in functional MRI of the human brain. Magn. Reson. Med. 30, 161-173 (1993)

17. J.S. Bendat and A.G. Piersol: Random Data - Analysis and measurement procedures. New York: John Wiley & Sons 1986

18. H. Caussinus: Models and uses of principal component analysis. In: J. De Leeuw (ed): Multidimensional data analysis. Leiden: DSWO Press 1986, pp. 149-178

19. H. Benali, I. Buvat, F. Frouin, J.P. Bazin and R. Di Paola: A statistical model for the determination of the optimal metric in Factor Analysis of Medical Image Sequences (FAMIS). Phys. Med. Biol. 38, 1065-1080 (1993)

20. P. Besse, H. Caussinus, L. Ferre and J. Fine: Principal component analysis and optimization of graphical displays. Statistics 19, 301-312 (1988)

21. J. Fine and A. Pousse: Asymptotic study of the multivariate functional model. Application to the metric choice in principal component analysis. Statistics 23, 63-83 (1992)

22. J. Fine: Asymptotic study of the multivariate functional model in the case of a random number of observations for each mean. Statistics 25, 285-306 (1994)

23. W.A. Edelstein, G.H. Glover, C.J. Hardy and R.W. Redington: The intrinsic signal-to-noise ratio in NMR imaging. Magn. Reson. Med. 3, 604-618 (1986)

24. A. Macovski: Noise in MRI. Magn. Reson. Med. 36, 494-497 (1996)

25. N.A.C. Cressie: Statistic for spatial data. New York: Wiley International Publication 1993

26. A.G. Journel and C.J. Huijbregts: Mining geostatistics. London: Academic Press 1978

27. D.F. Morrison: Multivariate statistical methods. Tokyo: McGraw-Hill 1978

28. J.V. Hajnal, R. Myers, A. Oatridge, J.E. Schwieso and I.R. Young: Artifacts due to stimulus correlation motion in functional imaging of the brain. Magn. Reson. Med. 31, 283-291 (1994)

29. J.L.R. Andersson: A rapid and accurate method to realign PET scans utilizing image edge information. J. Nucl. Med. 36, 657-669 (1995)

30. P.E. Danielsson and M. Hammerin: High accuracy rotation of images. CVGIP 54, 340-344 (1992)

31. A. Otsu: A threshold selection method from grey-level histogram. IEEE Trans. Systems Man. Cybernet. 8, 62-66 (1978)

# Jackknifing a Normal Database for Regional Cerebral Blood Flow SPECT Obtained Using Principal Components

Alexander S. Houston

Department of Nuclear Medicine, Royal Hospital
Haslar, Gosport, Hants, UK.

**Abstract.** A normal atlas for rCBF was created previously from 50 normal subjects using a mean image and several eigenimages to represent normal variation in rCBF SPECT images. The parameters of the atlas were optimized to differentiate between further normal subjects and patients with suspected dementia. These parameters included the optimal number of principal components. In this paper the Partial Correlations Test is used to determine the optimal number of principal components yielding similar results to that obtained experimentally. In order to determine the false positive rate, each image in the set is classified as normal or abnormal according to predefined criteria. This will be a biased classification as the image is included in the set used to define the normal atlas. The jackknife process is then applied to the normal database. This involves redefining the atlas by computing the mean image and eigenimages 50 times, missing out each individual in turn. The image of the individual is then reclassified on the basis of being excluded from the set. The results are similar to those obtained for images of a further 40 normal subjects obtained subsequently. The jackknife allows an unbiased estimation of the eigenimages which form the atlas. It is demonstrated that these vary very little from the originals, although there is some disagreement between the original and jackknifed eigenvalues.

## 1 Introduction

### 1.1 Original Concept

The design of a normal database of medical images requires two stages: (I) the acquisition of images from a representative sample of the normal population; and (II) the representation of these images in some data-reduced format. Stage I involves defining exclusion criteria for subjects likely to provide an image which, by some definition, could be described as abnormal. Images from subjects who are not thus excluded may then be acquired. It is important, as in all statistical applications of this nature, that the number of subjects is large and representative of the normal population. Stage II involves aligning and scaling the images in order that they may be compared with each other. Some form of data reduction is then necessary. It has been proposed [1] that the data is best represented as an atlas comprising a mean image and several eigenimages obtained from a principal component analysis (PCA) applied to the database of images. For a new image outside the normal database, a "nearest normal equivalent" (NNE) image is calculated automatically from the database and compared with the new image. A difference image is formed which is compared with a residual SD image obtained from the residuals of the images in the normal database to yield a significance image [1].

The concept is applied in this instance to regional cerebral blood flow (rCBF) SPECT images obtained using $^{99}Tc^m$-HMPAO. In this case the alignment technique should, in theory, account for anatomical differences among individuals in the database allowing the eigenimages to represent correlated normal variations in physiology.

## 1.2 Previous Work

In a previous paper Houston et al [2] have optimized several parameters of the atlas representation by seeking optimal separation of 40 normal controls and 200 patients suffering from dementia. The main conclusions were that, after image alignment and scaling to global counts in the region to be analyzed, either (a) the full image should be used for the atlas resulting in a mean and around four or five eigenimages; or (b) the cortical region alone should be used resulting in a mean and around four eigenimages. While this is important, it ignores the statistical information inherent in the normal database which, in itself, tells us much about optimizing the representation of the data. This paper examines the normal database using the Partial Correlations Test for optimizing the number of components [3], followed by the jackknife procedure [4, 5] applied to the results of the PCA.

## 1.3 Related Work

The original work of this nature applied to medical images was that of Barber [6] who formed eigenimages for a collection of normal brain images obtained from planar nuclear medicine. Several methods have evolved from PET imaging of the brain for evaluating the significance of changes in voxel values between and among different images. The most widely used of these is probably SPM (statistical parametric mapping) [7], which involves a univariate method of establishing a significant change in voxel values combined with a multivariate method of analyzing such changes. For the problem of representing a normal image database, a univariate approach for identifying abnormal voxels may not be adequate. An alternative method using a multivariate approach is the scaled subprofile model [8], which has the added advantage of an automatic scaling of the images. One problem with this method is that only images in the database may be scaled in this way and it is unclear how to scale images outside the database.

## 1.4 Restrictions on Sampling

One of the difficulties facing designers of normal image databases in medicine is the ethical issue involving the imaging of normal subjects. This is particularly true of nuclear medicine where the issue of radiation protection looms large. The result is that normal image databases will be neither as large nor as representative as desired. In this case the number of subjects included in the database was restricted to fifty. The question arises whether this sample is large enough to give unbiased estimates of the eigenimages. In this paper the jackknife technique is applied in an attempt to answer this question.

## 1.5 The Jackknife

Jackknifing has previously been applied to PCA by Reyment [9], Gibson et al [10] and McGillivray [11]. In particular, the latter computed eigenvector elements and their standard errors using this technique. The first stage of the jackknifing process is used in this paper to reclassify individuals in the normal database with a view to obtaining an unbiased estimate of the false positive rate. The jackknife is then used to re-compute the eigenimages and their eigenvalues together with the associated standard errors, thus providing unbiased estimates of the eigenvalues and eigenimage elements.

## 2 Methods

### 2.1 Construction of Normal Database

SPECT images of rCBF were obtained from 50 normal volunteers (30 male; 20 female) with an age range of 18-58 (median 28). Strict exclusion criteria were applied in their selection including no history of neurological disease, no previous head injuries involving concussion, and no active participation in boxing or undersea diving [12]. The acquisition procedure involved an intravenous injection of 600 MBq of $^{99}Tc^m$-HMPAO followed by acquisition of 64 projection images of matrix size 64x64 around one complete revolution using a Siemens ZLC7500 gamma camera interfaced to a Park Medical MICAS V computer system. The images are subsequently zoomed to 24 axial slices of matrix size 32x32 [1].

A reference image was selected from the normal database and all other images registered with respect to it using a 3D affine transform with twelve degrees of freedom [13]. The cortical region was defined on the reference image by a nuclear medicine physician and involved sixteen axial slices. Two sets of images were prepared: one set involving the entire image and the other with voxels values outside the cortical region set to zero. In both cases, the images were scaled to total (remaining) counts. Since around four principal components (PCs) were considered to be optimal for representing both sets [2], a mean image, four eigenimages and a residual SD image were extracted in each case.

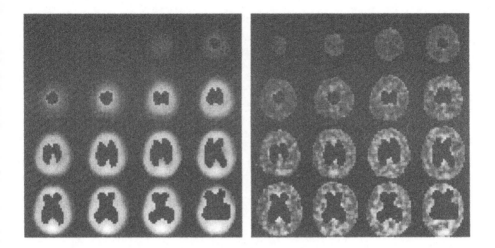

**Fig. 1.** The mean image (on left) and the residual SD image for the cortical atlas obtained using four PCs.

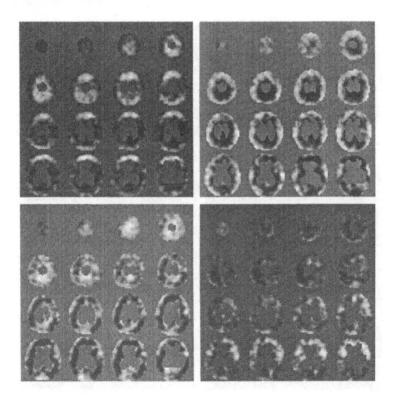

**Fig. 2.** The four eigenimages (first at top left; second at top right; third at bottom left) for the cortical atlas.

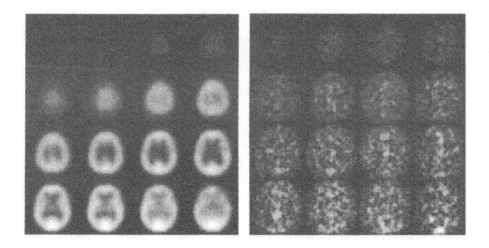

**Fig. 3.** The mean image (on left) and the residual SD image for the full image atlas obtained using four PCs.

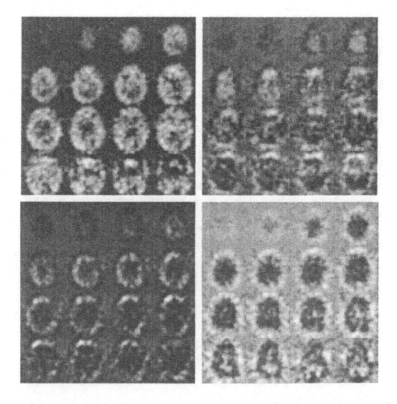

**Fig. 4.** The four eigenimages (first at top left; second at top right; third at bottom left) for the full image atlas.

The mean and residual SD image are shown in Figure 1 and the four eigenimages in Figure 2 for the atlas based on the cortical region. For the atlas based on the full image, the same 16 (of 24) axial slices of the equivalent images are shown in Figures 3 and 4. In order to retest the optimal number of PCs, alternative atlases containing between 0 and 10 eigenimages were generated for both sets.

## 2.2 Definition of Normality

For images obtained from a subject or patient outside the normal database, the NNE image, the difference image and the significance image are produced. The latter two images are calculated only for count deficient voxels in the cortex, since most relevant pathological conditions are associated with a reduced rCBF in this region. From results obtained previously [2], it would appear that a reasonable definition of abnormality in an image would be at least one deficit of 10 or more connected voxels at the 3 SD level to be present. Since these results were obtained for patients with dementia and may not be generally applicable, the number of connected voxels necessary to define abnormality has been redefined in this paper to cover the range from 1 to 12, although the 3 SD threshold has been retained. As well as new images, the images within the normal database may also be classified as normal or abnormal in this way. Since they belong to the normal database used to generate the PCs, this classification will be biased. An unbiased classification of each member of the normal database may be sought using the first stage of the jackknifing process.

## 2.3 Statistical Testing for PCA

Statistical tests exist for various aspects of a PCA [14]. For example, it is possible to test for the underlying assumption of multivariate normality, for complete independence of the variables (obviating the need for PCA), for sphericity, i.e. whether the variables are homoscedastic as well as independent, for covariance matrix equality, i.e. whether samples from different classes such as male and female belong to the same population, etc. One problem with the normal database described here is that the number of variables (voxel values), $p$, greatly exceeds the number of individuals (subjects), $n$. Although certain aspects of a PCA allow the roles of individual and variable to be exchanged, this is not the case for the some of these tests. Furthermore, even in cases where this is possible, the number of voxels to include is a problem as many have values of zero or close to zero. As a result, these issues have not yet been addressed.

## 2.4 Estimating the Number of PCs

The optimal number of PCs was retested using the Partial Correlations Test [3]. Let $\varepsilon_r$ be the $n \times p$ residual matrix after $r$ components have been extracted. Let $\mathbf{D} = \text{diag}(\varepsilon_r^T \varepsilon_r)$. Now let $\mathbf{R} = \mathbf{D}^{-1/2} \varepsilon_r^T \varepsilon_r \mathbf{D}^{-1/2}$ and let $r_{ij}$ represent the $(i,j)$th element of $\mathbf{R}$. Then the function given by $f_r = \Sigma\Sigma \, r_{ij}^2/p(p-1)$, where summation is over unequal (off-diagonal) values of $i$ and $j$, will lie in the interval $[0,1]$. As $r$ increases from 0, this function will reduce until the optimal number of components is reached, after which it will increase. When $p>n$, the residual matrix $\varepsilon^T$ may be used instead of $\varepsilon$, yielding the same result (although not necessarily the same values of $f_r$). This has been verified for the case of the cortical atlas. The analysis reported here was performed with this modification and the values of $f_r$ referenced and quoted from this stage onwards refer to those found using the modified analysis.

The value of $f_r$ was found for values of $r$ ranging from 0 to 10 for both the cortical and full image atlases.

## 2.5 Jackknifing the Normal Database

The first stage of the jackknife process as applied to PCA involves leaving each individual out of the normal database in turn and performing the PCA on the remaining 49 subjects. The omitted image was then reclassified as normal or abnormal while outside the normal database of 49 images, and this compared to its classification obtained within the original normal database of 50 images. This was done for both the cortical and full image atlases using four eigenimages. Classification was based consistently on the definition of abnormality as previously stated, i.e. at least one lesion of $N$ connected voxels at a threshold of 3 SDs with $N$ taking values ranging from 1 to 12.

In the above process, a set of eigenvalues and eigenimages was calculated for each of the 51 cases, i.e. the whole sample plus each case omitted in turn. Suppose that $\theta$ is a biased estimate of some parameter, e.g. a single eigenimage element. Then, if $\theta_n$ is the statistic calculated using the whole sample and $\theta_i$ is the statistic calculated with the $i$th individual removed, a set of $n$ partial estimates $\theta_i^* = n\theta_n - (n-1)\theta_i$ may be obtained . The jackknife estimator $\theta^*$ is simply the mean of the partial estimates. The variance of $\theta^*$ is given by $\Sigma(\theta_i^* - \theta^*)^2/n(n-1)$ where the summation is over $i = 1$ to $n$.

In the current example, $\theta$ may be an eigenvalue or the value of any element of an eigenimage obtained from the PCA. Since eigenvalues are measures of variance and since log-transformed variances perform better under jackknifing than actual variances [15, 16], it was decided to follow the example of Gibson et al [10] and convert the eigenvalues to their common logarithms prior to jackknifing. The jackknife estimator, $\theta^*$, and its standard error were calculated for the common logarithm of each of the first ten eigenvalues and also for each (non-transformed) element of the first ten eigenimages.

## 2.6 Application to a Normal Test Set

As part of trials involving boxers and divers, a further 40 normal subjects had rCBF SPECT imaging performed as previously described. These were all male and in the age range 18-29. The age and sex differences with respect to the normal database arise from the fact that these subjects were chosen specifically to match the boxers and divers for age and sex.

After image alignment and scaling, the image for each subject was classified as normal or abnormal using the cortical and full image atlases obtained for the full (50 subjects) normal database according to the definitions previously described.

# 3 Results

The results obtained using the Partial Correlations Test are shown in Table 1. Clearly, $f_r$ behaves as described reaching a minimum value at five PCs for the cortical atlas and four PCs for the full image atlas. This is very similar to the results obtained experimentally using dementia patients and further normal subjects and gives us reasonable confidence in our choice of four PCs for each.

The results of reclassification are shown in Table 2. The original results for individuals retaining membership of the reference set are compared with the results obtained after individual omission. The results obtained for the new set of 40 normal subjects are also included.

The first ten log-transformed eigenvalues and their jackknifed estimates are shown for both cortical and full image atlases in Table 3. The standard error of each jackknifed estimate is also shown. The first four jackknifed eigenimages are displayed in Figure 5 for the cortical atlas, and in Figure 6 for the full image atlas.

The jackknifed images in Figures 5 and 6 are almost identical in appearance to their original counterparts in Figures 2 and 4 respectively. It is therefore not surprising that inspection of the appropriate files indicate that the associated standard errors for the jackknifed eigenimage elements are very small. On the other hand, the log-transformed eigenvalues shown in Table 3, before and after jackknifing are often quite different.

| No. of PCs (r) | $f_r$ (x10$^{-2}$) for Cortex | $f_r$ (x10$^{-2}$) for Full Image |
|---|---|---|
| 0 | 1.234 | 1.987 |
| 1 | 0.996 | 0.845 |
| 2 | 0.853 | 0.686 |
| 3 | 0.725 | 0.570 |
| 4 | 0.660 | 0.564 |
| 5 | 0.628 | 0.573 |
| 6 | 0.659 | 0.609 |
| 7 | 0.694 | 0.675 |
| 8 | 0.742 | 0.741 |
| 9 | 0.792 | 0.815 |
| 10 | 0.885 | 0.884 |

**Table 1.** Partial correlation score ($f_r$) (x10$^{-2}$) for cortical and full image PCs.

| No. voxels | Cortex | | | Full Image | | |
|---|---|---|---|---|---|---|
| | Reference (50) | Reclassified (50) | New set (40) | Reference (50) | Reclassified (50) | New set (40) |
| ≥1 | 40 | 50 | 40 | 35 | 50 | 39 |
| ≥2 | 26 | 46 | 34 | 21 | 43 | 34 |
| ≥3 | 11 | 37 | 31 | 9 | 30 | 31 |
| ≥4 | 5 | 32 | 28 | 4 | 22 | 28 |
| ≥5 | 3 | 22 | 25 | 2 | 19 | 22 |
| ≥6 | 2 | 18 | 17 | 1 | 15 | 13 |
| ≥7 | 0 | 11 | 14 | 1 | 10 | 11 |
| ≥8 | 0 | 9 | 7 | 1 | 7 | 7 |
| ≥9 | 0 | 5 | 4 | 0 | 6 | 6 |
| ≥10 | 0 | 4 | 3 | 0 | 4 | 6 |
| ≥11 | 0 | 3 | 3 | 0 | 3 | 4 |
| ≥12 | 0 | 1 | 3 | 0 | 3 | 4 |

**Table 2.** Number of subjects classified as abnormal, i.e. with largest significant deficit greater than or equal to the specified number of connected voxels, for (a) the reference set; (b) the reclassified reference set based on omitting each case in turn; and (c) the new set. Total numbers in each group are shown in parenthesis. Results are shown for the cortical and full image atlases.

| PC No. | Cortex | | | Full Image | | |
|---|---|---|---|---|---|---|
| | Reference | Jackknife | Std Error | Reference | Jackknife | Std Error |
| 1 | -1.032 | -1.197 | 0.024 | -0.668 | -0.703 | 0.005 |
| 2 | -1.147 | -1.162 | 0.003 | -1.177 | -1.259 | 0.012 |
| 3 | -1.240 | -1.312 | 0.010 | -1.302 | -1.656 | 0.052 |
| 4 | -1.289 | -1.403 | 0.017 | -1.332 | -1.302 | 0.005 |
| 5 | -1.372 | -1.664 | 0.043 | -1.442 | -1.459 | 0.003 |
| 6 | -1.462 | -1.632 | 0.025 | -1.512 | -1.682 | 0.025 |
| 7 | -1.500 | -1.582 | 0.012 | -1.582 | -1.869 | 0.042 |
| 8 | -1.521 | -1.662 | 0.021 | -1.600 | -2.067 | 0.068 |
| 9 | -1.557 | -1.746 | 0.027 | -1.631 | -2.175 | 0.079 |
| 10 | -1.579 | -1.806 | 0.033 | -1.669 | -2.074 | 0.059 |

**Table 3.** The first ten log-transformed eigenvalues are shown beside the estimates obtained using the jackknife procedure together with the SEs of these estimates. Results for both the cortical and full image atlases are displayed.

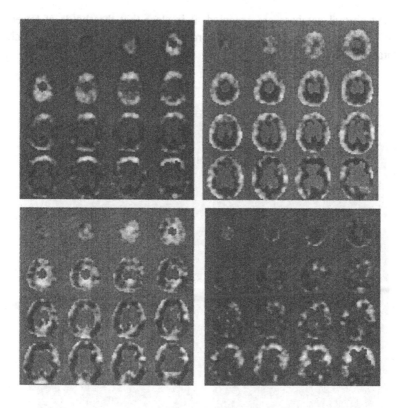

**Fig. 5.** The four cortical eigenimages obtained from jackknifing the normal database.

## 4 Discussion and Conclusions

The estimated number of PCs obtained using the Partial Correlations Test is in good agreement with that obtained experimentally when differentiating between patients with dementia and normal subjects outside the database. It is clear that either four or five PCs is optimal for both the cortical and full image atlases.

The results of reclassifying individuals in the normal database, omitting each image in turn, indicate that the number of abnormal cases found in the original analysis is, as expected, biased towards normality. This results from the fact that, in the original analysis, each case is included within the training set from which the eigenimages are formed and, as a result, plays a role in the definition of normality. Omitting each case in turn produces false positive rates which are reasonably consistent with those obtained for a new set of normal subjects. It may be argued that they are slightly lower than those of the new set and that this is slightly surprising given that the new set comprised young males only. In order to match the new set to boxers in particular, these young males were active participants in sports other than boxing and it is possible that sports such as rugby union and association football may also contain a risk element with regards to head injury. If the results of the reclassified normal database are accepted, it is clear that thresholds of fewer than eight or nine connected voxels will produce false positive rates which are unacceptably high.

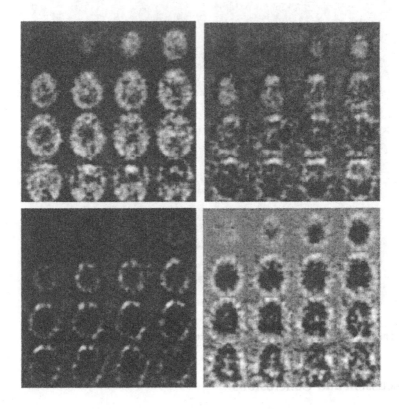

**Fig. 6.** The four full image eigenimages obtained from jackknifing the normal database.

The jackknifed eigenimages are remarkably similar, but not identical, to the eigenimages obtained directly from the PCA. This is encouraging as these images, along with the mean image, are the building blocks of the atlas. Jackknifing was not applied to the mean image as the mean is an unbiased estimate and is unchanged by jackknifing. The differences between the jackknifed eigenvalues and their original estimates, even after log-transformation, have not yet been fully explained. In particular, the ranking of the eigenvalues is affected by jackknifing, even among the first four PCs.

Gibson et al [10] noted the same phenomenon when performing a similar analysis on the physical characteristics of several species of the common myna. They concluded that it was due to the effect of outliers. In this study the principal differences among the first four PCs concern the first eigenvalue of the cortical atlas and the third eigenvalue of the whole image atlas. An analysis of the actual eigenvalues obtained from each of the 50 datasets with one image omitted revealed that one value for the first PC of the cortical atlas and two for the third PC of the whole image atlas lay outside a 5% limit of the original eigenvalue. In each case the corresponding eigenimage appeared slightly different from the original eigenimage but clearly this was insufficient to have a significant effect on the jackknifed eigenimage.

The re-ordering of the PCs that would be necessary if the jackknifed eigenvalue estimates are accepted is of some concern. The fact that the first four eigenimages appear in the same order for all 50 jackknifed samples in each atlas, as is indicated by the high degree of their similarity before and after jackknifing, implies that re-ordering should not be performed. In any case, PC ordering is used solely to determine whether or not an eigenimage should be included in the atlas and, for the cortical atlas with four PCs, a re-ordering based on jackknifed eigenvalues would make no difference.

The immediate task, which is progressing currently, is to explain the strange results obtained for jackknifed eigenvalues. If this is due to outliers, then jackknifing can serve the purpose of identifying these, allowing appropriate action to be taken.

In order to examine the full working database used for classification purposes, the jackknifing process must also be applied to the residual SD image. It is unclear, as yet, whether or not the elements of this image require a transformation prior to jackknifing. In view of previous comments regarding jackknifing variance estimates, some form of logarithmic transformation may be appropriate. Until the question of a suitable transformation has been resolved and jackknifing employed, the jackknifing task remains incomplete.

When jackknifing has been completed, it is possible to apply certain statistical tests to validate certain assumptions regarding the appropriate nature of the database [10, 16]. These include yet another method for determining which components are significant and methods for analyzing between-class differences for classes forming a subdivision of the database, e.g. male and female. The best use of these methods is currently under consideration.

Future work could involve proper statistical analysis of the underlying assumptions of the application of a PCA to the normal database and the use of other statistical testing as indicated in the paper. It may also be possible to relate the eigenimages to factors such as age and sex using some form of transformation. For univariate identification of abnormal voxels, SPM uses statistical testing based on the theory of Gaussian fields [6]. The extension of this method to multivariate identification of abnormal voxels could provide a more accurate way of combining connected voxels of known departure from normality. The validity of such an approach, however, is dubious.

Finally, the results of this analysis will form the basis of the design of a normal rCBF database for images obtained on a new dual-headed high-resolution gamma camera. It is primarily for this purpose that this task was undertaken.

# Acknowledgments

The author would like to thank Professor David Barber of the Royal Hallamshire Hospital Sheffield, England for the use of his image registration program. The author would also like to thank many others for interesting discussion and advice on this subject, most notably Paul Kemp, Roger Pethybridge, Murdo Macleod and Bob Appledorn.

# References

1    A.S. Houston, P.M. Kemp and M.A. Macleod: A method for assessing the significance of abnormalities in HMPAO brain SPECT images. Journal of Nuclear Medicine 35, 239-244 (1994)
2.   A.S. Houston, P.M. Kemp and M.A. Macleod: Optimization of factors affecting the state of normality of a medical image. Physics in Medicine and Biology 41, 755-765 (1996)
3.   W.F. Velicer: Determining the number of components from the matrix of partial correlations. Psychometrika 41, 321-327 (1976)
4.   M.H. Quenouille: Notes on bias in estimation. Biometrika 43, 353-360 (1956)
5.   M.G. Kendall and A. Stuart: The advanced theory of statistics. Vol. 2, 4$^{th}$ ed. London: Griffin 1979
6.   D.C. Barber: Digital computer processing of brain scans using principal components. Physics in Medicine and Biology 4, 223-228 (1976)
7.   K.J. Friston, A.P. Holmes, K.J. Worsley, J-P. Poline, C.D. Frith and R.S.J. Frackowiak: Statistical parametric maps in functional imaging: A general linear approach. Human Brain Mapping 2, 189-210 (1995)
8.   J.R. Moeller, S.C. Strother, J.J. Sidtis and D.A. Rotterberg: Scaled subprofile model: A statistical approach to the analysis of functional patterns in positron emission tomographic data. Journal of Cerebral Blood Flow and Metabolism 7, 649-658 (1987)
9.   R.A. Reyment: Phenotypic evolution in a cretaceous foraminifer. Evolution 36, 1182-1199 (1982)
10.  A.R. Gibson, A.J. Baker and A. Moeed: Morphometric variation in introduced populations of the common myna (acridotheres tristis): An application of the jackknife to principal components analysis. Systematic Zoology 33, 408-421 (1984)
11.  W.B. McGillivray: Size, sexual size dimorphism and their measurement in great horned owls in Alberta. Canadian Journal of Zoology 63, 2364-2372 (1985)
12.  P.M. Kemp, A.S. Houston, M.A. Macleod and R.J. Pethybridge: Cerebral perfusion and psychometric testing in military amateur boxers and controls. Journal of Neurology Neurosurgery and Psychiatry 59, 368-374 (1995)
13.  D.C. Barber: Registration of low resolution medical images. Physics in Medicine and Biology 37, 1485-1498 (1992)

14. A. Basilevsky: Statistical factor analysis and related methods: Theory and applications. New York: John Wiley & Sons 1994
15. R.G. Miller: The jackknife - A review. Biometrika 61, 1-15 (1974)
16. F. Mostellar and J.W. Tukey: Data analysis and regression: A second course in statistics. Reading, Massachusetts: Addison-Wesley 1977

# Generating 3-D Cardiac Material Markers Using Tagged MRI

William S. Kerwin and Jerry L. Prince

Department of Electrical and Computer Engineering
The Johns Hopkins University, Baltimore, MD 21218

**Abstract.** Tagged magnetic resonance imaging (MRI) has shown great promise in noninvasive analysis of heart motion. To replace implanted markers as a gold standard, however, tagged MRI must be able to track a sparse set of material points, so-called material markers, with high accuracy. This paper presents a new method for generating accurate motion estimates over a sparse set of material points using standard, parallel-tagged MR images. The tracked points are located at intersections of three tag surfaces, each of which is estimated using thin-plate splines. The intersections are determined by an iterative alternating projections algorithm for which a proof of convergence is provided. The resulting data sets are compatible with applications developed to exploit implanted marker data. One example from a normal human volunteer is shown in detail, and numerical results that include additional studies are discussed.

## 1 Introduction

Measurement of the three-dimensional (3-D) displacement of material points within the heart is fundamental to the understanding of cardiac mechanics. By tracking the movement of specific points within the myocardium, the complex motion of the heart muscle can be resolved and modeled. Clinically applicable techniques for material point tracking are also likely to prove diagnostically valuable for quantifying the degree and extent of ischemic heart disease. Because it is the principal powerhouse of the heart, motion studies typically address the left ventricle.

Until recently, material motion measurements of the left ventricle were obtained using implanted ultrasonic or radiopaque markers in conjunction with appropriate imaging modalities [1,2]. Such studies produce displacement data with accuracies on the order of 0.1mm [2], but the invasiveness of the implantation procedures limits their applicability. As a result, most studies have been performed on canine hearts with small numbers of markers in isolated regions. Also, the presence of the markers has an unknown effect on local myocardial properties.

The introduction of tagged MR imaging presented an opportunity for noninvasive measurements of material point motion [3]. MR tags are spatially modulated patterns of magnetization induced in tissue. The patterns move with the otherwise featureless tissue, giving a visual indication of motion in the images. Typically, MR tagging produces thin sheets of magnetically presaturated tissue orthogonal to the image plane. These "tag surfaces" result in a set of dark "tag lines" in the image that may be arranged in parallel, grid, or starburst configurations. Such magnetic markers, temporarily induced in the tissue, can easily be used on large numbers of human subjects without risk.

Many methods have been developed to extract motion information from tagged MR images. Those particularly relevant to this paper include Axel and Dougherty [4], Moulton et al. [5], and Radeva et al. [6]. Axel and Dougherty introduced the idea of tracking a 2-D grid of tag lines as it deforms in the image plane. Moulton et al. introduced the idea of using spline interpolation to reconstruct tag surfaces from tag lines and Radeva et al. developed a 3-D tag localization and tracking method using B-splines. These concepts of deforming grids, tag surface reconstruction and splines are used in our method as well. Motion estimation methods have also been presented by Denney and Prince [7], O'Dell et al. [8], and Young and Axel [9], among others.

The common characteristic of these past methods is the generation of a dense field of motion estimates throughout the left ventricle. These dense displacement estimates are fundamentally different from implanted marker data, which consist of a limited set of displacement measurements for specific material points in the left ventricle. There are, in fact, applications when such sparse data sets are preferable to dense ones. For example, Arts et al. [10] used data from implanted markers to optimize 13 parameters in a simulated heart model. These parameters define such aspects of motion as rotation and torsion and are determined using a least squares fit to the motion of a small number of implanted markers. To be used with such techniques, tagged MRI must produce a sparse motion estimate. Then, the techniques would take advantage of the noninvasive nature of tagged MRI.

The principal contribution of this paper is the presentation of a method to generate motion estimates over a sparse set of material points using a 3-D grid of applied tag surfaces. The grid is produced by inducing in the tissue three sets of parallel planar tags, oriented in orthogonal directions. The points we track are the intersections of these tag surfaces, which form a grid in space. In order to determine the intersections, a continuous representation of each tag surface is reconstructed from the image data using a thin-plate spline. The intersections of the resulting spline surfaces approximate the actual tag grid intersections. We believe that these grid points are ideally suited for accurate material point tracking since they are closest to the tag features being extracted from the images.

Tracking a tag surface intersection point is conceptually equivalent to implanting a marker at the initial intersection point and tracking the marker. Therefore, the data from our algorithm closely parallel implanted marker data, but have some important advantages. Like implanted markers, the tracked points are spaced a few millimeters apart in a regular pattern. However, hundreds of points can be tracked instead of a few dozen, the noninvasive procedure can be performed on large numbers of subjects, and because physical markers are not used, this approach has no effect whatsoever on heart motion.

This paper is organized as follows. Section 2 gives some background on tagged MRI, from basics on image acquisition to low-level image processing of tagged images, and concludes with an an overview of thin-plate splines. In Section 3, we describe both the reconstruction of tag surfaces using thin-plate splines and the estimation of spline surface intersection points. In Section 4, we show sequences of estimated ma-

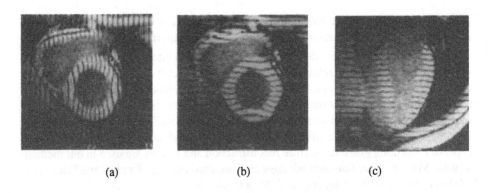

(a)  (b)  (c)

**Fig. 1.** Examples of tagged MR images: (a) short axis image with vertical tags; (b) short axis image with horizontal tags; and (c) long axis image with horizontal tags.

terial markers from an MRI experiment and comment on algorithm performance. The paper concludes in Section 5 with a brief discussion of the results.

## 2 Background

### 2.1 MR Tag Data

Motion of the left ventricle is observed by obtaining MR images at a series of time frames in the cardiac cycle. In our data sets, these images are typically spaced at regular intervals of approximately 30 msec. To facilitate motion tracking from the sequence of images, MR tagging is used to induce artificial magnetic features in the tissue. Using ECG gating, the tags are applied at end-diastole and images are obtained through end-systole, a duration of roughly 300 msec. Beyond end-systole, the tag patterns fade beyond recognition because of $T_1$ relaxation of the magnetization.

We use sets of parallel planar tags oriented orthogonal to the image planes as in O'Dell et al. [8]. These "tag planes" manifest themselves as dark bands called "tag lines" in the images. The tag lines are initially straight and parallel, but translate and bend as the heart contracts. Fig. 1 shows examples of such tagged MR images after the tags have been distorted somewhat by heart motion. In the figure, the first two images are short-axis (SA) views, in which the left ventricle appears as a ring-shaped object, and the third image is a long-axis (LA) view, in which the left ventricle appears as a cup-shaped object.

Sets of images are obtained spanning the entire left ventricle. SA image sets consist of stacks of images, from base to apex, as depicted in Fig. 2a. This figure also shows a "tag surface" (deformed tag plane) intersecting the stack of images, producing one tag line in each image. SA image planes are nominally separated by 5-8 mm and, typically, a stack has 6-9 images. In an LA image set, however, successive image planes are rotated by a fixed angle (nominally 30°) around the long axis of the heart, as depicted in Fig. 2b (this figure shows an angle of 60° between image planes for visual clarity).

Two SA image sets and one LA image set are obtained per time frame. As depicted in Fig. 1, the tag planes in the two SA image sets are rotated by 90 degrees with respect

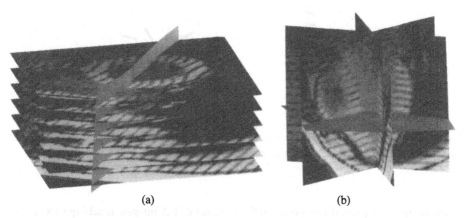

**Fig. 2.** Geometry of image planes: (a) stack of SA image planes intersected by a single tag surface; and (b) set of LA image planes intersected by a single tag surface.

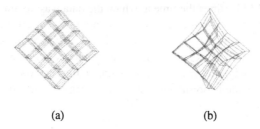

(a)           (b)

**Fig. 3.** Tag surfaces viewed as a regular material grid: (a) original grid; and (b) deformed grid after left ventricle contraction.

to each other, and the resulting geometry comprises three sets of mutually orthogonal tag planes. In combination, these tag planes define a regular 3-D grid induced in the tissue, as depicted in Fig. 3a. This regular grid is then deformed by heart motion as depicted in Fig. 3b. While Fig. 3 is conceptually valid, it is important to note that the tag planes are not applied all at once. Images are obtained in three separate series, each consisting of a sequence of 20 heartbeat breath-holds. Also, the image planes do not in general pass through an intersection point. Developing a method to determine these points, in fact, was the precise objective of the research we report in this paper.

Once the images have been acquired, the locations of tag lines corresponding to each tag surface are obtained using the semi-automated tag recognition routine developed by Guttman *et al.* [11]. This routine generates a set of equally spaced "tag points" along the center of a tag line. The spacing between points is selectable and is usually set to 1 mm. Only those points within the myocardium of the left ventricle are found and each tag line is indexed to identify which tag surface it corresponds to. Examples of tag point sets, corresponding to the individual tag surfaces depicted in Fig. 2, are shown in Fig. 4. The first set was obtained from the stack of SA images, resulting in a parallel pattern

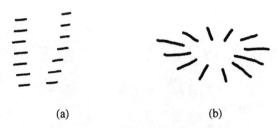

(a)                         (b)

**Fig. 4.** Tag line recognition results for the tag surfaces shown in Fig. 2: (a) tag points from the stack of SA images; and (b) tag points from the set of LA images.

of tag points. The second was obtained from the set of LA images, resulting in a spoke pattern of tag points.

The extracted tag points are organized into sets corresponding to particular tag surfaces at given times. Each set of points will be denoted $P_{j,k,t}$ where $j \in \{1, 2, 3\}$ identifies which of the three image sets the data came from, $k$ identifies which tag surface the data came from, and $t$ identifies the time at which the data was obtained. The complete tag surface, on which these points reside, will be denoted $S_{j,k,t}$. The tag points $\{\mathbf{p}_i\}_{i=1}^N$ within $P_{j,k,t}$ are of the form $(x_i, y_i, z_i)_{j,k,t}$, $i = 1, \ldots, N$ (where $N$ itself depends on $j$, $k$, and $t$), and are given in scanner coordinates. In scanner coordinates, the $z$-axis points down the bore of the magnet, the $y$-axis points up, and the $x$-axis points from right to left, to form a right-handed coordinate system. The origin of the coordinate system is the center of the bore.

## 2.2 Thin-Plate Splines

The thin-plate spline is a standard interpolating tool for reconstructing a surface from a scattered set of data samples, $(x_i, y_i, h_i)$. Each of these samples is interpreted as a height $h_i$ relative to the $xy$-plane located at the point $(x_i, y_i)$. The thin-plate spline is the shape that a thin metal plate of infinite extent would assume if deformed from a flat surface in the $xy$-plane to one that is tacked into position at the data points. Mathematically, the spline is given by the unique function $\hat{z}(x, y)$ that achieves $\hat{z}(x_i, y_i) = h_i$ and minimizes the total bending energy of the plate, given by

$$\iint_{R^2} \left( \left( \frac{\partial^2 \hat{z}}{\partial x^2} \right)^2 + 2 \left( \frac{\partial^2 \hat{z}}{\partial x \partial y} \right)^2 + \left( \frac{\partial^2 \hat{z}}{\partial y^2} \right)^2 \right) dx \, dy$$

The function that achieves this minimum is

$$\hat{z}(x, y) = a_0 + a_1 x + a_2 y + \sum_{i=1}^N w_i r_i^2 \ln r_i^2 \tag{1}$$

where $r_i = \|(x, y) - (x_i, y_i)\|$. The $N + 3$ coefficients $\{w_i\}_{i=1}^N$ and $\{a_j\}_{j=0}^2$ are found by setting

$$\hat{z}(x_i, y_i) = h_i, \quad i = \{1, \ldots, N\}$$

subject to the three additional constraints

$$\sum_{i=1}^{N} w_i = 0$$
$$\sum_{i=1}^{N} w_i x_i = 0$$
$$\sum_{i=1}^{N} w_i y_i = 0$$

This set of linear equations is easily solved for the unknown coefficients and, hence, the thin-plate spline. Details regarding the derivation of the thin-plate spline can be found in articles by Bookstein [12], or Meinguet [13].

Two properties of the thin-plate spline will prove useful. First, the thin-plate spline is invariant under rotations of the sample points $(x_i, y_i)$. Second, the thin-plate spline is invariant under translations of the coordinate origin. These properties mean that a change in the data coordinate system does not change the resulting spline surface if the direction of the $z$-axis is not changed. On the other hand, if the direction of the $z$-axis is changed, the two surfaces are unlikely to be the same.

## 3  Method

### 3.1  Tag Surface Reconstruction

The first step in finding the intersections of a deformed tag grid is to reconstruct the deformed grid from tag point data. This is done by individually reconstructing each tag surface, $S_{j,k,t}$, from its corresponding set of tag data, $P_{j,k,t}$, using a thin-plate spline. This interpolation method was chosen for several reasons. First, it has a physical interpretation not unlike the actual situation. When the heart contracts, the thin, essentially planar, surface of tagged tissue is subjected to deforming stresses. Second, the thin-plate spline has a very tractable, easy-to-code form. Third, it can be used with the irregular sampling patterns of tag line data. Fourth, it does not require boundary conditions, and fifth, it has the desirable characteristic of being continuously differentiable.

In order to evaluate the thin-plate spline, the tag points corresponding to a single surface must first be transformed from scanner coordinates into an appropriate frame of reference. In particular, the tag points must be put into the form $(x_i', y_i', h_i)$, where $h_i$ is the height of the surface above the $x'y'$-plane at the point $(x_i', y_i')$. Let the frame of reference be specified by the basis $\{\mathbf{e}_{x'}, \mathbf{e}_{y'}, \mathbf{e}_{z'}\}$ and origin o. Then each tag point, $\mathbf{p}_i$ is transformed into this frame by evaluating

$$x_i' = (\mathbf{p}_i - \mathbf{o}) \cdot \mathbf{e}_{x'}$$
$$y_i' = (\mathbf{p}_i - \mathbf{o}) \cdot \mathbf{e}_{y'}$$
$$h_i = (\mathbf{p}_i - \mathbf{o}) \cdot \mathbf{e}_{z'}$$

There are still several issues to consider before specifying the basis vectors and origin. For the thin-plate spline, choosing a frame of reference amounts to choosing the base vector $\mathbf{e}_{z'}$, which determines the direction in which the height is measured. All frames of reference that share this base vector are related by translations of the coordinate origin and rotations of the basis about the $\mathbf{e}_{z'}$ axis. As stated previously, surfaces generated by the thin-plate spline are unaffected by such transformations. Therefore, once $\mathbf{e}_{z'}$ has been specified, the choices of $\mathbf{o}$, $\mathbf{e}_{x'}$, and $\mathbf{e}_{y'}$ are arbitrary, as long as they define an orthonormal basis.

Some care must be taken in selecting $\mathbf{e}_{z'}$, however, because arbitrary choices can lead to singularities in the spline. We have chosen $\mathbf{e}_{z'}$ to be perpendicular to the ideal tag plane that would have been induced in the tissue, were it not for instrumentation error such as magnetic field inhomogeneities. This choice of $\mathbf{e}_{z'}$ maintains the analogy between tag surface deformation and the bending of a thin metal plate. The original tag plane is like the undeformed metal plate and the location of the deformed surface is measured as a height in its normal direction.

To complete the reference frame specification, we let the origin be the scanner origin $\mathbf{o} = (0, 0, 0)$, and set $\mathbf{e}_{x'}$ to be perpendicular to $\mathbf{e}_{z'}$ and $\mathbf{e}_{y'} = \mathbf{e}_{z'} \times \mathbf{e}_{x'}$. With this specification, conversion from scanner coordinates to this frame of reference is just a rotation $\mathbf{R}_j$ around the origin. The $j$ subscript indicates that there is one rotation operator for each of the three tag plane orientations.

Given our choice of reference frames, thin-plate splines are evaluated for every tag surface. All tag points corresponding to tag surface $S_{j,k,t}$ are rotated into the appropriate reference frame using

$$(x_i', y_i', h_i)_{j,k,t} = \mathbf{R}_j \mathbf{p}_i, \quad \mathbf{p}_i \in P_{j,k,t}, \ i = 1, \ldots, N$$

The complete rotated set of points is used to determine the $N + 3$ coefficients, $\{w_i\}_{i=1}^{N}$ and $\{a_j\}_{j=0}^{2}$, that define (1), the thin-plate spline equation. The spline reconstruction of tag surface $S_{j,k,t}$ will be denoted $\hat{z}_{j,k,t}(x', y')$.

A point $\mathbf{p}^j$ on the tag surface is found by selecting $x'$ and $y'$, evaluating the thin-plate spline, and rotating the point into scanner coordinates. That is,

$$\mathbf{p}^j = \mathbf{R}_j^{-1}(x', y', \hat{z}_{j,k,t}(x', y')) \tag{2}$$

Examples of thin-plate spline surfaces produced from tag data are shown in Fig. 5. Also, the tag surfaces shown in Fig. 2 are actually thin-plate spline reconstructions generated from tag point data. By generating thin-plate spline approximations of every tag surface at a given time, the complete deformed tag grid is reconstructed.

## 3.2 Tag Surface Intersections

Once the deformed tag grid has been reconstructed, the intersection points of the grid are found individually. This is done by selecting one thin-plate spline reconstruction from each of the three tag orientations and determining where the three surfaces intersect. An example of three intersecting surfaces is shown in Fig. 5c. An analytic solution for the intersection of three thin-plate splines is intractable because each spline equation may involve hundreds of individual logarithm terms. Therefore, an iterative approach is used to determine the intersection point.

The iterative approach we choose is a modification of alternating projections. In standard alternating projections, a chosen starting point is first projected onto one of the surfaces, that point is then projected onto a second of the surfaces, and that point to the third surface. The same series of projections is reapplied to the resulting point

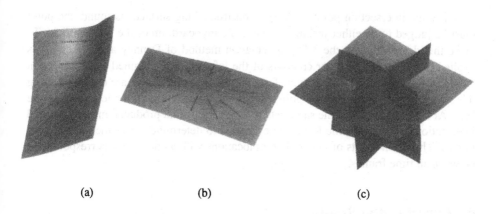

**Fig. 5.** Sample tag surface reconstructions: (a) tag surface from short axis images; (b) tag surface from long axis images; and (c) three tag surfaces forming an intersection.

and this iterative process is repeated until it converges. Denoting the three projection operators as $\mathbf{P}_1$, $\mathbf{P}_2$, and $\mathbf{P}_3$, the iterative scheme can be written

$$\mathbf{p}(m+1) = \mathbf{P}_3\mathbf{P}_2\mathbf{P}_1\mathbf{p}(m)$$

In our method, the same scheme is used, but the operator $\mathbf{P}_j$ is an oblique projection onto the thin-plate spline, $\hat{z}_{j,k,t}(x',y')$, corresponding to tag surface $S_{j,k,t}$. These oblique projections occur along $\mathbf{e}_{z'}$ in each corresponding reference frame. Henceforth, we will refer to these operators as simply projections. We will use the notation $\mathbf{e}_{z'}^j$ to denote the projection direction of $\mathbf{P}_j$. To perform the projection of a given point $\mathbf{p}$, it is first rotated into the reference frame giving

$$(x',y',z') = \mathbf{R}_j\mathbf{p}$$

Then, the spline is evaluated at $(x',y')$. The resulting point $(x',y',\hat{z}_{j,k,t}(x',y'))$ is rotated back into scanner coordinates using (2) to give $\mathbf{P}_j\mathbf{p}$. The algorithm is started with the point $\mathbf{p}(0) = (0,0,0)$ and stops when each projection in a given iteration moves the point by less than 0.01 mm.

For any three of these spline surfaces that intersect, we have found a sufficient condition for the convergence of this algorithm to the unique point of intersection. Suppose that for all three surfaces the following condition is met

$$\|\nabla\hat{z}_{j,k,t}(x',y')\| < \frac{1}{\sqrt{2}}, \quad \text{for all } x',y' \tag{3}$$

where $\nabla$ is the gradient operator in the $x'y'$-coordinate system. Then the intersection point is unique, and every sequence generated by the algorithm converges to that point. A proof of this statement is presented in the appendix. Condition (3) is easy to test by evaluating the gradient of the surfaces at many points, or testing the gradient during the iteration procedure. Of course, this is only a sufficient condition and the algorithm may converge even if it is not met.

Once the intersection point of three reconstructed tag surfaces is found, the point must be judged to be either inside or outside the myocardium of the left ventricle. To make this determination, the 3-D segmentation method of Denney and Prince [7] is applied to the inner and outer contours of the left ventricle obtained from images in the first time frame. All intersections found at the first time frame are evaluated using this segmentation and only those points within the myocardium of the left ventricle are kept. At subsequent times, the same sets of tag surfaces that produced intramyocardial intersections at the first time frame are evaluated to determine where the intersections moved. The result is sets of material point locations with a one-to-one correspondence between all time frames.

# 4 Experimental Results

## 4.1 Normal Human Study

Our method has been applied to several MR tagging studies, producing similar results. Here we present the detailed results of just one of these studies. A set of tagged MR images was obtained from a human volunteer with normal cardiac function. Seven SA image planes were acquired at an 8 mm separation. Six LA image planes were acquired 30° apart. The initial tag plane spacing was 6 mm in all cases. The time interval between successive image sets was 32.5 msec, and images were collected at ten time frames.

From this data set, our algorithm produced 401 material markers within the myocardium of the left ventricle. Fig. 6 depicts their locations at three times in the sequence. The markers have been rendered as spherical beads to emphasize the similarity between these results and those of implanted markers, which are often small metal balls. Two views are shown, demonstrating the 3-D nature of the results. The top set in the figure is viewed from the base toward the apex; the bottom set is viewed from the side, with the free wall on the left and septum on the right. The three time frames shown are, from left to right, at end-diastole, mid-systole and end-systole. The complete set of ten time frames was assembled into a movie depicting the contraction phase of the left ventricle.

Several observations can be made from Fig. 6. First, in the end-diastole, base-to-apex view, the fact that the points are the intersection points of a grid of tag planes is apparent. The regular pattern of material points is unmistakable. The base-to-apex views also demonstrate the twisting action of the contracting left ventricle. On the other hand, the side views (in Fig. 6) look "end on" at the tag surfaces showing nearly horizontal lines of material points. These lines move closer together by an average of 14% from end-diastole to end-systole, demonstrating a longitudinal shortening of the left ventricle during contraction. The slight bending of these same lines in the bottom left image of Fig. 6 also reveals that tag surfaces are not perfectly flat at the time of the first image. This bending may be the result of heart movement between application of the tag pattern and acquisition of the first set of images. More likely, the bending is the result of magnetic field inhomogeneities at the time of tag application.

322

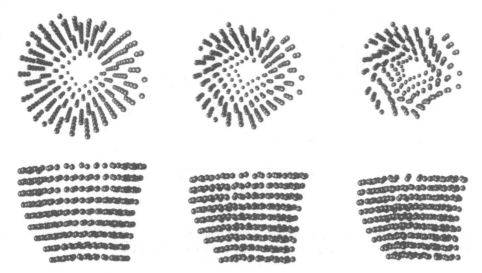

**Fig. 6.** Material point estimates for the left ventricle viewed from base to apex (top three) and from the side with the free wall on the left (bottom three). Three time frames are shown. From left to right these are 47, 177, and 307 msec after tag application.

## 4.2 Algorithm Performance

The algorithm was programmed in C and run on an IBM RS/6000 model 3AT workstation. The time required to find a complete set of intersections for all time frames was less than 5 minutes. Processing time was dominated by the calculation of thin-plate spline coefficients for tag surface reconstruction. Determining the set of spline coefficients for one tag surface averaged 550 msec. There are 30 to 40 tag surfaces comprising the complete grid, which means the time required to find all spline coefficients was approximately 20 seconds per time frame. By comparison, the time required to find several hundred intersections at a given time frame was on the order of 1 second.

To examine the convergence properties of the algorithm, we tested a data set for conformity to our sufficient condition (3). The data set we chose was a "high density" set, in which SA image planes were separated by only 5 mm. This data set, also from a normal human subject, was selected because the higher density of image planes provided more information for determining gradients. The LA image planes were separated by 30°, the tag planes were separated by 5.5 mm, and image sets were obtained every 35 msec for 10 time frames. We tested all tag surfaces reconstructed from this data set against the sufficient condition.

This test requires the gradient of the spline, which can be found by differentiating (1) to give

$$\frac{\partial}{\partial x'}\hat{z}_{j,k,t} = a_1 + 2\sum_{i=1}^{n} w_i(x' - x_i')(1 + \ln r_i^2)$$
$$\frac{\partial}{\partial y'}\hat{z}_{j,k,t} = a_2 + 2\sum_{i=1}^{n} w_i(y' - y_i')(1 + \ln r_i^2)$$
$$\|\nabla \hat{z}_{j,k,t}(x',y')\| = \sqrt{(\frac{\partial}{\partial x'}\hat{z}_{j,k,t})^2 + (\frac{\partial}{\partial y'}\hat{z}_{j,k,t})^2}$$

This equation was evaluated for all tag surfaces in the study, using a square grid of points in each of the reference frames. The points were spaced every 0.5 mm in the $x'$

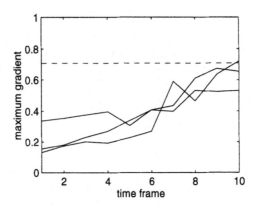

**Fig. 7.** Maximum gradient encountered versus time frame for each of three orientations of tag surfaces. The dashed line is the guaranteed convergence threshold of $1/\sqrt{2}$.

and $y'$ directions, and the grid extended at least 10 mm outside the bounds of the tag point data. Outside the range of data, thin plate splines become asymptotically smooth.

At each time frame, the maximum gradient was found for each of the three tag plane orientations. This maximum gradient is depicted as a function of time in Fig. 7; it increases with time because heart contraction distorts the tag surfaces. This figure shows that one of the orientations at time frame 10 does not meet the sufficient condition. Fortunately, the sufficient condition is very restrictive, and the algorithm is likely to converge even if it is not met. In fact, the algorithm will still converge if there exists an $\alpha \geq 0$ such that

$$\|\nabla \hat{z}_{j,k,t}(x',y')\| < \sqrt{\tfrac{1}{2} + \alpha}, \quad \text{for all } x', y'$$
$$\|\nabla \hat{z}_{l,k,t}(x',y')\| < \sqrt{\tfrac{1}{2} - \alpha}, \quad \text{for all } x', y', l \neq j$$

This more general sufficient condition guarantees convergence in the case of Fig. 7. We chose (3) for our sufficient condition because it is simple to test and it applies in most cases encountered to date. It also indicates to the user when there is a potential for nonconvergence, or nonuniqueness. Suspect points can be visually verified or simply thrown out.

We also monitored convergence of the algorithm by including a flag that identified when a threshold of 20 iterations was reached. The purpose of this flag was to prevent the algorithm from diverging or entering a cycle that never converged. To date, more than 28,000 intersections have been found by the algorithm, including those for the two studies presented here. The threshold of 20 iterations has never been reached.

## 5 Summary and Discussion

A technique for estimating material point motion in the left ventricular myocardium was presented. In contrast to other methods using tagged MRI, which produce dense motion estimates, our method intentionally generates motion estimates over sparse sets of material points. Our estimates are therefore akin to the implanted marker measurements commonly used in heart motion studies. Our estimates may be applied wherever implanted markers have been used. However, unlike implanted markers, our noninvasive method allows motion estimates to be generated for large populations of human subjects. Thus, techniques previously used with implanted markers can be used with our method to develop statistically significant estimates of the range of heart function.

Our method hinges on the ability to find the intersection point of three tag surfaces. We used thin-plate splines to reconstruct tag surfaces although any alternative surface formulation could easily be substituted. An alternating projection method then finds the intersection points. We provided a proof of convergence under conditions usually met in the real data, and a test for these same conditions. In a high-resolution study, this condition was met in all but one case, and an alternate condition revealed that convergence was guaranteed anyway. The convergence record of the algorithm is perfect to date.

On our workstation, the algorithm typically determined a complete set of intersection points in under 5 minutes, given a set of tag points from a tag recognition algorithm. However, the tag recognition program we used to preprocess the images requires user verification and correction. Thus, several hours were required to prepare a data set for use with our intersection algorithm. Work is in porgress to decrease the amount of user intervention required in tag line recognition.

We showed that the tag surfaces in the first set of images are not generally flat. Because little motion occurs between tag application and acquisition of the first image, this suggests the tag planes are not flat when applied. This is significant because some methods, such as that of Denney and Prince [7], assume the initial tag surfaces are perfectly flat. This should introduce additional errors into the resulting motion estimates.

Finally, we believe that the motion estimates for our sets of material points are generally more accurate than those obtained by other tagged MRI methods. Our principal reasoning is that the points we track are determined solely by the grid of tag surfaces. Thus the points are at the inherent resolution of the tag features. Also, our method allows motion data to be interpolated between image planes without knowing the underlying point-by-point motion. Our reconstructed tag surfaces can be tracked from one time frame to another without knowing which point on the former surface moved to which point on the latter. Future work is directed toward theoretically and experimentally quantifying the accuracy of our approach.

## Appendix - Proof of Convergence and Uniqueness

**Proposition.** Assume three surfaces, defined as in Section 3.1, satisfy (3) and intersect at a point $\mathbf{p}^*$. Then, $\mathbf{p}^*$ is the unique intersection point and the method of alternating projections, defined in Section 3.1, converges to that point.

*Sketch of Proof.* We assume the intersection point $\mathbf{p}^*$ is $(0,0,0)$. This can be done without loss of generality because changes in the coordinate origin do not change the thin-plate spline surfaces. Then, if $\mathbf{p}^j \neq \mathbf{p}^*$ is a point on the $j^{th}$ surface, we can write

$$\frac{|\mathbf{p}^j \cdot \mathbf{e}^j_{z'}|}{\sqrt{\|\mathbf{p}^j\|^2 - (\mathbf{p}^j \cdot \mathbf{e}^j_{z'})^2}} < \frac{1}{\sqrt{2}}$$

The left hand side of this inequality is the absolute value of the slope of the line connecting $\mathbf{p}^j$ to $\mathbf{p}^*$. The bound on this value is obtained from the intermediate value theorem, which says the slope of this line cannot exceed the maximum gradient of the surface. We can rewrite this as

$$(\mathbf{p}^j \cdot \mathbf{e}^j_{z'})^2 < \frac{\|\mathbf{p}^j\|^2}{3}, \quad \mathbf{p}^j \neq \mathbf{p}^* \tag{4}$$

To prove uniqueness, assume $\mathbf{p}' \neq \mathbf{p}^*$ is a second intersection point. Because this point is on all three surfaces, (4) holds for all $j$. Summing over $j$ gives

$$\sum_{j=1}^{3} (\mathbf{p}' \cdot \mathbf{e}^j_{z'})^2 < \|\mathbf{p}'\|^2$$

Because $\{\mathbf{e}^j_{z'}\}_{j=1}^3$ defines an orthonormal basis,

$$\sum_{j=1}^{3} (\mathbf{p}' \cdot \mathbf{e}^j_{z'})^2 = \|\mathbf{p}'\|^2 \tag{5}$$

and a contradiction results.

To prove convergence, we use the concept of strict monotonicity with respect to a map $c(\mathbf{p})$, where strict monotonicity means

$$c(\mathbf{P}_3\mathbf{P}_2\mathbf{P}_1\mathbf{p}) < c(\mathbf{p}), \quad \forall \mathbf{p}, \, \mathbf{p} \neq \mathbf{p}^* \tag{6}$$

Monotonicity has been explored by Meyer [14], among others. For a continuous operator with a unique solution, convergence is guaranteed if there exists a continuous, scalar function $c(\mathbf{p})$ that is radially unbounded and strictly monotonic. The operator $\mathbf{P}_3\mathbf{P}_2\mathbf{P}_1$ is continuous because the underlying spline surfaces are continuous. We choose

$$c(\mathbf{p}) = \max_j \{(\mathbf{e}^j_{z'} \cdot \mathbf{p})^2\}$$

This continuous function approaches infinity as $\mathbf{p}$ gets far from the origin and is therefore radially unbounded. To prove it satisfies (6) we can show, with some algebra, the following relations

$$\mathbf{e}^l_{z'} \cdot \mathbf{P}_j\mathbf{p} = \mathbf{e}^l_{z'} \cdot \mathbf{p}, \quad l \neq j \tag{7}$$

$$(\mathbf{e}^j_{z'} \cdot \mathbf{P}_j\mathbf{p})^2 < c(\mathbf{p}), \quad \mathbf{p} \neq \mathbf{p}^* \tag{8}$$

$$c(\mathbf{P}_j\mathbf{p}) \leq c(\mathbf{p}) \tag{9}$$

Equation (7) comes from the fact that $\mathbf{P}_j$ projects orthogonal to $\mathbf{e}^l_{z'}$. Inequality (8) comes from (5), (7) and the fact that $c(\mathbf{p}) \geq \frac{1}{3}\|\mathbf{p}\|^2$, and (9) comes from (7) and (8). From (7), (8) and (9), we find

$$(\mathbf{e}^j_{z'} \cdot \mathbf{P}_3\mathbf{P}_2\mathbf{P}_1\mathbf{p})^2 < c(\mathbf{p}), \quad \forall j$$

This leads to (6) and convergence is proven.

## Acknowledgements

The authors thank Elliot McVeigh for data and insight, Thomas Denney, Jr. for his segmentation program, and Gerard Meyer for consultation on algorithm convergence. This work was supported by an NIH grant (R01-HL45090; PI Elias Zerhouni), an NSF grant (MIP93-50336; PI Jerry Prince), and a Whitaker Foundation Graduate Fellowship, held by the first author.

# References

1. J. Park, D. Metaxas, and L. Axel. Analysis of left ventricular wall motion based on volumetric deformable models and MRI-SPAMM. *Medical Image Analysis*, 1(1):53–71, 1996.
2. A.S. Douglas, E.K. Rodriguez, W. O'Dell, and W.C. Hunter. Unique strain history during ejection in canine left ventricle. *Am. J. Physiol.*, 260 (Heart Circ. Physiol. 29):H1596–H1611, 1991.
3. E.A. Zerhouni, D.M. Parish, W.J. Rogers, A. Yang, and E.P. Shapiro. Human heart: tagging with MR imaging — a method for noninvasive assessment of myocardial motion. *Radiology*, 169:59–63, 1988.
4. L. Axel and L. Dougherty. Heart wall motion: improved method of spatial modulation of magnetization for MR imaging. *Radiology*, 172:349, 1989.
5. M.J. Moulton, L.L. Creswell, S.W. Downing, R.L. Actis, B.A. Szabo, M.W. Vannier, and M.K. Pasque. Spline surface interpolation for calculating 3-D ventricular strains from MRI tissue tagging. *Am. J. Physiol.*, 270 (Heart Circ. Physiol. 39):H281–H297, 1996.
6. P. Radeva, A. Amini, J. Huang, and E. Marti. Deformable B-solids and implicit snakes for localization and tracking of MRI-SPAMM data. In *Mathematical Methods in Biomedical Image Analysis*, pages 192–201. San Francisco, CA, June 1996.
7. T.S. Denney Jr. and J.L. Prince. Reconstruction of 3D left ventricular motion from planar tagged cardiac MR images: an estimation theoretic approach. *IEEE Transactions on Medical Imaging*, 14(4):625–635, December 1995.
8. W.G. O'Dell, C.C. Moore, and E.R. McVeigh. Displacement field fitting approach to calculate 3D deformations from parallel-tagged MR images. *J. Magn Reson. Imag.*, 3 (P):P208, 1993
9. A.A. Young and L. Axel. Three-dimensional motion and deformation of the heart wall: estimation with spatial modulation of magnetization – a model-based approach. *Radiology*, 185:241–247, 1992.
10. T. Arts, W.C. Hunter, A. Douglas, A.M.M. Muijtjens, and R.S. Reneman. Description of the deformation of the left ventricle by a kinematic model. *J. Biomech.*, 25(10):1119–1127, 1992.
11. M.A. Guttman, J.L. Prince, and E.R. McVeigh. Tag and contour detection in tagged MR images of the left ventricle. *IEEE Transactions on Medical Imaging*, 13(1):74–88, 1994.
12. F.L. Bookstein. Principal warps: Thin-plate splines and the decomposition of deformations. *IEEE Transactions on Pattern Analysis and Machine Intelligence*, 11(6):567–585, 1989.
13. J. Meinguet. Surface spline interpolation: Basic theory and computational aspects. In S.P. Singh et al., editor, *Approximation Theory and Spline Functions*, pages 227–142. D. Reidel Publishing Company, 1984.
14. G.G.L. Meyer. Convergence conditions for a type of algorithm model. *SIAM J. Control Optim.*, 15(5):779–784, August 1977.

# Identification of Myocardial Tags in Tagged MR Images Without Prior Knowledge of Myocardial Contours

Thomas S. Denney Jr.

Auburn University, Auburn, AL 36849, USA

**Abstract.** Magnetic resonance (MR) tagging has been shown to be a useful technique for non-invasively measuring the deformation of an *in vivo* heart. An important step in analyzing tagged images is the identification of tag lines in each image of a cine sequence. Most existing tag identification algorithms require prior knowledge of the myocardial contours. Contour identification, however, is time consuming and requires a considerable amount of user intervention. In this paper, a new method identifying tag lines is presented that does not require prior knowledge of the myocardial contours. The method is composed of three stages. First the tags are estimated across the entire region-of-interest (ROI) with a snake algorithm based on a maximum-likelihood (ML) estimate of the tag center. Next a maximum *a posteriori* (MAP) hypothesis test is used to detect tag centers inside the myocardium. Finally a pruning algorithm is used to remove detected tag line centers that do not meet a spatio-temporal continuity criterion. This method is demonstrated on data from an *in vivo* human heart.

## 1 Introduction

Magnetic resonance (MR) tagging [1, 2, 3, 4] has been shown to be a useful technique for non-invasively measuring the deformation of an *in vivo* heart. Tagged images appear with a spatially encoded pattern of lines called tag lines that move with the tissue and can be analyzed to reconstruct a three-dimensional (3-D) description of the heart's deformation during a portion of the cardiac cycle [4, 5, 3]. An important step in the reconstruction process is the identification of tag line position in each image of a cine sequence.

Several methods have been proposed for identifying tag lines in tagged images, but most require prior knowledge of the epicardial (outer) and endocardial (inner) contours of the left ventricle (LV). Guttman, et al. [6] used a template matching approach along with a least-squares error criterion. Contours are used in this approach to restrict the domain over which the template match is performed. Young and Axel [5], Amini, et al. [7, 8], and Kumar and Goldgof [9] used snakes to identify tag lines based on image intensity and spatial continuity constraints. Contours are used in these approaches to break the continuity constraints at the epicardial and endocardial boundaries. Contour identification, however, is a time consuming process and requires a considerable amount of user intervention. Typically 3-4 hours are required to process a 200 image study [10].

In this paper a new method for identifying tag lines is presented that does not require prior knowledge of the LV contours. The method is composed of three stages. First the tags are estimated across the entire region-of-interest (ROI) with a snake algorithm [11] based on a maximum-likelihood (ML) estimate of the tag center. Next a maximum *a posteriori* (MAP) hypothesis test is used to detect tag centers inside the myocardium. Finally a pruning algorithm is used to remove detected tag line centers that do not meet a spatio-temporal continuity criterion.

While this paper was in review, a snake-based contourless tag identification algorithm by Guttman, et al. [12] was brought to our attention. Our approach, however, differs considerably from the approach in [12] in the image forces used in the active contour algorithm. In addition, our approach uses an hypothesis test based on tag shape to differentiate between tag centers inside and outside the myocardium instead of the intensity thresholding method used in [12].

This paper is organized as follows. The tag estimation, detection, and pruning algorithms are developed in Section 2. In Section 3 these algorithms are demonstrated on data from an *in vivo* normal human heart. Conclusions and directions for future work are presented in Section 4.

## 2  Algorithm Development

Tags are flat saturation planes which are applied to the heart at end-diastole. As shown in Figure 5, images acquired on planes orthogonal to these tag planes show the tags as dark lines which are nearly straight in images taken shortly after end-diastole and are curved in later images. In this section we use *a priori* knowledge of the tagging process to derive a tag line model, which we then use to develop algorithms for estimating and detecting tag lines. We then use *a priori* knowledge of the spatial and temporal continuity of tag lines to develop an algorithm for removing false tag point detections due to noise.

### 2.1  Tag Line Model

It is known from the imaging protocol [13] that along a line perpendicular to the tag line, the tags have approximately a Gaussian profile as shown in Figure 1. We model this profile $s(x)$ as

$$s(x) = 1 - A(t)e^{-(4\ln 2)x^2/\text{FWHM}^2} , \tag{1}$$

where $0 \leq A(t) \leq 1$ is the tag amplitude, and FWHM is the full width at half maximum of the tag. The tag pattern amplitude is known to decay with time due to $T_1$ relaxation [1]. We model this decay as

$$A(t) = e^{-t/T_{1\text{nom}}} ,$$

where $T_{1\text{nom}}$ is the nominal $T_1$ of the myocardium listed in Table 1. The FWHM of the tag also changes with time due to contraction and expansion of the myocardium, but this effect is neglected in this analysis.

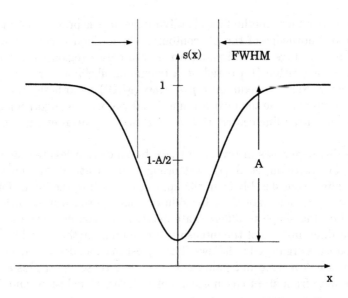

**Fig. 1.** Intensity profile of a tag along a line perpendicular to the tag line.

The intensity profile of a single tag in the myocardium consists of the signal from the myocardium $m_{\mathrm{myo}}(x)$ multiplied by the tag profile $s(x)$ plus noise. The intensity profile of a single tag $w(x)$ is modeled as

$$w(x) = m_{\mathrm{myo}}(x)s(x - \mu) + n(x)\,, \tag{2}$$

where $\mu$ is the position of the tag center. This position changes from time frame to time frame in a cine sequence due to the motion of the myocardium.

## 2.2  Tag Estimation

The problem of estimating tag lines consists of estimating the tag center at several points along the tag line from the image data. In the case of parallel vertical tags as shown in Figure 5, the tags are perpendicular to the image rows, so for each tag we estimate a tag center for each image row.

**Maximum Likelihood Estimate of the Tag Center** We first consider the estimation of the tag center $\mu$ from a set of $N_s$ image pixels along a line perpendicular to the tag line. These pixels can be stacked into an $N_s$-vector $\mathbf{w}$. These image pixels are samples of the intensity profile in Equation (2), so we can express them as

$$\mathbf{w} = \mathbf{S}(\mu)\mathbf{m}_{\mathrm{myo}} + \mathbf{n}\,, \tag{3}$$

where $\mathbf{m}_{\mathrm{myo}}$ and $\mathbf{n}$ are $N_s$-vectors of samples of the myocardium and noise signals respectively, and

$$\mathbf{S}(\mu) = \begin{bmatrix} s(-\mu) & & & \\ & s(\Delta - \mu) & & \\ & & \cdots & \\ & & & s((N_s - 1)\Delta - \mu) \end{bmatrix},$$

where $\Delta$ is the image pixel spacing. In MR images the myocardium signal can vary from subject to subject, from scan to scan, and even from time frame to time frame, so we model the myocardium signal vector $\mathbf{m}_{\mathrm{myo}}$ as a Gaussian random vector with mean $\mathbf{m}_{\mathrm{myo}} = \bar{m}_{\mathrm{myo}}\mathbf{1}$, where $\mathbf{1}$ is an $N_s$-vector of ones, and covariance matrix $\mathbf{C}_{\mathrm{myo}}(i, j) = \sigma^2_{\mathrm{myo}} \rho^{|i-j|}_{\mathrm{myo}}$. Values for $\bar{m}_{\mathrm{myo}}$ and $\sigma^2_{\mathrm{myo}}$ are estimated from the image data for each time frame in the sequence (see Section 3). The value of $\rho_{\mathrm{myo}}$ could in principle be estimated from the image data, but in practice, this value is chosen by the user and is listed in Table 1. The noise vector $\mathbf{n}$ is modeled as a zero mean white Gaussian vector with covariance $\sigma^2_n\mathbf{I}$. A value for $\sigma^2_n$ is estimated from the image data for each time frame in the sequence (see Section 3).

We formulate the estimation of the tag center $\mu$ from the data $\mathbf{w}$ as a maximum likelihood estimation problem. In this formulation, $\mu$ is considered to be an unknown parameter. An $N_s$-variate probability density function (PDF) is derived for $\mathbf{w}$ as a function of $\mu$, and the optimal tag center estimate $\hat{\mu}$ is the tag center that maximizes the PDF.

Given the above models for the myocardium signal, tag line, and noise, the observation vector $\mathbf{w}$ is a Gaussian random vector whose PDF is parameterized by $\mu$. The PDF of the observation vector is given by

$$f(\mathbf{w}; \mu) = \frac{1}{(2\pi)^{N_s/2}\sqrt{|\mathbf{C}_1(\mu)|}} \exp\left(-\frac{1}{2}[\mathbf{w} - \mathbf{m}_1(\mu)]^T \mathbf{C}_1^{-1}(\mu)[\mathbf{w} - \mathbf{m}_1(\mu)]\right), \tag{4}$$

where $|\cdot|$ denotes determinant, $\mathbf{m}_1(\mu)$ is the mean of $\mathbf{w}$ given by

$$\mathbf{m}_1(\mu) = \mathbf{S}(\mu)\mathbf{m}_{\mathrm{myo}},$$

and $\mathbf{C}_1(\mu)$ is the covariance matrix of $\mathbf{w}$ given by

$$\mathbf{C}_1(\mu) = \mathbf{S}(\mu)\mathbf{C}_{\mathrm{myo}}\mathbf{S}(\mu) + \sigma^2_n\mathbf{I}.$$

After taking the natural logarithm of $f(\mathbf{w}; \mu)$ and deleting constant terms, the maximum likelihood estimate of the tag center $\hat{\mu}$ is given by

$$\hat{\mu} = \arg\min_{\mu} L_1(\mu), \tag{5}$$

where

$$L_1(\mu) = \frac{1}{2}[\mathbf{w} - \mathbf{m}_1(\mu)]^T \mathbf{C}_1^{-1}(\mu)[\mathbf{w} - \mathbf{m}_1(\mu)] + \frac{1}{2}\ln|\mathbf{C}_1(\mu)| \tag{6}$$

where $\ln(\cdot)$ denotes natural logarithm. A plot of $L_1(\mu)$ for a 5-pixel neighborhood of a tag line in an *in vivo* heart image is shown in Figure 2.

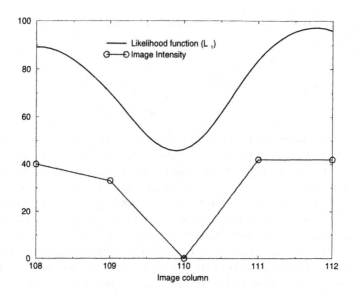

**Fig. 2.** A plot of the tag center log likelihood function $L_1(\mu)$ versus position (image column) for a 5-pixel neighborhood of a tag line in an *in vivo* heart image. The image pixel intensities are denoted by circles. The position where $L_1(\mu)$ is minimum is the maximum likelihood estimate of the tag center.

**Snake Algorithm** In principle, a tag line could be estimated by applying Equation (5) independently to each tag center in each tag line. Imaging artifacts and noise spikes, however, can cause large estimation errors, and since each tag line is estimated independently, there is nothing to prevent two tag lines from occupying the same physical position. For these reasons, we optimize Equation (6) for each tag center subject to spatial continuity constraints and a constraint on tag separation [14]. The resulting algorithm is similar to the snake-based tag estimation algorithms proposed by other researchers [14, 15, 5, 9]. The algorithm in this paper differs from these other snake-based algorithms in that we use a snake force based on the tag center likelihood function derived in the previous section.

We denote the vector of tag centers for the $j$th tag line as

$$\mathbf{t}_j = [\mu_{0\,j}\; \mu_{1\,j}\; \cdots\; \mu_{N_c-1\,j}]^T,$$

and define the optimal tag line as the tag line that minimizes the following energy function

$$E(\mathbf{t}_j) = \sum_{i=0}^{N_c-1} (1/\zeta)L_1^{i\,j}(\mu_{i\,j}) + \gamma E_{\text{sep}}(\mathbf{t}_{j-1}, \mathbf{t}_j, \mathbf{t}_{j+1}) + \alpha E_{\text{stretch}}(\mathbf{v}_j) + \beta E_{\text{bend}}(\mathbf{v}_j),$$

$$(7)$$

where $N_c$ is the number of centers in each tag line, $\gamma$, $\alpha$, and $\beta$ are user-specified weights, and $\mathbf{v}_j$ is the displacement of the tag line $\mathbf{t}_j$ from its previous position

$\mathbf{p}_j$ such that $\mathbf{t}_j = \mathbf{p}_j + \mathbf{v}_j$. $L_1^{ij}(\mu)$ is the likelihood function defined in (6) for the $i$th center on the $j$th tag line, and $\zeta$ is a normalizing factor defined as maximum value of $dL_1(\mu)/d\mu$ over all pixel positions in the image region of interest (ROI). $E_{\text{sep}}$ is a tag separation constraint, and $E_{\text{stretch}}$ and $E_{\text{bend}}$ are constraints on the stretch and bending of the tag line (see [11] for details).

Differentiating Equation (7) with respect to $\mathbf{t}_j$ and finite differencing the resulting partial differential equation (cf. [11]) yields the following iteration for the $j$th optimal tag line displacement

$$(\mathbf{I} + \tau\mathbf{A})\mathbf{v}_j^k = \mathbf{v}_j^{k-1} - \tau\mathbf{q}_j(\mathbf{t}_{j-1}, \mathbf{t}_j + \mathbf{t}_{j+1}), \qquad (8)$$

where $k$ is the iteration index, $\mathbf{A}$ is an $N_c \times N_c$ pentadiagonal matrix derived from the internal energy terms (cf. [11]), and $\tau$ is a step size. There is an Equation (8) for each tag line in the ROI, and these equations are solved simultaneously. The vector $\mathbf{q}_j$ contains "force" terms derived from the log likelihood function and the tag separation constraint. The $i$th component of $\mathbf{q}_j$ is

$$q_{j,i}(\mathbf{t}_{j-1}, \mathbf{t}_j, \mathbf{t}_{j+1}) = -(1/\zeta)\frac{d}{d\mu}L_1^{ij}(\mu_{ij}) \qquad (9)$$

$$-\gamma[(d_{\text{sep}} - \mu_{ij} + \mu_{ij-1})u(d_{\text{sep}} - \mu_{ij} + \mu_{ij-1}) \qquad (10)$$

$$+(d_{\text{sep}} - \mu_{ij} + \mu_{ij+1})u(d_{\text{sep}} - \mu_{ij} + \mu_{ij+1})], \qquad (11)$$

where $u(x) = 1$ for $x \geq 0$ and $u(x) = 0$ otherwise.

## 2.3 Tag Line Detection

In the tag estimation algorithm described above, a contiguous set of $N_c$ tag centers is estimated for each tag line across the entire ROI regardless of whether the centers are inside the myocardium or not. In this section we develop an algorithm to detect tag points that are inside the myocardium. This detection algorithm considers the following two hypotheses:

**Hypothesis 1:** Estimated center is part of a tag line in the myocardium.
**Hypothesis 0:** Estimated center is not part of a tag line in the myocardium.

We assume that the probability of each hypothesis is known and denote $P_0$ as the probability of Hypothesis 0 and $P_1$ as the probability of Hypothesis 1.

For Hypothesis 0 we assume that the estimated center $\hat{\mu}$ is located in non-myocardium tissue, which we will refer to as background tissue. Under Hypothesis 0, the observation vector $\mathbf{w}$ is modeled as

$$\mathbf{w} = \mathbf{m}_{\text{back}} + \mathbf{n}, \qquad (12)$$

where $\mathbf{m}_{\text{back}}$ is an $N_s$-vector of background signal samples, and $\mathbf{n}$ is the same noise vector described in Section 2.2. The background vector $\mathbf{m}_{\text{back}}$ is modeled as a random vector with mean $\mathbf{m}_{\text{back}} = \bar{m}_{\text{back}}\mathbf{1}$ and covariance matrix $\mathbf{C}_{\text{back}}(i,j) = \sigma_{\text{back}}^2 \rho_{\text{back}}^{|i-j|}$. Values for $\bar{m}_{\text{back}}$ and $\sigma_{\text{back}}^2$ are estimated from the image data for each time frame in the sequence (see Section 3).

The joint PDF of the observation vector conditioned on Hypothesis 0 is given by

$$f(\mathbf{w}|H_0) = \frac{1}{(2\pi)^{N_s/2}\sqrt{|\mathbf{C}_0|}} \exp\left(-\frac{1}{2}[\mathbf{w} - \mathbf{m}_{\text{back}}]^T \mathbf{C}_0^{-1}[\mathbf{w} - \mathbf{m}_{\text{back}}]\right), \qquad (13)$$

where $\mathbf{C}_0$ is the covariance matrix of $\mathbf{w}$ under Hypothesis 0 and is given by

$$\mathbf{C}_0 = \mathbf{C}_{\text{back}} + \sigma_n^2 \mathbf{I}.$$

The signal model under Hypothesis 1 (center is part of a tag line) is described in Section 2.2. The joint PDF of the observation vector conditioned on Hypothesis 1 is therefore given by

$$f(\mathbf{w}|H_1) = f(\mathbf{w}; \hat{\mu}), \qquad (14)$$

where $f(\mathbf{w}; \hat{\mu})$ is defined in Equation (4).

The maximum *a posteriori* (MAP) decision rule based on the PDF's defined in Equations (13) and (14) and the known probabilities $P_0$ and $P_1$ is to choose $H_1$ if

$$\frac{f(\mathbf{w}|H_1)}{f(\mathbf{w}|H_0)} > \frac{P_0}{P_1}, \qquad (15)$$

and $H_0$ otherwise. Taking the natural logarithm of both sides of (15) and cancelling terms results in the rule that an estimated tag center $\hat{\mu}$ is part of a tag line if

$$L_1(\hat{\mu}) > \eta(\mathbf{w}), \qquad (16)$$

where $\eta(\mathbf{w})$ is a data dependent threshold given by

$$\eta(\mathbf{w}) = \frac{1}{2}[\mathbf{w} - \mathbf{m}_{\text{back}}]^T \mathbf{C}_0^{-1}[\mathbf{w} - \mathbf{m}_{\text{back}}] + \frac{1}{2}\ln|\mathbf{C}_0| - \ln(P_0/P_1). \qquad (17)$$

Note that the prior probabilities $P_0$ and $P_1$ effectively bias the decision rule in favor of one hypothesis or the other. In practice, the log probability ratio $\ln(P_0/P_1)$ is chosen by the user as a tuning parameter.

Thus the tag detection algorithm consists of applying the decision rule given by Equations (16) and (17) to each center in a tag line estimated with the snake algorithm in Equation (8).

## 2.4 Removal of False Tag Points

With real image data, the tag detection rule in Equations (16) and (17) sometimes detects a false tag. These false tag detections usually occur in small, isolated clusters that spontaneously appear and disappear in time. As a result, we follow the MAP tag detection algorithm with pruning algorithm, which consists of two subroutines. The first, called removeShortRuns() deletes all tag points that appear in contiguous groups of less than $N_{\text{min}}$ in size. The second, called applyTemporalContinuity(), deletes all tag points who do not have a neighboring tag point in the same tag line within $\pm N_{\text{nbhd}}$ points in either the previous or next time frame. This allows the tag line to either grow or shrink by $N_{nbhd}$ points due to the expansion or contraction of the myocardium between time frames. After the tags have been estimated and detected, these subroutines are called for each time frame in the following order:

1. `removeShortRuns()`
2. `applyTemporalContinuity()`
3. `removeShortRuns()`

# 3  In Vivo Heart Experiment

## 3.1  Imaging

The LV of a normal human volunteer was imaged using a parallel planar tag imaging protocol [13]. The tag planes were separated in the reference state (end-diastole) by 6mm, which resulted in 12 tags across the LV. The resulting images are $256 \times 256$ with a pixel size of $h = 1.25$mm, a slice thickness of 8mm and are spaced 32.5ms apart for a total of 10 time frames through systole.

## 3.2  Algorithm Implementation

**Algorithm Overview** The tag estimation, detection, and pruning algorithms described in Section 2 were implemented as shown in Figure 3. First the user specified a rectangular region of interest (ROI) and a rectangular region over which the image noise statistics were computed (see below). These regions are shown in Figure 4a. The same regions were used for each time frame. The user also specified the initial alignment of the tag lines as shown in Figure 4b. This was the only user intervention required by the algorithm. At this point for each imaged phase (time frame) of the cardiac cycle, the algorithm first computed the image statistics (see below), ran the tag estimation algorithm and then ran the tag detection routine. Finally after all time frames were processed, the tag pruning algorithm was run over all time frames.

**Computation of Image Statistics** In order to run the tag estimation and detection algorithms, the mean and variance of the myocardium pixels ($\bar{m}_{myo}$, $\sigma^2_{myo}$) and background pixels ($\bar{m}_{back}$, $\sigma^2_{back}$) and the noise variance $\sigma^2_n$ must be computed for each image in the sequence. The noise variance was computed using the pixels enclosed by the rectangular region specified by the user as a sample and assuming a zero mean. The method used for computing the myocardium and background statistics was motivated by the observation that the tagged tissue is among the brightest tissues in the ROI. The myocardium and background statistics were computed by first performing a morphological closing operation over the ROI to remove the tag lines as described in [6]. The resulting pixel intensities were then sorted. $\bar{m}_{myo}$ and $\sigma^2_{myo}$ were set equal to the sample mean and variance of the brightest 50% of the pixel intensities. $\bar{m}_{back}$ and $\sigma^2_{back}$ were set equal to the sample mean and variance of the darkest 50% of the pixel intensities.

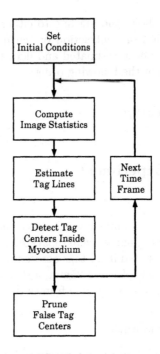

**Fig. 3.** Flow chart of the tag tracking and detection algorithm.

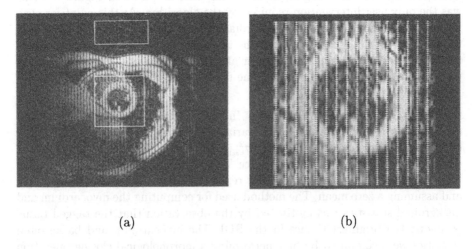

(a)                                         (b)

**Fig. 4.** (a) Region of interest (ROI) for both noise computation (upper box) and tag tracking (lower box). (b) Initial tag line alignment.

## 3.3 Results

The algorithm summarized in Figure 3 was run using the parameters listed in Table 1 on an image sequence taken from a single slice located near the base of the left-ventricle. Figure 5 shows two images from this sequence. Figure 6

| Tag Line Model Parameters | | |
|---|---|---|
| $A$ | tag amplitude | 1.0 |
| FWHM | tag full width at half maximum | 2.0 pixels |
| $\rho_{myo}$ | correlation of myocardium signal | 0.2 |
| $T_{1_{nom}}$ | nominal $T_1$ of the myocardium | 500 ms |
| Tag Tracking Parameters | | |
| $\alpha$ | snake continuity weight | 1000 |
| $\beta$ | snake bending weight | 10 |
| $d_{sep}$ | minimum tag separation | 1 pixel |
| $\tau$ | snake algorithm time step | 0.1 |
| $N_s$ | tag center neighborhood size | 5 pixels |
| Tag Detection Parameters | | |
| $\rho_{back}$ | correlation of background signal | 0.2 |
| $\ln(P_0/P_1)$ | log probability ratio | 0.0 |
| Tag Line Pruning Parameters | | |
| $N_{min}$ | spatial neighborhood size | 3 pixels |
| $N_{nbhd}$ | temporal neighborhood size | 1 pixel |

**Table 1.** Parameters used in tag tracking and detection experiment.

shows these same images overlaid with the results of the tag estimation algorithm. The position of tag centers outside the myocardium are primarily determined by the continuity and tag separation constraints. Note that the tag separation constraint keeps the tags from crossing one another. Also note that the algorithm estimates tags well at the myocardial boundaries even though the spatial smoothness constraints are enforced there. The results of the tag detection algorithm are shown in Figure 7. Most of the tag points inside the myocardium are preserved, and the false tag points occur in small, isolated clusters. The tag pruning algorithm results are shown in Figure 8. Most of the the false tag centers are removed while preserving the tag centers inside the myocardium. Note that the algorithm will preserve tag centers in any persistently tagged tissue as seen at the bottom of the images in Figure 8. MPEG loops of the full image sequences in Figures 6, 7 and 8 can be accessed at http://www.eng.auburn.edu/~tdenney/tagTracking.html.

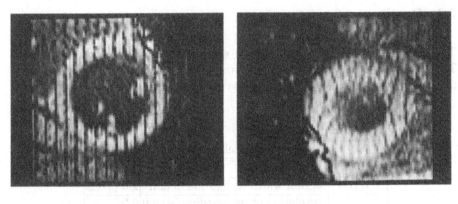

End-diastole (47 ms)                    End-systole (340 ms)

**Fig. 5.** Tagged images of the left ventricle of a normal human volunteer at two phases of the cardiac cycle.

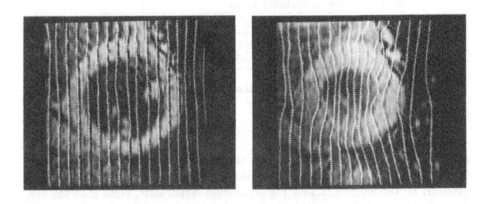

End-diastole (47 ms)                    End-systole (340 ms)

**Fig. 6.** Results of snake based tag tracking algorithm.

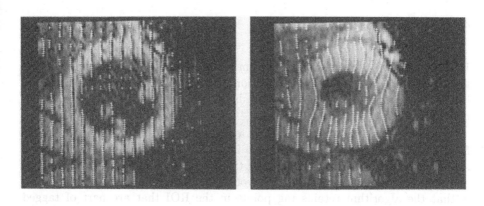

End-diastole (47 ms)                          End-systole (340 ms)

**Fig. 7.** Results of maximum *a posteriori* (MAP) tag detection algorithm.

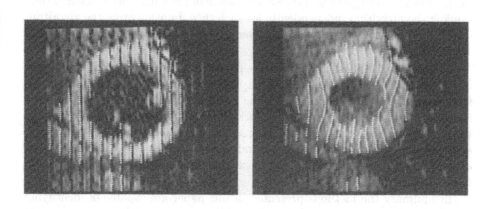

End-diastole (47 ms)                          End-systole (340 ms)

**Fig. 8.** Final result after temporal pruning algorithm.

# 4 Discussion

In this paper we presented an algorithm for estimating and detecting MR tag lines inside the myocardium without prior knowledge of the myocardial contours based on *a priori* knowledge of the tag shape and spatio-temporal continuity of the tag lines.

The algorithm was demonstrated on a single slice of a tagged image sequence from a normal human volunteer. Visual inspection of the results show that the algorithm does a good job of estimating tag line position inside the myocardium and removing tag points outside the myocardium. One side effect of this process is that the algorithm retains tag points in the ROI that are part of tagged non-myocardium tissue. This effect can be reduced somewhat by using a tighter ROI, but a more interesting alternative is to use these points in an algorithm that identifies the myocardial contours based on the spatio-temporal motion of the tag points.

The algorithm was also found to be relatively insensitive to the user-defined parameters in Table 1 such as $T_{1_{nom}}$ and the FWHM of the tag. A more thorough robustness study as well as a quantitative accuracy study will be addressed in future work.

While the experiments were performed on a single slice image sequence, the algorithm can be implemented on a multislice sequence by propagating the initial tag alignment and regions of interest to all slices in the multi-slice stack and then running the algorithm independently for each slice. Implementing the algorithm in this manner and performing tests over a large number of imaging studies is subject of future work.

At present, the algorithm assumes a parallel tag pattern like the one shown in Figure 5, but the methods presented in this paper could easily be extended for use in other radial [1] or grid [2] tag patterns. The algorithm also assumes that the images are acquired using a black blood imaging protocol [16]. In bright blood images, the relatively bright intensity of the blood pool could potentially skew the computation of myocardium and background statistics. Other methods of computing these statistics in both black and white blood images are currently under investigation.

In summary the methods presented in this paper are capable of identifying tag lines without prior knowledge of the LV contours and have the potential to reduce the amount of user intervention required to perform cardiac motion analysis and improve the clinical viability of MR tagging techniques.

# Acknowledgements

The author would like to thank Elliot R. McVeigh, PhD for making the *in vivo* human data available to him and for helpful discussions on MR tagging and tag identification.

# References

1. E.A. Zerhouni, D.M. Parish, W.J. Rogers, A. Yangand, and E.P. Shapiro. Human heart: tagging with MR imaging — a method for noninvasive assessment of myocardial motion. *Radiology*, 169:59–63, 1988.
2. L. Axel and L. Dougherty. MR imaging of motion with spatial modulation of magnetization. *Radiology*, 171:841–845, 1989.
3. W.G. O'Dell, C.C. Moore, W.C. Hunter, E.A. Zerhouni, and E.R. McVeigh. Displacement field fitting for calculating 3D myocardial deformations from parallel-tagged MR images. *Radiology*, 195:829—835, 1995.
4. T.S. Denney Jr. and J.L. Prince. Reconstruction of 3D left ventricular motion from planar tagged cardiac MR images: an estimation theoretic approach. *IEEE Transactions on Medical Imaging*, 14(4):625–635, December 1995.
5. A.A. Young, D.L. Kraitchman, L. Dougherty, and L. Axel. Tracking and finite element analysis of stripe deformation in magnetic resonance tagging. *IEEE Transactions on Medical Imaging*, 14(3):413–421, Septmeber 1995.
6. M.A. Guttman, J.L. Prince, and E.R. McVeigh. Tag and contour detection in tagged MR images of the left ventricle. *IEEE Transactions on Medical Imaging*, 13(1):74–88, 1994.
7. A. Amini, R. Curwen, R.T. Constable, and J.C. Gore. MR physics-based snake tracking and dense deformation from tagged cardiac images. In *AIII Spring Symposium Series. Applications of Computer Vision in Medical Image Processing*, March 1994.
8. P. Radeva, A. Amini, J. Huang, and E. Marti. Deformable B-solids and implicit snakes for localization and tracking of MRI-SPAMM data. In *Mathematical Models in Biomedical Image Analysis*, June 1996.
9. S. Kumar and D. Goldgof. Automatic tracking of SPAMM grid and the estimation of deformation parameters from cardiac MR images. *IEEE Transactions on Medical Imaging*, 13(1):122–132, 1994.
10. A. Bazille, M.A. Guttman, E.R. McVeigh, and E.A. Zerhouni. Impact of semi-automated versus manual image segmentation errors on myocardial strain calculation by MR tagging. *Investigative Radiology*, 29(4):427–433, 1994.
11. L.D. Cohen. Note on active contour models and balloons. *CVGIP: Image Understanding*, 53(2):211–218, 1991.
12. M.A. Guttman, E.A. Zerhouni, and E.R. McVeigh. Fast, contourless tag segmentation and displacement estimation for analysis of myocardial motion. In *Proc. SMR/ESMRMB*, volume 1, page 41, Nice, August 1995. SMR.
13. E.R. McVeigh and E. Atalar. Cardiac tagging with breath-hold cine MRI. *Magnetic Resonance in Medicine*, 28:318–327, 1992.
14. M.A. Guttman, E.A. Zerhouni, and E.R. McVeigh. Analysis and visualization of cardiac function from MR imgages. *IEEE Computer Graphics and Applications*, 17(1):30–38, January 1997.
15. D.L. Kraitchman, A.A. Young, C.-N. Chang, and L. Axel. Semi-automatic tracking of myocardial motion in MR tagged images. *IEEE Transactions on Medical Imaging*, 14(3):422–433, Septmeber 1995.
16. R.R. Edelman, D. Chien, and D. Kim. Fast selective black blood MR imaging. *Radiology*, 181(3):655–60, December 1991.

# An Autofocus Algorithm for the Automatic Correction of Motion Artifacts in MR Images

David Atkinson[1], Derek L. G. Hill[1], Peter N. R. Stoyle[2], Paul E. Summers[1], and Stephen F. Keevil[1].

[1] UMDS, Radiological Sciences, Guy's Hospital, London SE1 9RT, UK.
e-mail: d.atkinson@umds.ac.uk
[2] Defence Research Agency, St. Andrew's Road, Great Malvern. WR14 3PS, UK.

**Abstract.** We present the use of an entropy focus criterion to enable automatic focussing of motion corrupted magnetic resonance images. Our technique can determine unknown patient motion or use knowledge of motion from other measures as a starting estimate. The motion estimate is used to compensate the acquired data and is iteratively refined using the image entropy. Our entropy criterion focuses the whole image principally by favoring the removal of motion induced ghosts and blurring from otherwise dark regions of the image. Using only the image data, and no special hardware or pulse sequences, we demonstrate correction for arbitrary rigid-body translational motion in the imaging plane and for a single rotation. Extension to 3D and more general motion should be possible.

## 1 Introduction

Magnetic Resonance Imaging (MRI) is capable of sub-millimeter resolution, shows excellent contrast between soft tissues and does not subject the patient to ionising radiation. However, ghosting and blurring caused by patient motion can either reduce the diagnostic usefulness of the scan, necessitate a repeat scan, or in many paediatric studies require the use of general anaesthetics (with an increase in both cost and risk to the patient).

Existing techniques to reduce the effects of motion include navigator echoes, fast or modified acquisitions and post-processing. Navigator correction of translational displacements in the frequency encode direction is well established [1,2]. Correction of more complicated motion has been less successful and requires either further radio frequency (RF) pulses [3], phase retrieval algorithms [1], patient preparation with special markers [4] or the gradient control necessary for orbital navigator echoes [5].

Alternatively, the sensitivity to motion can be reduced by decreasing the total scan time although this often compromises the image resolution and quality. Furthermore, rapid acquisitions using single shot echo planar imaging (EPI) require specialized hardware.

The effects of unknown motion can also be reduced by acquiring data using a spiral k-space trajectory. This requires compliant hardware and complicated gradient programming (not always available). Radial-scan with projection reconstruction is an alternative to 2D Fourier reconstruction and can reduce motion-induced ghosting [6]. However, ghosting still exists and motion between read-outs leads to shifted projections and blurring.

Motion can be deduced using post-processing techniques that examine the k-space data or its 1D Fourier transform (hybrid space). Zoroofi *et al.* [7] combined phase retrieval and edge-detection to correct for motion in the phase-encode and read-out directions. Alternatively, interleaved spiral acquisitions may provide phase information about motion [8] at certain times during a scan. Both techniques suffer from the need to retrieve phase information from the data. As a further alternative, segments of k-space acquired while the patient is stationary between discrete movements can be identified from discontinuities in k-space [9]. This technique presumably will not work with continuous motion.

Post-processing of the image data has been demonstrated. Two acquisitions can be combined using a weighted average to reduce motion artifacts [10]. Alternatively, if two interleaved acquisitions are taken, ghosts due to quasi-periodic motion can be removed [11] by assuming that the motion is approximately periodic with respect to the acquisition order. The method of generalized projections uses a predefined region of image support prior to iterative image improvement [12]. This requires phase retrieval and a prior knowledge of the region of support, such as a motion-free image. Recently, a minimum energy method has been proposed [13] that iteratively determines and corrects for rigid body motion. This technique minimises the MR image energy outside of the object and also requires the image boundary to be found prior to motion correction.

Although motion degrades images, the mechanism is principally through the corruption of the phase of the received signal. No information is lost during rigid body translations and information is lost only at certain times during rotations. Following from the autofocus of radar images [14], the objective of this work was to develop an automatic post-processing technique that autofocuses an image using only the original real and imaginary data from a conventional scanner. No patient preparation, extra pulse sequences, edge detection, phase retrieval, or region of image support are needed. The algorithm developed can detect step, cyclic or generalized aperiodic motion to sub-pixel resolution. The methods presented here provide a new tool that can be used in isolation, or in combination with many of the motion correction techniques mentioned previously.

## 2 Method

### 2.1 Outline of Method

Patient motion is modeled as a series of displacements or rotation angles as a function of time - the motion trajectory. Time is discretized into nodes with the timing of each node corresponding to the acquisition of a k-space line. In this way, continuous movement is approximated in a piecewise constant or piecewise linear fashion. The starting estimate of the trajectory can be zero motion, or the output of some other motion measure such as navigator echoes. This estimate is modified with a trial motion, the acquired data is corrected for this motion and the resultant image quality is assessed using a focus criterion. Using an optimisation algorithm, the patient motion parameters that yield the best quality image are determined iteratively.

## 2.2 Compensation for Translational Motion

The effects of translational motion in the frequency encoding (FE) and phase encoding (PE) directions are compensated by applying phase shifts to the acquired k-space data [1,2]. The relation between acquired data $S_{aq}(u, v)$ and the corrected data $S_c(u, v)$ for the $u^{\text{th}}$ k-space point in the $v^{\text{th}}$ readout-line is,

$$S_c(u, v) = S_{aq}(u, v) \times$$
$$\exp\left\{-2\pi i \left[\frac{d_{\text{FE}}}{\text{FOV}_{\text{FE}}}\left(u - \frac{N_{\text{FE}}}{2}\right) + \frac{d_{\text{PE}}}{\text{FOV}_{\text{PE}}}\left(v - \frac{N_{\text{PE}}}{2}\right)\right]\right\} \quad (1)$$

where $d_{\text{FE}}$ and $d_{\text{PE}}$ are the displacements, $\text{FOV}_{\text{FE}}$ and $\text{FOV}_{\text{PE}}$ are the fields of view and $N_{\text{FE}}$ and $N_{\text{PE}}$ are the number of points in the FE and PE directions respectively. The indexing of $v$ is from 0 to $N_{\text{PE}}-1$ and $v \equiv N_{\text{PE}}/2$ corresponds to zero PE gradient, similarly for $u$. Only motion occurring between the acquisition of phase encode lines is compensated in the current implementation.

## 2.3 The Entropy Focus Criterion

Improvements to images degraded by incomplete and noisy data have been made using entropy maximisation, for example, see [15]. Entropy maximisation attempts to produce the smoothest image consistent with the data, this can prevent low brightness objects from being obscured by noise. The corruption of MR data by patient motion is not directly analogous to these situations [16] and following radar autofocussing work [14], we use entropy *minimisation* as a focus criterion. Entropy minimisation favors high contrast and we demonstrate its use to remove motion induced ghosts from low intensity regions of an image.

The entropy focus criterion $E$, used here is,

$$E = -\sum_{j=1}^{M} \frac{B_j}{B_{max}} \ln\left[\frac{B_j}{B_{max}}\right] \quad (2)$$

where $M$ is the number of image pixels ($128^2$ here) and $B_j$ is the modulus of the complex value of the $j^{\text{th}}$ image pixel, referred to in this work as the pixel 'brightness'. The image energy is constant under motion induced phase shifts and if all the image energy were in one pixel, we would have the largest possible pixel brightness $B_{max}$, given by;

$$B_{max} = \sqrt{\sum_{j=1}^{M} B_j^2}. \quad (3)$$

Using this scheme, $E = 0$ when all the image energy is located in a single pixel and the remaining pixels are black. When the $128 \times 128$ 'image' is uniformly gray, $B_j/B_{max} = 1/128$ for all pixels and the image entropy has the value $E = 621$.

This entropy criterion thus favors alterations to the data that tend to increase the number of dark pixels. Motion often has the opposite effect, creating ghosts and blurring in image regions that would otherwise be dark. Thus one might expect entropy minimisation to aid the search for a motion free image, though it is by no means clear that this will always be the case.

In Fig. 1 we plot the variation of entropy with simulated sinusoidal and step motion on a good quality image. In these examples, entropy always increases monotonically with the motion amplitude, indicating that it is a good focus criterion.

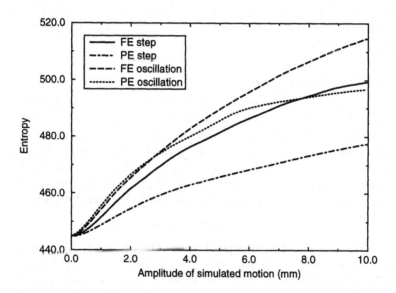

**Fig. 1.** The effect of simulated translational motion on image entropy. The step motions occur half way through the acquisition of k-space, oscillatory motion covers 3 cycles over the whole scan time.

## 2.4 Optimisation Strategy for In-Plane Translational Motion

The role of the optimisation strategy is to allow the iterative determination of the patient motion trajectory using the focus criterion as a measure of image quality. Minimisation of the focus criterion is multi-dimensional with translational motion possible in two dimensions and at any time during the acquisition. Our preliminary work indicates that finding the gross temporal features of motion before refining these features is a good search strategy.

The 128 readouts within the acquisition time are initially grouped into 16 intervals, each of 8 nodes. The interval nearest scan center (zero phase encode gradient) has trial displacements of $\{-Ns, -(N-1)s, \ldots, -s, s, \ldots, (N-1)s, Ns\}$ in both the FE and PE directions applied, where $s$ is a step size. Typically $N = 3$, giving 36 combinations of displacement to try for this interval. For each combination, the data is Fourier transformed to the image domain and the entropy calculated using equation (2). The combination giving the lowest image entropy is accepted and the motion curves are updated.

The algorithm then similarly considers each interval in turn to the end of the scan, after which it considers the remaining intervals from scan center to the start of the scan. Working outwards from the center of k-space (low image spatial frequency) is analogous to the use of multi-resolution search schemes in other areas of image processing. This process is repeated a second time and then the interval length is halved and the whole iteration procedure repeated. In this way the gross temporal features of the patient motion are determined first and subsequently refined. The algorithm halts after considering all the intervals with lengths of two nodes.

## 2.5 Compensation for Rotational Motion

Rotational motion part way through a scan causes a rotation of the corresponding section of k-space, for example, see [4]. If the image is to be reconstructed from k-space using the fast Fourier transform (FFT), the rotated data must be interpolated or 're-gridded' to lie on a regular Cartesian grid. To interpolate data we must chose a convolution kernel that is a balance between computational speed, accuracy and the introduction of extra image artifacts. We take from Marschner et al. [17] the separable windowed sinc kernel $h$ given by;

$$h(k) = [1 + \cos(\pi k/k_r)] \, \text{sinc}(4k/k_r) \tag{4}$$

where $k$ is the number of k-space points along the FE or PE direction from the k-space position being interpolated to the data point and $k_r$, the kernel 'radius' is 4.78. Because our focus criterion is sensitive to ghosts, we oversample the data (i.e. zero pad the image) to reduce post-aliasing effects. Using this kernel it takes less than 30 seconds to rotate an oversampled image ($256 \times 256$) on a Sparc Ultra 1-140 using un-optimised code. Our rotation of k-space rotates the image about its center, however, the true center of rotation will be nearer the point of contact of the head with the bed. Also, as the subject nods, this point of contact will move. To account for these effects, the rotated sections of k-space must have an unknown translational correction applied after the rotation correction.

For rotational motion, we have not yet developed an optimisation strategy other than to use the prior knowledge that the volunteer made a single "yes" type nod of between $-10°$ and $+10°$ within $\pm 10$ nodes of k-space center. All possible combinations of rotation angle (to an accuracy of $1°$) and time are applied to the data, followed by a simple gradient descent algorithm to find the translational correction for the unknown center of rotation.

## 2.6   Image Acquisition

All images were acquired on a Philips Gyroscan ACS-II MRI scanner operating at 1.5 T. The acquisition parameters were: spin-echo, TR=500 ms, TE=10 ms with a navigator echo at TE=50 ms, used as a control to determine motion, slice thickness 5 mm, sagittal orientation. In all cases, the PE gradient was decremented sequentially.

Each volunteer was first asked to lie still and imaged with the bed stationary. Images degraded by translational motion were then obtained by manually moving the scanner bed during a scan; this moves the volunteer in the cranio-caudal direction. Navigator echoes were taken to provide an independent estimate of the volunteer motion. The estimate was obtained using a least squared method that detects shifts in the navigator hybrid space [18]. Normally this gives motion in the FE direction only and there is no information about phase encode motion. Here we have designed the experiment such that the motion in the FE direction is the same as that in the PE direction. This is achieved by orienting both of the imaging gradients at 45° to the direction of bed motion.

For rotational motion, the volunteer was asked to count the gradient pulses (clearly audible) and perform a step nod at the $64^{th}$ imaging pulse. The nod moved his chin away from his chest.

In all cases the algorithm had no prior knowledge about the direction of translational motion. The autofocus algorithm treats motion in the FE and PE directions as independent. Except for the rotation case, the algorithm had no prior knowledge of whether the motion is step-like or more general. Some prior knowledge of the magnitude of the motion is currently required to set the step size $s$ if $N$ is to be kept low in order to constrain the amount of computer time required. However, with more complex optimisation strategies, this *a priori* knowledge may not be required. Only motion in the imaging plane is considered.

## 3   Results

Figure 2 presents the results for step motion at 45° to the imaging gradients. We show images of the volunteer stationary, corrupted by motion, after autofocussing and after navigator correction. The step size used was 0.63 mm (0.3 of a pixel size) and $N = 9$.

The step motion at a time near the acquisition of the center of k-space has caused blurring, ghosting and a double image to appear. After autofocussing, the image entropy reduces by 6.1% and after navigator correction, it decreases by 4.6% . Visually the navigator corrected, autofocussed and stationary images appear to be of similar quality, indicating that autofocus is effective. In Fig. 3 we plot the navigator and autofocus determined motion. In the optimisation process, all intervals are allowed to vary freely and the origin of displacement will be determined by some average position of the initially blurred image. Hence the origins of the FE, PE and navigator displacements will all be different for a given image. In Fig. 3, the origins of the FE and PE autofocus determined

Stationary · Motion corrupted

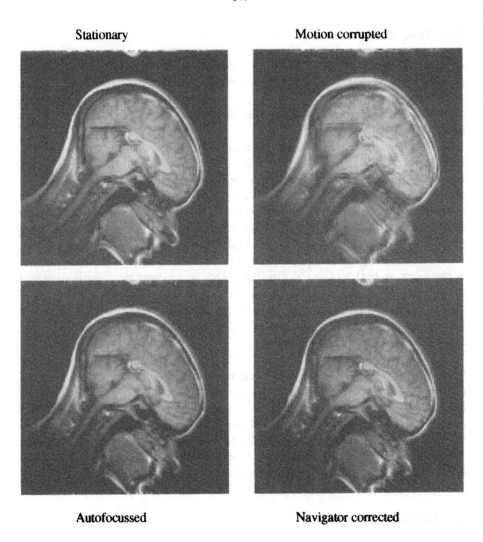

Autofocussed · Navigator corrected

**Fig. 2.** Volunteer stationary, with step motion near the center of k-space , after autofocus and after navigator correction. The read-out direction is horizontal in the images.

displacements have been shifted (but not scaled) to minimise the mean absolute difference (MAD) between the algorithm and navigator displacements. For motion in the FE direction the MAD is 0.2 mm and in the PE direction it is 0.9 mm. These compare well with a search step size $s$ of 0.63 mm. The program has tracked the FE motion very well. For the PE direction, there is some inaccuracy at times near the motion step and near the outer regions of k-space (near nodes 0 and 127).

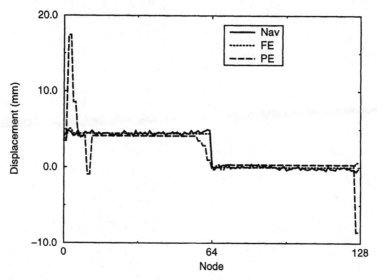

**Fig. 3.** Navigator and autofocus determined motion corresponding to Fig. 2.

Results on data from other volunteers (not shown here), moved in the PE direction only, indicate that the algorithm can fail to detect PE motion near the edges of k-space when this causes ghosts in the brain but not outside the head. By dividing the image into small regions and calculating the entropy in each region, we have observed that the presence or absence of ghosts in the brain has relatively little effect on the entropy. The algorithm performs the bulk of its focusing by removing ghosts and blurring from regions of the image that would otherwise be dark (i.e. the region outside the head, in the paranasal sinuses, oesophagus and bone).

Figure 4 is similar to Fig. 2 except that the motion is more general, the bed was moved throughout the scan. The step size $s$ was 0.63 mm and $N = 3$. Again clear improvements can be seen in image quality for both autofocus and navigator corrected images. The entropy reduction is 3.8% after autofocus and 3.7% after navigator correction.

**Stationary**

**Motion corrupted**

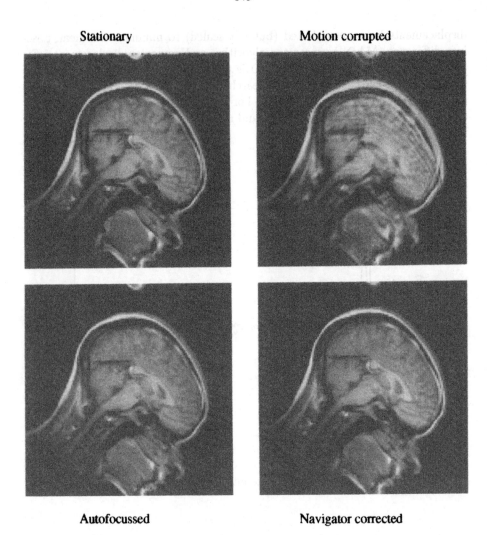

**Autofocussed**

**Navigator corrected**

**Fig. 4.** Volunteer stationary, with general motion over the whole acquisition, after autofocus and after navigator correction.

Figure 5 shows that again the program determined FE motion follows the navigator well (MAD of 0.52 mm), as has the PE motion (MAD 0.83 mm) although there are some deviations near the edges of k-space.

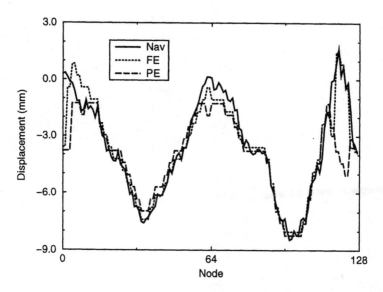

**Fig. 5.** Navigator and autofocus determined motion corresponding to Fig. 4

When searching phase encode line $v$ for the optimum displacement $d_{PE}$ in equation (1), the phase correction applied to the acquired data is equivalent for any value of $d_{PE}$ that yields the same phase correction, modulo $2\pi$. This means that the more extreme variations of PE displacement in Figs. 3 and 5 are actually equivalent to displacements closer to the navigator determined motion.

The use of entropy to correct for rotational motion is demonstrated in Fig. 6 with entropy being reduced by 1.5% . Clear focussing can be seen in the brain and around the nose. The neck still appears blurred and ghosted - presumably because the motion is not rigid-body in this region.

The examples presented above illustrate the operation of our algorithms. Navigator echo data was taken to validate the output from the algorithm. In practice, navigator echo information might be used to correct images for motion detected in the FE direction and an autofocus approach could be used to determine any additional, unknown, motion. To investigate this, we used the known navigator motion in the case of general motion (Fig. 4) to correct only for FE direction motion; the algorithm then searched for motion in the PE direction only. The detected PE motion trajectory was similar to before (MAD now 0.9 mm) and the image visually appears similar to the fully navigator corrected output. This demonstrates that autofocus can be used alone or in conjunction

Stationary　　　　　　　　　　Motion corrupted

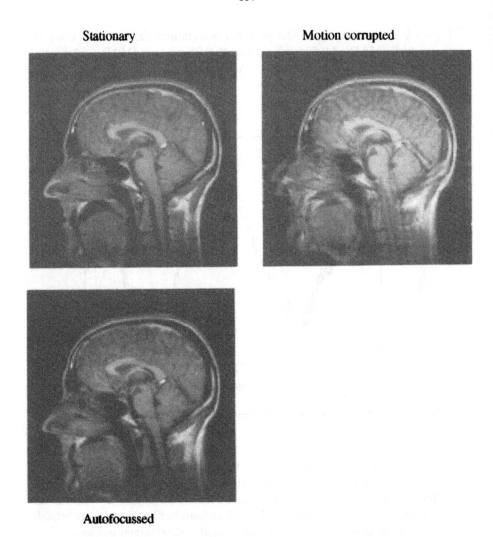

Autofocussed

**Fig. 6.** Volunteer stationary, with a single nod near the center of k-space and after focussing using the entropy focus criterion.

with navigator echoes to compensate for motion. Prior knowledge from other motion tracking sources might also be used. Searching for motion in only one direction reduces the search space and this took only 20 minutes on a Sparc Ultra 1-140 using un-optimised code, compared with 3.5 hours for the full 2D search.

# 4 Discussion and Conclusion

We have demonstrated the use of an entropy focus criterion to compensate for motion induced artifacts in an MR image. Our illustrative examples show reduced blurring and ghosting but in some cases there is a residual, un-corrected ghosting that is not present in the image of the volunteer lying still. These ghosts are also present in the navigator corrected data and hence we infer they are caused by uncorrected out of plane motion, or motion between an RF excitation and the subsequent readout.

The examples presented here demonstrate the concept of using entropy as a focus criterion in the improvement of MR images. The algorithms should be extendable to 3D volume acquisitions and more general rotational and translational motion. The amount of computer time will increase with the higher dimensional search space and we are currently devoting effort to reduce the optimisation time. The loss of data upon rotation is unavoidable with this type of acquisition sequence and may ultimately limit the types of motion for which correction is possible.

The autofocus method should also be applicable to other MR imaging sequences such as T2-weighted images, "fast" or "turbo" sequences, segmented EPI and half k-space acquisitions. Navigator correction of diffusion weighted images [20] is most effective when diffusion is measured in the phase encode direction. Autofocus techniques may be used to complement these navigator corrections for diffusion measurements in other directions. Correction of image artifacts due to other physical causes, such as timing errors in echo planar imaging that result in Nyquist ghosts, might also be compensated using autofocus methods.

The entropy focus criterion we chose to use in this work should be applicable whenever ghosts or blurring occur in regions of the image that would otherwise be dark. Studies in which $B_{max}$ of equation (2) is varied locally within an image indicate that we can make the focus criterion sensitive to contrast changes both within tissue regions and outside. A number of other contrast measures and focus criteria exist in the literature [14, 19, 21, 22] and these may also be beneficial to improving the effectiveness of autofocus techniques. This is the subject of on-going work.

In conclusion, we have demonstrated the use of an autofocus algorithm based on the minimisation of an entropy focus criterion to reduce motion induced blurring and ghosting in MR images. The algorithms were validated using independent navigator echo information and comparison with volunteers lying still. In practice, other motion measures such as navigator echoes can be used to quicken the search and improve its accuracy. We envisage that this type of autofocus algorithm will be used as a new tool in improving the quality of patient imaging. The technique does not require patient preparation, extra pulse sequences, complex gradient programming or specialized hardware. All that is required is the real and imaginary data from a conventional MRI scanner to achieve a reduction in motion induced blurring and ghosting.

# 5 Acknowledgements

We would like to acknowledge Dr. K. Hanson of Los Alamos National Laboratory and Dr. J.V. Hajnal of Hammersmith Hospital, UK, for useful discussions. We are also grateful to the anonymous volunteers, to Mr J.D. Cox and Mr D. Greenhaugh of the DRA for their support, and for the encouragement of Dr. D. Hawkes as Director of the Radiological Sciences Image Processing Group.

# References

1. R. L. Ehman and J. P. Felmlee: Adaptive Technique for High-Definition MR Imaging of Moving Structures. Radiology **173** (1989) pp. 225-263
2. H. W. Korin, F. Farzaneh, R. C. Wright, and S. J. Riederer: Compensation for Effects of Linear Motion in MR Imaging. Magn. Reson. Med. **12** (1989) pp. 99-113
3. K. Butts, A. de Crespigny, J. M. Pauly, and M. Moseley: Diffusion-Weighted Interleaved Echo-Planar Imaging with a Pair of Orthogonal Navigator Echoes. Magn. Reson. Med. **35** (1996) pp. 763-770
4. H. W. Korin, J. P. Felmlee, S. J. Riederer, and R. L. Ehman: Spatial-Frequency-Tuned Markers and Adaptive Correction for Rotational Motion. Magn. Reson. Med. **33** (1995) pp. 663-669
5. Z. W. Fu, Y. Wang, R. C. Grimm, P. J. Rossman, J. P. Felmlee, S. J. Riederer, and R. L. Ehman: Orbital Navigator Echoes for Motion Measurements in Magnetic-Resonance-Imaging. Magn. Reson. Med. **34** (1995) pp. 746-753
6. G. H. Glover and J. M. Pauly: Projection Reconstruction Techniques for Reduction of Motion Effects in MRI. Magn. Reson. Med. **28** (1992) pp. 275-289
7. R. A. Zoroofi, Y. Sato, S. Tamura, H. Naito, and L. Tang: An Improved Method for MRI Artifact Correction Due to Translational Motion in the Imaging Plane. IEEE Trans. Med. Imag. **14** (1995) pp. 471-479
8. R. Khadem and G. H. Glover: Self Navigation Correction for Motion in Spiral Scanning. Proc. Soc. Magn. Reson. (1994) pp. 346
9. M. L. Wood, M. J. Shivji, and P. L. Stanchev: Planar-Motion Correction Using k-space Data Acquired by Fourier MR Imaging. J. Magn. Reson. Imag. **5**(1) (1995) pp. 57-64
10. B. Madore and R. M. Henkelman: A New Way of Averaging With Applications to MRI. Med. Phys. **23**(1) (1996) pp. 109-113
11. Q. S. Xiang, M. J. Bronskill, and R. M. Henkelman: Two-Point Interference Method for Suppression of Ghost Artifacts Due to Motion. J. Magn. Reson. Imag. **3** (1993) pp. 900-906

12. M. Hedley, H. Yan, and D. Rosenfeld: Motion Artifact Correction in MRI Using Generalized Projections. IEEE Trans. Med. Imag. **10**(1) (1991) pp. 40-46

13. R. A. Zoroofi, Y. Sato, S. Tamura and H. Naito: MRI Artifact Cancellation Due to Rigid Motion in the Imaging Plane. IEEE Trans. Med. Imag. **15**(6) (1996) pp. 768-784

14. R. P. Bocker, and S. A. Jones: ISAR Motion Compensation Using the Burst Derivative Measure as a Focal Quality Indicator. Int. J. Imaging Systems and Technol. **4** (1992) pp. 285-297

15. S. F. Gull, and G. J. Daniell: Image Reconstruction from incomplete and noisy data. Nature **272** (1978) pp. 686-690

16. R. T. Constable and R. M. Henkelman: Why MEM Does Not Work in MR Image Reconstruction. Magn. Reson. Med. **14** (1990) pp. 12-25

17. S. R. Marschner and R. J. Lobb: An Evaluation of Reconstruction Filters for Volume Rendering. In: R. D. Bergeron and A. E. Kaufman. (eds.) Proc. Visualization '94. IEEE Computer Society Press, 1994, pp. 100-107

18. Y. Wang, R. C. Grimm, J. P. Felmlee, S. J. Riederer, and R. L. Ehman: Algorithms for Extracting Motion Information from Navigator Echoes. Magn. Reson. Med. **36** (1996) pp. 117-123

19. D. C. Noll, J. M. Pauly, C. H. Meyer, D. G. Nishimura, and A. Macovski: Deblurring for Non-2D Fourier Transform Magnetic Resonance Imaging. Magn. Reson. Med. **25** (1992) pp. 319-333

20. A. W. Anderson and J. C. Gore: Analysis and Correction of Motion Artifacts in Diffusion Weighted Imaging. Magn. Reson. Med. **32** (1994) pp. 379-387

21. A. Buffington, F. S. Crawford, S. M. Pollaine, C. D. Orth, and R. A. Muller: Sharpening Stellar Images. Science **200** (1978) pp. 489-494

22. F. Berizzi, and G. Corsini: Autofocusing of Inverse Synthetic Aperture Radar Images Using Contrast Optimization. IEEE Trans. Aerospace and Elec. Systems **32**(3) (1996) pp. 1185-1191

# Measurement of Global and Regional Cerebral Volume Changes by Integrating Boundary Shifts Between Registered Serial 3D MR Scans

Peter A. Freeborough and Nick C. Fox

Dementia Research Group, National Hospital for Neurology and Neurosurgery,
8-11 Queen Square, London WC1N 3BG, UK.

**Abstract.** A measure of regional and global cerebral volume change derived directly from registered repeat MR scans is proposed. This measure, the *boundary shift integral* (BSI), correlated closely with simulated volume change in brain ($r=1.000$) and ventricles ($r=0.999$). The BSI was used to determine brain volume loss in 21 control scan pairs and 11 scan pairs from Alzheimer's disease (AD) patients (1 year scan intervals). Loss in the AD group (mean 34.7cc) was widely separated from that in the control group (mean 1.8cc, SD 3.8cc). In contrast, the difference in segmented brain volumes in the AD group (mean 34.9cc) overlapped considerably with that of the control group (mean -2.9cc, SD 13.4cc). The RMS error between repeated measures of the brain BSI was 1.77cc. The ventricular BSI correlated closely with the difference in segmented ventricular volumes ($r=0.997$), with mean increases of 0.4cc (controls) and 10.1cc (AD). The BSI is both sensitive and highly reproducible.

## 1 Introduction

Magnetic Resonance (MR) is an imaging modality capable of resolving fine structural detail within the brain. It is sensitive to the subtle structural changes that are associated with many neurological conditions. Conventional volumetric measurements from MR images have allowed the size of specific cerebral structures to be compared. Measures of cerebral structures such as the temporal lobe, the hippocampus or the amygdala have been shown to discriminate Alzheimer's disease (AD) from normal aging [1-3]. Nonetheless these studies have tended to show overlap between subject groups, being confounded by the massive biological variability between normal subjects.

The comparison of serial scans circumvents problems of inter-subject variability as subjects are their own reference. However, whereas measures based on a single scan represent the accumulation of change since the onset of disease, measurement of change between serial scans represents only the change in the intervening interval; an interval which for clinical utility must be relatively small. These subtle changes may be difficult to detect by comparing conventional volumetric measures obtained from each scan independently.

Accurate registration of serial 3D MR scans permits the visualization of subtle changes within the brain [4-6]. Figs. 1a and 1b show baseline scans of a normal control and an AD patient respectively. Fig. 1c shows the difference between the baseline scan of the normal control and a registered repeat scan acquired approximately 1 year later; the difference is represented using a linear intensity scale where white represents an increase, mid-gray no change, and black a decrease in intensity. Note there is near complete cancellation of intensities within the brain, indicating little or no change over the interval. Correspondingly, fig. 1d compares the baseline scan of the AD patient to a repeat scan acquired after a similar interval; note there is significant loss of intensity (representing volume loss), particularly around the ventricular system, but also around the cortical surface.

Using this methodology patterns of loss have been observed in AD patients using scan intervals as short as 3 months [4].

We have previously shown a glch ' measure of cerebral volume change may be

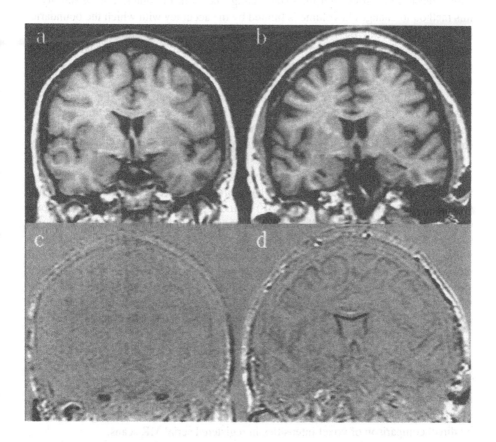

**Fig. 1.** Baseline scans from a normal subject (a) and an Alzheimer's disease patient (b). Repeat scans were acquired over one year later and registered to the baseline; the difference between the baseline and the repeat is shown in (c) and (d) respectively.

obtained by registration of repeat 3D MR scans of the same subject, followed by integration of the difference in voxel intensities over only those brain voxels which differ by more than a threshold figure [7,8]. Although a useful diagnostic marker, the approach implicitly assumes simplistic models for tissue loss and image formation, and hence does not yield a measure of the actual loss in volume. Furthermore, exclusion of intensity differences below the threshold level means the more subtle changes are not accounted for — these may be the very changes of interest.

In this paper, we develop and validate a novel method for measuring cerebral volume changes between registered repeat scans. We investigate the use of the method for measuring both global and regional changes in cerebral structure volumes.

## 2 Rationale

A change in the volume of a structure between two MR scans is conventionally measured by delineating its boundaries on each scan, determining the volume enclosed within those boundaries, and then subtracting one from the other. The sensitivity of this method to changes in volume is limited by the accuracy with which the boundaries of the structure can be identified. The identification of the boundaries of many structures (segmentation) often involves substantial user input or manual outlining, even where semi-automated methods are used; hence, the resulting volume estimates tend to be observer dependent.

An alternative approach, which is less dependent upon the accuracy of segmentation, is to register the scans accurately and compare the intensities of corresponding voxels. Using a partial volume model the volume of tissue lost may be calculated by subtracting the registered images from one another, dividing by the difference in intensity between tissue and its substitute (when tissue is lost) and then integrating (i.e. summing and then multiplying by the voxel size) this difference over the structure of interest. Hence a voxel that represented purely gray matter on the first scan and purely cerebrospinal fluid (CSF) on the second would count as a whole voxel of tissue loss whereas a voxel that had a change in signal intensity of half that amount (having gone from half gray matter and half CSF to purely CSF) would count as half a voxel of volume loss. This calculation is relatively simple if the structure to be measured is all of one known signal intensity and the tissue which replaces it when the structure atrophies is also all of one known intensity. In the case of cerebral atrophy white matter or gray matter may be replaced by CSF or dura and CSF, and hence the calculation of volume loss becomes problematic. Nonetheless this approach has been shown to be a useful diagnostic marker [7,8].

The difference in volume of a structure at two different time points equals the total volume through which the boundaries have shifted between those time points. The problem of knowing the exact intensity transition associated with loss of volume may therefore be avoided by measuring the total volume through which the boundaries of a structure shift. The methodology we propose is based on measuring this volume by direct comparison of voxel intensities in registered serial MR scans.

# 3 Measurement of Boundary Shifts

## 3.1 Registration

The repeat scan is registered to the baseline by determining the rotations and translations required to minimize the standard deviation of the ratio between corresponding voxels within the brain, while in parallel, determining spatial scaling factors so as to minimize the mean square distance between corresponding voxels on the surface of the cranium [4]. The method incorporates scaling factors based on the cranial surface so as to correct for changes in voxel size which may mimic tissue loss or 'gain'. Sinc interpolation is used for re-sampling. The procedure has been shown to achieve registration accurate to a fraction of a voxel [4].

## 3.2 Internal and Boundary Regions

We define the set of voxels corresponding to a given structure on the baseline and registered repeat scans using interactive morphology based procedures followed by manual editing where necessary [9,10]; we refer to these sets as $S_{base}$ and $S_{reg}$ respectively. We also utilize the morphological operator $B$, consisting of the origin and its 6 immediate neighbors in 3D. We define the internal region, $T$, as the intersection of $S_{base}$ and $S_{reg}$ eroded by an operator of size $N_e$, such that

$$T = \left(S_{base} \cap S_{reg}\right) \Theta \left(B \oplus B \oplus \cdots \oplus B\right) \qquad (1)$$

where $B$ occurs $N_e$ times on the right hand side.

Similarly we define a boundary region, $E$, as the set of voxels which are members of the union of $S_{base}$ and $S_{reg}$ dilated by an operator of size $N_d$, while also not being members of the interior set $T$, that is

$$E = \left(\left(S_{base} \cup S_{reg}\right) \oplus \left(B \oplus B \oplus \cdots \oplus B\right)\right) \cap T^C \qquad (2)$$

where $B$ occurs $N_d$ times on the right hand side.

## 3.3 Intensity Normalization

Due to variations in the scanner and the acquisition environment, the image intensities in a pair of repeat scans of a patient may not be directly comparable. Scaling image intensities on each scan to give the same mean over a structure or region which has not changed between the scans, to a first approximation, eliminates this variability.

We assume that tissue deeply within the brain (i.e. distant from the external boundary and any new internal boundaries associated with the opening of new spaces), has largely unchanged MR response. This requires, to a first approximation, that tissue lost within the brain is completely substituted by adjacent tissue, resulting in structural readjustment and a reduction in brain volume — this assumption is supported by the observation of volume loss in the degenerative dementias. We therefore normalize the intensities on each scan by dividing by the mean intensity of the brain interior region (**T**), yielding unit mean over this region.

## 3.4 Image Intensity Formation

The acquisition of true 3D MR scans can be described as the digitization of a non band limited continuous signal (i.e. the MR point response of brain tissue) by a device whose point spread function (PSF) is a sinc function. This can be modeled as a two stage process in which an ideal low pass filter is first applied to the signal (i.e. convolution with the sinc function) which is then multiplied by a perfect comb function (i.e. ideal sampling). As multiplication by a comb function in the time domain is equivalent to convolution with a comb function in the frequency domain, the power spectrum of the final signal consists of that of the intermediate low pass filtered signal plus non-overlapping high frequency duplicates. Perfect reconstruction of the intermediate low pass filtered signal from the samples is possible, and is achieved by removing the high frequency duplicates by convoluting the samples with a sinc function (i.e. ideal low pass filtering). We will refer to these continuous reconstructed low pass filtered signals, *after registration and intensity normalization*, as $i_{base}(x,y,z)$ and $i_{reg}(x,y,z)$ on the baseline scan and repeat scan respectively.

Note that the use of sinc interpolation within registration is consistent with this model (i.e. the frequency spectrum is maintained) and hence $i_{reg}(x,y,z)$ can be correctly calculated from the re-orientated repeat scan.

An important consequence of this model is that where the brain is unchanged between the baseline and repeat scans, $i_{base}(x,y,z)$ and $i_{reg}(x,y,z)$ should be identical, irrespective of difference in the orientation of the head within the scanner.

## 3.5 Boundary Shift Integral

Fig. 2 shows, at two different time points, the MR response *prior to sampling* (i.e. the low pass filtered point MR response) on a line through a boundary within the brain. Low pass filtering and the complexity of the boundary result in a response significantly different from a step function. We assume that the majority of cell loss is not adjacent to the boundary of the structure, and hence to a good approximation the boundary of the structure does not change its form; there is however a shift in the boundary associated with the volume loss. Therefore, in our one-dimensional example, in the neighborhood of the boundary there is a shifting of the point MR response along the line, and consequently an identical shift of the low pass filtered MR response. Hence if $i_{base}(x)$ is the low pass filtered point MR response along a line on the baseline scan and $i_{reg}(x)$ is the same response from a registered repeat scan on which there has been a reduction in the width of the structure leading to a boundary shift of $\Delta w$, (see fig. 2), then the responses must be related by

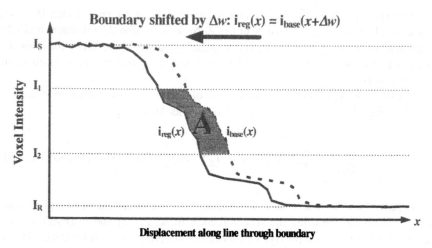

**Fig. 2.** Intensity profiles through a boundary on registered baseline and repeat MR scans

$$i_{reg}(x)= i_{base}(x+\Delta w) \tag{3}$$

If we assume $i_{base}(x)$ and $i_{reg}(x)$ to be monotonic, we can define the inverse functions $x_{base}(i)$ and $x_{reg}(i)$; hence

$$x_{base}(i)= x_{reg}(i)+\Delta w \tag{4}$$

A simple estimate of $\Delta w$ may be obtained as $x_{base}(I)-x_{reg}(I)$, where $I$ may be any value such that $I_R<I<I_S$, $I_S$ being the intensity within the bulk of the structure and $I_R$ the intensity at the other side of the boundary. A more robust estimate may be obtained by averaging the estimates of $\Delta w$ obtained over a range of $I$, such that

$$\Delta w = \frac{1}{I_1-I_2} \int_{I_2}^{I_1} \left(x_{base}(i) - x_{reg}(i)\right)di \quad \text{where} \quad I_R \le I_2 < I_1 \le I_S \tag{5}$$

This may alternatively be expressed as an integral with respect to $x$,

$$\Delta w = \frac{1}{I_1-I_2} \int_{boundary} \left(clip\left(i_{base}(x),I_1,I_2\right) - clip\left(i_{reg}(x),I_1,I_2\right)\right)dx \tag{6}$$

where, $\quad I_R \le I_2 < I_1 \le I_S, \quad clip(a,I_1,I_2) = \begin{cases} I_2 & a < I_2 \\ a & I_2 \le a \le I_1 \\ I_1 & a > I_1 \end{cases} \tag{7}$

One may confirm that equations 5 and 6 are equivalent by considering that both integrals evaluate the area labeled A in fig. 2. Note that while the minimum limits for the integration of equation 6 are $x_{reg}(I_1)$ to $x_{base}(I_2)$, outside these limits the integrand evaluates to zero and hence, for simplicity, we have extended the limits to cover the whole boundary.

If we now extend this analysis to three-dimensions, we may determine the total volume displaced over the boundary of a structure as $\Delta v$, where

$$\Delta v = \frac{1}{I_1 - I_2} \iiint_{\text{boundary}} \left( \text{clip}\left( i_{\text{base}}(x,y,z), I_1, I_2 \right) - \text{clip}\left( i_{\text{reg}}(x,y,z), I_1, I_2 \right) \right) dxdydz \quad (8)$$

This integral may be determined numerically by evaluating the integrand at small sampling intervals, requiring the reconstruction of $i_{base}(x,y,z)$ and $i_{reg}(x,y,z)$ at these intervals. However, for simplicity, we choose the sampling intervals for the evaluation of the integral to be the same as on the original scans. Hence we approximate $\Delta v$ by the *boundary shift integral* (BSI) which we define as:

$$\text{BSI} = \frac{K}{I_1 - I_2} \sum_{x,y,z \in \mathbf{E}} \left( \text{clip}\left( I_{\text{base}}(x,y,z), I_1, I_2 \right) - \text{clip}\left( I_{\text{reg}}(x,y,z), I_1, I_2 \right) \right) \quad (9)$$

where $K$ is the product of the sampling intervals in each dimension (i.e. the voxel volume), $\mathbf{E}$ is the set of voxels in the boundary region (see equation 2), and $I_{base}(x,y,z)$ and $I_{reg}(x,y,z)$ are the normalized voxel intensities on the registered scans. We refer to the range of the integral, $[I_1,I_2]$, as the *intensity window*, which we define in terms of its center $I_c=I_1/2+ I_2/2$, and width $I_w=I_1-I_2$.

Note that the approximation between the BSI and $\Delta v$ can be reduced to any desired level by sub-sampling the scans prior to evaluation. Hence, assuming consistent, noiseless scan acquisition, the BSI may be used to measure volume change to arbitrarily high levels of accuracy — the acquisition voxel size places a limit only in that it determines the accuracy with which the boundaries of one structure can be separated from those of another.

### 3.6 Parameter Selection

Evaluation of the BSI over any structure requires the appropriate selection of an intensity window, (i.e. $I_c$ and $I_w$), and sizes for the morphological operators (i.e. $N_e$ and $N_d$). The intensity window should be selected such that it is spanned by all of the intensity transitions associated with the boundaries of a structure — for typical structures within the brain this is complicated by adjacent structures having several different intensities and the structure itself being made up of tissues with differing intensities. Similarly, the morphological operator sizes should be ideally selected such that the boundary region includes the whole of the structure's boundary. However, maximizing the signal-to-noise ratio of the BSI, imposes counteracting constraints.

The intensity window should be made as wide as possible so as to maximize the number of contributing boundary voxels (i.e. signal); whereas the morphological operators should be made as small as possible, (while still covering the entire boundary), so as to minimize the number of contributing non-boundary voxels and to avoid extending the boundary region across more than one boundary.

The optimum set of parameters is primarily dependent upon the scan acquisition protocol, and the arrangement and intensity of adjacent tissue types with respect to the structure — none of which should vary substantially from patient to patient. We may therefore determine an optimum set for a given scan type and structure based upon a single subject.

This is performed by comparing simulated and measured volumes of loss over a range of parameter values. We simulate different volumes of loss in a given structure on a single scan, by spatially scaling the scan about the central point of the structure, by equal amounts in each dimension. This yields a series of new scans in each of which the volume of the structure has been artificially increased or decreased by percentages which are known exactly. The BSI may then be evaluated between each of the re-sampled scans and the original, and plotted against the known change in volume (i.e. the corresponding percentage of the structure's volume as obtained by segmentation). Typically, these plots are very linear over a wide range of parameter values, however the gradient of a linear fit to the points, which we refer to as the *gain* of the BSI, in general is less than the ideal of unity. We suggest this is due to difficulties in determining an intensity window which is spanned by all the intensity transitions around the structure's boundaries, this leads to some boundary shifts being unaccounted for. Similarly, where a structure is bordered by tissue of the same intensity, the BSI inevitably yields a gain of less than one, as shifting of the corresponding boundary cannot be detected by any intensity window. We select the optimum set of parameters as that which maximizes the gain of the BSI, although compromises must be made to obtain a sufficiently wide window ($I_w$) to ensure the measure is robust to noise. We assume the determined optimum parameters are valid for the given structure in all patients scanned using the same protocol.

### 3.7 Quality Control

Patient motion during the scan results in phase errors in the MR signal which are observed on the scans as motion artifact. The level of artifact may vary widely between scans — being dependent upon the stillness of the patient — and where there is significant artifact, registration accuracy will be reduced and the BSI will not represent a reliable measure of volume change. We assess the level of motion artifact in a scan according to the figure $m_0$ (see below); and discard scan pairs for which the mean $m_0$ is greater than a threshold figure.

One consequence of the motion related phase errors is increased noise in voxels displaced from the head in the phase encoding direction. We base our measure of motion artifact, $m_0$, on the level of this noise.

We define $S_0$ as the set of all voxels between the head and the edge of the scan along lines in the phase encoding directions. We determine $S_0$ automatically in 5 stages: 1) the scan is normalized by dividing each voxel intensity by the mean intensity over the brain (the brain having been previously identified for registration), 2) $S_0$ is initialized to the null set, 3) every coronal slice is scanned left-to-right and right-to-left and every voxel between the start of the row and the first voxel with intensity above 0.15 is added to $S_0$ (where no voxel above this threshold is found $S_0$ is unchanged), 4) $S_0$ is dilated 3 times by the operator $B$, and 5) $S_0$ is eroded 4 times by the operator $B$. As previously, the operator $B$ consists of the origin and its 6 neighbors in 3D. The level of motion artifact, $m_0$, is calculated as the mean voxel intensity over the set $S_0$.

In addition to motion, one would expect $m_0$ to be directly influenced by other sources of noise; thermal noise in particular. To assess the degree to which $m_0$ is dependent upon motion artifact we ranked 20 scans (acquired as described in section 4) according to a visual assessment of the severity of motion related 'ringing' artifact within brain. We compared our rankings with the $m_0$ figure obtained for each scan and found a rank correlation coefficient of 0.76; suggesting that $m_0$ is predominantly dependent upon the level of motion artifact.

## 4 Methods

Baseline and repeat $T_1$-weighted 3D MRI scans were acquired from 14 normal control subjects and 7 AD patients using a 1.5T GE Signa unit with a spoiled gradient echo technique (256*128*128 matrix; 24*24*19.2cm FOV; TR/TE/NEX/FLIP 35/5/1/35). Several subjects had further repeat scans, yielding a total of 22 control scan pairs and 15 AD scan pairs, all with scan intervals of 1 year (± 3 months).

In addition, in order to examine the reproducibility of the BSI, repeat MR scans of several subjects were acquired where on a subject's second visit two scans were obtained — so providing two baseline-repeat scan pairs spanning the same interval. This yielded 3 dual scan pairs from AD patients and 6 from controls.

The parameter selection procedure was performed for both whole brain BSI and ventricular system BSI. The procedures utilized a single control scan and 32 levels of simulated volume change (-8% to +8% in steps of 0.5%). The selected parameter sets were used in the following stages.

All baseline-repeat scan pairs were registered as previously described [4]. We calculated the motion artifact figure, $m_0$, and the residual registration error over the brain, $r_{err}$, where,

$$ r_{err} = \frac{\sum_{brain} |I_1(x,y,z) - I_2(x,y,z)|}{N_{vox}} \tag{10} $$

and $N_{vox}$ is the number of voxels corresponding to brain. The brain BSI and ventricular BSI were calculated between those scan pairs for which the mean $m_0$ was less than 0.047 (arbitrarily selected to reject only the most severe cases).

# 5 Results and Discussion

Fig. 3 shows the effect of the measurement parameters ($N_d$, $N_e$, $I_c$ and $I_w$) on the gain of the brain BSI. Initially we used a narrow intensity window and no dilations ($I_w$=0.05, $N_d$=0), and varied the size of the erosion operator ($N_e$) and the window center ($I_c$). With $N_e$=0 the gain was found to peak at 0.81 with $I_c$=0.55, for $N_e$=1 the gain peaked at 0.88 with $I_c$=0.6, but further increases in $N_e$ had no effect upon gain (fig. 3a). This suggests that with no erosion the inner border of the brain boundary region does not extend sufficiently into the brain, sufficient extension is obtained by use of an erosion operator with $N_e$=1, but further increases in $N_e$ have no benefit. Note that this inward extension of the boundary region also resulted in an increased $I_c$ at the peak — a consequence of a greater proportion of high intensity changes being included in the boundary region. We selected $N_e$=1 as optimum.

Using a narrow intensity window ($I_w$=0.05) and fixing $N_e$ at 1, we varied the size of the dilation operator ($N_d$) and the window center ($I_c$). With $N_d$=0 the gain was found to peak at 0.88 with $I_c$=0.6, for $N_d$=1 the gain peaked at 0.93 with $I_c$=0.5, but further increases in $N_d$ led to a reduction in gain (fig. 3b). This suggests that with no dilation the boundary region does not extend sufficiently away from brain, and that sufficient coverage requires a dilation operator with size $N_d$=1, however further increases in the size of the operator distort the measure by including boundaries not associated with brain. The increased outward extension of the boundary region also resulted in a decrease in $I_c$ at the peak — this is associated with a greater proportion of low intensity changes being included in the boundary region. We selected $N_d$=1 and $I_c$=0.5 as optimum.

Fixing $N_e$=1, $N_d$=1 and $I_c$=0.5, we varied the width of the intensity window, $I_w$, from 0.05 to 1.0 and found that gain steadily reduced with increasing $I_w$ (fig. 3c). This may have been predicted as increasing the intensity window width must result in a smaller proportion of the intensity transitions at the boundaries of the brain fully spanning the intensity window, leading to a reduction in gain. However, obtaining a measure robust to noise requires a wide window so that the range of intensities over which the boundary shift is averaged is large (fig. 2). We arbitrarily chose to trade 10% of the peak gain for an increased window size, and hence adopted $I_w$=0.5 giving a gain of 0.84.

Fig. 3d shows the brain BSI for different levels of volume change, evaluated using the selected parameters ($N_e$=1, $N_d$=1, $I_c$=0.5 and $I_w$=0.5). The relation closely approximates linearity (product-moment $r$=1.000).

Applying the same parameter selection procedure to the ventricular BSI we observed identical trends, resulting in the selection of $N_e$=1, $N_d$=1, $I_c$=0.6 and $I_w$=0.5, yielding a correlation of $r$=0.999 and predicted gain of 1.10. The optimum intensity window is higher than that obtained for brain as there is a greater proportion of white matter around the ventricular surface as compared to the brain surface as a whole (white matter appearing brighter than gray matter in $T_1$ MR scans). Note also that the predicted gain is greater than one, whereas we have argued that the BSI should generally yield a gain of less than one. We suggest that the prediction is actually an overestimate — a result of an underestimate in the segmented ventricular volume from which the volume of simulated atrophy is determined (by taking percentages). Our

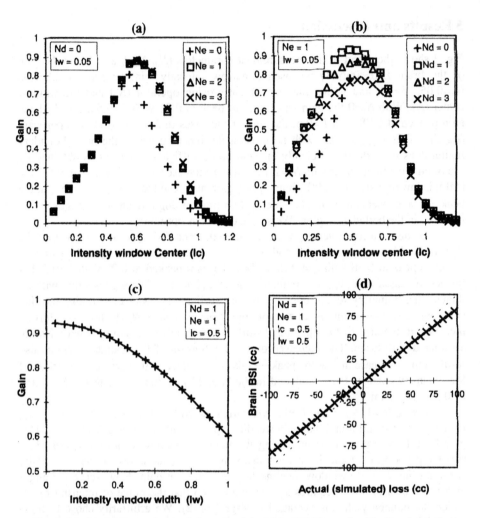

**Fig. 3.** (a), (b), (c) Dependence of the gain of the brain BSI (determined by the simulation procedure) on the measurement parameters ($I_c$, $I_w$, $N_d$, $N_c$); (d) the brain BSI plotted against simulated volume loss for the selected parameter set ($I_c$=0.5, $I_w$=0.5, $N_d$=1, $N_c$=1).

ventricular segmentation method is highly sensitive to the threshold selected to detect the boundary. We utilized a threshold of 0.5 of the mean brain intensity whereas the selection of $I_c$=0.6 suggests that this is not the center of the intensity transition and that hence we are underestimating our actual volumes of simulated atrophy. This does not undermine the parameter selection method as the optimum parameters will still correspond to the peak gain.

In the 22 control scan pairs we compared the motion artifact measure, $m_o$, to the residual registration mismatch and found a significant correlation (product-moment $r$=0.532, $p$=0.01), demonstrating motion artifact is a major source of noise for which we must control. We chose to reject only those scan pairs with the highest levels of motion artifact; we adopted a threshold $m_o$ of 0.047 leading to the rejection

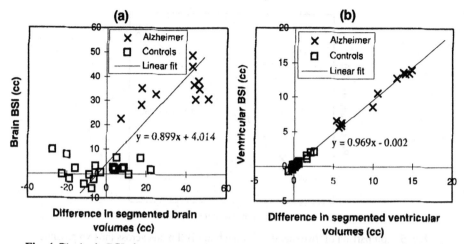

**Fig. 4.** The brain BSI plotted against difference in segmented brain volume (based on the same region definitions used to generate the boundary region) for 11 Alzheimer and 21 Control scan pairs (a); and the corresponding comparison of the ventricular BSI with difference in segmented ventricular volume (b). The linear fits were based on minimizing the error in the segmentation measure (x-axis).

of 4 AD and 1 control scan pair. In general we have found a larger prevalence of motion artifact in scans of AD patients. This reinforces the need to control for the artifact — to inhibit a possible causal relation between symptoms (i.e. forgetting to remain still) and the BSI. However, scan rejection in this manner is undesirable for routine clinical use, and we are currently investigating the use of head restraints and other devices to reduce patient motion.

For the remaining 21 control and 11 AD scan pairs, fig. 4a shows the brain BSI plotted against the difference in absolute segmented volumes (the latter being based upon the same region definitions used to generate the boundary region). The brain BSI in the AD group (mean 34.7cc, SD 7.3cc) was widely separated from that in the control group (mean 1.8cc, SD 3.8cc). In contrast, the difference in segmented volumes in the AD group (mean 34.9cc, SD 15.1cc) overlapped greatly with that in the control group (mean -2.9cc, SD 13.4cc). Note that while the BSI yielded much less group spread, the group means were similar to those obtained by segmentation. These reslts demonstrate that the BSI provides a measure substantially more accurate than the segmentation upon which it is based. Fitting a linear regression line (to minimize error in the segmentation measure) we obtained a gradient of 0.90; this compares to the gain of 0.84 predicted by the simulation procedure.

Fig. 4b similarly shows the ventricular BSI plotted against the difference in absolute segmented volumes. In contrast to their application to brain, there is very tight correlation between the two measures ($r=0.997$); the BSI indicated mean (±SD) increases in ventricular volume in the AD group of 10.1cc (±3.5cc) compared to 0.4cc (±0.7cc) in the control group. The ventricles are a simple structure with very sharp defining boundaries and may be accurately segmented by semi-automated methods. These results therefore further confirm that the BSI provides a linear measure of

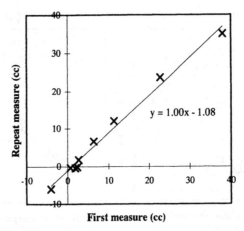

**Fig. 5.** Comparison of two measures of the brain BSI made across the two possible baseline-repeat scan pairs for the 9 subjects who had 2 scans on their second visit

volume change. Again fitting a linear regression line we obtained a line of gradient 0.97, which compares to the gain of 1.10 predicted by simulation.

The reproducibility of the brain BSI was assessed using those scans from the subjects who had two repeat scans on their second visit. The brain BSI's obtained between each of the repeat scans and the baseline are compared in Fig. 5. Each measure was influenced by patient positioning, scan acquisition, segmentation and registration as well as the quantification methodology. Despite this, the reproducibility was shown to be excellent. The RMS and absolute difference between the two measures were 1.77cc and 1.51cc respectively (compared to a mean brain volume of 1150cc).

Note that segmentation errors merely influence the sensitivity of the BSI (by distorting the boundary region) and do not introduce large biases as occurs when comparing absolute volumes. This is likely to be the predominant reason for the improved accuracy and reproducibility of the brain BSI.

The brain BSI was found to slightly underestimate volume change (gain less than unity). For complex structures with several defining boundaries it is unlikely that a single, sufficiently wide, intensity window will be spanned by all the possible intensity transitions at its boundaries; hence loss tends to be underestimated. The parameter selection procedure aims to assess and minimize the degree of underestimate by determining an intensity window which is spanned by most boundaries.

Although not demonstrated here, these methods may in principle be applied to structures which do not have definitive boundaries on all sides (e.g. cortical gyri) for which comparison of segmented volumes is clearly problematic. Note also that where a structure is bounded by regions both of higher and lower intensity, two intensity windows may be needed to account for the two possible directions of change. Validation of these methods is part of ongoing work.

# 6 Conclusions

We have proposed the BSI as a novel method for quantifying changes in cerebral volumes from registered repeat MR scans. We have found the method yields a highly reproducible and linear measure of volume change with levels of accuracy far higher than that of the segmentation on which it is based. We have demonstrated its application to obtaining both global and regional measures of loss. This methodology represents a powerful tool for the investigation of neurodegenerative disorders; potential applications include early diagnosis, monitoring progression and assessment of response to potential treatments.

**Acknowledgments:** We gratefully acknowledge support and advice from Dr. Martin Rossor (National Hospital for Neurology and Neurosurgery, London, UK) and Dr. Paul Tofts (Institute of Neurology, London, UK).

# References

1. C.R. Jack, R.C. Petersen, P.C. O'Brien, E.G. Tangalos: MR-based hippocampal volumetry in the diagnosis of Alzheimer's disease. Neurol 1992;42:183-188
2. C.A. Cuenod, A. Denys, J.L. Michot, P. Jehenson, F. Forette, D. Kaplan, A. Syrota, F Boller: Amygdala atrophy in Alzheimer's disease. An in vivo magnetic resonance imaging study. Arch Neurol 1993;50:941-945
3. S. Lehericy, M. Baulac, J. Chiras, L. Pierot, N. Martin, B. Pillon, B. Deweer, B. Dubois, C. Marsault: Amygdalohippocampal MR volume measurements in the early stages of Alzheimer disease. AJNR 1994;15:927-937
4. P.A. Freeborough, R.P. Woods, N.C. Fox: Accurate registration of serial 3D MR brain images and its application to visualizing in change in neurodegenerative disorders. J Comput Assist Tomogr 1996; 20:1012-1022
5. S.J. Nelson, B.S. Nalbandian, E. Proctor, D.B. Vigneron: Registration of images from sequential MR studies of the brain. Journal of Magnetic Resonance Imaging 1994;4:877-883
6. J.V. Hajnal, N. Saeed, A. Oatridge, E.J. Williams, I.R. Young, G.M. Bydder: Detection of subtle brain changes using subvoxel registration and subtraction of serial MR images. J Comput Assist Tomogr 1995;19:677-691
7. N.C. Fox, P.A. Freeborough, M.N. Rossor: Visualisation and quantification of atrophy in Alzheimer's disease. The Lancet 1996;348:94-97
8. P.A. Freeborough, N.C. Fox: Assessing patterns and rates of brain atrophy by serial magnetic resonance imaging: a segmentation, registration, display and quantification procedure. In: K.H. Hohne, R. Kikinis (eds.): Lecture Notes in Computer Science 1131 (Proc. VBC96). Berlin: Springer 1996, pp. 419-428
9. P.A. Freeborough, N.C. Fox, R.I. Kitney: Interactive algorithms for the segmentation and quantitation of 3-D MRI brain scans. Computer Methods and Programs in Biomedicine. In press.
10. K.H. Hohne, W.A. Hanson: Interactive segmentation of MRI and CT volumes using morphological operations. J Comput Assist Tomogr 1992;16:285-294

# Automatic Detection of Sulcal Bottom Lines in MR Images of the Human Brain

Gabriele Lohmann, Frithjof Kruggel, D. Yves von Cramon

Max-Planck-Institute of Cognitive Neuroscience, Inselstr. 22-26
04103 Leipzig, Germany
e-mail: {lohmann,kruggel}@cns.mpg.de

**Abstract.** This paper describes an automatic procedure for extracting sulcal bottom lines from MR (magnetic resonance) images of the human brain, which will serve as a tool for landmark extraction as well as for investigating the morphometry of sulci. The procedure consists of a sequence of several image processing steps, including morphological operators and a constrained distance transform which provides information about sulcal depth at each location.

## 1 Introduction

This paper describes an automatic procedure for extracting the bottom lines of the main cortical sulci from MR (magnetic resonance) images of the human brain. The sulci are deep narrow valleys or folds of the cortical surface.

The automatic detection of sulcal bottom lines is of interest for several reasons. Firstly, sulcal bottom lines are suited to serve as landmarks that can be used to reference brain locations in a way that is anatomically meaningful. Secondly, sulcal bottom lines allow us to represent an entire sulcus by a tree like structure of curves rather than of surfaces, and thus present a highly condensed representation of a prominent landmark.

Another aspect associated with the work reported here is that in the process of the extraction of sulcal bottom lines information about sulcal depth becomes available. This aspect may be relevant in studying interpersonal sulcal variability. It is, for instance, an ongoing question whether the interpersonal variability in sulcal patterns decreases with depth. The depth information made available by our method will hopefully help to address this issue from a new viewpoint.

Previous investigations of sulcal structure and interpersonal variability [1], [2], [3] were often based on manual segmentations and were therefore restricted to very few data sets. Automatic procedures for the identification of sulcal bottom lines have not been reported in the literature so far.

However, the automatic extraction of other prominent lines as landmarks from 3D data sets has received considerable attention. Particularly, the computation of curvature properties for the purpose of ridge line extraction should be mentioned. The methods described in [4],[5],[6],[7] fall into that category. Our approach differs in that it extracts lines of *maximal depth* as measured from the smoothed brain surface as opposed to lines of *maximal curvature*. Sulcal bottom lines do not usually coincide with lines of maximal curvature, so that ridge line extraction is not a viable approach to our problem.

The automatic extraction of sulcal structures has been the subject of several research projects either focusing on the extraction of sulcal skeletons [8] or sulcal surfaces [9],[10]. These techniques differ from ours in that they are not aimed at making depth information available.

Our bottom line extraction process consists of several steps beginning with a segmentation procedure to identify the sulcal interiors. We skeletonize the sulcal compartments to obtain medial surfaces which are then eroded until the bottom is reached. Finally, the resulting chains of bottom voxels are connected into a graph of polygons. In the following, each of these steps will be described in detail. The method reported here is an extension of our earlier work [11] improving it in both accuracy and computational efficiency.

## 2 Depth measurements

We start out with a white matter segmentation of the initial MR data set. To obtain the sulcus interior, we apply a 3D morphological closing filter using a sphere shaped structuring element of very large size, e.g. of radius 7 or larger. The difference between the binarized white matter image and the morphologically closed image yields the sulcal areas.

Once sulcal and white matter areas are labelled, depth measurements in the sulcal compartments are made. The technique used for this purpose is an adaptation of the constrained distance transform [12]. Each voxel which has been labelled as "sulcus interior" receives a depth label indicating its depth as measured from the idealized brain surface.

Standard distance transforms [13] require a binary image as input in which feature points are marked as "white" pixels. In the distance transformed image each "black" voxel receives a label indicating its distance from the nearest feature point.

Input images to constrained distance transforms may contain an additional third type of label which represent a class of "obstacle" points. The constrained distance transform attributes a distance label to each "black" voxel towards its nearest "white" voxel where the length is measured along paths that are forced to avoid voxels labelled as "obstacles". In the present case, the obstacle voxels are the ones that are labelled as "white matter". We now seek the lengths of shortest paths from each sulcal voxel towards the idealized surface which do not trespass white matter areas.

The distance transform is performed by moving two 3D filter masks over the image in two separate scans. The filter mask represents local distances which are propagated through the entire image as the algorithm progresses. Note that some voxels may be entirely surrounded by obstacle voxels so that no valid path to any feature voxel exists. Those voxels will of course remain unlabeled.

Shallow sulci can be eliminated by thresholding the output of the depth labeling procedure. Typically, we are only interested in sulci deeper than 4mm.

# 3  Extraction of sulcal medial surfaces

After the sulcal compartments have been identified, their medial surface is extracted. A large number of skeletonization algorithms have been reported in the literature, e.g. [14], [15],[16]. In our experiments we found that a modified version of Tsao's method [16] yielded the best results.

Tsao's algorithm performs a parallel deletion of directional border points where a voxel is a border voxel in a given principal direction (north, south, west, east, top, bottom) if its neighbour in that direction belongs to the background.

We modified this algorithm by changing the order in which points are considered for deletion. The basic idea[17] is the following: we first compute the distance transform of the image to be thinned such that each foreground voxel receives a label indicating its distance from the nearest background voxel. We then place all foreground voxels in an array and sort it by distance values. The points that receive the smallest distance values are the first to be considered for deletion, where the same deletion criteria and subcycle schedule as in Tsao's original algorithm is used. If no more points at this distance level can be deleted, we move on to the next higher distance value, and so on until all distance levels have been processed.

There are two prime advantages of this method over the original procedure. Firstly, by placing all foreground voxels into an array we do not need to scan the entire image for each deletion subcycle, and thus gain a considerable increase in computation speed. Secondly, by sorting this array according to distance values, we achieve a much better localization for the resulting skeleton as skeletal voxels are forced to reside on local maxima of the distance transform. Figure 1 shows two slices of a thinning result.

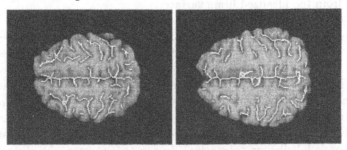

Figure 1: 3D Thinning: axial slices

# 4  Extraction of sulcal bottom lines

The next step consists in reducing the medial surface such that only its bottom line remains. We use a modification of the thinning algorithm to achieve this. The basic idea is to remove voxels at progressively deeper levels while leaving voxels at the sulcus ends unchanged.

As before, we place all foreground voxels belonging to the medial surface into an array. Note that each voxel in this array already has a depth label obtained in a previous step. We now use this labeling to sort the array by depth and begin by deleting voxels at the smallest depth level. Points are deletable if they are topologically simple, and if they are not endpoints, where end points are characterized by the fact that there are no more than two non-zero 26-adjacent voxels.

In contrast to our thinning procedure, deletion is now performed sequentially rather than in parallel as only sequential deletion is guaranteed to preserve topology. A pseudo-code version of the algorithm is given below:

```
BottomLine(image)
{
  copy medial surface voxels into array;
  sort array by depth;
  for (depth d = 1 to maxdepth) {
    ndelete = 1;
    while (ndelete > 0) {
      ndelete = 0;
      for (all voxels v in array at depth d) {
        if (not EndVoxel(v) and SimplePoint(v)) {
          Delete(v);
          ndelete = ndelete + 1;
        }
      }
    }
  }
}
```

The above procedure reduces sulcal medial surfaces to sulcus bottom lines so that at the end of this stage only one-voxel thick chains of foreground voxels remain.

We now transfer the binary raster image into a graph structure by first creating a node for each foreground voxel specifying its voxel address and its depth. We then establish links between nodes such that each node is connected to all its 26-adjacent neighbouring nodes. We thus obtain an undirected graph with a symmetric arc relation where adjacent nodes are linked in both directions. Lastly, spurious branches are pruned in a final postprocessing step.

# 5 Experiments

The method was applied to seven T1 weighted MRI data sets from three different MR scanners. The same set of parameters was used for all data sets. The results were checked manually by two human experts (neurologists) doing random checks. The results were found to be correct in almost every case. The only errors that were found are related to the following systematic problem.

The algorithm blindly interprets every cavity or indentation within the white matter as a sulcus. Therefore, structures such as the basal ganglia and the ventricles are filled with a "sulcus" line unless those structures have been masked out beforehand. For the same reason, the Cisterna pontis and Cisterna vallecula cerebri are also wrongly interpreted as "sulci" causing a conglomeration of lines around the brain basis connecting the two hemispheres. In our experiments, we used a visual editor to manually break and remove such obviously incorrect lines. With the exception of those systematic errors, the results were found to be correct.

Figure 2 shows some bottom lines resulting from one such experiment, indicating how the verification was done: the mouse cursor is linked to the sagittal, coronal and axial slices of the data set so that a mouse click onto a node in the graph automatically positions the cursor to the corresponding location in the MR data set, so that the expert can assess the correctness of the location of a node.

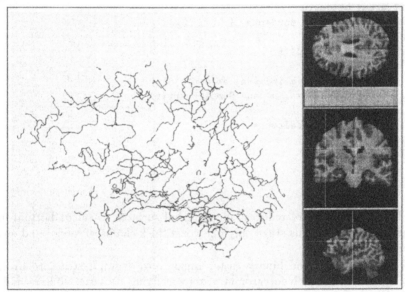

Figure 2: Sulcus bottom lines

# 6   Conclusion

A new method for the extraction of sulcal bottom lines was presented. The method is essentially parameter free with the exception of two thresholding parameters for the postprocessing step and another threshold applied to the depth labelled image to exclude shallow sulci. All three thresholds are uncritical in the sense that standard settings can be adopted.

Our method will serve both as a tool for landmark extraction as well as a tool for investigating the morphometry of sulci. Future work will focus on a classification of sulcus types and on studying interpersonal variability of sulcal structures. The depth information provided by this tool will play a central role in this work. In particular, we hope that this method will help to clarify to question of whether or not interpersonal variability decreases with depth.

# References

1. M. Ono, S. Kubik, C.D. Abernathy. *Atlas of the cerebral sulci*. Georg Thieme Verlag, Stuttgart, New York, 1990.
2. T. Paus, F. Tomaiuolo, N. Otaky, D. MacDonald, M. Petrides, J. Atlas, R. Morris, A.C. Evans. Human cingulate and paracingulate sulci: pattern, variability, asymmetry, and probabilistic map. *Cerebral Cortex*, 6:207–214, Mar/Apr 1996.
3. P.M. Thompson, C.Schwartz, R.T. Lin, A.A. Khan, A.T. Toga. Three-dimensional statistical analysis of sulcal variability in the human brain. *The Journal of Neuroscience*, 16(13):4261–4274, 1996.
4. J. Declerck, G. Subsol, J.-P. Thirion, N. Ayache. Automatic retrieval of anatomical structures in 3D medical images. In N. Ayache, editor, *Computer Vision, Virtual Reality and Robotics in Medicine*, pages 153–162, Nice, France, April 1995. Springer Lecture Notes, 905.
5. A. Guéziec, N. Ayache. Smoothing and matching of 3-d space curves. *International Journal of Computer Vision*, 12(1):79–104, 1994.
6. O. Monga, S. Benayoun. Using partial derivatives of 3d images to extract typical surface features. *Computer vision and image understanding*, 61(2):171–189, March 1995.
7. J.P. Thirion, A. Gourdon. The marching lines algorithm: new results and proofs. *Technical Report No. 1881*, April 1993.
8. R.L. Ogniewicz, G. Szekely, O. Kübler. Detection of prominent boundary points based on structural characteristics of the hierarchic medial axis transform. In H. (Hrsg.) Pöppl, S. H.; Handels, editor, *15. DAGM-Symposium, Mustererkennung 1993*, pages 321–331. Springer Verlag, 1993.
9. Yaorong Ge, J.Michael Fitzgerald, Benoit M. Dawant, Jun Bao, Robert M. Kessler, Richard A. Margolin. Accurate localization of cortical convolutions in MR brain images. *IEEE Transactions on Medical Imaging*, 15(4):418–428, Aug. 1996.
10. M. Valliant, C. Davatzikos, R.N. Bryan. Finding 3D parametric representations of the deep cortical folds. In *Proc. Mathematical Methods in biomedical image analysis (MMBIA 96)*, pages 151–157, San Francisco, CA, June 1996. IEEE Computer Society.
11. G. Lohmann, F. Kruggel. Extracting lines of maximal depth from MRI images of the human brain. In *Proc. Intern. Conf. on Pattern Recognition*, Wien, Aug. 1996.
12. P.W.Verbeek, L. Dorst, B.J.H.Verwer, F.C.A. Groen. Collision avoidance and path finding through constrained distance transformation in robot state space. In *Proc. Intelligent Autonomous Systems*, pages 634–641, Amsterdam, The Netherlands, Dec. 1986.
13. G. Borgefors. Distance transforms in arbitrary dimensions. *Computer Vision, Graphics, and Image Processing*, 27:321–345, 1984.
14. T.C.Lee, R.L.Kashyap, C.N. Chu. Building skeleton models via 3-d medial surface axis thinning algorithms. *Computer Vision, Graphics, and Image Processing*, 56(6):462–478, 1994.
15. R.L. Ogniewicz, M. Ilg. Voronoi skeletons: theory and applications. In *Proc. Computer Vision and Pattern Recognition (CVPR 92)*, pages 63–69. Computer Society Press, 1992.
16. Y.F. Tsao, K.S. Fu. A parallel thinning algorithm for 3d pictures. *Computer Graphics Image Proc.*, 17:315–331, 1981.
17. G. Malandain. personal communication, July 1996.

# Segmentation and Interpretation of MR Brain Images Using an Improved Knowledge-Based Active Shape Model

Nicolae Duta[2], Milan Sonka[1]

[1] Department of Electrical and Computer Engineering
[2] Department of Computer Science, The University of Iowa, Iowa City, IA 52242

**Abstract.** An improvement of the *Active Shape* procedure introduced by Cootes and Taylor is presented. The new automated brain segmentation and interpretation approach incorporates *a priori* knowledge about neuroanatomic structures and their specific structural relationships to provide robust segmentation and labeling.

The method was trained in 8 MR brain images and tested in 19 brain images by comparison to observer-defined independent standards. Neuroanatomic structures in all images from the test set were successfully identified. The presented method is applicable to virtually any task involving deformable shape analysis.

## 1  Introduction

The goal of our work reported here is to improve the *Active Shape* procedure introduced by Cootes and Taylor [1,2] to find new examples of previously learned shapes using the point distribution models. This approach is particularly useful in medical image analysis since human organs are not rigid and the variations in shape and appearance are difficult to model.

Automatic detection of brain structures is motivated by an ongoing effort to advance knowledge about relationships between anatomy and mental diseases in human brains. To date, most of the image segmentation in neuroscientific studies that utilize CT, MR, or PET rely on manual tracing. Despite the substantial interest and effort in the development of automated methods to identify brain structures, no reliable automated tools are available to date. The automated brain segmentation and interpretation approach described below represents a novel approach that incorporates *a priori* knowledge about neuroanatomic structures and their specific structural relationships to provide robust segmentation and labeling.

## 2  PDM Approach to MR Brain Image Interpretation

In many areas of image segmentation and interpretation, reliable a priori knowledge is available to help guide the image analysis process. For instance, in brain imaging, the image data are routinely represented in a normalized Talairach space. Consequently, approximate positions of individual neuroanatomic structures can be determined. Knowledge about their sizes, shapes, gray level appearance, etc. can be acquired from a training set of examples.

## 2.1 Knowledge-Based Point Distribution Model

In order to improve the shape model and to take advantage of the available a priori knowledge, three additional features characteristic to MR brain images were included in the model: Gray-level appearance, border strength, and average position. In the implementation described below, we also used the implicit knowledge about object context representing inter-relationships of several objects and the fact that all objects of interest were always present in the image we search, a condition not applicable generally but appropriate for our application.

**Gray-level appearance** is calculated in neighborhoods around each of the shape model points. It is determined for every shape model point $j$ of each training image along a profile $g_j$ of a constant length, centered at the point $j$. Since the profiles vary with gray level scaling, derivatives of the gray levels along each profile are determined and normalized.

**Border strength** is determined for each border segment of the model. Every two consecutive model points that lie on the object boundary define a border segment. To compute its strength, a local filtering is applied to each clique on that border segment. The filter is based on a pair of close parallel profiles.

**Average position** of each shape model point that is calculated in the image coordinates is also incorporated in the model.

Our **knowledge-based shape model** combines generally applicable parameters of the point distribution model and the knowledge-specific parameters appropriate for the image segmentation task in question. As such, the complete model is composed of:

1. The eigenvectors corresponding to the largest eigenvalues of the covariance matrix describing the *Allowable Shape Domain* [1,2].
2. The average gray level appearance values for each point of the model.
3. The average border strength for corresponding border segments and the parameters of the mask (width, length) for which the strength was computed.
4. The average position of the points of the average shape.
5. Connectivity information (the number of shapes, point ordering along contours).

## 2.2 Searching for Objects: Model Fitting

The searching procedure developed for our PDM approach to image segmentation and interpretation is based on the model fitting strategy that substantially differs from the *Active Shape Procedure* of Cootes and Taylor. The difference is twofold. First, our search is entirely model driven meaning that segmentation hypotheses are not influenced by possibly misleading image data and do not use any preprocessing. At each step of the fitting process, several model location hypotheses are considered and evaluated. Second, an outlier detection and re-placement procedure has been developed to detect misplaced points and infer their new positions. The outlier detection improves robustness and accuracy of the shape model fitting process. The searching procedure consists of the following steps: 1) Model fitting using linear transforms, 2) model fitting using piecewise linear transforms, 3) outlier removal, 4) final point adjustment, 5) final outlier removal.

**Model Fitting Function** As a result of the hypotheses generation processes, shape model locations are sequentially hypothesized. In order to evaluate the model location hypotheses, a *fitness function* is needed to assess the agreement between the image data and the particular model instance. We have designed a *fitness function* $F = F_B/(F_{GA})^2$ that consists of two components:

1. *Fitness of the gray level appearance* $F_{GA}$ is determined as the average squared Euclidean distance between the actual gray level appearance and the mean gray level profile incorporated in the shape model.
2. *Fitness of the border* $F_B$ is calculated as the ratio between the aggregate response of all four point cliques along the contour and the maximum possible response (twice the number of cliques).

**Model fitting using linear transforms** Shape instance hypotheses specify the locations of all model points within the analyzed image. The hypotheses are generated using affine transformations and are applied to the model average position. All generated hypotheses are sequentially evaluated using the model fitting function $F$ and the best fit is determined.

**Model fitting using piecewise linear transforms** Since non-rigid objects or object with inter-subject variability are discussed here, rigid linear transforms do not account for any potential deformations of the expected shape. Therefore, affine transforms are applied to subsets of 5–7 consecutive model points.

**Outlier removal** Under unfavorable circumstances, the previous step may in-troduce incorrectly determined vertices – **outliers**. This may happen if a sub-shape fitted by the previous step exhibits weak edges or if there exists another border of similar properties in the neighborhood. In the existing literature deal-ing with point distribution models, no outlier detection has been introduced. Typically, when using PDM's, shapes that do not correspond to the allowed shape at any stage of the detection process are rejected (Fig. 1).

To treat the problem of outliers in a systematic fashion, an approach to outlier detection and position adjustment was developed. The misplaced points are identified using the information about the relative positions of the shape model vertices that are implicitly included in the shape model. Let $z = (x', y')^T$ be the model point positions after the piecewise linear transforms were applied and the resulting shape was aligned with the shape average. According to the shape model, the hypothesized shape should satisfy $z = \bar{x} + Pb$ where $\bar{x}$ is the average shape, $P$ is the matrix of the first $t$ eigenvectors, and $b$ is a vector of

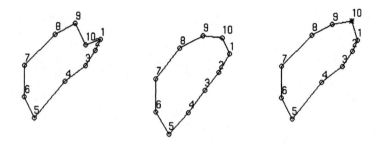

**Fig. 1.** Example of a shape hypothesis rejected by the Cootes' ASM procedure (left). Note the one outlier responsible for rejection (marked by 10). The same shape hypothesis after our outlier removal and adjustment steps (right, adjusted vertex marked by *). The average shape is shown in the middle.

weights. Therefore,

$$b_j = \sum_{i=1}^{n} P_{i,j}(z_i - \bar{\mathbf{x}}_i) = \sum_{i=1}^{n} v_{i,j} \tag{1}$$

where

$$|v_{i,j}| = |P_{i,j}(z_i - \bar{\mathbf{x}}_i)| \tag{2}$$

is the absolute variation induced by point $i$ in parameter $b_j$. Let the percentage of variation induced by point $i$ in parameter $b_j$ be defined as

$$V_{i,j} = \frac{|v_{i,j}|}{\sum_{i=1}^{n} |v_{i,j}|} \cdot 100 \tag{3}$$

and let the maximum percentage of variation induced by point $i$ in any of the parameters $b_j$ be defined as

$$u_i = \max_{j=1..t} V_{i,j} \tag{4}$$

If all the points were to generate an equal amount of variation, then all the percentages $u_i$ were approximately $100/n$, $n$ being the number of object points. However, since outliers may be present, larger variation may be associated with some points – the outliers. A point is considered to be an outlier if the percentage of variance generated by its position in any of the parameters $b_i$ of the model is more than 4× greater than the average amount of variation. If several outliers are present, the variance is distributed among them and (perhaps) the well placed points. As a result, it is difficult to identify outliers if more than a few occur simultaneously. Once such misplaced points are detected, they must be moved to a new position that can be inferred from the alignment of the rest of the shape instance with the average shape.

**Final point adjustment** Some of the shape model points may have been declared outliers in the previous step. Consequently, their position may have been

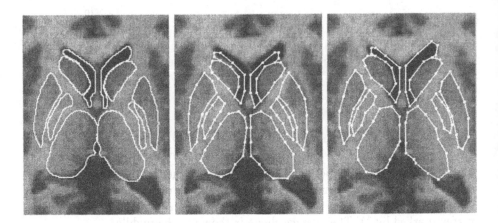

**Fig. 2.** Example of automated brain image segmentation and interpretation. From left to right: Manual tracings. Initial average position of the shape model. Automated segmentation.

adjusted solely considering the average shape appearance and not considering the image data. Therefore, they must be subjected to the position optimization step to better correspond with the image data.

**Final outlier removal** Resulting from the previous steps or newly introduced during the final point adjustment, outliers may remain present in the shape model. Following the same outlier detection procedure applied in the first outlier removal step, the outliers are identified and removed, no adjustment is attempted in this final step of model fitting.

## 3 Experimental Methods

The method presented above was employed to design a PDM shape model for ten neuroanatomic structures: left/right ventricles, left/right caudate nucleus, left/right putamen, left/right globus pallidus, left/right thalamus.

The knowledge-based PDM image interpretation method was tested in in vivo MR brain images. The image set consisted of individual T1-weighted contiguous MR images of the human brain, imaged in the coronal plane and acquired from a GE 1.5 Tesla Signa scanner with in-slice resolution of $256 \times 256$ pixels, slice thickness 1.5 mm, and a field of view of 26 cm. The images were acquired from 27 subjects and "normalized" using a three-dimensional proportional Talairach grid system.

Observer-defined contours identified by a neuroanatomist were available for all the images in the brain data set. However, a subset of 8 images from this set, called the training set, served for the shape model construction. The remaining 19 images formed the test set that was used for validation.

Performance of the PDM approach to image interpretation was assessed in the test set by quantitatively comparing the labels, areas, and border positions of identified neuroanatomic structures with those determined by the observer-defined independent standard. Signed area error, labeling error and border positioning error were used as measures for comparing the observer-defined and computer-determined contours of neuroanatomic structures. The calculated indices were identical to those previously employed in [3].

## 4 Results

The PDM approach to brain image segmentation and interpretation correctly interpreted the brain neuroanatomic structures in all images from the test set. Fig. 2 shows the observer-traced and computer-detected contours. In the test set, the neuroanatomic structures were identified with the signed percent area error of $12 \pm 5\%$ and labeling error of $7 \pm 3\%$. Border positioning errors were quite small, with the average border positioning error of $0.8 \pm 0.1$ pixels, and maximum border positioning error of $4.3 \pm 1.2$ pixels. The detection time was about 3 minutes using a combination of C and MATLAB running on an HP 750 workstation.

## 5 Conclusion

A new fully automated segmentation and interpretation method has been presented in which a novel outlier-detection approach was successfully utilized. Compared to our previously-reported brain image segmentation and interpretation approach [3], our new method described here offers comparable segmentation and interpretation performance while the speed of the interpretation process has increased thirty times.

## Acknowledgments

The authors wish to express their thanks to Nancy Andreasen, M.D., Ph.D., Michael Flaum, M.D., Rajprabhakar Rajarethinam, M.D.; and Ted Cizadlo, M.S. for providing both original and manually-traced MR brain data utilized in the presented study. Computer facility support of Prof. George Stockman after N. Duta moved to the Michigan State University is also gratefully acknowledged. This work was supported in part by the NSF grant IRI 96-16747.

## References

1. T F Cootes, A Hill, C J Taylor, and J Haslam. Use of active shape models for locating structures in medical images. *Image & Vision Computing*, 12(6):355–366, 1994.
2. T F Cootes, C J Taylor, D H Cooper, and J Graham. Active shape models – their training and application. *Computer Vision and Image Understanding*, 61:38–59, 1995.
3. M Sonka, S K Tadikonda, and S M Collins. Knowledge-based interpretation of MR brain images. *IEEE Trans. Med. Imaging*, 15:443–452, 1996.

# Gaussian Random Fields on Sub-Manifolds for Characterizing Brain Surfaces*

Sarang C. Joshi, Ayananshu Banerjee, Gary E. Christensen John G. Csernansky,
John W. Haller, Michael I. Miller, and Lei Wang

Washington University, St. Louis, Missouri 63130.

**Abstract.** This paper provides analytical methods for characterizing the variation of the shape of neuro-anatomically significant substructures of the brain in an ensemble of brain images. The focus of this paper is on the neuro-anatomical variation of the "shape" of 2-dimensional surfaces in the brain. Brain surfaces are studied by building templates that are smooth sub-manifolds of the underlying coordinate system of the brain. Variation of the shape in populations is quantified via defining Gaussian random vector fields on these sub-manifolds. Methods for the empirical construction of Gaussian random vector fields for representing the variations of the substructures are presented. As an example, using these methods we characterize the shape of the hippocampus in a population of *normal* controls and *schizophrenic* brains. Results from a recently completed study comparing shapes of the hippocampus in a group of matched schizophrenic and normal control subjects are presented. Bayesian hypothesis test is formulated to cluster the normal and schizophrenic hippocampi in the population of 20 individuals.

## 1   Introduction

We have been studying brain anatomy in humans, as imaged via MRI-MPRAGE sequences by representing the typical global structures via the construction of templates, and their variabilities by the definition of probabilistic diffeomorphic transformations applied to the templates[1, 2, 3, 4, 5]. The transformations are defined by diffeomorphisms $h : \Omega \leftrightarrow \Omega$ of the coordinate system of the template defined as $\Omega$. The dimension of the transformation,

$$h : x = (x_1, x_2, x_3) \in \Omega \mapsto h(x) = (h^1(x_1), h^2(x_2), h^3(x_3)) \in \Omega ,$$

is roughly equivalent to the number of voxels in the volume, thereby accommodating a very fine variation in anatomy. The transformation $h$, mapping the coordinate system of the template to that of the target is estimated using the procedure developed in [5, 6].

We have been using these transformations to study the "shape" of neuro-anatomically significant substructures in the brain by representing them as smooth sub-manifolds of the template and using the maps to transform the sub-manifolds from the template to the target. Using these transformations we have been quantifying the variation of the shape in a population by empirically building Gaussian random fields on these sub-manifolds that characterize the population.

## 2   Gaussian Fields on 2-D Sub-Manifolds.

### 2.1   Constructing 2-D Brain Sub-Manifolds.

We begin with whole brain volumes generated via MRI MP-RAGE imaging consisting of $256^2 \times 160$ voxels as shown in Figure 1. The neuro-anatomical substructure of interest is carefully hand-segmented in a MR data set. Figure 1 shows the MR brain volume and the manual segmentation of the hippocampus. Using these contours a triangulated graph representing the surface of the substructure is generated using the Marching Cubes algorithm[7]. The bottom left panel of Figure 1 shows a the triangulated graph representing the hippocampal surface.

The surface $\mathcal{M}$ representing the neuro-anatomically significant substructure is assumed to be a smooth two-dimensional differential sub-manifold of $\Omega \subset \mathbb{R}^3$ of class two ($C^2$), i.e., each point $x \in \mathcal{M}$ has a neighborhood $U$ diffeomorphic to an open subset $D$ of $\mathbb{R}^2$, $U \subset \mathcal{M} \underset{\phi^{-1}}{\overset{\phi}{\rightleftharpoons}} D \subset \mathbb{R}^2$ , where $\phi$ is a diffeomorphism at least twice differentiable. Each pair $(U, \phi)$ is called a coordinate neighborhood or a local chart.

A second order local chart is established at each point in the surface by locally approximating

$$\phi^{-1} : (u, v) \in D \to \phi^{-1}(u, v) = x(u, v) \in \mathcal{M} \tag{1}$$

by up to the quadratic terms in it's Taylor series following the procedure developed in [8].

With the template surface represented as a smooth $C^2$ sub-manifold of $\Omega$ we can use the diffeomorphic transformations generated following [5, 6], to study the surface in ensembles of brain data. Let $h : \Omega \leftrightarrow \Omega$ represent the diffeomorphism mapping the template to the target. As the diffeomorphism maps the underlying coordinate system of the template to that of the target we define the surface of interest in the target brain as the image of the template surface under $h$:

* This work was supported in part by the NIH grants RR01380, RO1-MH52158-01A1, ARO DAAL-03-86-K-0110, NSF grant BIR-9424264 and a grant from the Whittaker Foundation.

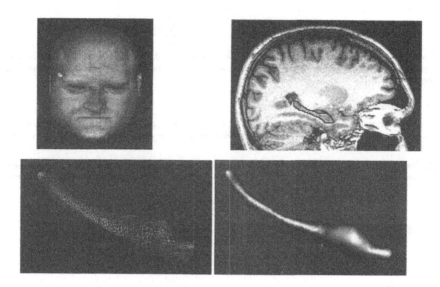

**Fig. 1.** The top left shows a whole MRI-MPRAGE image volume. The top right panel shows a section through the brain delineating the surface of the hippocampus. The bottom left panel shows the triangulated graph representing the hippocampal surface. Top right panel shows the rendering of the hippocampal surface represented as a smooth manifold.

$$\mathcal{M}^d = h \circ \mathcal{M} = \{h(x) : x \in \mathcal{M}\} \ .$$

As $h$ is a diffeomorphism of $\Omega \leftrightarrow \Omega$ than by theorem (5.5), Pg. 78 of Boothby [9], $\mathcal{M}^d$ is also a smooth sub-manifold of $\Omega$.

### 2.2 Gaussian fields on 2-D Sub-Manifolds.

To study the variation of the sub-manifolds we represent the sub-manifolds in the ensemble as a deformation around the template. Define the diffeomorphisms $\{h_i, i = 1, \cdots, N\}$ mapping the template volume on to each of the $N$ studies. The sub-manifold in each of the targets is defined as the image of the template under the transformation $h_i$, the corresponding deformation field is given by

$$u_i(x) = h_i(x) - x, x \in \mathcal{M} \ .$$

We assume that these deformation fields are realization from a Gaussian random vector field on the sub-manifold $\mathcal{M}$. These Gaussian fields then completely characterize the variation of the sub-manifold. For this define the inner product on the Hilbert space $\mathcal{H}(\mathcal{M})$ to be

$$\langle f, g \rangle = \int_{\mathcal{M}} f^1(x) g^1(x) d\nu(x) + \int_{\mathcal{M}} f^2(x) g^2(x) d\nu(x) + \int_{\mathcal{M}} f^3(x) g^3(x) d\nu(x) \ ,$$

where $d\nu$ is a measure on the oriented manifold (see [9] ).

**Definition 1.** The random field $\{U(x), x \in \mathcal{M}\}$ is a Gaussian field on a manifold $\mathcal{M}$ with mean $\mu_u \in \mathcal{H}(\mathcal{M})$ and covariance operator $K_u(x, y)$ if $\forall f \in \mathcal{H}(\mathcal{M})$, $\langle f, \cdot \rangle$ is normally distributed with mean $m_f = \langle \mu_u, f \rangle$ and variance $\sigma_y^2 = \langle K_u f, f \rangle$

Note that the Gaussian field is completely specified by it's mean $\mu_u$ and the covariance operator $K_u(x, y)$. We shall construct the Gaussian random fields $\{U(x), x \in \mathcal{M}\}$ as a quadratic mean limit using a complete $\mathbb{R}^3$-valued orthonormal basis $\{\phi_k, k = 1, 2, \cdots\}, \phi_k$ is $\mathbb{R}^3$-valued, spanning the space of square integrable vector fields on $\mathcal{M}$. The quadratic mean Gaussian field $\{U(x), x \in \mathcal{M}\}$ is defined to be the quadratic mean limit as

$$U(x) \stackrel{\text{q.m}}{=} \sum_{k=1}^{\infty} Z_k \phi_k(x) \ ,$$

with $\{Z_k, k = 1, \cdots\}$ are independent, Gaussian random variables with fixed means $E\{Z_k\} = \mu_k$ and variances $E\{|Z_k|^2\} - E^2\{Z_k\} = \sigma_k^2$. The Gaussian field is completely specified by it's mean and covariance operator,

$$E\{U(x)\} = \sum_{k=1}^{\infty} \mu_k \phi_k(x) \ , \ K_U(x,y) = \sum_{k=1}^{\infty} \sigma_k^2 \phi_k(x) \phi_k^T(y) \ .$$

It will be assumed that the means and variances decay quickly enough so that the quadratic mean limit exists, minimally requiring that the field have a covariance $K_U$ with finite trace, $\sum_k \sigma_k^2 < \infty$, and the mean is square integrable, $\sum_k |\mu_k|^2 < \infty$

### 2.3 Empirical construction of covariance

We now present results on using eigen methods[10, 11, 12] for generating the covariance empirically. This is principle component analysis used in classical statistics. For this we establish the principle components on square integrable vector fields on surfaces.

**Theorem 2.** *Let $U(x), x \in \mathcal{M}$ be a zero mean Gaussian random vector field on a manifold $\mathcal{M}$ with covariance $K_U(x,y)$. The set of orthonormal functions, $\{\phi_i(x), i = 1, \cdots, N, x \in \mathcal{M}\}$, that minimize the mean squared error*

$$\arg\min_{\phi_i} \ E\{\int_{\mathcal{M}} ||U(x) - \sum_{i=1}^{N} Z_i \phi_i(x)||^2 d\nu(x)\} \ , \tag{2}$$

*where $Z_i = \int_{\mathcal{M}} U^T(x)\phi_i(x)d\nu(x)$ , and $d\nu$ is the measure on the manifold $\mathcal{M}$, satisfy the integral equation*

$$\lambda_i \phi_i(x) = \int_{\mathcal{M}} K_U(x,y)\phi_i(y)d\nu(y) \ . \tag{3}$$

Given a family of maps $\{u^i, i = 1, \cdots N\}$ mapping the template sub-manifold $\mathcal{M}$ to $N$ studies, the empirical estimate of the covariance operator of the sample is given by

$$\hat{K}_U(x,y) = \frac{1}{N} \sum_{i=1}^{N} u_i(x)u_i(x)^T$$

We now numerically compute the eigen functions and eigen values of the empirical covariance $\hat{K}_U(x,y)$. Algorithm for generating the eigen functions becomes:

1. Let $\{\phi^{(i)}, i = 1, \cdots, N\}$ be vectors of length $3M$ with $\phi_k^{(i)} = \phi_i(x_k)$, $\Lambda$ be a diagonal matrix of size $3M \times 3M$ with $\Lambda_{3j,3j} = \Lambda_{3j+1,3j+1} = \Lambda_{3j+2,3j+2} = \nu(y_j)$, and $\hat{K}_U$ be a $3M \times 3M$ symmetric matrix with $\hat{K}_{i,j} = \hat{K}_U(x_i, x_j)$. The system of linear equations in theorem 2 becomes $\lambda_i \phi^{(i)} = \hat{K}\Lambda\phi^{(i)}$ ,$i = 1, \cdots, N$ .
2. The eigen basis $\{\phi^{(i)}, i = 1, \cdots, N\}$ are generated by diagonalizing the matrix $\hat{K}\Lambda$. Define the $3M \times N$ matrix $U$ with entries $U_{i,j} = \frac{1}{\sqrt{N-1}} u_j(x_i)$ $j = 1, \cdots, N$ . As $\Lambda$ is a diagonal matrix with positive elements on the diagonal $\lambda_i \sqrt{\Lambda}\phi^{(i)} = \sqrt{\Lambda}UU^T\sqrt{\Lambda}\sqrt{\Lambda}\phi^{(i)}$ .
3. Define $\bar{\phi}^i = \sqrt{\Lambda}\phi^i$. Then $\bar{\phi}^i$ satisfy $\lambda_i \bar{\phi}^{(i)} = (\sqrt{\Lambda}U)(\sqrt{\Lambda}U)^T \bar{\phi}^{(i)}$ .
4. The matrix $(\sqrt{\Lambda}U) \in \mathbb{R}^{3M \times N}$ using Singular Value Decomposition (SVD)[13] can be factored as the product $OWV$ where $O \in \mathbb{R}^{3M \times N}$ is an orthogonal matrix whose columns are the eigenvectors of $(\sqrt{\Lambda}U)(\sqrt{\Lambda}U)^T$ and $W^2$ is a diagonal matrix of the respective eigenvalues.
5. The eigen maps $\{\phi^i, i = 1, \cdots, N\}$ are given by

$$\sqrt{\Lambda}^{-1}O \ .$$

The eigen basis computed characterize the variation of the "shape" of the surface $\mathcal{M}$ in the population.

## 3 Characterizing a 2-D Brain Sub-Manifold: The Hippocampal Surface

We now present results on the shape of the hippocampus from a study directed by Dr. John Csernansky and Dr. John Haller of the Department of Psychiatry at Washington University [14, 15]. A MR data set was carefully hand-segmented to generate the hippocampus. Figure 1 shows the MR brain volume and the manual segmentation of the hippocampus. This segmentation provides the template hippocampus $\mathcal{M}_0$, represented as a smooth $C^2$ sub-manifold of $\Omega$ following the procedure outlined in Section 2. From the template hippocampus $\mathcal{M}_0$, the diffeomorphic maps were generated to map the hippocampus in an ensemble of 20 brain volumes. The template hippocampus was transformed onto the family of 20 targets. The target hippocampus is defined as the image of the template hippocampus $\mathcal{M}_0$, under the transformation $h$ mapping the template brain volume to the target. Shown in Figure 2 are three rendered surfaces embedded in the three target volumes $h_i \circ \mathcal{M}_0, i = 1, \cdots 4$. These surfaces were generated by transforming the template hippocampus through the volume transformations carrying the template onto the targets.

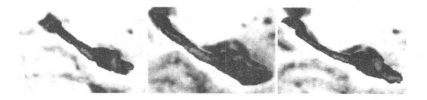

**Fig. 2.** The figure shows three rendered surfaces in three of the the the target volumes of the template hippocampus deformed under the transformations.

### 3.1 Mean Hippocampus of the Population

To statistically quantify shape variation of the hippocampus in the population we first construct the Mean or the composite Hippocampus representing the population under study. As proven in Grenander and Miller [16] , under small deformation assumptions, the empirical average of the family of maps $\{h_i, i = 1, \ldots, N\}$ provides the minimum mean-squared error (M.M.S.E.) estimate of the deformation and is the minimum energy representation of the ensemble of brain data. The mean transformation and the mean hippocampus becomes

$$\bar{h} = \frac{1}{N} \sum_{i=1}^{N} h_i \quad , \quad \bar{\mathcal{M}} = \bar{h} \circ \mathcal{M}_0$$

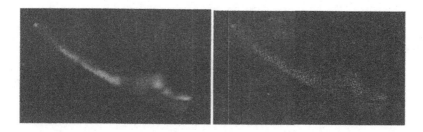

**Fig. 3.** Left panel shows the mean hippocampus of the population of 20 studies. The right panel shows the triangulated graph representing the template hippocampus.

Shown in left panel of Figure 3 is the image of the template hippocampus under the mean transformation $\mathcal{M} = \bar{h} \circ \mathcal{M}_0$. This represents the mean of the population. Shown in Figure 3 is the smooth structure and the associated triangulated graph.

### 3.2 Bayes testing on shape variation between populations.

To quantify the shape variation in the population we use the empirical eigen basis described in section 2.3. Using the procedure outlined in section 2.3 we compute the empirical covariance and it's eigen functions from the 20 deformation fields. To visualize the eigen shapes $\mathcal{E}^k, k = 1, \cdots, N$ of the hippocampus we construct the new surfaces relative to the mean $\bar{\mathcal{M}}$, $\mathcal{E}^k = \{x + (\lambda_i^2)\phi_i(x) : x \in \bar{\mathcal{M}}\}$. Shown in Figure 4 are the first six eigen shapes of the hippocampus generated from the 20 maps. The eigen basis computed characterize the "shape" of the hippocampus

We now set up the problem for testing the statistical hypotheses about the shape of the hippocampus in the two populations *Normals* and *Schizophrenics*. To test the null hypothesis $H_0$, meaning a normal hippocampus, against the alternative hypothesis $H_1$, we need to calculate the likelihood ratio

$$L(u) = \frac{P_1(u)}{P_0(u)} \ .$$

We the expand the deformation field $u$ in the eigen functions $\phi_i$ as $u_N(x) = \sum_{k=1}^{N}(Z_k)\phi_k(x)$ . We assume that the deformation fields $\{U_{norm}, U_{schiz}\}$ are Gaussian random fields with means $\{\bar{u}_{norm}, \bar{u}_{schiz}\}$ and covariance $K_U(x, y)$. In general this will not be true. We are currently analyzing more brains to determine the different covariances empirically. Under this assumption the expansion coefficients $Z_k$ are independent Gaussian random variables with probability densities given by:

$$p_1(Z_1, \cdots, Z_N) = \Pi_{i=1}^N \frac{1}{\sqrt{(2\pi\sigma_i^2)}} e^{-\frac{(z_i - \hat{z}_i^{schiz})^2}{2\sigma_i^2}} \qquad p_0(Z_1, \cdots, Z_N) = \Pi_{i=1}^N \frac{1}{\sqrt{(2\pi\sigma_i^2)}} e^{-\frac{(z_i - \hat{z}_i^{norm})^2}{2\sigma_i^2}} ,$$

where $\sigma_i^2$ are the eigen values of the covariance $K_U(x, y)$ shown in the left panel of Figure 5 and $\bar{Z}_i^{schiz} = \frac{1}{10} \sum_{k=1}^{10} (Z_i^k)_{schiz}$ $\bar{Z}_i^{norm} = \frac{1}{10} \sum_{k=1}^{10} (Z_i^k)_{norm}$ . The log-likelihood ratio $\Lambda_N = \log L_N(u)$ is given by

$$\Lambda_N = \sum_{i=1}^N -\frac{(Z_i - \bar{Z}_i^{schiz})^2}{2\sigma_i^2} + \frac{(Z_i - \bar{Z}_i^{norm})^2}{2\sigma_i^2} . \tag{4}$$

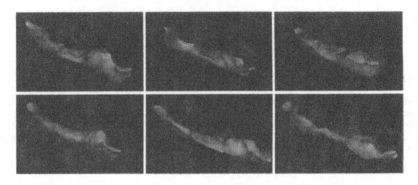

**Fig. 4.** This figure shows the first six eigen shapes of the hippocampus generated from a population of twenty maps.

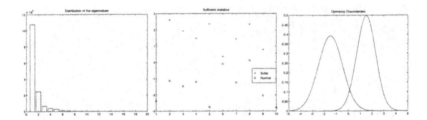

**Fig. 5.** The left panel shows the distribution of the eigen values of the covariance generated from a population of twenty maps. The middle panel shows the sufficient statistics $\Lambda$ plotted for the normal (o) and the schizophrenic (+) studies. The right panel shows the operating characteristics the test statistics $\Lambda$.

The Bayes hypothesis test for this population becomes:

$$\Lambda_N \underset{H_1}{\overset{H_0}{\lessgtr}} 0$$

We now compute the sufficient statistics for the 10 normal and 10 schizophrenic subjects under study. The middle panel of Figure 5 shows the plot of the sufficient statistics for the populations using 10 eigen basis. The schizophrenics are plotted with a "+" and the normals with a "o". Having introduced the statistics $\Lambda$ above to cluster the two groups we now study the probability of miss classification. We do this by finding the probability density of the test statistics $\Lambda$. As $\Lambda$ is a linear combination of Gaussian random variables $Z_i$, $\Lambda$ itself is Gaussian distributed under the two hypothesis. Under $H_0$, $\Lambda$ is Gaussian distributed with mean $\mu_0$ and variance $\sigma_0^2$ and under $H_1$ it is Gaussian distributed with mean $\mu_1$ and variance $\sigma_1^2$. The right panel Figure 5 shows the plot of the two Gaussian distribution and summarizing the operating characteristics the test statistics $\Lambda$.

## 4  Summary

The experiment and results presented are limited because the sample size studied which consisted of only 10 pairs of schizophrenics and controls. The other important comment is that the hypothesis test statistics were generated from the same data set as the one used to learn the covariance structure of the deformation fields. This study illustrates the mathematical methods for studying shape of brain sub-manifolds. In particular we examine the vector fields describing the shape variation as Gaussian fields. The mean and covariance operators are used to characterize the populations.

# References

1. M.I. Miller, G.E. Christensen, Y. Amit, and U. Grenander. Mathematical textbook of deformable neuroanatomies. *Proceedings of the National Academy of Science*, 90(24), December 1993.
2. G. Christensen. *Deformable Shape Models for Anatomy*. Ph.D. Dissertation, Department of Electrical Engineering, Sever Institute of Technology, Washington University, St. Louis, MO, Aug 1994.
3. G. E. Christensen, R. D. Rabbitt, and M.I. Miller. 3D brain mapping using a deformable neuroanatomy. *Physics in Medicine and Biology*, 39:609–618, 1994.
4. U. Grenander and M. I. Miller. Representations of knowledge in complex systems. *Journal of the Royal Statistical Society B*, 56(3):549–603, 1994.
5. Sarang C. Joshi, Michael I. Miller, Gary E. Christensen, Ayananshu Banerjee, Thomas A. Coogan, and Ulf Grenander. Hierarchical brain mapping via a generalized dirichlet solution for mapping brain manifolds. In *Proc. of the SPIE's 1995 International Symposium on Optical Science, Engineering, and Instrumentation:Vision Geometry IV*, volume 2573, pages 278–289, San Diego, CA., August 1995.
6. G. E. Christensen, S. C. Joshi, and M. I. Miller. Volumetric transformation of brain anatomy. *IEEE Transactions on Medical Imaging*.
7. M. Claudio and S. Roberto. Using marching cubes on small machines. *Graphical Models and Image Processing*, 56:182–3, 1994.
8. Sarang C. Joshi, Jing Wang, Michael I. Miller, David Van Essen, and Ulf Grenander. On the differential geometry of the cortical surface. In *Proc. of the SPIE's 1995 International Symposium on Optical Science, Engineering, and Instrumentation:Vision Geometry IV*, volume 2573, pages 304–311, San Diego, CA., August 1995.
9. W. M. Boothby. *An Introduction to Differentiable Manifolds and Riemannian Geometry*. Academic Press, 1986.
10. T.F. Cootes, C.J. Taylor, D.H. Cooper, and J. Graham. Active shape models—their training and application. *Computer Vision and Image Understanding*, 61(1):38–59, 1995.
11. Alan Yuille and Peter Hallinan. *Active Vision*, chapter Deformable Templates. MIT Press, Cambridge, MA, 1992.
12. Paul D. Sampson, Fred L Bookstein, Florence H. Sheehan, and Edward L Bolson. *Eigen Shape Analysis of Left Ventricular Outlines From Contrast Ventriculograms*, pages 211–233. Plenum Press, New York, 1996.
13. G. H. Golub and C. F. Van Loan. *Matrix Computations*. The Johns Hopkins Univ. Press, Baltimore, 1983.
14. John W. Haller, Gary E. Christensen, Sarang Joshi, , John W. Newcomer, Michael I. Miller, John C. Csernansky, and Michael W. Vannier. Hippocampal mr imaging morphometry by means of general pattern matching. *Radiology*, 199(3):787–791, June 1996.
15. John W. Haller, A. Banerjee, Gary E. Christensen, Sarang Joshi, Michael I. Miller, Michael W. Vannier, and John C. Csernansky. 3d hippocampal volumetry by high dimensional transformation of a neuroanatomical atlas. *Radiology*, submitted June 1996.
16. U. Grenander and M. I. Miller. Anatomically complex probability measures for medical imaging. *IEEE Transactions on Medical Imaging*.

# Fuzzy Logic Approach to 3D Magnetic Resonance Image Segmentation

Yutaka Hata[†], Syoji Kobashi[†], Naotake Kamiura[†] and Makoto Ishikawa[‡]

[†] Department of Computer Engineering, Himeji Institute of Technology
2167, Shosha, Himeji, 671-22, JAPAN
[‡] Ishikawa Hospital
784, Bessho, Bessho-cho, Himeji, JAPAN

## Abstract

This paper proposes an approach of fuzzy logic to 3D MR image segmentation. We show a fuzzy knowledge representation method to represent the knowledge needed to segment the target portions, and apply our method to 3D MR human brain image segmentation. In it we consider position knowledge, boundary surface knowledge and intensity knowledge. They are expressed by fuzzy if-then rules and compiled to a total degree as the measure of segmentation. The degree is evaluated in region growing technique and which segments the whole brain region into the left cerebral hemisphere, the right cerebral hemisphere, the cerebellum and the brain stem. The experimental result on 36 MR voxel data shows that our method extracted the portions precisely.

## 1. Introduction

Medical imaging[1-5] has evolved at an explosive rate in the past few years. In the context of medical imaging, fuzzy logic technique[2-7] appears as a powerful framework since it provides tools adapted to this task. Its main properties are: 1. It provides a way to represent and manipulate imprecise and uncertain information. 2. It will be able to demonstrate knowledge of Medical doctors. 3. It is well adapted to image processing since the natural spatial interpretation of fuzzy logic leads to efficient representations of imprecise or implicit structures or classes in pictures.

This paper proposes an approach of fuzzy logic to 3D MR image segmentation. First, we show a method to represent the knowledge needed to segment the target portions. The method employs fuzzy knowledge representation to express human knowledge and uses fuzzy if-then rules to segment them. Next, we apply our fuzzy segmentation method to 3D MR human brain image segmentation. In it we consider position knowledge, boundary surface knowledge and intensity knowledge. They are expressed by fuzzy if-then rules and compiled to a total degree as the measure of the segmentation. The degree is evaluated in region growing technique. Finally our method segments the whole brain region into the left cerebral hemisphere, the right cerebral hemisphere, the cerebellum and the brain stem. An experimental result on 36 MR voxel data shows that our method extracted the target portions precisely for all data.

## 2. Knowledge Representation by Fuzzy if-then Rule

For the convenience of the reader, a brief summary of some of the relevant aspects of the theory of fuzzy sets and the linguistic approach is presented[6, 7]. The symbol U denotes a universe of discourse. If A is a finite subset of U whose elements are $u_1$, ... , $u_n$. A is expressed as A = {$u_1$, ... ,$u_n$}. A finite fuzzy subset A of U is a set of ordered pairs: A = {($u_i$, $\mu_A(u_i)$)}; $u_i \in$ U, where the $\mu_A(u_i)$ represent membership functions, which indicate the degree of membership. The $\mu_A(u_i)$ are assumed to lie in the interval [0,1], with 0 and 1 denoting no membership and full membership, respectively. Let $\mu_A(X)$ be a membership function for the element $x \in X$ with respect to the fuzzy subset A. The MAX $\vee$ and MIN $\wedge$ are defined as, $\mu_A(x) \vee \mu_B(x) = \max(\mu_A(x), \mu_B(x))$ and $\mu_A(x) \wedge \mu_B(x) = \min(\mu_A(x), \mu_B(x))$. We will use fuzzy subsets to represent linguistic variables. Informally, a linguistic variable, L, is a variable whose values are words or sentences in a natural language or in a subset of it. Fuzzy inference plays an important role in our approach, which is the fuzzy if-then statement: if A then B, in which A (the antecedent) and B(the conclusion) are fuzzy subsets rather than propositional variables. The conditional statement "if X is A then Y is B" is represented by the fuzzy relation R and defined as follows: $\mu_R(u,v) = \min(u_A(u), u_B(v))$; $u \in$ U and $v \in$ V. If R is a fuzzy relation from U to V, and x is a fuzzy subset of U, then the fuzzy subset y of V which is induced by x is denoted by y =xoR and defined as follows: $\mu_y(v) = \max_{u \in U} \min(u_x(u), u_R(u, v))$.

When R = A $\rightarrow$ B and x = A we obtain : Y = X o(A$\rightarrow$ B) = B as an exact identity.

Next we describes a knowledge representation method based on fuzzy logic. The fuzzy if-then rule methods employ some information obtained by our cognitive information such as "this is on that", "this is near to that" and so on. Here, we show a method to segment the portions by fuzzy if-the rules. Our method represents the entire knowledge residing within a collection of if-then rules and can employ the following three items for the segmentation :

Item 1. Position (destination) knowledge
Item 2. Boundary surface knowledge
Item 3. Intensity (gray level) data (raw image)

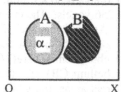 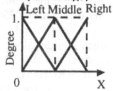 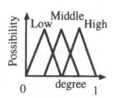

Figure 1 An example.         Figure 2 Membership functions.

Here we consider a segmentation of regions A and B shown in Figure 1. We can derive the following knowledge;

Knowledge 1. Region A is located on the left.
Knowledge 2. Region B is located on the right.

Then, we can derive the following fuzzy if-then rules for any point.

If the location of the point is left-hand side then the point is in Region A
If the location of the point is right-hand side then the point is in Region B.

These rules are derived from the destination knowledge. We can compile the Knowledge 1 to the following three fuzzy if-then rules. Here, Right, Middle and Left membership functions and High, Middle and Low membership functions are shown in Figure 2. Let $\mu_A(x)$ denote the degree of region A for point x. Then,

If the location of x is Right then $\mu_A(x)$ is Low,

if the location of x is Middle then $\mu_A(x)$ is Middle,

if the location of x is Left then $\mu_A(x)$ is High.

Note that the set of rules is not unique, we can arrange the other rules. Figure 3 represents the max-min inference mechanism. Considering a point, $\alpha$, we obtain the conclusions of three rules and compile their conclusions into a result $\mu_A(\alpha)$. The result expresses "a point $\alpha$ is Region A with relatively high degree". In the similar way to the above case, we can derive the if-then rules for Knowledge 2. On Items 2 and 3, we can employ the similar way of the above case and also use many image

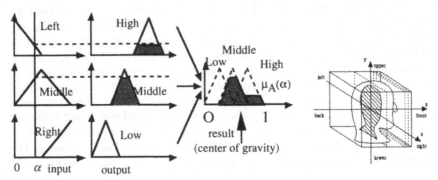

Figure 3 Fuzzy inference mechanism.          Figure 4 Coordinate system.

## 3. Brain MR Image Segmentation Based on Fuzzy Logic

We used MR images obtained from 1.5T MR unit (Sigma Advantage 5.x, General Electric) using a circularity polarized head coil as both transmitter and receiver. The image acquisition method was coronal three-dimensional Spoiled Gradient Echo (SPGR). TR was 14 msec; TE was 3 msec; and flip angle was 20 degree. Field of view was 220mm. Matrix was 256 by 256. This generated 124, 1.5mm-thick, contiguous section images; giving voxel dimensions of $0.86 \times 0.86 \times 1.5 mm^3$. We construct the voxel data, which consisted of $124 \times 256 \times 256$ voxels. The intensity of all intracranial structures ranged between 0 and 255. Assume that the 124 two-dimensional MR images are arranged in order along the z-axis as shown in Figure 4. The interesting portions in this paper are: the left cerebral hemisphere(LCH for short), the right cerebral hemisphere(RCH), the cerebellum(CB) and the brain stem(BS). For a given 3D MR image we extract the target areas, the white matter and the gray matter, based on the region growing algorithm[1]. For the obtained brain data, assume the center of gravity of the brain region as the origin and its coordinate system is shown in Figure 4. We mainly describe a method to extract the target portions. We consider the following items for the segmentation.

(i) Position knowledge
(ii) Boundary knowledge: (ii)-1 : Adjacency, (ii)-2 : Euclidean distance
(iii) Intensity knowledge

*(i) Position knowledge representation* : For each axis of x, y and z, Table 1 tabulates which location every portion belongs to. This table shows that LCH is located at x = left, y = upper and z = any place( * denotes any place), etc. According to Table 1, we can make a fuzzy knowledge table shown in Table 2. In it, N, Ze and P express Negative, Zero and Positive membership functions, respectively, in Figure 5. The

horizontal axis is correspond to arrows, x, y, or z, in Figure 4. The membership functions VH, H, L and VL are shown in Figure 6.

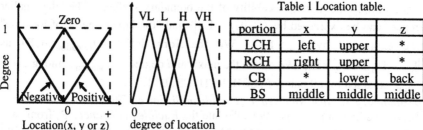

Table 1 Location table.

| portion | x | y | z |
|---|---|---|---|
| LCH | left | upper | * |
| RCH | right | upper | * |
| CB | * | lower | back |
| BS | middle | middle | middle |

Figure 5 Location membership functions

Figure 6 Output membership functions

Table 2 A knowledge table on the portions.(N: Negative, Ze: Zero, P: Positive, VH: Very High, H: High, L: Low, VL: Very Low)

| portion | x | | | y | | | z | | |
|---|---|---|---|---|---|---|---|---|---|
| | N | Ze | P | N | Ze | P | N | Ze | P |
| $\mu_{LCH}$ | VH | L | VL | L | H | VH | VH | VH | VH |
| $\mu_{RCH}$ | VL | H | VH | L | H | VH | VH | VH | VH |
| $\mu_{CB}$ | VH | VH | VH | VH | H | VH | VH | H | VL |
| $\mu_{BS}$ | VL | VH | VL | VH | H | VL | VL | VH | L |

The notation $\mu_X$ denotes the membership function of the portion X. Table 2 means that , for example, considering x-axis of the left cerebral hemisphere, we can derive the following rules: If x=N(left) then $\mu_{LCH}$ = VH, if x=Ze(middle) then $\mu_{LCH}$ = L , if x=P(right) then $\mu_{LCH}$ = VL. For a given voxel whose location is (a, b ,c), a fuzzy inference result, $U_{LCH}$, is obtained via a min-max inference,

$$U_{LCH}(a) = [a \wedge N \wedge VH] \vee [a \wedge Ze \wedge L] \vee [a \wedge P \wedge VL].$$

The center of gravity, $g_{LCH}(a)$, of $U_{LCH}$ is obtained. We can also obtain $g_{RCH}(a)$, $g_{CB}(a)$ and $g_{BS}(a)$ for a of (a, b, c). Similarly, we can obtain the values, $g_{LCH}(b)$ and $g_{LCH}(c)$, for b and c of (a, b, c), respectively. Finally, we determine a degree $L_{LCH}(a,b,c) = g_{LCH}(a) \wedge g_{LCH}(b) \wedge g_{LCH}(c)$, for the voxel as the degree for the left cerebral hemisphere. Similarly, the degrees $L_{RCH}(a,b,c)$, $L_{CB}(a,b,c)$ and $L_{BS}(a,b,c)$, for the other portions are also obtained. Thus we can determine a set $[L_{LCH}(a,b,c), L_{RCH}(a,b,c), L_{CB}(a,b,c), L_{BS}(a,b,c)]$ for every voxel. For every voxel, we determine which portion the voxel belongs to.

**Case 1**; When only one degree, $L_P$, of the set is lager than 0.5, we determine the voxel belongs to the portion "p".

**Case 2**; When two or more degrees are lager than 0.5, we do not determine which portion the voxel belongs to. We accommodate the determination with the result obtained from the fuzzy rule-based inferences.

*(ii) -1 Boundary Surface Knowledge : Adjacency:* Consider the portion A and portion B; A, B ∈ {LCH, RCH, CB, BS}. The difference between $L_A$ and $L_B$ can serve as an indicator of the boundary surface between their portions. Let the degree,

$D_{Location}(A, B)$, denote the membership value on the location of the boundary surface between portions A and B. Both the smaller difference and the lager degree of location imply the higher possibility of the boundary surface. The "the smaller difference" can be expressed by $(1 - |L_A - L_B|)$ and "the larger degree of location" can be expressed by $L_A \times L_B$. We therefore define $D_{Location}(A, B)$ as $(1 - |L_A - L_B|) \times L_A \times L_B$ We obtain the maximum degree, $P_{Location}$, among every $D_{Location}$ obtained for all pairs of {LCH, RCH, CB, BS}.

*(ii) -2 Boundary Surface Knowledge: Euclidean distance* : There exists the narrow part between adjacent portions. We calculate the *Euclidean distance, $\varepsilon$*, from each of voxels to the outside of the brain region (i.e., background region). In the standard fuzzy inference based on the knowledge that the voxel is closer to the boundary surface as the possibility becomes higher, the following rules hold: If the Euclidean distance is H then the possibility is HI, if the Euclidean distance is M then the possibility is MI, if the Euclidean distance is L then the possibility is LO. A result obtained by the inference is denoted by $R_\varepsilon$. The center of gravity, $P_{Distance}$, is a degree of the boundary surface with respect to the *Euclidean distance.*

*(iii) Intensity knowledge* : The boundary surface mainly consists of the gray matter. We therefore consider a fuzzy inference on intensity in the same way to case, (ii)-2. If the intensity is L then the possibility is HI, if the intensity is M then the possibility is MI, if the intensity is H then the possibility is LO. The result obtained by the inference is denoted by $R_I$. The center of gravity, $P_{Intensity}$, is a degree of boundary surface with respect to intensity. Here we obtain a total degree from all inference results. For every voxel we calculate a total degree,

$$P = \sum_{pair\ i=1}^{6} P_{Location}(A, B) \times \omega_i^\alpha \times P_{Location} + \sum_{pair\ i=1}^{6} P_{Location}(A, B) \times \omega_i^\beta \times P_{Distance}$$

$$+ \sum_{pair\ i=1}^{6} P_{Location}(A, B) \times \omega_i^\gamma \times P_{Intensity}.$$

Table 3 The weight table.

| Pair $i$ | portion A | portion B | $\omega_i^\alpha$ | $\omega_i^\beta$ | $\omega_i^\gamma$ |
|---|---|---|---|---|---|
| 1 | LCH | RCH | 1 | 1 | 0 |
| 2 | LCH | CB | 0 | 1 | 1 |
| 3 | LCH | BS | 1 | 1 | 0 |
| 4 | RCH | CB | 1 | 1 | 1 |
| 5 | RCH | BS | 1 | 1 | 0 |
| 6 | CB | BS | 1 | 1 | 0 |

$P_{Location}(A, B) = P_{Location}(B, A)$, therefore, we can consider all cases with Table 3. Here we briefly show our algorithm.

Step 1: For each of portions, starting voxels are determined as the voxels obtained by Case 1.

Step 2: Extract each portions by including smaller P as ROI.

Step 3: When the whole brain region is fulfilled by Step 2, we can obtain the left cerebral hemisphere, the right cerebral hemisphere, the cerebellum and the brain stem from the brain region.

## 4. Experimental Results and Conclusions

We applied our method to 36 MR voxel data. Figure 7 shows an example of the raw MR images, the segmented images and the 3D visualization. Our method can segment all data correctly. It required about three minutes on each MR voxel data on IRIS Indigo2 (IRIX 5.3, 150Mz, Memory 128M). This paper proposed a fuzzy expert system for segmentation of the brain portions. It employs three knowledge : Position, Boundary surface and Intensity and can segment the whole brain region into the left cerebral hemisphere, the right cerebral hemisphere, the cerebellum and the brain stem. In the future, it remains to enhance the processing time and to extract the smaller portions such as the hippocampus, the sulci and so on.

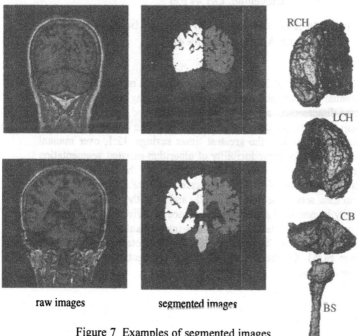

raw images        segmented images

Figure 7 Examples of segmented images.

### Related Publications and References

1. J.K.Udupa and G. T. Herman: "3D Imaging in Medicine," CRC Press, (1991).
2. L.O. Hall, A.M. Besaid, et al, "A comparison of neural network and fuzzy clustering techniques in segmenting magnetic resonance images of the brain," IEEE Trans. on Neural Networks, vol. 3, no. 5, pp. 672-682 (1992).
3. I. Bloch: "Information Combination Operators for Data Fusion: A Comparative Review with Classification," IEEE Trans. SMC, Part A, vol. 26, pp. 52-67 (1996).
4. I. Bloch: "Fuzzy Classification for Multi-Modality Image Fusion," IEEE Tint. Conf. on Image Processing, Austin, vol. I, pp. 628-632 (1994).
5. C.-W. Chang, G. R. Hillman et. al : "Fuzzy Rule-Based System for Labeling the Structures in 3D Human Brain Magnetic Resonance Images", Proc. of the 5th IEEE International Conference on Fuzzy Systems, pp. 1978-1982 (1996).
6. L.A. Zadeh: "Fuzzy sets and Applications," John Wiley and Sons, Inc. (1987).
7. W. Pedrycz: "Fuzzy Control And Fuzzy Systems," Research Studies Press Ltd. (1993).

# Comparison of Traditional Brain Segmentation Tools with 3D Self-Organizing Maps

David Dean[1], Krishnamurthy Subramanyan[2], Janardhan Kamath[2],
Fred Bookstein[3], David Wilson[2], David Kwon[4], and Peter Buckley[4]

[1] Department of Neurological Surgery
[2] Department of Biomedical Engineering
[4] Department of Psychiatry
Case Western Reserve University
Cleveland, OH 44106

[3] Institute of Gerontology, University of Michigan
Ann Arbor, Michigan 48109

**Abstract.** Algorithm-assisted 3D MR brain segmentation may be significantly faster than manual methods and produce visually pleasing results. We tested two- and three-dimensional region growing (2DRG and 3DRG) and self-organizing map (SOM) algorithms for segmentation of the cerebral ventricles. The SOM algorithm provides the greatest times savings, 12:1, over manual segmentation. Concern for reproducibility of algorithm-assisted segmentation motivated an intra-operator comparative study of these and manual segmentation methods. One of us, DK, segmented the cerebral ventricles from 5 3D MR-scan data sets three times manually and with the three algorithms. When variability is measured as the shape variance of derived landmarks sets, the three algorithm-assisted methods show less intra-operator variability than manual segmentation. The 2DRG and 3DRG segmentations show more variability than SOM. Of the 4 methods, SOM segmentation requires the fewest operator decisions.

## 1 Introduction

It would be useful to obtain accurate and reproducible surface representations of the cerebral ventricles, a space within the brain filled with cerebrospinal fluid (CSF). We have previously segmented the ventricular brain surface from 3D MR-scans manually to make shape comparisons between schizophrenic patients and controls via a 3D deformable wire-frame template (Dean *et al.* [2]). In this note we document our implementation of three algorithm-assisted segmentation methods, and a validation study of that software. The primary goal of this validation study is to determine whether these three algorithm-assisted segmentation procedures demonstrate intra-operator reproducibility on a par with manual segmentation (*cf.* Chalana and Kim [1]).

The landmarks, depicted in Figure 1, are extremal point landmarks (i.e., poles, tips, grooves, etc.) found recurrently on the surface of the cerebral ventricles. Following segmentation these landmarks were identified manually, by mouse, on each segmented 3D ventricular image. These landmarks form the basis of the intra-operator segmentation variability study reported in section 4.

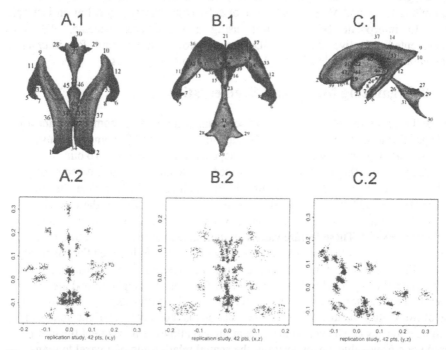

**Fig. 1.** The upper panel, A1-C1, presents curvature extrema landmarks (numbered). The lower panel, A2-C2 presents a 60-shape Procrustes fit coordinate scatterplot for 42 of the 48 landmarks depicted (without: 7-10, 36-37). Abbreviation key: Ant = Anterior, Ext = External, For = Foramen, Front = Frontal, Inf = Inferior, Int = Internal, Lat = Lateral, Med = Medial, Occ = Occipital, Sup = Superior, Temp = Temporal, Vent = Ventricle, r = Right, l = Left, Intsect = Intersection.

| Fig. 1. Landmark Key | | |
|---|---|---|
| 1. r_AntLatFrontPole | 17. r_SupAntForMonro | 33. l_MedNotchLatCrestIntsect |
| 2. l_AntLatFrontPole | 18. l_SupAntForMonro | 34. r_MidSupIntCrest |
| 3. r_AntMedFrontPole | 19. InfAntForMonro | 35. l_MidSupIntCrest |
| 4. l_AntMedFrontPole | 20. r_SupPosForMonro | 36. r_LatTorsionMax |
| 5. r_LatTempPole | 21. l_SupPosForMonro | 37. l_LatTorsionMax |
| 6. l_LatTempPole | 22. InfPosForMonro | 38. r_AntMidVentPole |
| 7. r_MedTempPole | 23. Ant3rdVent | 39. l_AntMidVentPole |
| 8. l_MedTempPole | 24. AntInf3rdVent | 40. Pos3rdVent |
| 9. r_OccPole | 25. PosSup3rdVent | 41. r_SupMidLatForMonro |
| 10. l_OccPole | 26. AntInf4thVent | 42. l_SupMidLatForMonro |
| 11. r_InfExtNotch | 27. PosSup4thVent | 43. r_InfMidLatForMonro |
| 12. l_InfExtNotch | 28. r_ForLuschka | 44. l_InfMidLatForMonro |
| 13. r_MidInfIntCrest | 29. l_ForLuschka | 45. r_Lat3rdVent |
| 14. l_MidInfIntCrest | 30. ForMagendie | 46. l_Lat3rdVent |
| 15. r_AntInfMedFrontPole | 31. Ant4thVent | 47. r_Lat4thVent |
| 16. l_AntInfMedFrontPole | 32. r_MedNotchLatCrestIntsect | 48. l_Lat4thVent |

## 2 Region-growing Segmentation

Region growth algorithms provide a very fast method for segmentation. A good example is Joliot and Mazoyer's [3] use of a 3D connectivity algorithm on isotropic slices to interpolate between slices using a shape-based scheme. We have implemented adaptive 2D and 3D region growth algorithms for interactive segmentation of the cerebral ventricles using multiple seed points.

## 3 Self Organizing Map-based Segmentation

Our Self-Organizing Map (SOM) brain segmentation procedure combines intensity and spatial information. Kohonen's [4] implementation of self organizing sensory maps was applied to bat sonatotopy and image pattern recognition. To our knowledge ours is the first truly volume-based segmentation method based upon Kohonen's SOM neural network approach. For each voxel, its Euclidean Distance $X_d$ $(x*x+y*y+z*z)^{\frac{1}{2}}$ from the "origin" (the anterosuperior corner of the volume in standard orientation) , together with the voxel's grayscale (u), is used to create a feature: $(u^2+X_d^2)^{\frac{1}{2}}$. These feature values are normalized to maximum 1 and input to a "resonator," the first layer of a two layer network. Distances between the voxels are used to limit the search for similar voxels to a "neighborhood" of known dimensions within the volume. Voxels of similar intensity far from the neighborhood are ignored. The location and relative extent of these neighborhoods together constitute one of two feature vector elements. The other one is the gray level of the voxels in each neighborhood. The neural network approach allows us to segment the brain based upon gray-value, voxel position, the spatial relationship of a voxel to many neighbors, and a comparison of many neighbors' gray values (the texture).

The SOM two layer network in Figure 2 is generated in two passes. The first pass identifies where connections between layers A and B, "synapses", should exist. The second pass identifies feature clusters which are fed into the graphics engine for anatomic labeling by the end user. The first pass in SOM generation begins with Layer A processors referred to as "resonators". Layer A processors are assigned a set of connections, referred to as "synapses", with layer B processors referred to as "neurons". On the first pass this assignment is random. Each of the layer B processors forms it own dendritic tree according to a weighted sum of inputs from processors in layer A as well as from neighboring processors in layer B. The normalized feature data being fed to the Level A processors is modulated by a sigmoidal function. Only the highest scoring features can activate layer B processors. Thus, synapses between level A neurons and level B resonators are graded such that the "weaker" connections are parsed. The strength of an input is $W_{rl}*V_l$ where $V_l$, is the activity of an axon and $W_{rl}$ expresses the "strength" of the synapse of neuron "r's" axon "l". The sign of $W_{rl}$, generated in the sigmoidal function, indicates the excitatory or inhibitory state of the synapse. By comparing the output of all the processors in layer B, the winner is identified. Once the winner is identified, its synaptic strengths, i.e., $\Delta W_{rl}$, are positively accentuated, and its neighbors are negatively inhibited. By doing so, we increase the chance of forming topographically related groups, and of abstracting major identifiable features while eliminating small fluctuating errors. As more and more synapses are parsed, attenuation occurs more rapidly and the appropriate position for each voxel in the SOM is adopted more quickly. The process continues until the generated resultants of all the layer B processors show ascending or descending order in their response to incoming data. When the iterations are stopped, each layer B processor has a group of voxels which spatially represent related and internally homogenous structures.

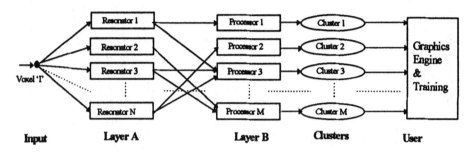

**Fig. 2.** The SOM network has two layers of processors. The resulting feature clusters are back-projected onto the original volume image. The user recognizes anatomical shapes in the back-projected data and can rapidly label features as anatomically significant objects.

A second pass through the data produces feature clusters. In this second pass the "tuned" resonators produce a characteristic output. As characteristic values, i.e., "tuned" frequencies, become known neuron processor-resonator "synapses" between layers A and B are assigned. The resulting synapses and feature clusters (combined spatial and grayscale information) are saved as a self-organized map.

## 4 Validation Study Results

To validate each segmentation method's reproducibility the same operator segmented 5 3D MR brain scan data sets (cases) three times (replications) manually and with each of the three algorithms. It is useful to first consider the variance of the three replications for each combination of case and method. This variation is quantified as the variance of "shape" of the manually detected landmarks shown in Figure 1, as assessed by Procrustes analysis (Dean *et al.* [2]).

Panel B of Figure 1 shows a Procrustes fit coordinate scatterplot of 42 landmarks across all 60 data sets (5 scans segmented 3 times via 4 methods). The six most variable landmarks, 7-10 and 36-37, were far noisier than the other 42 so they were deleted and the fit was recalculated. Figure 3 shows the variability at each landmark over all 3 replications for each combination of algorithm and case. Note that the line representing SOM is most often at bottom, whereas that for Alice (TM), the manual segmentation software, is often at the top. Figure 3 is consistent with the net "error variance" found for each method, from lowest to highest: SOM (0.000224), 2DRG (0.000287), 3DRG (0.000311), Alice (0.000429).

# landmark-specific error variances by method

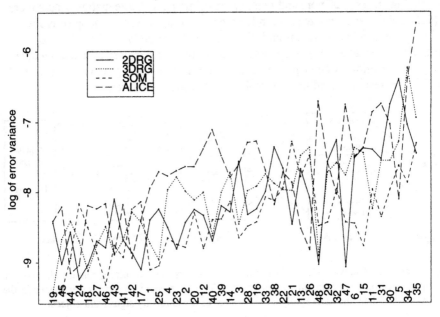

landmarks (sorted by sum of error variances)

**Fig. 3.** Variance at each landmark obtained from one user digitizing 5 data sets three times using Alice (TM) software (manual segmentation), and 2DRG, 3DRG (two and three dimensional region growing), and SOM (self organizing maps) algorithms independently.

Figure 4 is a landmark by landmark view of whole sample averages by algorithm (top) and by case (bottom). The overlapping symbols indicate little difference between the algorithm-assisted methods. Only 3 landmarks (46, 38, 31) have more inter-methodological variance than within case variance. Of the 42 analyzed, the noisiest landmarks (5, 11, 34) show distinctly more variation across cases. Summing separate ANOVA models for main effects of case variation versus algorithm, the sum of squares for the former is 0.095, 0.022 for the latter, and 0.020 for interaction between case and algorithm.

## 5 Conclusions

This study found that intra-operator variation in segmentation via 3 algorithm-assisted methods was less variable than manual work. All 4 segmentation methods provide surfaces from which we are locating "the same points", as the variance found over manual and algorithm-assisted segmentation replications was considerably less than that over cases at almost every landmark. We conclude that manual and algorithm-assisted segmentation differ in the resulting intrinsic variance of subsequently acquired shape information. SOM is the most favorable from this point of view. Manual segmentation requires many human decisions based on an 8 bit screen rendering and mouse effectuation of this low resolution rendering. SOM segmentation requires fewer operator decisions, with those remaining benefitting from direct processing of the images full grayscale range and spatial resolution.

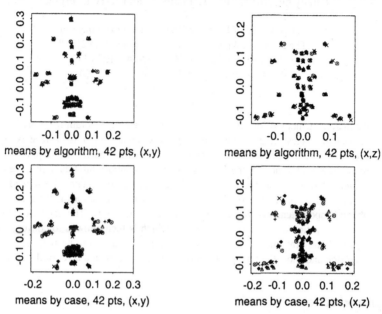

means by algorithm, 42 pts, (x,y)

means by algorithm, 42 pts, (x,z)

means by case, 42 pts, (x,y)

means by case, 42 pts, (x,z)

**Fig. 4.** Case variance averaged across segmentation methods and replications (bottom) swamps segmentation method variance averaged across cases and replications (top). Upper Panel: X=manual, ⊙=2DRG, Δ=3DRG, +=SOM; Lower Panel: symbols change for each case.

This project has succeeded in a frontal challenge on the interplay of algorithms and landmark protocols (dependence of landmark locations on segmentation algorithms, and variation over algorithms in the variance of those derived data). This could justify tests of SOM-based segmentation of other structures with less clear boundaries than the ventricles (e.g., cerebral cortex, basal ganglia, heart ventricle, liver, prostate, and various tumors).

## References

1. Chalana, V., Kim, Y.: A methodology of Image Segmentation Algorithms on Medical Images. In (M.H. Loew and K.M. Hanson, eds.) SPIE MI'96 **2710-20** (1996) 178-189.
2. Dean, D., Buckley, P., Bookstein, F., Kamath, J., Kwon, D., Friedman, L., and Lys, C.: Three Dimensional MR-based Morphometric Comparison of Schizophrenic and Normal Cerebral Ventricles. In (K.-H. Höhne and R. Kikinis, eds.) Visualization in Biomedical Computing '96. Lecture Notes in Computer Science. **1131** (1996) 363-372.
3. Joliot, M., Mazoyer, B.M.: Three-dimensional segmentation and interpolation of magnetic resonance brain images. IEEE Trans. Med. Imaging **12** (1993) 269-277.
4. Kohonen, T.: Physiological interpretation of the self-organizing map. Neural Networks **6** (1993) 895-905.

# Finding the Brain Cortex Using Fuzzy Segmentation, Isosurfaces, and Deformable Surface Models

Chenyang Xu[1], Dzung L. Pham[1,2], and Jerry L. Prince[1]

[1] Department of Electrical and Computer Engineering,
The Johns Hopkins University, Baltimore, MD 21218
[2] National Institutes of Health, NIA/GRC/LPC,
4940 Eastern Avenue, Baltimore, MD 21224

**Abstract.** A method for finding the cortical surface of the brain from magnetic resonance images using a combination of fuzzy segmentation, isosurface extraction, and a deformable surface is presented. After MR images are acquired and preprocessed to remove extracranial tissue, fuzzy membership functions for gray matter, white matter, and cerebrospinal fluid are computed. An iterative procedure using isosurfaces of filtered white matter membership functions is then used to obtain a topologically correct estimate of the cortical surface. This estimate forms the initialization of a deformable surface, which is then allowed to converge to peaks of the gray matter membership function. We demonstrate the results of each step and show the final parameterized map of the medial layer of the cortex.

## 1 Introduction

Recent advances in medical imaging of the brain allow anatomical information derived from high resolution imaging modalities such as magnetic resonance imaging (MRI) and computed tomography (CT) to be fused with physiological information. These advances have placed a priority on obtaining accurate reconstructions of the cortical surface, not only to provide valuable information on the geometric and anatomical properties of the brain but for other purposes as well. For example, the location of functional activity obtained from positron emission tomography (PET), functional magnetic resonance imaging (fMRI), and other methods can be mapped to the extracted cortical surface, providing a better understanding of brain function and organization [1]. The surfaces can also be warped to other cortical surfaces for the purposes of image registration [2,3] or atlas labelling [4].

Geometrically, the human cerebral cortex is a thin folded sheet of gray matter (GM) that lies inside the cerebrospinal fluid (CSF) and outside the white matter (WM) of the brain. Reconstruction of the cortex is problematic, however, due to its highly convoluted surface. Recently, there has been a considerable amount of work in this area of research. Many methods have employed deformable surfaces, which are synthetic surfaces that move and conform to object boundaries. While deformable surface models have been highly successful in extracting the shapes of simple objects, they suffer from an inability to converge to highly complex structures without an initialization that is already close to the desired result. In their work, Sandor and Leahy [4] largely ignored this problem and were primarily concerned with extracting only the outer cortex. MacDonald *et al.* [2]

improved convergence of their deformable surfaces by constraining the solutions of their model. Dale and Sereno [1] performed a three-step flood-filling algorithm on the white matter, and used the tessellated white matter surface as an initialization for their deformable surface.

In this paper, we present a method for extracting the medial layer surface of the cortex from MR images of the brain. A novel approach is used to provide a proper initialization for a deformable surface based on isosurfaces of a fuzzy segmentation. The deformable surface is then applied to obtain a parameterized surface representation of the medial layer of the cortex.

## 2 Methods and Results

Our technique consists of four major steps: 1) data acquisition and preprocessing, 2) fuzzy segmentation, 3) initial surface estimation, and 4) refinement using a deformable surface. Results of applying each procedure to a sample data set are shown.

### 2.1 Data acquisition and preprocessing

Data was acquired on a GE Signa 1.5 Tesla MR scanner using a Spoiled GRASS (SPGR) imaging protocol with a pulse repetition time of 35 ms, pulse echo time of 8 ms, and tip angle of 45 degrees. The image size was 256×240, zero padded to 256×256 with pixel dimensions of 0.9375×0.9375 mm. 124 axial slices were acquired with a slice thickness of 1.5 mm.

The acquired images were stacked to form a volume and then preprocessed to remove skin, bone, fat and other extracranial tissue. This can be achieved using automated methods [4] or by manual tracing. In this paper, the extracranial tissue removal was accomplished using a semi-automated software package developed by Christos Davatzikos and Jerry Miller [1]. Fig. 1a shows one slice from a sample data set after this procedure.

### 2.2 Fuzzy segmentation

There has been a trend in the recent literature favoring the use of fuzzy segmentations over hard segmentations in defining anatomical structures [5]. Fuzzy segmentations retain more information from the original image than hard segmentations by taking into account the possibility that more than one tissue class may be present in a single voxel. This circumstance often occurs when imaging very fine structures, resulting in partial volume averaging. Small errors in the data acquisition or segmentation will also be less of a factor in fuzzy segmentations since this will only alter the membership function by some fractional number while in a hard segmentation, small errors might change the entire classification.

We applied the fuzzy c-means (FCM) algorithm [6] to the preprocessed brain volume, resulting in fuzzy membership functions for GM, WM, and CSF tissue classes

---

[1] Department of Radiology and Radiological Science, Johns Hopkins University School of Medicine.

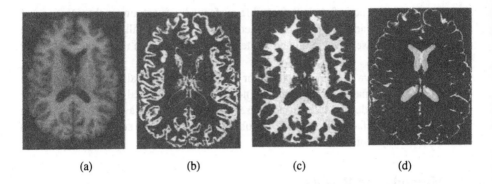

(a)                    (b)                    (c)                    (d)

**Fig. 1.** (a) Sample slices from acquired MRI data set. Membership functions: (b) GM, (c) WM, and (d) CSF.

(i.e., $K=3$). The resulting membership functions for one slice in the brain volume are shown in Fig. 1b-d. Fig. 1b is the GM membership function, Fig. 1c is the WM membership function, and Fig. 1d is the CSF membership function. Pixel locations with high intensity values reflect a high membership value for that class. The membership functions were used exclusively for all subsequent processing.

### 2.3 Initial estimation of the cortical surface

In order to use a deformable surface to extract the surface of the cortex, a proper initialization is required. The initialization must be sufficiently close and isomorphic (i.e., have an equivalent topology) to the medial layer surface of the GM. The first requirement stems from the fact that deformable surfaces have difficulty finding concave surfaces such as the cortex [7]. Deformable surface initializations are typically computed by using a simple geometric object (e.g., a sphere or ellipsoid) or by manual interaction. For the cortex, however, it is difficult to define a simple geometric object that would allow a deformable surface to converge to deep sulci (or gyri). On the other hand, manual initializations for three-dimensional data are labor intensive and time consuming. For the second requirement, we assume the extracted cortex should be topologically equivalent to a sphere.

Because voxels at the GM-WM interface will contain both GM and WM, the membership functions computed in Section 2.2 can be used to estimate the location of the GM-WM interface by computing an isosurface at a threshold value of 0.5. Isosurfaces, however, are in general topologically unconstrained [8], hence special care is required in order to satisfy the isomorphism constraint.

The topology of a surface can be summarized by its Euler characteristic, $X$, which can be computed by [9]

$$X = V - E + F \qquad (1)$$

where $V$ is the number of vertices, $E$ is the number of the edges, and $F$ is the number of faces. A value of $X$ equal to two indicates that the surface is topologically equivalent to a sphere. The existence of handles (like that of a coffee cup) in the surface reduces

| # Vertices | $\chi$ | # meshes |
|------------|--------|----------|
| 356,814 | −462 | 1 |
| 178 | 2 | 1 |
| 51 − 124 | 2 | 6 |
| 21 − 50 | 2 | 45 |
| 6 − 20 | 2 | 507 |

| # iterations | $\chi$ |
|--------------|--------|
| 0 | −462 |
| 1 | −26 |
| 2 | −12 |
| 3 | −6 |
| 4 | 0 |
| 5 | 2 |

(a)            (b)

**Table 1.** (a) Euler characteristic of resulting surface after each iteration, (b) Size and Euler characteristics of meshes from original isosurface.

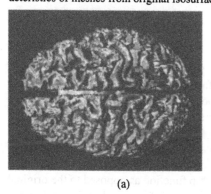 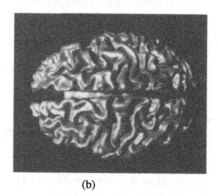

(a)            (b)

**Fig. 2.** (a) Isosurface of WM membership function, (b) topologically correct surface.

the value of $\chi$ [8]. We found that handles on the surface can be removed by performing successive median filters on the WM membership function and recomputing the isosurface.

In addition to the topology problem, the output from an isosurface algorithm on the WM membership function usually contains many small meshes which correspond to voxels that have been corrupted by noise and other artifacts. These meshes are physically not connected to the real WM outer surface, therefore, we designed an efficient algorithm that separates the meshes by their vertex connectivity, and outputs only the largest mesh.

Our automatic procedure for computing an initial estimate of the cortical surface can be summarized by the following:

1. Compute an isosurface on WM membership function.
2. Extract only connected surface with largest number of vertices.
3. Compute $\chi$.
4. If $\chi$ is not equal to 2, then apply a median filter to the WM membership function, recompute the isosurface on the filtered data, and go to Step 2.

We now provide some results from our sample data set. Isosurfaces were generated using the Visualization Data Explorer software from IBM which uses the ALLIGATOR algorithm [10]. Median filtering was performed using a $3 \times 3 \times 3$ kernel. Table 1a shows the number of surfaces and their $\chi$ values before any median filtering has taken place. The one mesh which is clearly much larger than all other meshes represents a topologically incorrect estimate of the GM-WM interface. Table 1b shows how the $\chi$ of the resulting surface increases after each iteration and eventually converges to the desired value of two. Figure 2a shows the result of the isosurface algorithm on the original WM membership function at a threshold of 0.5. Multiple surfaces and topological inconsistencies are present. Figure 2b shows the final, topologically correct surface after six iterations of our procedure. We see that although we have not yet applied the deformable surface model, many of the prominent geometrical characteristics of this cortical surface are already apparent.

## 2.4 Refinement of the cortical surface

After obtaining an initial estimate of the cortical surface which is topologically correct, the surface requires refinement. The initial surface is a smoothed version of the GM-WM interface. Using deformable surfaces, it is possible to have this initial surface move towards the desired surface (i.e., the medial layer surface of the GM). The main problem here lies in defining the external forces.

Two ideas were incorporated into the standard deformable surface model [11] in order to make the initial surface converge to the cortical surface. For the external force, the gradient was computed on the GM membership function as opposed to the original image. The gradient of the GM membership is well suited for providing forces directed towards the center of the GM. In addition, because the initial surface is known to lie inside the desired surface, a pressure force [12] was incorporated in order to resist the tendency of the deformable surface to shrink, which is a well known problem associated with the elastic internal force. Use of the pressure force also helps the surface conform to concave regions of the GM.

Fig. 3a shows the result of the final deformed surface on our sample data set. Fig. 3b shows a cross-section of the final deformed surface superimposed on the corresponding axial MR slice. Fig. 3c shows a magnified region of the same slice. These figures show that most of the complex sulci and gyri were extracted by the deformable surface. However, some structures still were not fully found.

## 3 Discussion and Conclusions

The presented method for finding the cortical surface in MR data has the potential to preserve even the deepest folds in the cortex using deformable surface models. Several possibilities exist, however, for further improvement. First, more sophisticated segmentation algorithms are available which take into account the spatial dependence of image intensities and MRI artifacts, such as intrascan intensity inhomogeneities. In order to take full advantage of our method, however, a fuzzy segmentation output is required. Second, an improvement in the initial cortical surface may be obtained by using a different isosurface threshold, or by computing an isosurface on a function of the membership functions. Finally, an external force model which is better suited to pulling the deformable surface towards concave regions is desirable.

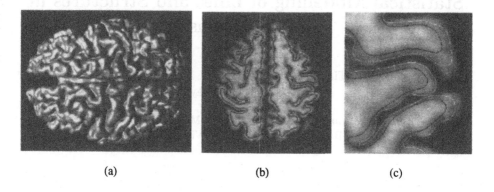

(a)                             (b)                             (c)

**Fig. 3.** (a) Final deformable surface. (b) Cross section of the final deformable surface overlaid on top of the MRI image. (c) A magnified view of a sub-region of (b). The initial position and the final position of the deformable surface are plotted in black and white, respectively.

## Acknowledgements

The authors would like to thank Dr. R. Nick Bryan for his support of this work.

# References

1. A. M. Dale and M. I. Sereno. Improved localization of cortical activity combining EEG and MEG with MRI cortical surface reconstruction: A linear approach. *J. Cogn. Neuroscience*, 5(2):162–176, 1993.
2. D. MacDonald, D. Avis, and A. C. Evans. Multiple surface identification and matching in magnetic resonance images. In *SPIE Proc. VBC '94*, volume 2359, pages 160–169, 1994.
3. G. E. Christensen et al. Topological properties of smooth anatomic maps. In *Information Processing in Medical Imaging*, pages 101–112, 1995.
4. S. Sandor and R. Leahy. Towards automated labelling of the cerebral cortex using a deformable atlas. In *Information Processing in Medical Imaging*, pages 127–138, 1995.
5. E. L. Chaney and S. M. Pizer. Defining anatomical structures from medical images. *Seminar in Radiation Oncology*, 2(4):215–225, October 1992.
6. J. C. Bezdek, L. O. Hall, and L. P. Clarke. Review of MR image segmentation techniques using pattern recognition. *Med. Phys.*, 20:1033–1048, 1993.
7. C. Davatzikos and R. N. Bryan. Using a deformable surface model to obtain a shape representation of the cortex. *IEEE Trans. Med. Imag.*, 15, Dec. 1996. To appear.
8. A. van Gelder and J. Wilhelms. Topological considerations in isosurface generation. *ACM Trans. on Graphics*, 13:337–375, 1994.
9. M. K. Agoston. *Algebraic Topology — A first course.* Marcel Dekker, Inc., New York, 1976.
10. A. D. Kalvin et al. Constructing topologically connected surfaces for the comprehensive analysis of 3D medical structures. In *SPIE Proc. Medical Imaging V: Image Processing*, volume 1445, pages 247–258, February 1991.
11. T. McInerney and D. Terzopoulos. A dynamic finite element surface model for segmentation and tracking in multidimensional medical images with application to cardiac 4d image analysis. *Comp. Med. Imag. Graph.*, 19(1):69–83, 1995.
12. L. D. Cohen. On active contour models and balloons. *CVGIP: Image Understanding*, 53(2):211–218, March 1991.

# Statistical Modelling of Lines and Structures in Mammograms *

Reyer Zwiggelaar[1][**], Tim C. Parr[1], Caroline R. M. Boggis[2], Susan M. Astley[1], and Christopher J. Taylor[1]

[1] Wolfson Image Analysis Unit, University of Manchester, Manchester, UK
[2] Greater Manchester Breast Screening Service, Withington Hospital, Manchester, UK

**Abstract.** Computer-aided mammographic prompting systems require the reliable detection of a variety of signs of cancer. The emphasis of the work described is the correct classification of linear structures in mammograms. Statistical modelling, based on principal component analysis (PCA), has been developed for describing the cross-sectional profiles of linear structures, the motivation being that the shapes of intensity profiles may be characteristic of the type of structure. PCA models have been applied to whole mammograms to obtain images in which spicules, linear structures associated with stellate lesions, are emphasised. The aim is to improve the performance of automatic stellate lesion detection by concentrating on those structures most likely to be associated with lesions.

## 1 Introduction

The UK Breast Screening Programme alone generates 1.5 million mammograms per annum. Potential malignancies can be detected from subtle abnormalities in radiographic appearance but it is known that radiologists fail to detect a significant proportion of these abnormalities and that their performance would improve if they were prompted with the possible locations of abnormalities [1].

In this study we concentrate on the detection of linear structures associated with stellate lesions. An example of such an abnormality is shown in Fig. 1a. We will show that it is possible to extract the linear structures which are most likely to be spicules. Our approach is based on the idea that the shapes of the cross-sectional profiles of linear structures may be characteristic of the type of structure. We have developed statistical models, based on principal component analysis (PCA) describing the shape of cross-sectional profiles of linear structures. Our various PCA models can be used to determine the probability that a particular type of linear structure (e.g. a spicule) is present at any given location in the image. The resulting probabilities can be used to obtain an odds-ratio

---

* The work presented in this paper is part of the Prompting Radiologists In Screening Mammography (PRISM) project and is funded by EPSRC.
** email: reyer@sv1.smb.man.ac.uk

image which can be used analogously to a line strength image as the basis for modelling and classifying spatial patterns of linear structures for application in the detection of stellate lesions and similar abnormalities [2–5].

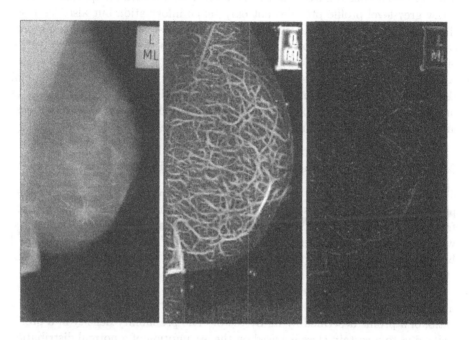

**Fig. 1.** a. Typical example of the (annotated) linear structures associated with a spiculated lesion in a mammogram (mdb181lm from the MIAS database [6]), b. The line strength image resulting from applying the line operator to the mammogram, c. Odds-ratio image resulting from applying (2) and the described approach to the mammogram

## 2 Modelling Linear Structures

To apply the PCA profile model to every pixel in a mammogram a sequence of steps must be taken.

### 2.1 Detecting Linear Structures and Extracting Profiles

Firstly, a detection technique for linear structures has to be applied to the mammogram, resulting in three values for every pixel: the line strength, orientation and scale. We detect linear structures in mammograms using a non-linear directional line operator - a detailed description can be found in [7], which also provides a comparison with other line detection methods.

Once the linear structures were detected, a random selection was labelled by an expert radiologist into anatomically distinct classes: *ducts, edges, fibrous tissue, skin folds, spicules, vessels* and *others* (a detailed description of the selection process can be found in [8]). Cross-sectional profiles were obtained. The profiles were corrected for background slope and transformed to a logarithmic intensity scale. Instead of using the cross-sectional profiles directly it is also possible to use information derived from them. The motivation for such an approach is that a raw grey-level profile provides not only shape information but also describes the local background grey-level and structure contrast. The shape of the profile can be described by the normalised (with respect to the mean) first derivative of the profile or by direct normalisation with respect to the standard deviation. Although the background grey-level value might not be related to the shape of the profile the mean value can give some information as particular classes of profiles are more likely to be present at certain anatomical regions of the breast area which might have a characteristic background grey-level value.

## 2.2 Principal Component Analysis and Profile Classification

The principal components of a set of observation vectors (e.g. the grey-level profiles) are the characteristic vectors of the covariance matrix ($C_i$) constructed from the data set. The characteristic values describe the variances associated with the principal components. The dimensionality of the data set can be reduced by ignoring the principal components with low (or zero) characteristic values; the weights of the prical components are given by $b_j = P^T (x_j - m)$.

We investigated the extent to which profiles could be classified as belonging to a particular anatomical class by determining the probability, and resulting odds-ratio, of a profile described by its $b_j$ vector. The probability density of a profile belonging to a certain class is based on the assumption of a normal distribution and uses the Mahalanobis distance given by $\delta_{ij} = (m_i - b_j)^T C_i^{-1} (m_i - b_j)$, the resulting probability density is

$$p_{ij} = \frac{1}{(2\pi)^{n/2}|C_i|^{1/2}} \exp\left(\frac{-\delta_{ij}}{2}\right). \tag{1}$$

The resulting odds-ratio of class/not-class probability densities is given by

$$R_{ij} = \frac{p_{ij}}{\sum_{n \neq i} p_{nj}}. \tag{2}$$

Based on the odds-ratio every profile can be classified into the most likely class by thresholding. In this case we are most interested in classifying all the profiles into being spicules/non-spicules and in obtaining a Receiver Operating Characteristic (ROC) curve for this particular problem.

## 3 Linear Structure Classification

We have assessed if principal component models provide a useful description of grey-level profiles and if the derived models can be used for profile classification. The total number of linear structures were 318 comprising 46,968 profiles. The results in this section are all based on a leave-one-image-out analysis. This means that the PCA model and the mean and covariance were determined from all the profiles except for those in one mammogram. The results were applied to the profiles present in the one mammogram which was left out of the training set. This was repeated for each mammogram in turn.

For the PCA model based on the raw profile the first principal component explains 96% of the training set variance and mainly describes the background grey-level. The cumulative variance associated with the first five principal components are respectively: 96.5%, 98.7%, 99.1%, 99.4% and 99.6%. This indicates that over 99% of the variance is described by the first three principal components.

For the other PCA models the trend is that the more the model relies on the shape of the profiles the more principal components are needed to describe 99% of the variation, for example for the model based on the normalisation with respect to the standard deviation the first principal component describes 19.4% of the variation and 26 principal components are needed to describe 99% of the variation.

ROC results for the spicule class are shown in Fig. 2; curves obtained using different PCA models. This shows that the raw profile can be used for classification purposes; the effects background grey-level and local contrast will, however, be compounded with shape. Both the direct normalised and first derivative profiles still retain information about the local contrast. Pure shape information described by normalised first derivative profiles cannot be used for classification purposes; this is probably due to the amplification of noise. However, pure shape information provided by normalisation with respect to the standard deviation provides useful discrimination. Additional discrimination can be obtained from the mean, standard deviation and width of the profiles.

Similar results were obtained for the other anatomical classes. These showed that for vessels the background grey-level decreased the classification accuracy, which is probably due to the fact that these linear structures can be present in all regions of the breast (i.e. on a variety of backgrounds) and that the pure shape information alone gave the best classification results indicating that the profile shape must be similar at a range of scales. For ducts there did not seem to be much discrimination power in the shape of the profiles (possibily because of the wide range of profile shapes for the ducts annotated in the mammograms) but that the background grey-level and local contrast do provide classification information.

## 4  Spicule Strength Images

The PCA model based on the normalisation with respect to the standard deviation has been used to generate images in which pixel intensities are related to the likelihood of the pixel belonging to a given class (in this case spicules) of linear structure. Results are illustrated for a mammogram (mdb181lm) from the MIAS database [6].

The first step is to detect the linear structures; the resulting line strength image is shown in Fig.1b. A simple threshold has been applied to the line strength

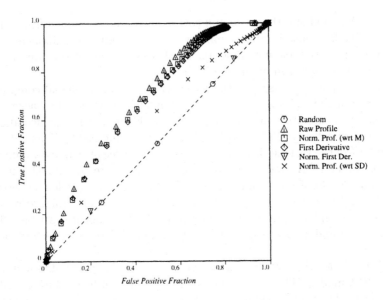

**Fig. 2.** Spicule profile classification for various PCA models

image to select a limited number of pixels which are more likely to form the backbone of the structures.

For each of the remaining pixels a profile was extracted from the original mammogram. Each profile was converted to its corresponding vector $\mathbf{b}_j$ using the PCA model. The probability density $(p_{ij})$ associated with class $i$ corresponding to a vector $\mathbf{b}_j$ is given by (1). and the odds-ratio is determined by (2). The resulting spicule/non-spicule odds-ratio image for the example image is shown in Fig. 1c. This shows that most of the linear structures which are situated around the spiculated lesion have a high probability of being spicules, whilst a majority of the linear structures which are not spicules have a lower probability and could be removed from the mammogram. This can be directly compared to the line strength image which shows that a large number of non-spicule linear structures have been removed.

## 5 Conclusions

An automated technique for detecting specific types of linaer structure in digital mammograms has been described. We have demonstrated how principal component analysis can be used to successfully model the shape of the cross-sectional intensity profiles of the anatomically different linear structures.

A leave-one-image-out classification experiment demonstrated anatomical classification with a significantly better than random correct classification for the spicule profiles. The potential of this technique for discriminating between ducts and vessels to reduce the number of false positives generated by automated micro-calcification detection algorithms is clear. A correct classification rate of

80% for spicules/non-spicules could be achieved (at a false positive percentage of ~55%), which will clearly be useful for the verification of potential spiculated lesions and architectural distortions. In similar experiments, not reported in detail here, good classification results have also been obtained for vessels and ducts. The detection and classification of ducts is likely to provide useful information for automated techniques attempting to locate the nipple.

A comparison of Figs 1a and 1c provides a qualitative demonstration of the achievement of our objective; similar results have been achieved for a number of images. Visual inspection of the images indicates that the linear structures associated with spiculated lesions have been preserved whilst a substantial number of other structures have been removed. When comparing Figs 1b and 1c it should be clear that the number of non-spicule linear structures has been reduced whilst the spicules themself are less affected.

In summary, the algorithms presented in this paper provide an automatic technique for locating and successfully classifying anatomically important linear structures of which spicules were used as an example. Such classification can be employed to verify automatically detected potential abnormalities such as microcalcification clusters, stellate lesions and architectural distortions. In addition, the technique can be used to provide strength images relating to specific classes of abnormality; spicule strength images can then be used to improve the accuracy of spiculated lesion detection algorithms [2–5].

# References

1. I.W. Hutt. *The Computer-aided Detection of Abnormalities in Digital Mammograms*. PhD thesis, The University of Manchester, UK, 1996.
2. W.P. Kegelmeyer Jr. Computer detection of stellate lesions in mammograms. *Proceedings of SPIE*, 1660:446–454, 1992.
3. N.J. Cerneaz and J.M. Brady. Finding curvilinear structurs in mammograms. *Lecture Notes in Computer Science*, 905:372–382, 1995.
4. N. Karssemeijer and G.M. te Brake. Detection of stellate distortions in mammograms. *IEEE Transactions on Medical Imaging*, 15(5):611–619, 1996.
5. T.C. Parr, S.M. Astley, C.J. Taylor, and C.R.M. Boggis. A statistical representation of pattern structure for digital mammography. *Excerpta Medica*, 1119:357–360, 1996.
6. J. Suckling, J. Parker, D. Dance, S. Astley, I. Hutt, C. Boggis, I. Ricketts, E. Stamatakis, N. Cerneaz, S. Kok, P. Taylor, D. Betal, and J. Savage. The mammographic images analysis society digital mammogram database. In Dance Gale, Astley and Cairns, editors, *Digital Mammography*, pages 375–378. Elsevier, 1994.
7. R. Zwiggelaar, T.C. Parr, and C.J. Taylor. Finding orientated line patterns in digital mammographic images. In *Proceedings of the 7th British Machine Vision Conference*, pages 715–724, Edinburgh, UK, 1996.
8. R. Zwiggelaar, T.C. Parr, C.R.M. Boggis, S.M. Astley, and C.J. Taylor. Statistical modelling of lines and structures in mammograms. *Proceedings of SPIE*, 3034:to appear, 1997.

# A Thinning Algorithm to Extract Medial Lines from 3D Medical Images*

Kálmán Palágyi and Attila Kuba

Department of Applied Informatics, József Attila University
H-6701 Szeged P.O.Box 652, Hungary

**Abstract.** This paper presents an efficient parallel algorithm for thinning elongated 3D binary objects (e.g., bony structures, vessel trees, or airway trees). This algorithm directly extracts medial lines (i.e., without creating medial surface). One iteration step consists of 12 subiterations (instead of 6, which is the usual case) according to the selected 12 deletion directions. Our topology preserving algorithm gives satisfactory results for synthetic data tests and for MR angiography brain studies.

## 1 Introduction

The skeletonization provides shape features that are extracted from binary image data. Its goal is to reduce the volume of elongated objects to their skeletons in a topology preserving way [1]. In the 3D Euclidean space, the skeleton can be defined as the locus of the centers of all the maximal inscribed spheres that touch the boundary of the object at least in two points. Thinning is a frequently used method for extracting skeletons in discrete spaces. Border points of the binary object that satisfy certain topological and geometric constraints are deleted in iteration steps until there are no more deletable points left. (Deletion means, that object elements are changed to background elements).

Thinning operation can be applied in medical image processing, too, and some important applications have been appeared. Van den Elsen et al. [2] extracted ridge–like features in their medical image registration method. They used 3D thinning to eliminate unwanted thick ridges and blobs. Thinning provides relevant information and reduces the feature search space of the geometric model to be evaluated. Gerig et al. [3] used 3D thinning for symbolic description of cerebral vessel tree.

In this paper, a new 3D thinning algorithm is proposed for extracting medial lines. Our noise–tolerant algorithm preserves topology and our test results have shown, that it provides a good approximation to the "true" Euclidean skeleton.

## 2 Basic definitions

In this section, the necessary definitions are given. We use the notations introduced by Kong and Rosenfeld [1].

---

* This work was supported by OTKA "Medical Image Registration" grant.

A *3D binary (26,6) digital picture* $\mathcal{P}$ is a quadruple $\mathcal{P} = (\mathbf{Z}^3, 26, 6, B)$, where each element in $\mathbf{Z}^3$ is called *point* of $\mathcal{P}$. A point in $B \subseteq \mathbf{Z}^3$ is called *black point*; a point in $\mathbf{Z}^3 \backslash B$ is called *white point*. Picture $\mathcal{P}$ is called *finite* if $B$ is a finite set. Value 1 is assigned to each black point; value 0 is assigned to each white point. Two black points are *adjacent*, if they are *26–adjacent*; two white points are *adjacent*, if they are *6–adjacent*, see Fig. 1.

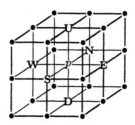

**Fig. 1.** The considered adjacencies in $\mathbf{Z}^3$. Points marked by **U**, **N**, **E**, **S**, **W**, and **D** are 6–adjacent to the point $p$; points 6–adjacent to $p$ and points marked by "•" are 26–adjacent to the point $p$;

The transitive closure of the 26–adjacency is called *26–connectivity* relation. Equivalence classes of $B$ under 26–connectivity are called *black 26–components* or *objects*. A singleton black component is called *isolated point*. A black point is called *border point*, if it is 6–adjacent to at least one white point. A border point $p$ is called **U**–*border point*, if the point marked by **U** in Fig. 1 is white. (We can define **N**–, **E**–, **S**–, **W**–, and **D**–border points in similar way.)

An iterative thinning algorithm deletes some border points that satisfy certain deletion conditions. The entire process is repeated until there are no more black points to be changed. Each thinning algorithm should satisfy the requirement of topology preservation. Kong and Rosenfeld [1] discussed some definitions of topology preservation of 3D thinning operations. Ma [4] established sufficient conditions for 3D parallel thinning operations to preserve topology. Topology preservation is not the only requirement to be complied with. Additional conditions have been stated to supply the skeleton.

CRITERION 2.1 [5, 6]. A 3D operation can be regarded as a *thinning algorithm*, if it fulfils the following three conditions.

1. Topology is preserved.
2. Isolated points and curves remain unchanged.
3. A black cube of size $2 \times 2 \times 2$ is changed after applying the algorithm.

A few 3D thinning algorithms have been developed so far. Most of them is *border sequential* [6, 7, 8]. Each iteration step is divided into more successive subiterations. Only a certain type of border points can be deleted during a subiteration. The subiterations are executed in parallel (i.e., all points that satisfy the actual deletion conditions are deleted simultaneously) and the deletion conditions depend on the $3 \times 3 \times 3$ neighbourhood of the points.

Some algorithms have been developed for generating *medial surface* [7]. Others produce medial surface and *medial lines*, too [6, 8]. Generally, the extraction of medial lines consists of two phases. During the first phase, the medial surface is to be extracted from the original object. The second phase results in the medial lines from the medial surface. The two–phase method is noise sensitive since it produces unwanted parasitic line segments (see later).

## 3  The new thinning algorithm

In this section, a new algorithm is described for thinning 3D binary $(26, 6)$ images.

Our 12–subiteration border sequential 3D thinning algorithm directly creates medial lines, i.e., without extracting medial surface. The new value of each point depends on its $3 \times 3 \times 3$ neighbourhood. This dependence is given by a set of $3 \times 3 \times 3$ lattice point configurations. Only deletion conditions are used (i.e., black points can be changed but white points remain the same). The deletion condition assigned to a subiteration is described by a set of masks (or matching templates). A black point is to be deleted, if and only if its $3 \times 3 \times 3$ neighbourhood matches at least one element of the given set of masks.

The masks are constructed according to the 12 deletion directions **US**, **NE**, **DW**, **UW**, **SE**, **DN**, **UN**, **SW**, **DE**, **UE**, **NW**, and **DS**. It means that these directions correspond to the directions of the 12 non–opposite pairs of 6–neighbours.

The masks, assigned to the direction **US**, give the condition to delete certain U–border points or S–borders points. The masks of **NE** are to delete certain N– or E–border points, etc. The 12 masks denoted by $\mathcal{M}_{\mathbf{US}}$ are assigned to the direction **US**, see Fig. 2. Deletion conditions of the other 11 subiterations can be derived from the appropriate rotations and reflections of masks $\mathcal{M}_{\mathbf{US}}$.

Let $\mathcal{P} = (\mathbb{Z}^3, 26, 6, B)$ be the finite 3D picture to be thinned. Since the set $B$ is finite, it can be stored in a finite 3D binary array $X$. (Outside of this array every point will be considered as 0 (white).) Denote $\mathcal{D}_i$ the $i$th deletion direction of the sequence of directions $\langle \mathbf{US}, \ldots, \mathbf{DS} \rangle$, for $i = 1, 2, \ldots, 12$. Suppose, that the subiteration that corresponds to the deletion direction $\mathcal{D}_i$ results picture $\mathcal{P}' = (\mathbb{Z}^3, 26, 6, B')$ from picture $\mathcal{P}$. Denote $\mathcal{T}(X, \mathcal{D}_i)$ the binary array representing the picture $\mathcal{P}'$. We are now ready to present our thinning algorithm formally.

ALGORITHM 3.1 for thinning the picture $\mathcal{P} = (\mathbb{Z}^3, 26, 6, B)$
  **Input:** binary array $X$ representing the picture $\mathcal{P}$
  **Output:** binary array $Y$ representing the thinned picture
  *begin*
  $Y = X$;
  *repeat*
    *for* $i = 1$ *to* 12 *do*
      $Y = \mathcal{T}(Y, \mathcal{D}_i)$;
  *until* no more points to be deleted;
  *end.*

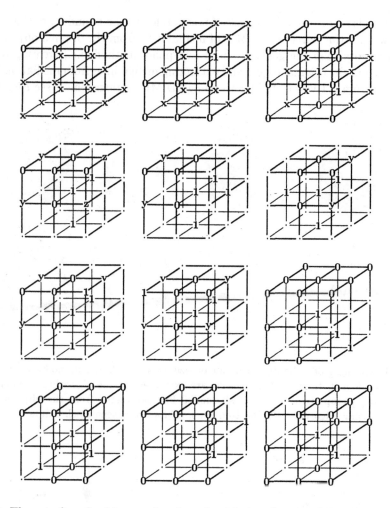

**Fig. 2.** The set of masks $\mathcal{M}_{\mathbf{US}}$ assigned to the deletion direction **US**. Notations: "." ("don't care") which matches either **0** or **1**; at least one point marked by "**x**" is **1**; at least one point marked by "**y**" and at least one point marked by "**z**" are **0**; and the values of the two points marked by "**v**" are different (one of them must be **0** and the other one must be **1**).

The masks $\mathcal{M}_{\mathbf{US}}$ can be very easily implemented. It can be described by a Boolean function of 26 variables requiring 187 logical "or" and "and" operations and 24 "not" operations (without optimization) [9]. It have been shown in [9], that Algorithm 3.1 is a 3D thinning algorithm in the sense of Criterion 2.1.

## 4 Discussion

We have tested Algorithm 3.1 with noisy and noise–free images as well, in order to estimate its noise sensitiveness (see Fig. 3). This example shows, that our algorithm is stable even in the case of noise added to the boundary of the object. It shows also that direct extraction of medial lines from the original object gives better results than the generally used two–phase method (i.e., creating medial surface from the original object and extracting medial lines from medial surface).

Algorithm 3.1 was tested for thinning 3D MR angiographies (see Fig. 4).

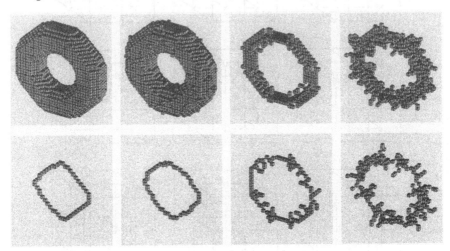

**Fig. 3.** Thinning of a 3D digital donut of size $32 \times 32 \times 9$ and its noisy version (top left two images); their medial surfaces are extracted by the algorithm of Gong and Bertrand [7] (top right two images); medial lines extracted from the objects above them by using Algorithm 3.1 (bottom row). (Cubes represent black points.)

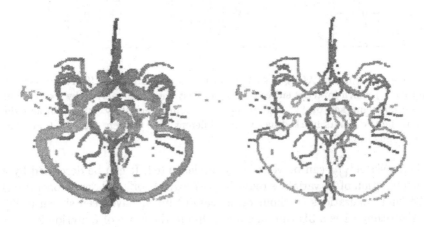

**Fig. 4.** Thinning of a 3D MR angiography image by using Algorithm 3.1. The original top–down projection of the thresholded image of dimensions $256 \times 256 \times 124$ (left); the thinned projection (right). The authors wish to acknowledge the UMDS Image Processing Group, London for the image.

# 5 Conclusions

A parallel algorithm has been presented for thinning 3D binary objects. It directly extracts medial lines by applying iteration steps consisting of 12 subiterations. The algorithm allows easy implementation. According to the experiments made on synthetic images, our algorithm provides a good approximation of the "true" Euclidean skeleton. It gives more stable and uniform (symmetric) medial lines than other algorithms, even in noisy cases.

# Acknowledgements

We are grateful to Dr Derek Hill, Radiological Sciences, UMDS, Guy's Hospital for supplying the image data for Fig. 4.

# References

1. T.Y. Kong, A. Rosenfeld: Digital topology: Introduction and survey. Computer Vision, Graphics, and Image Processing 48, 357–393 (1989)
2. P.A. van den Elsen, J.B.A. Maintz, E.J.D. Pol, and M.A. Viergever: Image fusion using geometrical features. In R.A. Robb (ed.): Visualization in biomedical computing. volume 1808 of Proc. SPIE. Bellingham, WA: SPIE Press 1992, pp. 172–186,
3. G. Gerig, Th. Koller, G. Székely, Ch. Brechbühler, and O. Kübler: Symbolic description of 3–D structures applied to cerebral vessel tree obtained from MR angiography volume data. In H.H. Barrett and A.F. Gmitro (eds.): Information Processing in Medical Imaging, Proceedings of 13th International Conference, IPMI'93. Lecture Notes in Computer Science 687. Berlin: Springer 1993, pp. 94–111
4. C.M. Ma: On topology preservation in 3D thinning. CVGIP: Image Understanding 59, 328–339 (1994)
5. A. Rosenfeld: A characterization of parallel thinning algorithms. Information Control 29, 286–291 (1975)
6. Y.F. Tsao, K.S. Fu: A parallel thinning algorithm for 3–D pictures. Computer Graphics and Image Processing 17, 315–331 (1981)
7. W.X. Gong, G. Bertrand: A simple parallel 3D thinning algorithm. In Proceedings of the 10th International Conference on Pattern Recognition. 1990, pp. 188–190
8. T. Lee, R.L. Kashyap, and C. Chu: Building skeleton models via 3–D medial surface/axis thinning algorithms. CVGIP: Graphical Models and Image Processing 56, 462–478 (1994)
9. K. Palágyi, A. Kuba: A topology preserving 12-subiteration 3D thinning algorithm. Internal report, Department of Applied Informatics, József Attila University (1996)

# Setting the Mind for Intelligent Interactive Segmentation: Overview, Requirements, and Framework

Sílvia D. Olabarriaga * and Arnold W.M. Smeulders

University of Amsterdam, Department of Computer Science
Kruislaan 403, 1098 SJ Amsterdam, The Netherlands
Email:{silvia,smeulders}@wins.uva.nl

**Abstract.** It is widely recognized that automatic segmentation is hard, leading to the state where user intervention cannot be avoided. In this paper we review existing literature and propose a systematic approach for the integration of automatic and interactive segmentation methods into one unified process. A framework and requirements for intelligent interactive segmentation are formulated, and an example is presented.

## 1 Introduction

Image segmentation is an important step in the analysis of medical images, being roughly based on homogeneity and discontinuities in the image function. Some segmentation algorithms combine both sources of information [1], or consider it at different scales [2], but most rely on visual evidence[2] of the represented objects. Such evidence is not always present, especially in medical imaging modalities where noise or 3D reconstruction impose severe limits on image quality and cause these algorithms to fail. For this reason interactive techniques have received increasing attention due to the promise of being a practical solution in terms of reliability for use in the clinic. In this paper we review the existing literature and present a systematic approach for intelligent interactive segmentation (*IIS*). We characterize situations for user intervention, formulate requirements for tools, and propose a framework for the design of *IIS* techniques. We conclude with a case where this framework was used.

## 2 Review of Interaction in Segmentation Algorithms

Interaction as an additional source of information for segmentation has been used for a long time[3]. A simple example is fully manual segmentation, which is

---

* Permanent affiliation: Instituto de Informática, Universidade Federal do Rio Grande do Sul, Porto Alegre, Brazil. Grant 200146/95.5 from CNPq (Brazilian Council for Scientific and Technological Development)

[2] Any type of image-derived data that can indicate the location of regions (e.g. statistical features) or the presence of boundaries (e.g. gradient).

time-consuming, tedious, and provide results heavily dependent on the operator's skills and mood. Other examples in the literature can be broadly organized into three categories, depending on *when* user intervention occurs:

*At the beginning of segmentation,* to provide initial parameter values such as a seed, points in the contour, or a threshold level (e.g. [4]). The automatic process must be repeated with other parameters if the result is not correct.

*At the end of segmentation,* to confirm or correct the output of an automatic method: user input is taken literally and combined with previous results. The final segmentation is thus generated by two different processes, in part manual and in part automatic, impinging discontinuity on subsequent measurement of the object's features (e.g. curvature at points in the contour).
A variation is interactive postprocessing: the image is presegmented at several resolutions [5] or confidence levels [6], each one leading to a result or "alternative." The user interactively selects parts from different alternatives to compose the desired output. The user can only choose among alternatives generated with automatic methods, leading to higher objectivity in the segmentation results. However, the success of interaction heavily depends on the success of presegmentation and on the degree of user knowledge about the method itself.

*During segmentation,* to adjust parameters or supply information to help the algorithm converge to a desired solution. Visual feedback is available, and the user may stop the process, adjust parameters, and resume it at any desired state. Current trends in interactive segmentation such as "deformable boundary" and "live wire" techniques display these ideas.
In live-wire (e.g. [7] and [8]) the user indicates one boundary point and drags the cursor. The algorithm finds the best contour between the initial point and the current mouse position, and displays the resulting line; the user may confirm it or move the mouse to obtain a better delineation. The method dynamically updates the objective criteria for "best contour" based on the selected edge.
In deformable contour (e.g. [9], [10], [11], and [1]) the initial boundary drawn by the user evolves towards a balance of forces derived from the image (e.g. gradient), geometric expectations (e.g. smooth curvature), and the user input. The final result is a compromise between all the forces along the whole contour, assuring high degree of objectivity.

In the examples above user input is explicit (parameters or image elements) with the exception of live-wire and deformable contours, where it is used to derive parameter values instead. In all cases the semantics of interaction is strongly related to the segmentation method, and not to *what* is wrong in the results. There are thus limited possibilities for learning, a necessary condition to make the segmentation tools more "intelligent." The goal is to develop efficient, precise, and objective tools by attaching more semantics to user interventions, so that the algorithm can more easily learn from them and react accordingly.

# 3 Characterization of the Intervention

We assume that the user is capable of prompt judgment of (1) where is the true border of the entity and (2) which type of insertion or correction is needed. The user knows what to do, the only remaining difficulty being how to efficiently convey the message to the algorithm. It is thus important to characterize the types of user input useful in the segmentation process, and support each one with a specific interaction tool. There are at least two orthogonal dimensions for the characterization of user intervention: (1) the reason why the automatic segmentation method failed so far and (2) the type of geometry of the segmented object. Note that this characterization refers to *data features* only and is not (yet) related to any particular segmentation procedure.

## 3.1 Reasons for Failure of Automatic Methods

We have identified four major causes for an automatic method to yield a different segmentation result than desired, which suggest different user actions:

1. Local visual evidence is too low, and the desired result cannot be picked with the current setting of parameters to the segmentation algorithm. Solution: local tuning of parameters guided by the user. Action: *"tune."*
2. Visual evidence is absent. No segmentation method could provide a solution, unless the missing border can be extrapolated from evidence elsewhere. Solution: a trained observer with insight on the object's anatomy or some shape model could provide missing data. Action: *"fill."*
3. Visual evidence is overrun by a neighboring object and the segmentation algorithm deposits the border at the wrong place. Solution: a trained operator could indicate the presence of more than one structure and the frontiers between them. Actions: *"cut"* or *"reposition border."*
4. Visual evidence deviates from what the computational model can handle. The patient might have a different anatomy than foreseen, or the recording is not ideal, or the model is just not complete. At any rate, the segmentation algorithm will fail even when some form of visual evidence is there. Solution: the operator could indicate another model to be used, or even correct the results manually, with the onus of introducing discontinuities. Action: *"fix."*

Note: the first cause could be considered as a special case of the fourth (part of the contour is always missing), and the third, as a special case of the second (lack of local visual evidence is due to the interference from another structure).

## 3.2 Types of Geometry

In medical imaging objects of interest are usually three-dimensional (3D) structures, although they might be depicted in different dimensions in the acquired images. The complete 3D-shape, however, might be irrelevant for some applications and the object may be represented with some simplified geometry. Different types of geometry suggest specific user actions and segmentation algorithms, and as such should be supported by a corresponding set of interaction tools with proper visual representation, feedback, and behavior. Geometry types of 3D-objects can be characterized as follows, with the purpose of designing tools with a large degree of application independency:

1. *point:* seen as an object of arbitrary scale without inner structure; only the position is relevant (e.g. the heart may be a point in a total body scan);
2. *line:* mostly, the object's axis (1D) is relevant (e.g. blood-vessels); some shape regularity is assumed for cross-sections;
3. *surface:* only the enclosing surface (2D) of the object is relevant (e.g. the heart outer wall);
4. *volume:* the outer surface and the inner structure are relevant (e.g. brain).

## 4  Requirements for *IIS*

Apart from being robust and predictable in terms of reliability, the following requirements are posed on (*IIS*) tools:

1. Data provided by the user should be used to derive model parameters and not directly as a literal part of the output. This guarantees that a *uniform process* generates segmentation results, with important implications for measurement continuity.
2. Segmentation results should be *locally invariant to user intervention,* being reproducible under predictable limits of variations. This is achieved by searching for a local optimum in the segmentation quality, which is a measured value derived from the image data, the segmentation result, a priori parameter settings, and parameter values derived from the interaction.
3. Interventions should have high *semantics* (small action = big impact into the desired direction). It requires the user to be able to predict the impact of her or his actions on the segmentation results, and it guarantees efficiency to the interaction.
4. User input should be *generalizable* to allow inference for neighboring or similar elements; that is, it should be possible to "learn" from user input. This requires parameters derived from user input to be used as a priori values in the next segmentation task, guaranteeing efficient interaction.

We suggest *IIS* to be implemented as the local steering of parameters for an otherwise automatic segmentation method to arrive at an uniform process to segment the image, which is simultaneously close to the interaction and to the original result where the interaction was absent.

## 5  Design of *IIS* Tools

As suggested in Sect. 4, tools should be specific for the action that the user wants to perform; it is wrong to make one universal editing tool as it will display nonspecific performance. Each of the situations characterized in Sect. 3 leads to a different type of extension to the segmentation method and to a corresponding interaction tool. As a conclusion, a system for intelligent interactive segmentation should provide at least $4 \times 4$ tools (see Tab.1) which express the combination of features in two dimensions: the reason for failure (tune, fill, cut, and fix), and the type of geometry (point, line, surface, and volume).

**Table 1.** Matrix of *IIS* Tools for 3D Objects

|  | Point | Line | Surface | Volume |
|---|---|---|---|---|
| Tune (locally low) |  |  |  |  |
| Fill (locally absent) |  | study-case |  |  |
| Cut (interference) |  |  |  |  |
| Fix (model deviates) |  |  |  |  |

### 5.1 An Example of IIS tool

We applied the framework to one study-case so far: the segmentation of an aortic aneurism in CT images[3]. The problem was considered a case of local absence of visual evidence, although it could also be approached as interference from neighboring objects: sometimes there is no image contrast between the spine and the aorta lumen (outer contour in Fig. 1 - left), and simple automatic segmentation methods like thresholding fail (see Fig. 1 - right).

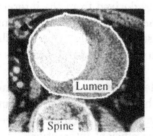 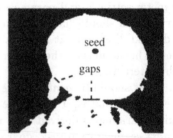

**Fig. 1.** Partial CT image with visible cross-sections of aorta and spine. *Left:* histogram-equalized image with lumen contour *Right:* thresholded image.

To correct this result the user points directly on the thresholded image to indicate gap positions and a seed inside the lumen (see Fig. 1 - right). The IIS

---

[3] $512 \times 512$, 126 slices orthogonal to the spine in the abdomen, 16 bits/voxel, provided by the Imaging Center Utrecht, The Netherlands.

algorithm delineates the complete boundary by growing from the seed outwards while searching for the existing visual evidence of contour. We use a region-growing algorithm combined with a "balloon" [10] with the following modification: the weight for the image-derived force is reduced where a gap has been pointed out by the user. The curvature-smoothing force naturally interpolates the boundary in the gap areas.

The type of geometry corresponds to a line-like object with variable, round-like, cross-sections. The approximate location of gaps can be easily propagated to the neighboring cross-sections, as well as the seed for region-growing. This example fits in the framework as shown in Tab.1 and is currently under development; it could not be compared to other techniques yet.

# 6 Conclusions

A framework to *IIS* has been presented, which provides a systematic approach to medical image segmentation. We have formulated the problem in terms of requirements, thus also providing guidelines for development of *IIS* tools which have been followed in a study-case, and one of the suggested IIS tools is now under development. Experimental results are still needed for a better evaluation.

# References

1. A. CHAKRABORTY, L.H. STAIB, and J.S. DUNCAN. Deformable boundary finding in medical images by integrating gradient and region information. *IEEE Trans. Medical Imaging*, 14(6):859–870, 1996.
2. M.J. McAULIFFE and et.al. Scale-space boundary evolution initialized by cores. In *Vis. Biomedical Computing*, pages 173–182, 1996.
3. J. UDUPA. Interactive segmentation and boundary surface formation for 3D digital images. *Computer Graphics and Image Processing*, 18.213–235, 1982.
4. G.J. SIVEWRIGIIT and P.J. ELLIOT. Interactive region and volume growing for segmenting volumes in mr and ct images. *Medical Informatics*, 19(1):71–80, 1994.
5. F. FONTANA and et.al. Multiseed interactive segmentation using different perspective angles for histological structures. *Proc. of the SPIE*, 1898:247–251, 1993.
6. D.V. BEARD and et.al. Interacting with image hierarchies for fast and accurate object segmentation. *Proc. of the SPIE*, 2167:10–17, 1994.
7. A.X. FALCAO and et.al. User-steered image segmentation paradigms: live wire and live lane. Technical Report 213, MIPG - University of Pennsylvania, 1995.
8. W.A. BARRET and E.N. MORTENSEN. Fast, accurate, and reproducible livewire boundary extraction. In *Vis. Biomedical Computing*, pages 183–192, 1996.
9. M. KASS, A. WITKIN, and D. TERZOPOULOS. Snakes: active contour models. *International Journal of Computer Vision*, 1(4):321–331, 1987.
10. L.D. COHEN. Active contour models and balloons. *CVGIP: image understanding*, 53(2):211–218, 1991.
11. M. WORRING and et.al. Parameterized feasible boundaries in gradient vector fields. *Computer vision and image understanding*, 63(1):135–144, 1996.

# Segmentation of Cerebral Vessels and Aneurysms from MR Angiography Data

Dale L. Wilson and J. Alison Noble

Department of Engineering Science, Oxford University, Parks Rd, Oxford OX1 3PJ.

**Abstract.** A three-dimensional representation of cerebral vessel morphology is essential for neurologists treating cerebral aneurysms. However, current imaging techniques cannot provide such a representation: slices of MR angiography (MRA) data can only give two-dimensional descriptions, and ambiguities of aneurysm position and size arising in X-ray projection imaging can often be intractable. To overcome these problems, we have established a new, fully automatic, statistically based algorithm for segmenting the three-dimensional vessel information from time of flight (TOF) MRA data. We introduce a mixture distribution for the data, motivated by a physical model of blood flow, that is used in a two stage segmentation algorithm. In the first stage we apply an expectation maximisation (EM) algorithm as a statistical classifier. We then utilise structural criteria in the second stage to refine the initial segmentation. We present results from applying our algorithm to two real data sets, containing both vessel and aneurysm structures.

## 1 Introduction

Increasingly, imaging is being applied in minimal invasive surgery to provide two-dimensional and three-dimensional visualisation of vascular structures to assist clinicians in pre-operation planning, real-time operating room decision-making, and post-operation monitoring. One emerging area of interest is in quantitative image processing techniques that can aid in the development of new and safer methods of endovascular treatment for intracranial saccular aneurysms. Safe embolisation of an aneurysm depends on accurate delivery of the embolic material (in order to avoid inducing stroke), and also on the accurate assessment of the size, location, and shape of aneurysms so that reliable occlusion can be achieved. The task of the clinician during the procedure involves the manipulation of objects in a highly complex three-dimensional environment, usually being guided by two-dimensional information.

The work described here is part of an on-going effort to improve on current practice, by providing true, three-dimensional, quantitative measurements and displays of vasculature using a combination of angiographic imaging modalities. In particular, this paper is concerned with a model-based method for segmentation of arteries and complex pathologies from MR angiography (MRA) data, to obtain a three-dimensional representation of the cerebral vasculature.

The model we have chosen is used as a statistical classifier in a modified expectation maximisation (EM) algorithm. Previous work using the EM algorithm as a classifier has been on the identification of cerebral tissues from MR image data (proton density, T1, and T2 weighted) with bias field correction [9], and without [5, 6, 7]. Our application is novel in that we use the classification technique to characterise vasculature (blood vessels) by their blood flow properties, rather than their chemical properties. Prior work on vessel extraction from MRA data has been based on geometric methods that use, for example, tubular models of cerebral vessel shape [1, 4], or differential characteristics [8] to extract vessel networks. In our work we introduce a model for the intensity distributions that are represented in time of flight (TOF) MRA data, and use a robust approach for estimating this model, that is more accommodating to statistical variations in the data.

## 2 The new segmentation algorithm

Our new algorithm for vessel extraction from TOF MRA data is computed in two stages. In the first stage we use a variant on the traditional EM algorithm to classify vessel voxels, on the assumption that all voxels are independent. Based on this initial segmentation, we then estimate the two thresholds necessary to perform hysteresis thresholding. The high threshold for hysteresis is a function of the distribution parameters estimated in the first stage. The low threshold is chosen on the a priori assumption that there will be vessel voxels representing slower flow close to the initially segmented fast flow voxels. Below we outline details specific to each step of the algorithm.

**2.1 Choice of mixture distribution:** Given an appropriate mixture distribution over a number of classes for a set of data, the EM algorithm provides a method for estimating the distribution parameters by maximising the likelihood of the distribution [2]. Using these estimated parameters, classification of each data point is achieved by choosing the class for which the conditional probability of belonging to that class is maximised.

A typical histogram shape for TOF MRA data is bi-modal (see Figure 1), where the low intensity peak consists mainly of background tissue (outside the head), and the cerebrospinal fluid surrounding the brain tissue, and the high intensity peak corresponds to voxels in the brain tissue, eyes, skin, and bone. Vessel voxels lie at the upper tail of this high intensity peak. This suggests that a mixture model of three class-conditional distributions, two Gaussians and a uniform distribution, is appropriate. The uniform density is given by $1/I$, where $I$ is the total number of intensity levels. In our case $I - 2^{12}$. Hence, the mixture distribution is defined by

$$p(x) = \omega_0 \frac{1}{I} + \sum_{k=1}^{2} \omega_k \frac{1}{\sqrt{2\pi\sigma_k^2}} \exp\left[-\frac{1}{2}\left(\frac{x-\mu_k}{\sigma_k}\right)^2\right], \tag{1}$$

where $\omega_k$ is the proportion of each class $k$, and $\mu_k$ and $\sigma_k$ are the mean and standard deviation of the Gaussian classes respectively.

**2.2 Initialisation and stopping criteria for the EM algorithm:** The model in Equation (1) has seven unknown parameters that must be given initial values. Since the data histogram is bi-modal, the two Gaussian means, $\mu_1$ and $\mu_2$, can be initialised as the intensity values at each of the peaks. Let $I_{min}$ be the intensity corresponding to the minimum frequency (of voxels) between the two peaks. Each Gaussian variance is set to be

$$\sigma_k^2 = \left(\frac{\mu_k - I_{min}}{2}\right)^2.$$

We know a priori that the proportion of vessel voxels is very small, so $\omega_0$ is initially set to a small arbitrary value (0.04). There are less obvious differences between the two

Gaussian proportions, so the distribution with the highest variance is given proportion 0.50, and the other distribution is given 0.46, to satisfy $\sum_{k=0}^{2} \omega_k = 1.0$.

We evaluate convergence of the EM algorithm by computing $\sum_{k=0}^{2} |\omega_k^{new} - \omega_k^{old}|$, which quantifies the change in proportion parameters between iterations. The algorithm is terminated when this measure reaches zero.

**2.3 High threshold selection:** Our choice of mixture distribution is interesting in that the voxels whose conditional probability of coming from the uniform class is higher than the conditional probability of coming from the other two distributions are also those voxels above a certain intensity threshold. Namely, voxel $i$ comes from the uniform class if $\omega_0 p(x_i|0) > \omega_k p(x_i|k)$, for $k = 1, 2$. This can be restated as

$$\omega_0 \frac{1}{I} > \omega_k \frac{1}{\sqrt{2\pi\sigma_k^2}} \exp\left[-\frac{1}{2}\left(\frac{x_i - \mu_k}{\sigma_k}\right)^2\right],$$

or rearranging,   $x_i > \mu_k + \sigma_k \sqrt{2 \ln\left(\frac{\omega_k}{\sigma_k} \frac{I}{\omega_0 \sqrt{2\pi}}\right)}.$   (2)

The Gaussian class that gives the largest value for the right hand side of Equation (2) determines the threshold value for vessel selection. Note that the right hand side is the mean of class $k$ adjusted by the scaled standard deviation for that class.

**2.4 Refining the segmentation using local connectivity:** Slow blood flow at vessel walls and turbulent flow within aneurysms produce lower intensities in TOF MRA. Hence, the threshold defined in Equation (2) may not be sufficient to select all of the vessel segments required. Voxels in missed segments may be recovered using local neighbourhood information based on the following assumption: if a voxel has sufficiently high intensity, and it is close to previously segmented vessel voxels, it has a high probability of being a vessel voxel. We establish this neighbourhood connection by applying three-dimensional hysteresis thresholding (with 27-connectivity) within a user-defined elliptic cylinder that excludes the skull and skin.

The high threshold used in the hysteresis processing is the threshold selected using Equation (2). To find the low threshold we analyse the distribution of intensity levels at increasing distances away from the initial segmentation. By computing a three-dimensional distance transform for the initial segmentation [3], we can calculate a histogram for each set of voxels in the original data that corresponds to each distance transform value. We then use the EM algorithm to fit the same three-class mixture distribution to every one of these histograms to estimate a threshold for the uniform distribution at each distance value. This procedure is performed up to a distance of 70 voxels. Using this method the threshold has a high value initially, then decreases to a minimum at some small distance, then increases again with increasing distance. We choose the minimum value as the low threshold in the hysteresis thresholding, on the assumption that the intensities of the brain tissue class at this distance give the best representation of the intensity distribution of this tissue type. We select a number of the largest connected components as the final segmentation, to remove the small pockets of incorrectly chosen voxels.

## 3   Results

In this section we present the results of applying our segmentation algorithm to two real TOF MRA volumetric images, which were collected using a 1.5T Siemens Magnetom Vision magnetic resonance machine. Each set consists of 37 (364 × 512 pixel, 12 bit) transaxial slices. The slice thickness is 1.4 mm, and the pixel size is 0.319 × 0.319 mm². Both sets were acquired with TR= 39 ms, TE= 7 ms, and a flip angle of 20°. The algorithm has been implemented in C, and runs (non-optimised) in under 5 minutes on a SUN Ultra 1.

**3.1 Data set A:** The initial model parameters were automatically estimated from the bi-modal intensity-frequency graph of the data, as described in Section 2. The initial and final mixture distribution estimates are plotted over the data histogram in Figures 1(a) and (b) respectively. Convergence of the EM algorithm took 68 iterations in this case. The final percentage of vessel voxels was estimated at approximately 0.3%, which is a significant change from the initial estimate of 4.0%.

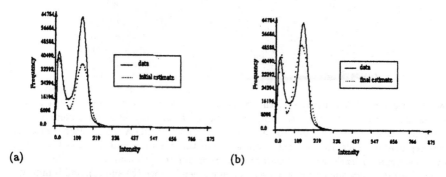

(a)                                    (b)

**Fig. 1.** Plots showing the frequency of intensities in the data, with (a) the initial estimate for the mixture distribution, and (b) the final estimate for the mixture distribution after applying the EM algorithm.

A surface-rendered display of the segmentation at this stage of the algorithm is shown in Figure 2(a), where it can be seen that some of the skin voxels have been erroneously classified as vessel voxels. These are removed by only selecting those vessel voxels inside the pre-defined elliptic cylinder for further hysteresis thresholding. After hysteresis thresholding, using the approach of Section 2.4, the two largest connected components were selected as the final estimate of the arterial structure. The final segmentation results are shown in Figures 2(b) and (c). For this data set the carotid and cerebral arteries form one component, and the vessels stemming from the basilar artery form another. This is because the flow in the posterior communicating arteries is very slow, and therefore these parts of the circle of Willis do not appear in the MRA scan. The anterior communicating aneurysm, indicated by the arrows, can be seen clearly in both figures.

**3.2 Data set B:** The results of applying the algorithm to a second data set B are shown in Figures 2(d) and (e). As for set A, the basilar and carotid vessel trees are separated. A carotid artery aneurysm can be seen in Figure 2(e), as indicated by the arrow. In the first stage of the segmentation process, the EM algorithm converged after 42 iterations, giving an estimated percentage of vessel voxels as approximately 0.2%.

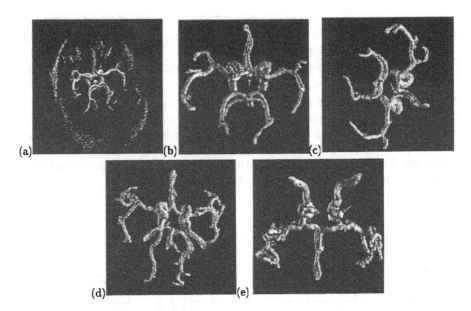

**Fig. 2.** Surface-rendered displays of the vessel voxels (a) extracted from data set A after the first stage of our algorithm, (b) and (c) extracted from data set A after completion of the segmentation algorithm, and (d) and (e) extracted from data set B after completion of the segmentation algorithm. Each picture within the pairs (b) and (c), and (d) and (e) shows the same patient's vessel structure, but from different viewing angles. The anterior communicating artery aneurysm of patient A can be seen in both (b) and (c), and is indicated by arrows. In (d) all extracted vessels are shown, whereas in (e) only the carotid circulation arteries are displayed, so that the internal carotid aneurysm of patient B can be seen. The aneurysm in (e) is indicated by an arrow.

**3.3 Error assessment:** We evaluated our vessel extraction algorithm by comparing the automatic segmentation of data set A with a tediously obtained manual segmentation. It was found that over 92% of the automatically segmented vessel voxels also appeared in the manual segmentation, but that there were more than twice as many voxels selected in the manual segmentation than in the automatic segmentation. In this comparison the automatic segmentation failed to select many voxels under the low threshold, implying that further improvement on the segmentation may be needed. This will be a subject of future work.

## 4 Discussion and future work

In this paper we have defined a model for the expected distributions found in cerebral TOF MRA data, and developed a fully automatic statistical segmentation algorithm that uses this model to extract vessels from the data. The results have shown that this algorithm can provide an accurate initial estimation of cerebral vessels and aneurysms.

By basing the algorithm on intensity levels, we are essentially applying a global flow measure as an indicator for vessel or aneurysm voxels. Because the flow may be slow or turbulent in small or complicated vessels and large aneurysms, the corresponding intensities at these points will be low, and may actually be similar in intensity to other brain matter. This implies that intensities in TOF MRA data cannot be used alone for quantifying vessel structure. We have assumed that one cannot impose a geometrical structure upon the vessels or aneurysms when solely using TOF MRA data. However, future work will involve introducing such structure assumptions with the aid of other types of data, such as phase contrast MRA or contrast-agent computed tomography images, which could provide more information about slow and turbulent flow regions.

Our three-dimensional representations of the cerebral vessels and aneurysms have already been used in the planning of cerebral endovascular procedures, by providing a more informative display of aneurysm position and the surrounding vessels. We intend to extend this application in the clinical domain, by using these three-dimensional vessel volumes to determine optimal viewing directions for X-ray angiography of aneurysms and vessels during clinical procedures.

**Acknowledgements:** The authors wish to thank James Byrne, for providing data, and continuing support, Dermot Dobson for helping to overcome data transfer problems, and Jacques Feldmar for many helpful discussions. DLW is supported by the Commonwealth Scholarship Commission and the Australian Federation of University Women (QLD).

# References

1. S. Aylward, E. Bullitt, S. Pizer, and D. Eberly. Intensity ridge and widths for tubular object segmentation and description. In *IEEE/SIAM Proc. Workshop on Math. Methods in Biomed. Image Anal.*, pages 131–138, San Francisco, California, June 1996.
2. C.M. Bishop. *Neural Networks for Pattern Recognition.* Clarendon Press, Oxford, 1995.
3. G. Borgefors. Distance transformations in digital images. *Comp. Vis. Graph. Im. Proc.*, 34:344–371, 1986.
4. E. Bullitt, A. Liu, S. Aylward, M. Soltys, and J. Rosenman. Methods of intracerebral vascular display. *Amer. J. Neuroradiol.*, 1996. To appear.
5. R. Guillemaud and M. Brady. Enhancement of MR images. In *Visualisation in Biomed. Comp.*, pages 107–116, Hamburg, Germany, September 1996.
6. Z. Liang, R.J. Jaszczak, and R.E. Coleman. Parameter estimation of finite mixtures using the EM algorithm and information criteria with application to medical image processing. *IEEE Trans. Nuclear Sc.*, 39(4):1126–1133, 1992.
7. Z. Liang, J.R. MacFall, and D.P. Harrington. Parameter estimation and tissue segmentation from multispectral MR images. *IEEE Trans. Med. Im.*, 13(3):441–449, 1994.
8. V. Prinet, O. Monga, C. Ge, X.S. Loa, and S. Ma. Thin network extraction in 3D images: application to medial angiograms. In *Int. Conf on Patt. Recog.*, August 1996.
9. W.M. Wells, W.E.L. Grimson, R. Kikinis, and F.A. Jolesz. Adaptive segmentation of MRI data. *IEEE Trans. Med. Imaging*, 15(4):429–442, 1996.

# Computation of Efficient Patient Specific Models From 3-D Medical Images: Use in Virtual Endoscopy and Surgery Rehearsal

S. Aharon, B.M. Cameron, and R.A. Robb

Biomedical Imaging Resource
Mayo Foundation Clinic
Rochester, MN U.S.A.

**Abstract.** Virtual reality environments provide highly interactive, natural control of the visualization process, significantly enhancing the scientific value of the data produced by medical imaging systems. Due to the computational and real time display update requirements of virtual reality interfaces, however, the complexity of organ and tissue surfaces which can be displayed is limited. In this paper, we present a new algorithm for the production of a polygonal surface containing a pre-specified number of polygons, from patient or subject specific volumetric image data, selected to optimize the trade-off between surface detail and real time display rates of anatomic models. To illustrate the utility of these models we also present a brief overview of their application in virtual endoscopy and surgery rehearsal.

## 1  Introduction

Virtual reality (VR) can bring an intimacy to the exploration and analysis of 3-D medical image data by separating the user from the traditional computer interface and from physical realities; allowing the user to study the data at any scale or orientation and to manipulate it in a natural fashion without having to study the process required to produce and display the images. This highly interactive interface would facilitate control over a three dimensional scene by responding to natural human gestures and language with visual, tactile and auditory cues in real time. This novel perspective on, exploration of and interaction with 3-D imagery enhances the value of the data produced by medical imaging systems.

While currently available rendering algorithms can generate photorealistic images from the volumetric data produced by medical imaging systems, the algorithms can not sustain real time display rates. Thus the complexity of the data must be reduced to fit within the limitations of the available hardware. In this paper, we present a method for the production of efficient geometric (polygonal) surfaces from volumetric data. We define an efficient geometric surface to be a surface containing a pre-specified number of polygons that accurately reflect the size, shape and position of the modeled object while being sufficiently small to permit real time display rates on modern workstations. To illustrate the utility of these models, we will present a brief overview of their application in virtual endoscopy and surgery rehearsal.

# 2 Modeling Algorithm

The generation of polygonal surfaces occurs in 4 phases: segmentation, surface detection, feature extraction and polygonization. The volumetric data is segmented into objects of interest using 3-D region growing, mathematical morphology, and/or multispectral analysis [1]. Surface detection is based on thresholding. Feature extraction involves determination of local surface curvature for the object. The calculation is done locally, using the sum of values in a 26-connected neighborhood, centered on each voxel in the binary object. The curvature calculation transforms the binary object into a set of surface curvature weights which represent how much the local surface curvature deviates from being flat. By eliminating those voxels where the surface is locally flat, the number of voxels that have to be tiled can be reduced without eliminating structural detail.

Our tiling algorithm is based on the "growing cell structures" [2] and the "growing neural gas" [3] algorithms of Fritzke. The algorithm is based on the successive addition of new nodes (units) to an initially small 2D Kohonen network [4] by evaluating local statistical measures gathered during previous adaptation steps. The network is adapted to a set $S$ of sample vectors by a Competitive Hebbian Learning (CHL) model [5], which involves the addition of new edges, or connections, to the network. To define the topological structure of the network, we define a set of unweighted edges $E$ among pairs of nodes. An edge aging scheme is used for removing obsolete edges during the adaptation. We consider a polygon $p$ to be defined by 3 nodes which are connected by three edges. A surface is defined by the set of all polygons $P$.

The tiling algorithm starts with three nodes $a$, $b$ and $c$ at random positions $v_a$, $v_b$ and $v_c$ in $R^3$. It then generates an input sample signal $s$ according to $S$, and finds the nearest node $n_1$ and the second nearest node $n_2$, which will be referenced to as the best matching units ($bmus$). The node $n_1$ and its direct topological neighbors (the direct topological neighbors of a given node $n$ is a set of all the nodes which are connected to it by a single edge), are moved towards $s$ by fractions $\varepsilon_b$ and $\varepsilon_n$, respectively, of the total distance. We increment by one the age of all edges emanating from $n_1$, and add the squared distance between the input signal and $n_1$ to a local error variable.

If $n_1$ and $n_2$ are connected by an edge, set the age of this edge to zero. If such an edge does not exist, create it. If a new edge was created, add all the possible polygons resulting from this additional edge (this step will insure a triangulated network and will prevent creation of holes).

We then remove edges with an age larger than $a_{max}$ and remove all the polygons which include this edge. If this results in points having no emanating edges and/or edges which belong to zero polygons, we remove them as well.

If the number of input signals generated to this point is an integer multiple of a parameter $\lambda$ (a user defined parameter which determines the add node frequency, hence the number of adaptation steps used to train the network before adding a new node), we insert a new node by determining the node $q$ with the maximum accumulated error, then inserting a new node $r$ halfway between $q$ and its direct neighbor $f$ with the largest error variable.

We insert edges connecting the new unit $r$ with units $q$ and $f$, and remove the original edge between $q$ and $f$, adding further edges and polygons to rebuild a structure consisting only of 2D simplices (triangles). The error variables of $q$ and $f$ are decreased by multiplying them with a constant $\alpha$ (empirically found to be 0.5 for most of the cases). The error variable of $r$ is initialized with the new value of the error variable of $q$.

At this point, all error variables are decreased by multiplying them with a constant $d$ (empirically found to be 0.995 for most of the cases). If the pre-specified net size (i.e., number of polygons) is not yet reached, generate a new input sample signal and repeat the process.

Initially the network is defined from three nodes and the edges which form a single triangle. During the adaptation, each addition and/or removal of a node or an edge is followed by additional supplementation or removal of nodes and edges in order to preserve the two-dimensionality of the network and to keep a triangulated network connection. During the process new nodes and edges (hence new polygons) are added to the network until a pre-specified number of polygons is reached. The overall network nodes and connections (edges) define the requested triangulated polygonal surface(s).

The insertion of edges between the nearest and second-nearest nodes with respect to an input vector are necessary to close (fill) holes and to merge split parts of a single network. The holes or network splitting could be created due to the removal of nodes, edges and polygons during the tiling procedure.

Since the connections between the nodes are added in an arbitrary order, a post-processing step is required to re-organize the polygonal surface in such a way that all the polygon normals will be pointing to the outside (or inside) of the volume defined by the object surface(s). This results in a smooth and realistic surface display using current VR rendering tools. The polygon normals are organized to point outside (or inside) using a method presented by Hoppe [6].

Figure 1 compares three models computed with our growing net algorithm with different numbers of polygons. It can be seen that even with a relatively small number of polygons (1500) the main surface details are captured in the model.

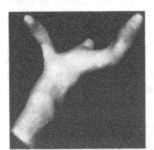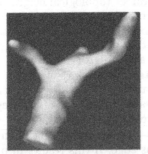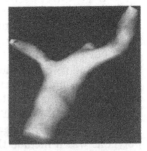

**Fig. 1.** Models computed with the new growing net algorithm of superior vena-cava, from the National Library of Medicine's Visible Human Male data set. From left to right, 8,000 polygonal surface, 4,000 polygonal surface and 1,500 polygonal surface.

Depending on the size and complexity of the surface and the number of polygons desired, the algorithm (O (n log n)) requires on the order of 3 minutes on an SGI Indy-class workstation to compute a surface of 2000-3000 polygons. The majority of the time is spent searching for the best matching units while adapting the Kohonen network. We are examining different methods to optimize the search for the best matching units, such as using the K-d tree algorithm.

The algorithm can, in principle, be extended to reconstruct surfaces with different levels of detail on the same surface. We are also working on developing an automated method to find the best network parameters as a function of the size of the data and the requested number of polygons.

## 3 Applications

The applications presented here are exemplary. They illustrate the use of 3-D biomedical images and patient specific models in support of specific clinical goals and are current works in progress.

At the center of Fig. 2 is shown a transparent rendering of a torso model of the Visible Human Male – VHM. This torso model has been used to develop and evaluate virtual endoscopic procedures applied to a variety of intra-parenchymal regions of the body. Surrounding the torso in Fig. 2 are several virtual endoscopy views which are single frames captured from fly-through movie sequences of the stomach, colon, spine, esophagus, airway, and aorta of the VHM. These visualizations illustrate the intra-parenchymal surface detail that can be interactively visualized with virtual endoscopy. Also illustrated in the simulated endoscopic views are different types of navigation guides superimposed upon the display to help the user interactively determine body orientation and precise anatomical localization while performing the virtual endoscopic examination.

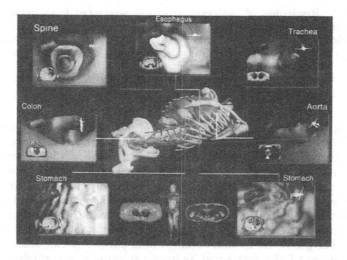

**Fig. 2.** Montage of virtual endoscopic views inside various segmented organs of the Visible Human Male. Center shows full 3D transparent model of torso. Small icons superimposed upon each endoscopic view include body orientation, 3D location, and 2D level/position.

Figure 3 illustrates volume renderings (left and center) of segmented anatomic structures from a spiral CT scan of a patient with colon cancer and polyps. Different ways of digitally analyzing the patient polyp with virtual endoscopy is shown. The upper right panel shows an enhancement of the polyp against the luminal wall. Such enhancement is possible only with virtual endoscopy, since the polyp itself can be digitally segmented and processed (e.g., brightened) as a separate object. The lower right panel illustrates the capability for "virtual biopsy". Both geometric and densitometric measures may be obtained numerically from the segmented polyp (density measures can be computed from the original image data).

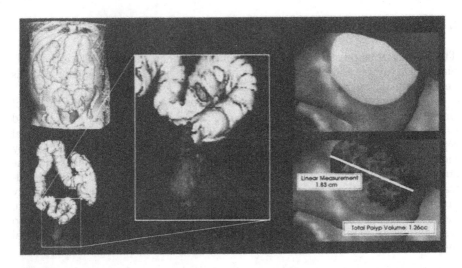

**Fig. 3.** Left: Renderings of anatomic structures segmented from spiral CT scan of patient with colon cancer. Right: Enhanced visualization of polyp, which was segmented and modeled separately from the colon wall. Measurement of diameter and volume of polyp, also of dense vascular bed, illustrates capability for "virtual biopsy".

The urologic surgeon can use displays of modeled prostate glands and surrounding regions in a real-time virtual environment to critically study the anatomic relationships pre-operatively. Virtual endoscopy can be performed in the bladder, urethra, and prostate gland itself for detailed visualization of shapes, sizes and contours, particularly relative to the tumor and critical structures like the seminal vesicles and neuro-vascular bundles. Segmentation and modeling of the VHM prostate gland and adjacent anatomy from the MRI sections was one of the first "proofs-of-concept" for helpful 3-D visualization of prostate anatomy in patients. The geometric models obtained from patient specific scans are faithful representations of the segmented anatomic structures, accurately reproducing their shape, size and location. Figure 4 shows a detailed model of the VHM prostate and models from two cancer patients. The patient-specific models can be studied independently, within the framework of the VHM pelvic model, or with the patient's own pelvic girdle if it is available for CT scan data (CT scan data and MRI scan data can be accurately registered into 3D space before providing the visualizations [1]). Virtual endoscopy can be performed on these patient specific models to precisely visualize the interior of the tumor relative to critical anatomic structures, such as the urinary sphincter, seminal vesicles and neuro-vascular bundles helping to define appropriate surgical margins to reduce the risk of post-operative complications (such as incontinence or impotence).

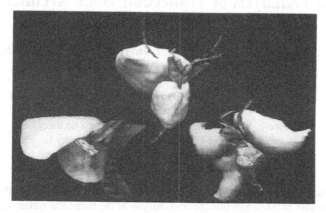

**Fig. 4.** Several models of prostate glands and adjacent structures (bladder, rectum, urethra, etc.) computed from MRI scans of Visible Human Male (top) and of two actual prostate cancer patients (bottom). Bright regions in models are patient prostate cancer.

## 4   Summary

We have presented a new method for the production of efficient 3D geometric (polygonal) surfaces containing a pre-specified number of polygons from volumetric medical data. We define these surfaces as efficient ones since they accurately reflect the size, shape and position of the modeled objects yet contain a small number of adapted polygons sufficient to optimize the trade-off between surface detail and real-time display rates. These efficient models can be used in various medical applications such as computed endoscopy, surgery planning and rehearsal, and as a powerful education tool for teaching anatomy.

**Acknowledgments** The authors are grateful to their colleagues in the Biomedical Imaging Resource for their contributions to this work. They are also grateful to the National Library of Medicine for the use of the Visible Human Data sets.

## References

1. R.A. Robb, "Surgery simulation with ANALYZE/AVW: a visualization workshop for 3-D display and analysis of multimodality medical images", Proc. of Medicine Meets Virtual Reality II, San Diego, CA, 1994
2. B. Fritzke, "Let it grow - self organizing feature maps with problem dependent cell structure", Proc. of the ICANN-91, Helsinki, 1991
3. B. Fritzke, "A growing neural gas network learns topologies.", in Advances in Neural Information Processing Systems 7, Eds. G. Teasauro, S. Touretzky and T.K. Leen. MIT Press, Cambridge MA, 1995
4. T. Kohonen, Self-organization and associative memory (3rd Ed), Springer-Verlag, Berlin, 1989
5. T.M. Martinetz, "Competitive Hebbian Learning rule forms perfectly topology preserving maps", In CANN'93: International Conference on artificial Neural Network, Amsterdam, Springer, 1993, 427-434
6. H. Hoppe, "Surface reconstruction from unorganized points", Doctoral Dissertation, University of Washington, 1994

# In Vivo Analysis of Trabecular Bone Architecture

W. J. Niessen[1], A. M. López[2], W. J. van Enk[1], P. M. v. Roermund[3]
B. M. ter Haar Romeny[1], M. A. Viergever[1]

[1] Image Sciences Institute, Utrecht University Hospital, Room E.01.334, Heidelberglaan 100,
3584 CX Utrecht, the Netherlands
[2] Computer Vision Center, Universitat Autònoma de Barcelona
[3] University Cluster of Orthopedics, Utrecht University Hospital

**Abstract.** Trabecular morphology has structural trends which are strongly correlated with physical function. In vivo analysis of the trabecular pattern has the potential to predict and treat malgrowth of bone owing to altered loading conditions in an early phase. Using multiscale texture analysis we determine the orientation trend of the trabecular network from CT images. First studies show that the obtained orientations in healthy individuals agree with histomorphometric studies. In vivo analysis of trabecular microstructure, to monitor development and progress of bone diseases as *e.g.* osteoporosis, is severely limited since high resolution CT and MR systems achieve at best resolutions in the order of the size of individual trabeculae.

## 1   Introduction

Bone structure and mass are strongly correlated with mechanical loading. External forces shape bone, while bone structure and mass determine bone strength. We propose in vivo analysis of trabecular morphology for two reasons. Firstly, external forces cannot be measured in vivo, therefore altered loading conditions are only apparent after the shape of the bone is affected. The orientation of the trabecular pattern gives insight in the main routes of stress. In vivo analysis of this pattern enables to predict changed loading conditions in an early phase to limit the extent of malgrowth. Secondly, bone diseases as *e.g.* osteoporosis become only relevant in the case of fracture. If the (often symptomless) underlying structural changes in trabecular morphology can be quantified, treatment can be started and monitored.

In section 2 we briefly describe trabecular bone morphology, and the relation of mechanical loading to the routes of stress. In section 3 we introduce the structure tensor which is applied to analyze oriented textures. It describes the local orientation by deriving an *angle* image which is supplied by a *confidence* estimate. Eigenvalue analysis of the structure tensor can also determine whether the local structure is platelike or rodlike. In section 4 we present results on 3D CT data.

## 2   Trabecular bone

Human bone can be classified as compact (cortical) or trabecular, depending on its relative density [7]. Most bones have both types, the compact part appears as a dense shell of the bone, in contrast with the mesh appearance of the trabecular part, which covers the interior side of the shell. Bone is a living tissue that is continuously remodeled by actions of building cells (osteoblasts) and eroding cells (osteoclasts). Forces acting upon the bone play an important role in sculpting the internal structure and external shape.

Extensive histomorphometric studies, *e.g.* [3,18,7] have given considerable insight in trabecular bone structure. In healthy bone it consists of a connected network of platelike and rodlike elements, with a typical diameter of 100-300 $\mu m$ and marrow spacings of 200-2000 $\mu m$. In order to visualize these structures in vivo, dedicated computed tomography methods are required [2,6,9,13]. However, the trabecular pattern is already visible at lower resolutions, which can be appreciated from conventional CT and MR images with a typical resolution of 1-4 $mm^3$.

As early as the end of the previous century relations between structural parameters and bone strength have been observed. According to the trajectory theory of Meyer and Culman [12]: "routes of stress coincide with trabecular patterns", while Wolff's law states that [19]: "the internal structure and external shape of a bone develop in response to the change in function and forces acting upon it". The routes of stress are artistically visualized for the ankle in Fig. 1 and for the femur in Fig. 2.

Some studies have already revealed relations between structure and mechanical loading. Gibson [7] showed that mechanical loading conditions influence trabecular geometry. Radiographic studies of the distal radius of children by Korstjens *et al.* [11] show that prevalence of trabeculae oriented perpendicular to the long axis of the radius decreases with age. Since the routes of stress appear at scales which are considerably higher than the individual trabeculae and vary within the human skeleton, we apply a multiscale texture analysis method based on the structure tensor [10,15,1].

A number of theoretical studies have fitted 3D models to the trabecular network in prepared specimens. Gibson [7] concludes that at low densities the trabecular network consists of rods while at larger densities the trabecular elements are platelike. Anisotropic loading conditions lead to anisotropic structures. Fazzalari *et al.* [4] consider surface to volume relations to conclude that the trabecular structure may consist of either a plate and rod network or a connected rod network. Osteoporosis appears to erode platelike trabecular structures and even remove plates and rods [14]. Since the structure tensor can determine whether the local structure is platelike or rodlike it enables a quantitative comparison over time.

## 3 Methods

Image analysis tools have been applied to obtain objective meaningful features of an oriented texture in 2D images [10,15] and, in general, $n$ dimensional images [1,8]. In the case of oriented textures, the most meaningful features are the *angle image* and the *confidence image*, that together constitute the so-called *intrinsic images* of the textured image [15]. In our work we model the trabecular pattern as an oriented texture.

The angle image specifies the dominant orientation at each point. To compute this orientation, it is sufficient to analyze the behavior of the image gradient in a given neighborhood. We assume that, at a given point, there is a single dominant orientation at most. Notice that the gradient of a function points into the direction of maximum change, and the dominant orientation is perpendicular to this direction. Two observations are crucial:

- The word *dominant* means dominant within a given neighborhood (window) of size $\sigma_I$ centered at a given point $\mathbf{x} \in \mathbb{R}^n$, *i.e.* $\mathcal{W}(\mathbf{x}; \sigma_I)$. The parameter $\sigma_I$ is known as integration scale.
- Since textured images are *views of a world scene L*, a measurement of $L$ at $\mathbf{x}$ is necessarily performed using an operator of a certain size $\sigma_D$ which is known as the differentiation scale.

To obtain derivatives of $L$ in a well-posed fashion we use concepts of linear scale space theory. In this framework differentiation is defined as convolution with derivatives of Gaussians [5]:

$$\frac{\partial}{\partial x}L(\mathbf{x}; \sigma_D) = L(\mathbf{x}) * \frac{\partial}{\partial x}G(\mathbf{x}; \sigma_D) \tag{1}$$

where the $n$-dimensional Gaussian is defined as:

$$G(\mathbf{x}; \sigma) = \frac{1}{(2\pi\sigma^2)^{\frac{n}{2}}} e^{-\frac{\|\mathbf{x}\|^2}{2\sigma^2}} \tag{2}$$

For simplicity we first consider the 2-dimensional case. In this case the dominant orientation at each point of the image will be given by an angle in $[-\frac{\pi}{2}, \frac{\pi}{2})$ (we are interested in the orientation, not in the specific direction; opposite directions should be identified). This yields a 2-dimensional array of angles that we coin the *angle image*.

To summarize, the steps to compute the angle $\theta(\mathbf{x}; \sigma_I; \sigma_D)$ are:

*i)* compute the gradients $\nabla L(\mathbf{y}; \sigma_D) \ \forall \ \mathbf{y} \in \mathcal{W}(\mathbf{x}; \sigma_I)$.
*ii)* determine the dominant orientation of these gradients: $\alpha(\mathbf{x}; \sigma_I; \sigma_D)$ by averaging the squared vectors [10,15]:

$$2\alpha(\mathbf{x}; \sigma_I; \sigma_D) = \sum_{\mathbf{y} \in \mathcal{W}(\mathbf{x}; \sigma_I)} w_{\mathbf{y}} l_{\mathbf{y}}^2 e^{\imath 2\theta_{\mathbf{y}}} \tag{3}$$

where $w_{\mathbf{y}}$ is a weighting factor, $l_{\mathbf{y}} = \|\nabla L(\mathbf{y}; \sigma_D)\|$, and $\theta_{\mathbf{y}}$ denotes the angle between the X-axis and the gradient direction.
*iii)* determine the dominant direction, which is perpendicular to the dominant gradient orientation.

This reasoning is equivalent [8] to the eigenvalue analysis of the so-called *structure tensor*, which generalizes to $n$ dimensions. The structure tensor can be represented by means of a symmetric and semi-positive definite $n \times n$ matrix

$$\mathbf{M}(\mathbf{x}; \sigma_I; \sigma_D) = \mathcal{W}(\mathbf{x}; \sigma_I) * (\nabla L(\mathbf{x}; \sigma_D)\nabla L(\mathbf{x}; \sigma_D)^T) \tag{4}$$

where $\mathcal{W}(\mathbf{x}; \sigma_I)$ is convolved elementwise with the matrix. A suitable choice for the window is a Gaussian profile, *i.e.* $\mathcal{W}(\mathbf{x}; \sigma_I) = G(\mathbf{x}; \sigma_I)$. This choice implies that neighbors are weighted as a function of their distance.

The orientation $\alpha(\mathbf{x}; \sigma_I; \sigma_D)$ of step *ii)* above is given by the eigenvector which corresponds to the highest eigenvalue of $\mathbf{M}(\mathbf{x}; \sigma_I; \sigma_D)$. However, we have assumed that every point has a preferred orientation. To check this assumption we introduce a confidence (or coherence) measure to a given orientation; we associate a value $\mathcal{C}(\mathbf{x}; \sigma_I; \sigma_D) \in [0, 1]$ to the angle $\theta(\mathbf{x}; \sigma_I; \sigma_D)$, which can be computed from the eigenvalues of the structure tensor [1,8]. In the two dimensional case, for example, similarity of the two eigenvalues of the structure tensor implies isotropy and, as a result $\mathcal{C}(\mathbf{x}; \sigma_I; \sigma_D)$ should be close to zero. A logical choice is a measure which checks whether the difference in eigenvalues ($\lambda_\triangle$) exceeds a predefined threshold $c$, which is characteristic for $\lambda_\triangle$ in the trabecular pattern: $\mathcal{C} = 1 - e^{-\frac{(\lambda_\triangle)^2}{2c^2}}$.

Eigenvalue analysis of the structure tensor also gives insight in the local structure. Rodlike structures yield two large and one small eigenvalue, while platelike structures yield one large and two small eigenvalues.

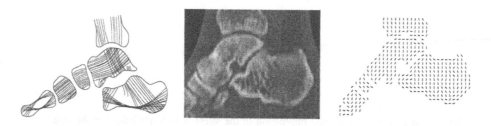

**Fig. 1. Left:** Redrawn version of D'Arcy Thompson's [17] diagram of the stress lines in the human foot. The sketched orientations have been confirmed by histomorphometric studies. **Middle:** High resolution sagittal CT slice of the ankle. Resolution = $425 \times 425 \ \mu m$. Slice thickness is 1 $mm$. **Right:** Trabecular orientation for $\sigma_I = 4$ and $\sigma_D = 0.5$ pixels.

## 4  Results

In Fig. 1 we plot the sagittal component of the orientation of the trabecular pattern for an in vivo ankle CT image. In the tibia the orientations agree very well. In Fig. 2 we plot the coronal component of the orientation of the trabecular pattern at two integration scales for the femur CT image. Since in large parts the orientation is not very accurately known we used the confidence image to select only the vectors for which $\mathcal{C} > 0.5$, where $c$ has been selected upon inspecting the trabecular pattern in the femoral neck. Cortical bone has significant influence on the estimation of the trabecular orientation, especially for higher scales. The orientation in the femoral neck corresponds qualitatively with the orientations in the artistic impression.

In Fig. 2 we plot the regions in which the pattern is rodlike and platelike. Note, however, that the resolution of the images is insufficient to quantify the shape of individual trabeculae.

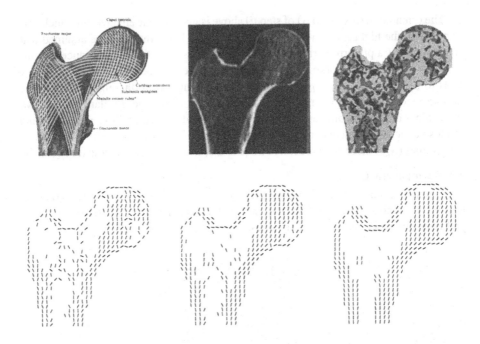

**Fig. 2. Top row left**: An artistic impression of the stress trajectories based on the orientation field observed in the trabecular patterns in the head of the femur. Reproduced from [16] with permission from the publisher. **Top row middle**: CT slice of dry femur. Resolution = 245× 245 $\mu m$. Slice thickness is 0.5 $mm$. **Top row right**: Upon inspecting the relative eigenvalues, platelike (one high eigenvalue; dark area) and rodlike (two high eigenvalues; bright area) regions can be identified. The grey area represents either a smooth (all eigenvalues are small) or noisy (all eigenvalues are large) region. Note that all these measures are relative, but they can be useful in follow-up studies. **Bottom row**: Trabecular orientation for three different integration scales. We used $\sigma_I = 2$ (left), $\sigma_I = 4$ (middle), and $\sigma_I = 8$ (right) respectively, while $\sigma_D = 0.5$ pixels. Vectors are plotted for which the confidence $C > 0.5; c = 1000$ Hounsfield units.

## 5 Discussion

We have presented the feasibility of in vivo studies of the trabecular orientation pattern. CT studies show strong correlation between the obtained orientations and data from histomorphometric studies. This shows the potential to detect altered loading conditions in an early phase, so treatment can be started to limit the extent of malgrowth.

A drawback of the presented method is that at one location only a single preferred orientation is present. We are currently considering texture autocorrelation to study multiple preferred orientations. However, these methods are more expensive from a computational point of view.

The presented method is also capable of analyzing the local architecture. However, to quantify structural changes at the level of individual trabeculae in *e.g.* osteoporosis resolutions of at least $100 \times 100 \times 100\ \mu m$ are required. An MR study on the finger [9] shows that for the extremities these resolutions become in reach.

# References

1. J. Bigun, G. Granlund, and J. Wiklund. Multidimensional orientation estimation with applications to texture analysis and optical flow. *IEEE Transactions on Pattern Recognition and Machine Intelligence*, 13(8):775–790, 1991.
2. E. P. Durand and P. Rüegsegger. Cancellous bone structure: Analysis of high resolution CT images with the run length method. *Journal of Computer Assisted Tomography*, 15(1):133–139, 1991.
3. E. D. Dyson, C. K. Jackson, and W. J. Whitehouse. Scanning electron microscope studies of human trabecular bone. *Nature*, 225:957–959, 1970.
4. N. J. Fazzalari, D.J Crisp, and B. Vernon-Roberts. Mathematical modeling of trabecular bone structure: the evaluation of analytical and quantified surface to volume relationships in femoral head and iliac crest. *Journal of Biomechanics*, 22(8):901–910, 1989.
5. L. M. J. Florack, B. M. ter Haar Romeny, J. J. Koenderink, and M. A. Viergever. Scale and the differential structure of images. *Image and Vision Computing*, 10(6):376–388, 1992.
6. T. K. F. Foo, F. G. Shellock, C. E. Hayes, J. F. Schenck, and B. E. Slayman. High-resolution MR imaging of the wrist and eye with short TR, short TE, and partial echo acquisition. *Radiology*, 183(1):277–281, 1992.
7. L. J. Gibson. Mechanical behavior of cancellous bone. *Journal of Biomechanics*, 18(5):317–328, 1985.
8. B. Jähne. *Spatio-Temporal Image Processing*. Lecture Notes in Computer Science 751. Springer Verlag, Berlin-Heidelberg, 1993.
9. H. Jara, F. W. Wehrli, H. Chung, and J. C. Ford. High-resolution variable flip angle 3D MR imaging of trabecular microstructure in vivo. *Magnetic Resonance in Medicine*, 29:528–539, 1993.
10. M. Kass and A. Witkin. Analyzing oriented patterns. *Computer Vision, Graphics, and Image Processing*, 37:362–385, 1987.
11. C. M. Korstjens, W. G. M. Geraets, F. C. van Ginkel, B. Prahl-Andersen, P. F. van der Stelt, and A. H. Burger. An analysis of the orientation of the radiographic trabecular pattern in the distal radius of children. *Growth, Development and Aging*, 58(4):211–221, 1994.
12. H. Meyer and M. Culman. Die architektur der spongiosa. *Arch. Anat. Physiol.*, 47(1):615–628, 1867.
13. R. Müller and P. Rüegsegger. Three dimensional finite element modeling of non-invasively assessed trabecular bone structures. *Journal of Medical Engineering Physics*, 17:126–133, 1995.
14. A. M. Parfitt. Trabecular bone architecture in the pathogenesis and prevention of fracture. *American Journal of Medicine*, 82:68–72, 1987.
15. A. R. Rao and B. Schunck. Computing oriented texture fields. *Graphical Models and Image Processing*, 53(2):157–185, 1991.
16. W. Spalteholz. *Atlas of Human Anatomy*. Scheltema & Holkema NV, Amsterdam, 1967. 16th edition, revised by R. Spanner.
17. D. W. Thompson. *On Growth and Form: abridged edition*. Cambridge University Press, London, 1917. ed. J. T. Bonner, 1961.
18. W. J. Whitehouse. The quantitative morphology af anisotropic bone. *Journal of Microscopy*, 101:153–168, 1974.
19. J. Wolff. Ueber die innere architektur der knochen. *Virchow's Arch.*, 50(1):389–453, 1870.

# Automatic Measurement of Vertebral Shape Using Active Shape Models

Paul P. Smyth[1], Christopher J. Taylor[1] and Judith E. Adams[2]

[1] Department of Medical Biophysics, University of Manchester, M13 9PT, U.K.
[2] Department of Diagnostic Radiology, University of Manchester, M13 9PT, U.K.

**Abstract.** In this paper, we describe how Active Shape Models (ASMs) have been used to accurately and robustly locate vertebrae in noisy lateral Dual Energy X-ray Absorptiometry (DXA) images of the spine. Vertebrae were located using either separate models for each vertebra, or a combined model of the whole spine. The combined model was found to be more robust. We show that ASMs allow normal vertebrae to be located as accurately as by human operators. We measure the performance of ASMs in locating fractured vertebrae of osteoporotic patients. We also describe how model parameters may be used to estimate how accurately a vertebra had been locatated, in order to detect vertebrae for which search had failed.

## 1 Introduction

Osteoporosis is a disease which affects many women after the menopause, leading to bone loss and fractures. Vertebral fractures are a good early indicator of osteoporosis, and are used to evaluate drug efficacy in trials. Rapid and reproducible measurement of vertebral deformity would help improve tests of efficacy.

Dual Energy X-ray Absorptiometry (DXA) scanners, which digitally image the whole spine, have recently become available for measuring fractures [4]. Vertebral fracture assessment is performed by marking six points on each vertebra manually, then calculating vertebral heights as measures of fracture. This method is laborious and takes up to 15 minutes per patient.

Locating variably shaped objects in a noisy environment is best tackled using flexible template models. Considerable attention has been given to development of such models in the literature, and these are summarised in [1]. Obtaining models specific to the objects of interest is particularly important. Active Shape Models (ASMs) [1], which combine explicit models of object boundaries and grey-level appearance surrounding the boundaries, allow *only* anatomically plausible interpretations. We have compared the accuracy of ASM search with that of the manual method for a large set of DXA scans of normal subjects. ASM location accuracy was also measured for scans of individuals with clinically significant fractures.

In segmentating medical images, one would often like to automatically estimate the segmentation accuracy. If we could predict the reliability of measurements based on a vertebra's segmentation, unreliable measurements could be excluded from subsequent analyses. We have attempted to find simple measures related to segmentation accuracy. We show that our measures can be used to detect cases which have been poorly segmented.

## 2   Active Shape Models

Active Shape Models (ASMs) combine models of shape and grey-level appearance to search for objects in images [1]. They are generated from labelled training images containing the objects of interest.

Shape is described by a Point Distribution Model (PDM), which is generated by performing principal component analysis on labelled landmark points over the training examples. The PDM represents shape in terms of a mean shape and a set of linearly independent modes describing the variation in the training examples. A subset of the modes describes the training set shapes to a given accuracy. A new shape can be generated by adding a weighted sum of the modes of variation to the mean shape, and this shape will be similar to those observed in training.

Grey-level appearance is modelled by analysing the grey-level image profile perpendicular to the object contour at each landmark point. This model is similar to that for shape, using principal component analysis. Details of the training and use of these combined grey-level and shape models are given in [3].

ASMs can be used to locate the modelled object in new images. An initial approximation is projected into the image and refined iteratively. The grey-level landscape around the current position of each landmark point is probed for grey-level evidence which best matches its profile model. A better position is suggested for each landmark point. The PDM then attempts to deform to fit to these new positions, within the constraints imposed by its modes of variation. This process is repeated until convergence. Because the PDM imposes global shape constraints, only objects of similar shape to those observed in the training set will be located.

## 3   Methods

78 lateral spine DXA images of normal women were obtained using a commercial DXA scanner. The external contours of ten vertebrae (from T7 to L4) were marked by the author (PPS) on each image on the advice of an experienced radiologist (JEA).

Moderately good initialisation of the model was useful for eliminating complete search failures. The operator roughly marked a point at the top of vertebra T7, one at the top of T12, and one at the bottom of L4 (taking $\approx$ 10 secs). The model was then initialised from these points, and search started. An example initial model position, and the search process through to convergence are shown in figure 1. To investigate the effect of having used a complete spine model, search was repeated using ten separate vertebral models. The top and bottom of *each* vertebra were marked to initialise search.

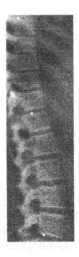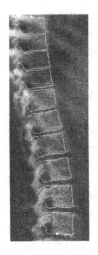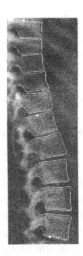

**Fig. 1.** ASM search, initialised from 3 manually marked points.

Additionally, 32 lumbar DXA scans, covering the lowest four visible vertebrae, were acquired from patients with vertebral fractures. Vertebral contours
were marked, and an ASM trained from these, and 70 normal contours. Search
was initialised from two manually marked points, corresponding to the top of L1
and bottom of L4.

## 4 Comparing Manual and ASM Accuracy

### 4.1 Method

To compare the accuracy of segmentation achieved using ASM search with manual methods, 40 of the 78 images were marked up by 4 operators using the standard six point method, in which the four vertebral corners and two midpoints
were marked. Cross-validation search experiments were performed to provide an
upper bound on the errors to be expected from the ASM in clinical use. The
ASM was trained on all examples except one. Its performance was then tested
on the excluded example. This train-and-test process was repeated with each
training example left out in turn. Each search experiment was performed 20
times, with the position of the 3 manual start points varied similarly to that of
human operators. Search experiments were also carried out for an ASM trained
from 32 fracture and 70 normal scans. Results are presented for the 32 fracture
scans.

### 4.2 Accuracy, Failure Rate and Precision

In the manual experiments the variance in point placement was measured between 4 operators for each of the 6 points marked. For the ASM experiments
the manually annotated outline was taken as truth. Accuracy was measured as

the rms point-to-line error from points on the manual annotation to the ASM contour.

In the automatic search experiments, precision was measured from the distribution of deviations from ground truth contour. Complete search failures were also detected as those cases outside the main distribution of deviations.

## 4.3 Results

**Table 1.** Manual and ASM accuracy (pixels rms), precision (pixels), and failure rate (%), broken down by vertebral level, for normal subjects.

| Vertebra | Manual Accuracy | Full-spine ASM Accuracy | Precision | Failure % | Separate ASMs Accuracy | Precision | Failure % |
|---|---|---|---|---|---|---|---|
| T7 | 1.66 | 1.60 | 0.17 | 0.8 | 2.44 | 0.42 | 1.5 |
| T8 | 1.28 | 0.98 | 0.11 | 2.1 | 1.62 | 0.30 | 2.1 |
| T9 | 1.15 | 0.98 | 0.12 | 3.4 | 1.51 | 0.22 | 0.5 |
| T10 | 1.17 | 1.08 | 0.14 | 2.3 | 1.69 | 0.24 | 0.3 |
| T11 | 1.18 | 1.10 | 0.21 | 3.7 | 1.61 | 0.24 | 2.1 |
| T12 | 1.11 | 1.02 | 0.24 | 5.0 | 1.15 | 0.20 | 5.7 |
| L1 | 1.12 | 1.17 | 0.26 | 5.3 | 1.03 | 0.14 | 0.8 |
| L2 | 1.13 | 1.09 | 0.25 | 5.5 | 0.95 | 0.11 | 0.4 |
| L3 | 1.15 | 1.08 | 0.25 | 6.0 | 1.01 | 0.13 | 0.5 |
| L4 | 1.47 | 1.61 | 0.28 | 2.2 | 1.15 | 0.20 | 5.7 |

Table 1 summarises the results for normal vertebrae. ASM search using a full-spine model was as accurate as human operators. Search using separate vertebral models performed as well as the spine model in the lower spine, where vertebrae are more visible, but worse for the less visible thoracic vertebrae. The decreased robustness using separate ASMs for each vertebra demonstrates that the shape constraints exploited by the full-spine model improve search performance. Overall precision was very good, and the failure rate was low.

**Table 2.** ASM accuracy (pixels rms), precision (pixels), and failure rate (%), broken down by vertebral level, for subjects with vertebral fractures.

| Vertebra | Accuracy | Precision | Failure % |
|---|---|---|---|
| L1 | 2.28 | 0.24 | 9.7 |
| L2 | 2.00 | 0.17 | 7.6 |
| L3 | 2.24 | 0.17 | 2.5 |
| L4 | 2.41 | 0.46 | 14.7 |

The accuracy, precision and failure rate of automatic ASM search for the fractured lumbar vertebra test set are shown in table 2. The accuracy is worse than for the normal vertebrae, as the training set was smaller than for the normal vertebrae, whilst the shape variability was greater. The model was therefore less able to generalise to unseen cases. Experiments with more examples are now being performed. Precision for all vertebrae was good.

Overall, these results suggest that accuracy similar to that of human operators can be achieved by an automatic system. More work is required on fractured vertebrae, but the performance already achieved would be useful in clinical practice and may improve on the best manual results given more training data.

## 5 Automatic Assessment of Segmentation Accuracy

In image search, a fitness measure, describing the match of the image evidence to each landmark's grey-level model is locally minimised. This is represented [2] by a factor model $f = \sum_{i=1}^{i=t} \frac{b_i^2}{\lambda_i} + \sum_{j=1}^{j=n} \frac{r_j^2}{v_j}$, where $b_i$ is the $i$th of $t$ model parameters, $\lambda_i$ is the $i$th mode's eigenvalue, and $r_j$ is the residual for the $j$th of $n$ modelled pixels, whose variance is $v_j$. We hypothesise that this measure shall be related to the accuracy of segmentation, and the visibility of a structure.

ASMs contain separate grey-level models for the profiles around *each* landmark point, so the fits for each landmark must be combined. A fit for each vertebra was calculated by adding each profile's fit measure. This process assumes the profiles to be independant.

To examine how the fit measure varied as search accuracy worsened, we repeated our previous search experiments, but introduced bad search solutions by restricting shape model modes. We also correlated manual error (representing how visible the vertebrae inherently were) with the fit value. ASM location error was relatively strongly related to grey-level fit value, while the correlation of manual accuracy with fit was weak ($r \approx 0.2$).

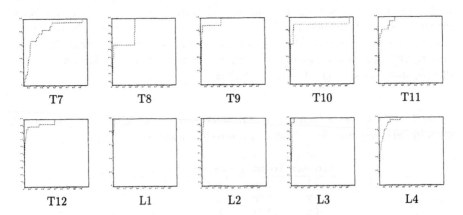

**Fig. 2.** ROC curves for detection of poorly located cases by grey-level fit, for vertebrae T7 to L4. Vertical axis is true positive fraction (0-1), horizontal axis is false positive fraction (0-1)

As there was good correlation between ASM accuracy and grey-level fit, the ability of fit to be used to detect poor segmentations automatically was investigated using ROC analysis. The ROC curves in Figure 2 show the proportion of sucessfully detected poor segmentations (chosen to be those with error > 3 pixels) against the proportion of false positives as the threshold on fit was varied for each vertebra.

The detection of poor segmentations was best for vertebrae L1-L3, which were clearly visible, while it was less effective in the thoracic spine, which was often noisy. The ability to detect bad segmentations seems to be related to the visibility of the vertebra, suggesting that poorly visible training examples are corrupting the grey-level models, making poor segmentations indistinguishable from poorly visible training examples. Training the grey-level model from selected training examples may improve the model.

## 6    Conclusions and Further Work

We have shown that ASM search is an accurate and robust tool for automatically analysing DXA spine images. It performed as well as manual observers at locating the vertebrae from T7-L4. It was fast, taking approximately 30 seconds to analyse a scan that would take a human operator up to 15 minutes. It accurately located the *full* vertebral contour, rather than just six points. We have compared separate and combined vertebral search strategies, and found that the interdependencies modelled in the combined strategy improve vertebral location.

We have presented preliminary results for the detection of fractured vertebrae, indicating that more training is necessary before fractured vertebrae can be located as accurately as normals but the results would already be clinically useable.

A grey-level fitness measure was used to detect poor segmentations, and worked well if the structures used in training were well visualised.

We intend to train the model using a large number of full-spine DXA images containing fractures, and then to perform fracture classification based upon the parameters of the shape model. Development into a working clinical system should then follow.

## References

1. T. F. Cootes, A. Hill, C. J. Taylor, and J. Haslam. The use of active shape models for locating structures in medical images. *Image and Vision Computing*, 12(6):276–285, July 1994.
2. T. F. Cootes, G. Page, C. Jackson, and C. J. Taylor. Statistical grey-level models for object location and identification. In 6$^{th}$ *British Machine Vison Conference*, pages 533–542, Birmingham, England, Sept. 1995. BMVA Press.
3. T. F. Cootes, C. J. Taylor, D. H. Cooper, and J. Graham. Active shape models - their training and application. *Computer Vision and Image Understanding*, 61(1):38–59, Jan. 1995.
4. P. Steiger, S. Cummings, H. Genant, H. Weiss, and the Study of Osteoporotic Fractures Group. Morphometric x-ray absorptiometry of the spine: Correlation in vivo with morphometric radiography. *Osteoporosis Int*, 4:238–244, 1994.

# A Hybrid Approach for the Detection of Small Airways Disease from Computed Tomographic Images

Guang-Zhong Yang and  David M Hansell
Department of Imaging, Royal Brompton Hospital
London SW3 6NP, U.K.

**Abstract** Bronchiolar obstruction is commonly manifested in Computed Tomographic (CT) images as areas of decreased attenuation relative to adjacent normal lung parenchyma. The certain identification of such areas is difficult in practice, particularly if such areas are poorly marginated. This paper presents a novel approach to the enhancement of feature differences between normal and diseased lung parenchyma so that reliable visual assessment can be made.

## 1. Introduction

Small airways disease may occur as a result of direct lung injury (for example, following viral lower respiratory tract infections, toxic fume inhalation or mineral dust exposure) or in association with a diverse range of lung disorder. In clinical practice the detection of small airways disease is difficult. Because these small airways normally contribute minimally to total airflow resistance, conventional tests of lung function are insensitive except in advanced cases and for this reason the small airways have been described as the "silent zone" of the lungs. Although lung biopsies have been suggested for the definitive diagnosis of small airways disease, they are rarely undertaken in practice. As a result, there has been interest in non-invasive tests for the detection of obliterative bronchiolitis, one of the "purest" forms of small airways disease.

To elucidate the CT features of small airways disease, this paper presents a wavelet feature enhancement technique which enhances the subtle density differences in the lung parenchyma of high resolution CT images. The aim of this technique is twofold. Firstly, it provides a means of enhancing feature differences between normal and abnormal lung parenchyma and thus improves the accuracy of diagnosis. Secondly, it serves as a basis for the automatic quantification of the extent of small airways disease.

The main steps of the proposed technique include the following procedures: structural filtering/wavelet decomposition, feature localization, wavelet reconstruction, structure enhancement, and image classification. The purpose of the structural filtering/wavelet decomposition step is to remove vessels of the lungs so that the areas within can be classified into two distinctive regions corresponding to normal and abnormal lung parenchyma. The filtered result also serves as a basis for quantifying the extent of air-trapping for later studies. The proposed operator is a hybrid structure filter as it combines the strength of grey-scale morphological operators and that of linear image filters so that intrinsic subtle attenuation differences between normal and abnormal parenchyma are well preserved during the process.

## 2. Hybrid Structural Filtering

The proposed hybrid structural filtering technique is an extension to the conventional grey-scale morphological filters, which have been introduced by using the concept of the *top surface* of a set and the related concept of the *umbra* of a surface.[1][2] In practical implementation, grey-scale dilation and erosion can be accomplished by using *min* and *max* operations. That is, given an input image $f(x)$ and a structuring element $k(x)$, grey-scale dilation of $f$ by $k$ can be calculated by

$$(f \oplus k)(x) = \max_{x-z \in D_f, \ z \in D_k} \{f(x-z)+k(z)\} \tag{1}$$

where $D_f$ and $D_k$ are the domains of $f$ and $k$, respectively. Similarly, grey-scale erosion of $f$ by $k$ can be obtained by

$$(f \ominus k)(x) = \min_{x+z \in D_f, \ z \in D_k} \{f(x+z)-k(z)\}. \tag{2}$$

In morphology, erosion followed by dilation (*opening*) has some important practical applications. The initial erosion removes small light details and darkens the image, whereas the subsequent dilation increases the brightness of the image without reintroducing the details removed by erosion, and thus leaves larger bright features relatively undisturbed. Though useful for the current application of removing pulmonary vessels within the CT lung images, the opening operation can introduce severe problems especially when noise is present. This is due to the fact that the opening process is a biased point estimator for signals embedded in noise and in our case it may undermine the subtle attenuation differences between normal and affected lung parenchyma.

To circumvent the problem encountered by the conventional grey-scale morphological filtering process, a novel hybrid approach has been developed. In essence, it is based on the modification to Eqs. (1) and (2) by redefining the *min* and *max* operators so that they take into account local intensity distributions. The new method is termed a *hybrid structural filter* in that it combines the strength of morphological filters in selectively removing small structural elements while preserving discontinuities such as edges, and the ability of conventional linear filters in dealing with image noise. Unlike the simple *min* and *max* operations adopted by conventional grey-scale morphology, we base our erosion and dilation processes on the underlying structure of the image. For image pixels covered by the structural element $k(x)$, a classification process is first employed to see if the pixels can be separated into two distinctive classes. Should this be the case, dilation or erosion is applied. Otherwise, the value of the centre pixel is replaced by the result of local linear or nonlinear filtering.

The classification process uses mean pixel intensity and gradient strength within the domain of the structure element $k(x)$. Denote $p_{mean}$, $g_{mean}$, $p^{(+)}_{mean}$, and $p^{(-)}_{mean}$ as follows:

$$p_{mean}(x) = \underset{x+z \in D_f, \ z \in D_k}{mean} \{f(x+z)\}$$

$$g_{mean}(x) = \underset{x+z \in D_f, \ z \in D_k}{mean} \{\nabla|f(x+z)|\}$$

$$p^{(+)}_{mean}(x) = \underset{x+z \in D_f, \ z \in D_k}{mean} \{ f(x+z) \mid f(x+z) \geq p_{mean}\}$$

and

$$p_{mean}^{(-)}(x) = \underset{x+z\in D_f, \ z\in D_k}{mean} \{ f(x+z) \mid f(x+z) < p_{mean} \}$$

i.e., $p_{mean}$ and $g_{mean}$ stand for the mean intensity and gradient strength of pixels within $D_k$ offset by vector $x$. Whereas $p^{(+)}{}_{mean}$ and $p^{(-)}{}_{mean}$ represent the mean of pixels with intensity values greater or less than $p_{mean}$ respectively. The erosion operator $\ominus$ is subsequently defined as

$$(f \ominus k)(x) = \begin{cases} p_{mean}^{(-)}, & if \ g_{mean} < \alpha\left( p_{mean}^{(+)} - p_{mean}^{(-)} \right) \\ p_{mean}, & if \ g_{mean} \geq \alpha\left( p_{mean}^{(+)} - p_{mean}^{(-)} \right) \end{cases} \tag{3}$$

where $\alpha$, ranging from 0 to 1.0, is a user defined parameter and its value is selected depending on the noise level of the image. Commonly, the noisier the image, the smaller the $\alpha$ value. If $\alpha$ is equal to zero, only local smoothing is applied.

The proposed method relies on the difference between $(p^{(+)}{}_{mean} - p^{(-)}{}_{mean})$ and $g_{mean}$ to justify the significance of distinctive pixel intensity distributions. A large difference between $(p^{(+)}{}_{mean} - p^{(-)}{}_{mean})$ and $g_{mean}$ suggests a good separation between the high and low pixel intensity classes. This applies to region borders as well as areas with noise spikes, and the value of the pixel under consideration is replaced by $p^{(-)}{}_{mean}$. A small difference between $(p^{(+)}{}_{mean} - p^{(-)}{}_{mean})$ and $g_{mean}$, however, indicates uncertainty about the separation and thus a smoothing process is applied and the pixel value is replaced by $p_{mean}$. For an ideal step edge without noise, the end results of applying the proposed erosion scheme and the traditional method are similar. When noise is present, however, the drawback of underestimating the intrinsic signal structure is minimised by using the new technique. When several steps of the erosion process are applied to a noisy image, the earlier steps are more biased towards smoothing, whereas the latter steps are more concentrated on erosion, a feature that is important for the robustness of the proposed technique. As in traditional morphology, dilation is defined as the dual of erosion.

## 3. Feature Localization via Wavelet Analysis

In order to restore possible structural distortions introduced by the hybrid filter, a feature localisation process based on wavelet reconstruction of feature extrema is used. Denote $f(x_1, x_2)$ as the original image, and $h(x_1, x_2)$ as the result after hybrid structure filtering. The proposed matching algorithm is based on a comparison of local maxima across all dyadic scales of $W_{2^j} f(x_1, x_2) = \left( W_{2^j}^{(1)} f(x_1, x_2), W_{2^j}^{(2)} f(x_1, x_2) \right)$ and $W_{2^j} h(x_1, x_2) = \left( W_{2^j}^{(1)} h(x_1, x_2), W_{2^j}^{(2)} h(x_1, x_2) \right)$. That is, within a small neighbourhood $\Omega$, a maximum in $W_{2^j} f(x_1, x_2)$ is preserved and its modulus value replaced if a matching candidate in $W_{2^j} h(x_1, x_2)$ can be found with similar magnitude and orientation values. Otherwise, it is discarded.

Denote $M_{2^j} f(x_1, x_2)$ and $A_{2^j} f(x_1, x_2)$ as the moduli and angles of wavelet coefficients. For a given pixel at $(x_{1(0)}, x_{2(0)})$ in $W_{2^j} f(x_1, x_2)$ that belongs to set $\partial_{M_{2^j} f(x_1, x_2)}$, which is defined to include all wavelet maxima of $f(x_1, x_2)$ at scale $2^j$, the matching algorithm searches within $W_{2^j} h(x_1, x_2)$ so that the following function is maximized

$$\Pi_{2^j}(x_1,\ x_2) = \Pi_{M_{2^j}(x_1,\ x_2)} \cdot \Pi_{A_{2^j}(x_1,\ x_2)}$$
$$\cdot\ \cos^{2n}\!\left(A_{2^j}\ f\!\left(x_{1(0)},\ x_{2(0)}\right) - A_{2^j}\ h\!\left(x_1,\ x_2\right)\right)$$

(4)

where

$$\Pi_{M_{2^j}(x_1,x_2)} = \exp\left\{-\ \frac{\left|M_{2^j}\ f\!\left(x_{1(0)},\ x_{2(0)}\right) - M_{2^j}\ h\!\left(x_1,\ x_2\right)\right|}{\beta}\right\}$$

and

$$\Pi_{A_{2^j}(x_1,\ x_2)} = \cos^2\!\left\{A_{2^j}\ f\!\left(x_{1(0)},\ x_{(0)}\right) - \theta\right\}\exp\left\{-\ \frac{\left|\left(x_1 - x_{1(0)},\ x_2 - x_{2(0)}\right)\right|}{\gamma_1}\right\}$$
$$+\ \sin^2\!\left\{\left(A_{2^j}\ f\!\left(x_{1(0)},\ x_{2(0)}\right) - \theta\right\}\exp\left\{-\ \frac{\left|\left(x_1 - x_{1(0)},\ x_2 - x_{2(0)}\right)\right|}{\gamma_2}\right\}$$

In the above equations $n$ is a positive integer, $\beta$, $\gamma_1$, and $\gamma_2$ are user defined control parameters, $\theta$ is the angle that vector $(x_1 - x_{1(0)},\ x_2 - x_{2(0)})$ makes with the horizontal axis, $(x_{1(0)},\ x_{2(0)}) \in \partial_{M_{2^j} f(x_1,\ x_2)}$ and $(x_1,\ x_2) \in \partial_{M_{2^j} h(x_1,\ x_2)}$.

The matching criterion defined in Eq. (4) consists of three terms; the first term $\Pi_{M_{2^j}(x_1,\ x_2)}$ ensures that the matched wavelet maxima have similar moduli. The smaller the scaling factor $\beta$, the closer the moduli will be. The second term $\Pi_{A_{2^j}(x_1,\ x_2)}$ indicates that the searching direction in $\Omega(x_{1(0)},\ x_{2(0)})$ should be along the direction defined by $A_{2^j}\ f(x_{1(0)},\ x_{2(0)})$. When a maximum is deviated from the searching direction, a smaller weighting factor is given. The control parameters $\gamma_1$ and $\gamma_2$ are uesd to control this anisotropic nature of the function. In general $\gamma_1 > \gamma_2$ and the larger the difference, the stronger the anisotropism. Eq. (4) also ensures that $\Pi_{A_{2^j}(x_1,\ x_2)}$ decays with distance, and thus it gives preferences to pixels that are close to $(x_{1(0)},\ x_{2(0)})$. The third term of Eq. (4) simply demands that the local orientation of matched maxima should be similar, the larger the integer value $n$, the stronger the restriction.

Since any sequence of two dimensional functions is not a priori the dyadic wavelet transform of some two-dimensional images,[3][4] the data resulted from feature localization cannot be directly inverse-transformed. In order to be a dyadic wavelet transform, such a sequence must satisfy the *reproducing kernel equations* and based on this the inverse-transform can be approximated by iterative convex projections of the feature localized image sequence onto the dyadic wavelet transform space.

## 4. Results and Conclusions

Figure (1) demonstrates the processing results of a test case using the proposed technique. The original CT image is displayed in (a) showing subtle and poorly marginated attenuation differences within the lung parenchyma due to obliterative

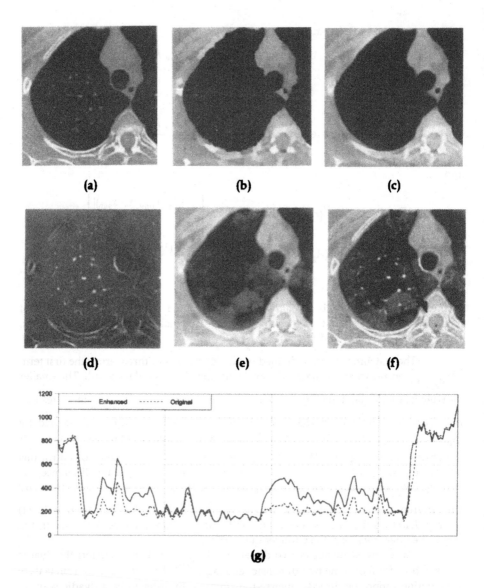

**Figure 1.** (a) The original CT image showing attenuation differences within the lung parenchyma due to obliterative bronchiolitis. (b) The result of hybrid filtering. (c) The result of applying the wavelet feature registration and reconstruction. (d) The difference between (a) and (c) with darker grey shades represent negative values and brighter grey shades indicate positive values. (e) The enhancement result of (c). (f) The final result when the difference image (d) is added to (e). (g) Pixel intensity profile along the line delineated in (f).

bronchiolitis. Figure (1b) is the hybrid filtering result of (a). It shows that the pulmonary vessels within the lung have successfully been removed while the intrinsic density differences of the lung parenchyma are retained. The result of applying the wavelet feature registration and reconstruction algorithm to (b) is given in (c). Figure (1d) is the difference between (c) and the original CT image (a). It is evident from (d) that the filtered structures are pulmonary vessels, the trachea wall, the rib and spine structures. The intensity differences in the lung parenchyma are almost uniformly zero. This represents an important feature of the algorithm in that it does not affect the intrinsic signal in the lungs and ensures that the subsequent classification process is accurate. The enhancement result of Figure (1c) is illustrated in (e), showing a marked improvement in contrast within the lung parenchyma. The final result when the difference image shown in (d) is added to Figure (e) is shown in Figure (1f). To allow for a more quantitative visual assessment of the enhancement result, Figure (g) illustrates the pixel intensity profile along the line delineated in (f).

Detecting small airways disease is difficult in clinical practice. Thus far, no single test has yet been devised that can accurately and reproducibly detect obliterative bronchiolitis over a wide range of severity. The use of high resolution CT imaging, combined with the proposed image enhancement and classification technique, holds the potential for providing a robust, and sensitive solution to detecting and quantifying the presence and extent of small airways disease. Because the density differences between normal and abnormal areas of lungs in patients with obliterative bronchiolitis are sometimes extremely subtle, our proposed method is expected to be of clinical value. Technically, the proposed hybrid structure filtering technique represents a novel and robust approach to image feature identification. Combined with the wavelet reconstruction algorithm, this method may be applicable to other clinical problems, for example subtle infiltration of the liver and other solid organs which may result in minimal density changes.

# References

1.      R. Haralick, S. Sternberg, and X. Zhuang, "Image Analysis Using Mathematical Morphology," *IEEE Trans Pattern Analysis and Machine Intelligence*, vol. 9, no. 4, pp. 691-696, 1987.

2.      J. Serra, *Image Analysis and Mathematical Morphology: Theoretical Advances*, vol. 2. New York: Academic Press, 1988.

3.      S. Mallat, "A theory for multiresolution signal decomposition: the wavelet representation," *IEEE Trans Pattern Analysis and Machine Intelligence*, vol. 11, pp. 674-693, 1989.

4.      S. Mallat and S. Zhong, "Characterization of signals from multiscale edges," *IEEE Trans Pattern Analysis and Machine Intelligence*, vol. 14, pp. 71-732, 1992.

# Computer Simulation of Convection and Diffusion Effects on Velocity Estimations from X-Ray Contrast Density Time Curves

SuiPing Huang[1], Brian E. Chapman[2], Joseph B. Muhlestein[3,6], Duane D. Blatter[5] and Dennis L. Parker[1,2,4]

Departments of Physics[1], Medical Informatics[2], Medicine[3], Radiology[4]
University of Utah, Salt Lake City, Utah 84132
and Radiology[5] and Cardiology[6] LDS Hospital Salt Lake City, Utah 84143

**Abstract.** The problem of velocity measurement in X-ray angiography using the leading edge of the contrast bolus is considered. The velocity obtained from the ratio of the temporal derivative to the spatial derivative of the contrast concentration curves is shown to reflect the **transport velocity**, which is the basis for an estimate of the true blood velocity in X-ray angiography. The contrast distribution along the vessel cross section affects the value of transport velocity. Under laminary flow conditions, the measured transport velocity of the leading edge has been found to be between the average and the peak (central) fluid velocities. Simulation studies of the bolus in laminar flow through a straight tube are presented in this paper to provide further proof of the higher transport velocity of the bolus leading edge. The simulation studies confirm observations made previously from X-ray images of contrast passage through simple tubes.

## 1 Introduction

Blood flow measurement is very important not only in hemodynamic studies but also in related disease diagnoses. At present, Digital Subtraction Angiography (DSA) is a popular tool in vascular disease diagnoses and appears to be the least invasive method capable of providing accurate quantitative studies of blood flow in small vessels. Almost all of the current techniques for blood flow measurements from DSA[1-3] are based upon the detection of the motion of an injected radi-opaque contrast material. However, most results show a consistent overestimation in determination of the true blood flow.

In this study, we consider the problem of the local velocity determination from the average contrast concentration curve as a function of position and time. We have previously developed a method to determine bolus transport velocity based upon the ratio of the temporal and spatial derivatives of the bolus concentration curves[4]. In this paper, we review the theory of the bolus transport velocity measurement and the method of the convective diffusion simulation. A simulation study was performed and results are presented to verify the predictions and the experimental results obtained previously.

## 2 Theory

Our theory of velocity measurement from bolus concentration curves has been published previously[4]. For completeness, we present an abbreviated derivation. The contrast bolus moving in the blood vessel abides by the law of Conservation of Mass (equation of continuity): $\frac{\partial \rho}{\partial t} + \nabla \cdot (\rho \vec{q}) = 0$. In cylindrical coordinates $\rho(r, x, t)$ is the local bolus concentration, $\vec{q}(r,x,t)$ is the local bolus velocity vector, and x is the axis of the local cylindrical coordinate system which is oriented along the vessel centerline. In the case of steady state laminar flow (a simplified mode) $q_r \approx 0$ and $q_\theta \approx 0$, so the continuity equation can be written as:

$$\frac{\partial(\rho(r, x, t)q_x(r, x, t))}{\partial x} + \frac{\partial \rho(r, x, t)}{\partial t} = 0 \tag{1}$$

Because the X-ray images are already projections of the contrast concentration through the vessel, it is convenient to consider the integral of Eq. (1) over the vessel lumen in a plane perpendicular to the flow direction. Here we define the one dimensional transport velocity and mean concentration as:

$$V_T(x, t) \equiv \frac{\int_0^R \rho(r, x, t)q_x(r, x, t)2\pi r dr}{\int_0^R \rho(r, x, t)2\pi r dr}, \quad C(x, t)) \equiv \frac{\int_0^R \rho(r, x, t)2\pi r dr}{\pi R^2} \tag{2}$$

Integrating both terms in Eq.(1) over the vessel lumen cross section we find that the one dimensional transport velocity $V_T(x, t)$ can be obtained after simple transformations:

$$V_T = -\frac{\partial C}{\partial t} \Big/ \frac{\partial C}{\partial x} - C \cdot \frac{\partial V_T}{\partial x} \Big/ \frac{\partial C}{\partial x} = V_D + \Delta V \tag{3}$$

Where $V_T$ is the transport velocity, $V_D \equiv -\frac{\partial C}{\partial t} \Big/ \frac{\partial C}{\partial x}$ is the derivative velocity which can be measured from C(x,t), and $\Delta V \equiv -C \cdot \frac{\partial V_T}{\partial x} \Big/ \frac{\partial C}{\partial x}$ can be considered to be the error between $V_D$ and $V_T$. That is, $\Delta V$ is the difference between the true transport velocity and the measurable velocity estimate, $V_D$.

There is a simple situation in which this error term $\Delta V$ can be estimated: when there is simple laminar flow and the effects of diffusion can be neglected. In our experiments, the bolus usually has a clear leading edge. To simplify the following analysis, we consider only measurements made on the bolus leading edge. In the case of a compact bolus injection and where the effects of diffusion can be ignored, we have demonstrated previously[4], that:

$$V_T = V_D + \frac{\Delta V_D}{2} = V_D - \frac{C}{2} \cdot \frac{\partial V_D}{\partial x} \Big/ \frac{\partial C}{\partial x} \tag{4}$$

In this expression, we find the correction, $\Delta V_D$, is exactly double that desired, that is $\Delta V = \Delta V_D/2$. All terms on the right hand of Eq. (4) are measurable and the result is an accurate estimate of the transport velocity in the region of the leading edge in the case of an initially compact and uniformly distributed bolus.

## 3  Simulation Method

Bolus dispersion under fully developed laminar flow through a straight circular tube has a great deal of theoretical interest and practical important in chemical and mechanical engineering [5-6]. Taylor first used the convection-diffusion equation to describe this problem in 1953[5]. In this simulation study, we use their methods to investigate the properties of the bolus transport velocity. One recent method[6] is capable of solving the convection-diffusion equation at both short times and high Peclet numbers, Pe (defined as Pe=RU0/D), which match the conditions of our simulations and prior experiments.

Because of its simplicity, accuracy and more efficient numerical computation, the method of Takahashi, *et al* [6] was chosen and is described briefly in their notations as follows.

When a bolus of contrast material is injected into a straight tube of circular cross-section with fully developed laminar flow, it is diluted with flow in the tube. The local concentration $\rho(r, x, t)$ of contrast bolus moving in the tube can be described by the convection-diffusion equation:

$$\frac{\partial \rho}{\partial t} = D\left(\frac{\partial^2 \rho}{\partial r^2} + \frac{1}{r}\frac{\partial \rho}{\partial r} + \frac{\partial^2 \rho}{\partial x^2}\right) - U_0\left(1 - \frac{r^2}{R^2}\right)\frac{\partial \rho}{\partial x} \tag{5}$$

where D is the diffusion coefficient, $U_0$ is the center velocity and R is the radius of tube.

In dimensionless form, with the definitions of Takahashi *et al*: $\theta \equiv \dfrac{\rho}{\rho_0}$, $P_e \equiv \dfrac{RU_0}{D}$,

$X \equiv \dfrac{x}{R}$, $y \equiv \dfrac{r}{R}$, $\tau \equiv \dfrac{Dt}{R^2}$. equation (5) can be written as:

$$\frac{\partial \theta}{\partial \tau} = \frac{\partial^2 \theta}{\partial y^2} + \frac{1}{y}\frac{\partial \theta}{\partial y} + \frac{\partial^2 \theta}{\partial x^2} - P_e(1 - y^2)\frac{\partial \theta}{\partial X} \tag{6}$$

With the boundary and initial conditions:

$$\frac{\partial}{\partial y}\theta(X, 0, \tau) = \frac{\partial}{\partial y}\theta(X, 1, \tau) = 0, \ \theta(X, y, 0) = 1$$

The scheme of the numerical method is:

I) Move the local concentration of $\theta(X, y, 0)$ to a new position at local transport velocity $P_e(1 - y^2)$ in a small enough time $\Delta\tau$ to get a pure convection solution.

II) Let radial and axial diffusion take place on the solution of step (I) according to the analytical solution of equation(6) with $P_e$ equal to zero. The analytical solution can be obtained by the method of separation of variables:

$$\theta(y, X, \Delta\tau) = \sum_{n=0}^{\infty} \frac{J_0(\lambda_n y)e^{-\lambda_n^2\Delta\tau}}{J_0^2(\lambda_n)\sqrt{\pi\Delta\tau}} \int_{-\infty}^{\infty}\int_0^1 \theta(\eta, \xi, 0)J_0(\lambda_n\eta)\eta e^{-\frac{(X-\xi)^2}{4\Delta\tau}} d\eta d\xi \quad (7)$$

Where $\lambda_n$ is the nth non-negative zero of $J_1(r)$, that is: $J_1(\lambda_n) = 0$, n=0,1,2,3....

III) Repeat step(I) and (II) until the desired value of $\tau$ is reached.

The mass balance technique for checking the computing error was adopted in the implementation of this simulation study with mass balance error within ±1 %. The transport velocity by definition (3) can be obtained with known local concentration $\theta(X, y, \tau)$ and local fluid velocity profile $P_e(1 - y^2)$.

## 4   Simulation Results

Our simulation results of the evolution of the bolus profile in the axial direction are quite similar to those in previous studies[5-6], especially for Peclet numbers greater than 1000. All the bolus profiles experience a transition from convective to diffusive dispersion for arbitrary Peclet numbers. The results presented in Fig. 1 are an example for Pe=100.

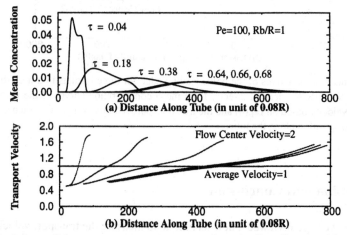

**Fig. 1.** Evolutions of the mean concentration curve along the flow direction (a) and the corresponding transport velocity (b) for a bolus which initially fully occupied the tube cross section with Pe=100.

The transport velocity of the leading edge was found to be consistently higher than the average velocity of fluid flow. For an initially concentrated bolus which is uniformly distributed over the cross section of the tube, the distribution of the bolus mean concentration becomes highly asymmetric early in the convective dispersion process($\tau$=0.04), especially for larger Peclet numbers. Simulations also show that the initial bolus profile at time of injection could affect the following bolus profiles and the peak of mean concentration curves could move faster or slower than the average fluid velocity depending on the initial bolus profile. During the final steady state, the peak of the mean concentration curve moves at the average velocity, and thus can be an ideal quantity for blood flow measurement. Our derivative method works well for transport velocity measurements of the bolus leading edge in the presence of diffusion effects. Fig. 2 shows such an example comparing the derivative velocities with the true transport velocity derived by definition of (3).

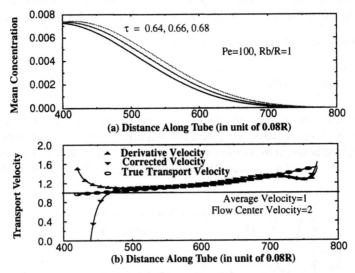

**Fig. 2.** (a) Concentration curves of the bolus leading edge for three instants in time. (b) Plots of the derivative velocity $V_D$ derived directly from mean concentration curves of the leading edge, the corrected velocity based on Eq.(4) and the true transport velocity computed from definition (3) as a function of position along the tube.

## 5 Discussion and Conclusion

In this paper, we have reviewed a new technique to measure the transport velocity of the bolus leading edge. We have used simulation methods to verify the prediction and experiment results. From these studies, we believe that the derivative method can be used to obtain an estimate of the contrast bolus transport velocity. For the bolus leading edge, we have shown that the transport velocity increases from the average to the maximum fluid velocity as a function of position from the bolus peak to the bolus leading edge and that measurements made near the bolus center should yield values closer to the average velocity. Unfortunately, the derivative method that we have presented loses all accuracy near the bolus center because the spatial and temporal derivatives of contrast density approach zero.

Our observations and simulation studies indicate that the velocities obtained from this technique are consistently higher than the average flow velocity. This is due to the fact that the bolus, itself, is transported at a rate higher than the average velocity in the bolus leading edge. This fact may provide an explanation for the velocity overestimation error which can occur in bolus tracking techniques[1-3]. Our simulation study provides an excellent confirmation that the measurements of velocity from the bolus leading edge will be between the peak and average fluid velocity. However, the work presented here is preliminary and our theoretical analysis and numerical simulation have been highly simplified. We believe that an improved understanding of these phenomena can be obtained through the application of the convection-diffusion theory considering curvature, pulsation and other complicated factors. The proposed technique may ultimately be of value in velocity determinations in short vessel segments where there is no existing method to obtain a velocity from other types of bolus tracking methods. Further work will be necessary to find an accurate relationship between the measured transport velocity and the more physiologically significant average velocity.

## Acknowledgments

The authors thank HongYue Dai, Andy Alexander, Craig Goodrich, and Rudy Van Bree for helpful discussions. This work was supported in part by a grant from Siemens Medical Systems and NIH grant R01 HL48223.

## References

1.    C. G. Shaw, D. B. Plewes, "Pulsed-injection method for blood flow velocity measurement in intraarterial digital subtraction angiography," *Radiology* 160, 556-559 (1986)

2.    D. J. Hawkes, A. M. Seifalian, A. C. F. Colchester, N. Iqbal, C. R. Hardingham, C. F. Blandin and K. E. F. Hobbsl, "Validation of volume blood flow measurements using three-dimensional distance-concentration functions derived from digital X-ray angiograms," *Invest. Radiol.* 4, 434-442 (1994)

3.    D. L. Parker, D. L. Pope, R. E. Van Bree, and H. W. Marshall, "Three-dimensional reconstruction of moving arterial beds from digital subtraction angiography". *Computers and Biomedical Research* 20,166-185(1987)

4.    S.P. Huang, R.J. Decker, K. C. Goodrich, D.J. Parker, J.B. Muhlestein, D.D. Blatter, and D.L. Parker. "Velocity measurement based on bolus tracking with the aid of 3D reconstruction from DSA". Submitted to *Medical Physics.*

5.    G. I. Taylor, "Dispersion of soluble matter in solvent flowing slowly through a tube," *Proc. Roy. Soc. (London)* 219A, 186-203 (1953)

6.    T. Korenaga, F. Shen, T. Takahashi, "A numerical solution for the dispersion in laminar flow through a circular tube". *Canadian J. Chem. Eng.* 68, 191-196 (1990)

# A Comparison of Retrospective Intensity Non-uniformity Correction Methods for MRI

John G. Sled, Alex P. Zijdenbos, Alan C. Evans

McConnell Brain Imaging Centre, Montréal Neurological Institute, McGill University, Montréal, Canada

**Abstract.** Intensity non-uniformity is an artifact often seen in MRI data that can significantly degrade automatic segmentation and prevent quantitative analysis. Using simulated MRI data, we have quantitatively compared the performance of three methods of correcting for intensity non-uniformity. In this analysis, novel stereotaxic space techniques were employed so that all three methods were fully automatic and capable of correcting volumes of any pulse sequence. Our results, based on correcting simulated T1, T2, and proton density (PD) weighted MRI scans with various levels of noise and non-uniformity, showed no method to be superior in all categories. However, the N3 technique distinguished itself for uniformly good performance without the limitation of assuming a sophisticated model of the data.

## 1 Introduction

An artifact often seen in MRI is for the signal intensity to vary smoothly across the image. Variously referred to as RF inhomogeneity, shading artifact, or intensity non-uniformity, it is usually attributed to such factors as poor radio frequency (RF) field uniformity, eddy currents driven by the switching of field gradients, and patient anatomy both inside and outside the field of view.

In the past, much of the effort on the correction of intensity non-uniformity (INU) has been directed at reducing the extreme variations seen in surface coil images. However, recent interest in automatic segmentation has driven expectations of better uniformity for routine volume acquisitions. While the intensity variations of 10%–30% often seen in clinical scanners have little impact on visual diagnosis, the performance of automatic segmentation techniques which assume homogeneity of intensity within each class can be significantly degraded by clinically acceptable levels of intensity non-uniformity. As automated methods are increasingly used to process large volumes of data for clinical trials, there is a need for an accurate, automatic, inexpensive, and robust means of correcting for this artifact [4].

We compare three non-uniformity correction methods for the task of removing typical levels of non-uniformity from volumetric scans of the human head. The methods are referred to respectively as the expectation maximization (EM) [9], white matter (WM) [3], and non-parametric (N3) [7] methods. All three are fully automated, 3D implementations formulated to detect and remove a multiplicative INU field by iterative approximation.

# 2 Methods

To facilitate automatic training of the classifiers which the EM and WM methods rely on, all volumes were first resampled into a standardized 3D, so-called stereotaxic, coordinate system [2, 8]. For this work we constructed 3D tissue probability maps (TPMs) of grey matter, white matter, and cerebrospinal fluid (CSF) based on the classification of 53 normal subjects [11].

A classifier training set was created for each individual brain by randomly selecting voxels in stereotaxic space corresponding to voxels in the TPM thresholded at the 90% level. This approach allowed automatic training of the classifier regardless of the volume's pulse sequence [6]. In addition, non-brain tissues were removed automatically using a standard brain mask derived from an average of normal brains defined in stereotaxic space.

The WM method terminates after two iterations, while the EM and N3 methods terminate when the coefficient of variation of the ratio between consecutive field estimates, calculated at all intracranial voxels, drops below a threshold of 0.001.

**Expectation Maximization Method (EM):** This methods iterates between a classification stage, designed to remove anatomical features from the image, and a filtering stage that smoothes the field estimate [9]. The filtering is done with a Gaussian filter whose kernel is truncated to remain within the volume of interest. A Bayesian classifier was used in this implementation. Wells et al. have since described an implementation [10] based on a Parzen window classifier.

Our experiments, not shown here, on simulated data with various widths of the smoothing kernel suggested that a Gaussian kernel with full width at half maximum (FWHM) of 30mm was nearly optimal. While the results produced with a 30mm kernel appeared visually "lumpy", larger kernels produced a significant edge artifact.

**White Matter Method (WM):** This method is a revised version of that described in [3]. It relies on an artificial neural network classifier [12] trained using TPMs to identify white matter in the brain region. Partial volume voxels are then eliminated from the white matter region using gradient information. Tensor cubic B splines are used to fit a smooth 3D field to the remaining white matter voxels and extrapolate this field to the rest of the volume. Once estimated, the non-uniformity field is used to correct the original volume and the process is repeated once.

**Non-parametric Method (N3):** Like the EM method, the N3 method alternates between estimating intensities of the uncorrupted volume and smoothing the estimate of the field. Unlike the EM method, this method does not rely on explicit tissue classification and can be applied to an image regardless of the distribution of tissues present. It does, however, require an estimate of the extent of the histogram blurring that intensity non-uniformity causes. The estimate of histogram blur was fixed throughout our analysis, irrespective of the type of volume. Smoothing was the same for the N3 and WM methods. The distance between basis functions used throughout is 200mm, significantly larger than the 30mm kernel used by the EM method. This greater degree of smoothing was possible because splines are less sensitive to boundaries.

## 3   Simulated MR Volumes

Non-uniformity correction methods such as those described here can be validated with real data using subjective measures of image quality and by assessing the reduction of variability in tasks such as segmentation. However, the large number of uncontrolled factors in such experiments have confounded attempts to evaluate and optimize algorithm performance. In particular, partial volume effects, true anatomical variability, and an unknown non-uniformity field prevent a sensitive analysis of methodological parameters. These issues were circumvented in our analysis by the use of an MR simulator which incorporates realistic models for noise and partial volume. Slices through simulated T1, T2, and PD volumes are shown in Fig. 1.

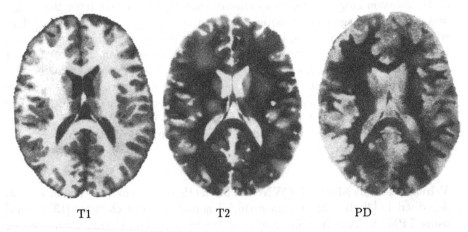

|  | | |
|---|---|---|
| T1 | T2 | PD |

**Fig. 1.** Simulated T1, T2, and PD weighted volumes. Non-uniform sensitivity of the reception coil was simulated causing the intensity to drop off at the bottom left. The noise distribution has a standard deviation 3% of the mean intensity of white matter.

The simulations used in this analysis were constructed using the method described in [7]. These simulations employ random small scale variations of the true signal intensity within each tissue class to produce an intensity histogram similar to that of real data. We used a number realizations of this "pseudo-anatomy" in our experiments to assess accuracy and avoid bias in our results. An issue for this analysis was whether there was an implicit field within the anatomical model that favoured a particular method. We addressed this by deriving the simulations from an anatomical model based on a discrete classification of each voxel as a particular type of tissue.

## 4 Experiments

Simulated MR volumes like those shown in Fig. 1 were used to evaluate the performance of the three methods at various levels of noise and non-uniformity. Correction performance was computed in terms of the coefficient of variation in the ratio of the estimated non-uniformity field to the known field imposed during simulation. This error measure is insensitive to global scale factors. It should be noted that zero estimation error is not achievable for these experiments since even if an algorithm were insensitive to the low spatial frequency components of the pseudo-anatomy and partial volume, there is still a low frequency component to the broad-band Gaussian noise that is indistinguishable from intensity non-uniformity.

*Sensitivity to Noise Level* A noise distribution with standard deviation 3% of the mean intensity of white matter is typical of 3D gradient-echo T1 weighted volumes. We chose a comparable level of noise for T2 and PD volumes and termed this 3% noise. The non-uniformity field used in these experiments is typical of the fields seen in real data, varying in magnitude by ±10% within the brain region.

The results of experiments on simulated T1 and PD data with varying noise level are shown in Figs. 2a and 2c. Also shown is the so-called baseline level of INU present before correction. Results above this line indicate that the method has made the INU worse. To estimate the intersubject variability in these results the experiments were repeated for four realizations of the pseudo-anatomy. This variability is reflected in the error bars shown in Fig. 2. All three methods performed similarly on T2 data, so this graph is not shown.

*Sensitivity to Non-uniformity Magnitude* A similar set of experiments was conducted for increasing levels of non-uniformity using the same shape of the non-uniformity field, but different magnitudes. We denote 50% INU as a multiplicative field that varies between 0.75 and 1.25. The results of these experiments experiments are shown in Figs. 2b and 2d. Also shown is the baseline for each level of non-uniformity. As before, the results for T2 data did not differentiate the methods so this graph is not shown.

## 5 Discussion

While no method distinguished itself on T2 scans, the results for T1 scans and to a lesser extent PD scans clearly differentiated the three methods. This fact can be rationalized from their respective designs. Consider the WM method, which relies on segmenting the white matter from the rest of the brain. On T1

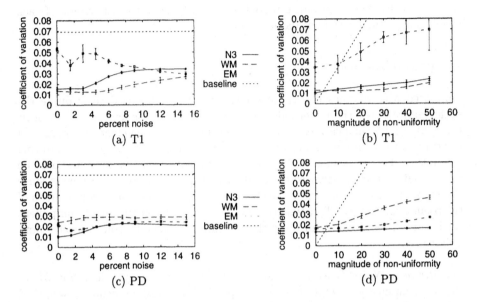

**Fig. 2.** A comparison of the three non-uniformity correction methods using simulated T1 and PD weighted data. (a) and (c) are for increasing noise level; (b) and (d) are for increasing levels of intensity non-uniformity. The lines on these graphs pass through the mean of four trials using different realizations of the pseudo-anatomy while the error bars are at ±1 standard deviation.

weighted volumes where the contrast between white matter and other tissues is greatest the WM method gave the best performance. Whereas on PD weighted volumes, where contrast is low, the performance of the WM method is relatively poor. Overall this method performed well by improving uniformity for all but the smallest fields and having little sensitivity to increasing noise.

Unlike the WM method, the contrast seen in T1 scans works against the EM method. In principle the EM method has an advantage over the WM method in that, by using the whole volume, it is less affected by noise. However, a number of authors have described this method as overly sensitive to the training of its classifier [1, 5]. Our experience has been that the method makes excessively large corrections to voxels that fall outside the classifier's tissue model. These outliers may dominate the correction process and cause poor results. If one trains the classifier on samples of pure tissue, or 90% pure as in our experiments, and the intensity distributions of the different classes are well resolved, as is the case in T1 scans, then regions of partial volume will produce intensities outside the tissue model and receive extreme corrections. In addition, as the level of noise increased the EM method performed better on T1 scans. This is due to the greater variability in the training data and reduced contrast in these images. Similarly, on PD weighted scans, with less contrast, the method performed better. Overall, the performance of this method was erratic.

The N3 method, besides performing well in all categories, has the significant advantage of not requiring stereotaxic space nor prior knowledge of the tissue classes present. Given the modelling assumptions of the WM method and the erratic results for the EM method on T1 scans, the N3 method is most attractive for it robustness and potentially broader range of applications.

# References

1. C. Brechbuhler, G. Gerig, and G. Szekely. Compensation of spatial inhomogeneity in MRI based on a parametric bias estimate. In *Forth International Conference on Visualization in Biomedical Computing*, pages 141–146, 1996.
2. D. L. Collins, P. Neelin, T. M. Peters, and A. C. Evans. Automatic 3D intersubject registration of MR volumetric data in standardized Talairach space. *J. Comput. Assist. Tomogr.*, 18(2):192–205, 1994.
3. B. M. Dawant, A. P. Zijdenbos, and R. A. Margolin. Correction of intensity variations in MR images for computer-aided tissue classification. *IEEE Trans. Med. Imag.*, 12(4):770–781, Dec. 1993.
4. A. C. Evans, J. A. Frank, J. Antel, and D. H. Miller. The role of MRI in clinical trials of multiple sclerosis: Comparison of image processing techniques. *Annals of Neurology*, 1996. In press.
5. R. Guillemaud and M. Brady. Enhancement of MR images. In *Forth International Conference on Visualization in Biomedical Computing*, pages 107–116, 1996.
6. V. Kollokian. Performance analysis of automatic techniques for tissue classification in magnetic resonance images of the human brain. Master's thesis, Concordia University, Montreal, QC, Nov. 1996.
7. J. G. Sled, A. P. Zijdenbos, and A. C. Evans. A non-parametric method for automatic correction of intensity non-uniformity in MRI data. *IEEE Trans. Med. Imag.*, 1996. (submitted).
8. J. Talairach and P. Tournoux. *Co-planar Stereotaxic Atlas of the Human Brain: 3-Dimensional Proportional System - an Approach to Cerebral Imaging*. Thieme Medical Publishers, New York, NY, 1988.
9. W. M. Wells III, W. E. L. Grimson, R. Kikinis, and F. A. Jolesz. Statistical intensity correction and segmentation of MRI data. In *VBC, Proceedings of the SPIE*, volume 2359, pages 13–24, 1994.
10. W. M. Wells III, W. E. L. Grimson, R. Kikinis, and F. A. Jolesz. Adaptive segmentation of MRI data. *IEEE Trans. Med. Imag.*, 15(4):429–442, 1996.
11. A. Zijdenbos, A. Evans, F. Riahi, J. Sled, H.-C. Chui, and V. Kollokian. Automatic quantification of multiple sclerosis lesion volume using stereotaxic space. In *Forth International Conference on Visualization in Biomedical Computing (VBC)*, Hamburg, Germany, 1996.
12. A. P. Zijdenbos, B. M. Dawant, R. A. Margolin, and A. C. Palmer. Morphometric analysis of white matter lesions in MR images: Method and validation. *IEEE Trans. Med. Imag.*, 13(4):716–724, 1994.

# A Robust and Efficient Algorithm for Image Registration [*]

B. C. Vemuri[1], S. Huang[1], S. Sahni[1], C. M. Leonard[2],
C. Mohr[2],T. Lucas[2], R. Gilmore[3] and J. Fitzsimmons[4]

[1]Department of Computer & Information Sciences
[2]Department of Neuroscience, [3]Department of Neurology
[4]Department of Radiology
University of Florida, Gainesville, Fl 32611

**Abstract.** Image registration is a very important problem in medical image processing. In this paper, a hierarchical optical flow motion model is used to solve the registration problem. We develop a novel numerical algorithm to achieve robust and efficient 3D/2D image registration. Motion estimation examples on synthetic & real data with performance comparison to competing ones are presented.

## 1 Introduction

Image registration is a very common and important problem in diverse fields such as medical imaging, computer vision, art, entertainment etc. The problem of registering two images, be they 2D or 3D, is equivalent to estimating the motion between them. We treat the problem of registering two images as equivalent to computing the flow field between the data sets. A large body of literature exists on registration methods for medical image data. Methods based on registering common features between datasets e.g., surfaces, contours etc. have been proposed in literature [2, 5, 8]. The accuracy of registration in these approaches is partially dictated by the accuracy of the feature detector. *In this paper, we propose a registration method that is robust and fast and is applicable directly to the volume data.*

Some algorithms in the recent past have used the direct approach, and The technique in [6] uses the concept of maximizing mutual information and reported results are quite impressive however, there is no provision for handling local motions in this method. In [3], a novel approach is described wherein the registration is modeled by a viscous fluid flow model expressed as a PDE. The reported cpu times for registration are however slow. Thirion [10] introduced an interesting demon-based registration that can be viewed as being similar to the fluid-based algorithm when the elastic filter in the later is repalced by a Gaussian.

In our approach, we use the hierarchical motion model to compute the registration. This model consists of globally parameterized motion flow models at one end of the "spectrum"and a local motion flow model at the other end. The global

---

[*] This work was supported in part by the grant NIH-R01-LM05944.

motion model is defined by associating a single global motion model with each patch of a recursively subdivided input image. Whereas, in the local flow model, the flow field is not parameterized. The flow field corresponding to the displacement at each pixel/voxel is represented by a B-spline basis. The unknown flow field may be estimated at each pixel/voxel via a numerical iterative minimization of a nonlinear objective function. In this paper, our main contributions are: (a) A new formulation of the hierarchical flow field computation model based on the idea of precomputing the Hessian at the optimum prior to knowing the optimum, (b) Development of a new and robust numerical solution technique using a modified Newton iteration. (c) A novel application namely, a volumetric flow-based registration of MRI data.

The rest of the paper is organized as follows, in section 2, we describe the glboal/local flow field motion model briefly. Section 3 contains the numerical algorithm used for computing the registration. In section 4, we present several examples of implementation results. Section 5 contains the conclusions.

## 2 Local/global Motion Model

The optical flow computation model[1, 4] is very general especially when set in a hierachical framework [9]. In this framework, at one extreme (local motion), each pixel/voxel is assumed to undergo an independent displacement. Thus producing a vector field of displacements over the image. At the other extreme, we have the global motion wherein the flow field model is expressed parametrically by a small set of parameters e.g., rigid motion, affine motion etc.

A general formulation of the image registration can be posed as follows: Given a pair of images (possibly from a sequence) $I_1$ and $I_2$, we assume that $I_2$ was formed by locally displacing the reference image $I_1$ as given by: $I_2(x_i + u_i, y_i + v_i) = I_1(x_i, y_i)$. The problem is to recover the displacement field $(u, v)$ for which the maximum likelihood solution is obtained by minimizing the error given by: $J\{E_{ssd}(\hat{\mathbf{T}})\} = E\{(I_m(\mathbf{X}_i, \hat{\mathbf{T}}) - I_2(\mathbf{X}_i))^2\}$. Where $E_{ssd}(\hat{\mathbf{T}})$ is the expectation of squared difference, $I_m(\mathbf{X}_i, \hat{\mathbf{T}}) = I_1(x_i + \hat{u}_i, y_i + \hat{v}_i)$, and $\hat{\mathbf{T}}$ is the estimated motion parameters.

We represent the displacement fields $u(x, y)$ and $v(x, y)$ by B-splines with a small number of control points $\hat{u}_k$ and $\hat{v}_k$ as in [9]. The displacement at a pixel location $i$ is given by $u(x_i, y_i) = \sum_k \hat{u}_k w_{ik} = \sum_k \hat{u}_k B_k(x_i, y_i)$ and $v(x_i, y_i) = \sum_k \hat{v}_k w_{ik} = \sum_k \hat{v}_k B_k(x_i, y_i)$, where the $B_k(x_i, y_i)$ are the *basis functions* with finite support.

When a global motion model is used to model the motion between $I_1$ and $I_2$, it is possible to parameterize the flow by rigid, affine, quadratic and other types of transformations. We employ the affine flow model in this paper which is given by

$$\begin{bmatrix} u(x,y) \\ v(x,y) \end{bmatrix} = \begin{bmatrix} t_0 & t_1 \\ t_3 & t_4 \end{bmatrix} \begin{bmatrix} x \\ y \end{bmatrix} + \begin{bmatrix} t_2 \\ t_5 \end{bmatrix} - \begin{bmatrix} x \\ y \end{bmatrix} \tag{1}$$

where, the parameters $\mathbf{T} = (t_0, ..., t_5)^T$ are called *global motion parameters*. To compute an estimate of the global motion, we first define the spline control vertices $\hat{\mathbf{u}}_{\mathbf{j}} = (\hat{u}_j, \hat{v}_j)^T$ in terms of the global motion parameters

$$\hat{\mathbf{u}}_{\mathbf{j}} = \begin{bmatrix} \hat{x}_j & \hat{y}_j & 1 & 0 & 0 & 0 \\ 0 & 0 & 0 & \hat{x}_j & \hat{y}_j & 1 \end{bmatrix} \mathbf{T} - \begin{bmatrix} \hat{x}_j \\ \hat{y}_j \end{bmatrix} \equiv \mathbf{T}_{\mathbf{j}}\mathbf{T} - \hat{\mathbf{X}}_{\mathbf{j}}. \tag{2}$$

We then define the flow at each pixel by interpolation using our spline representation. The error criterion $J\{E_{ssd}(\hat{\mathbf{T}})\}$ becomes

$$J\{E_{ssd}(\hat{\mathbf{T}})\} = E\{(I_1(\mathbf{X}_i + \sum_j w_{ij}(\mathbf{T}_{\mathbf{j}}\mathbf{T} - \hat{\mathbf{X}}_{\mathbf{j}})) - I_2(\mathbf{X}_i))^2\}. \tag{3}$$

Extending from 2D affine model to other 2D/3D models is quite straightforward and will not be discussed here.

## 3 Numerical Solution

We now describe a novel adaptation of an elegant numerical method by Burkardt and Diehl [7] which is a modification of the standard Newton method for minimizing our nonlinear error term $J\{E_{ssd}\}$. The modification invovles precomputation of the Hessian matrix at the optimum without starting the iterative minimization process. *Our adaptation of this idea to the framework of optical flow computation with spline-based flow field representations is new and invovles nontrivial derivations of the gradient vectors and Hessian matrices.*

In the following, we will essentially adopt the notation from [7] to derive the modified Newton iteration and develop new notation as necessary. The primary structure of the algorithm is given in the following iteration formula

$$\hat{\mathbf{T}}^{k+1} = \hat{\mathbf{T}}^k - \mathbf{H}^{-1}(\hat{\mathbf{T}} = \hat{\mathbf{T}}^* = \mathbf{T})g(\hat{\mathbf{T}}^k). \tag{4}$$

Where $\mathbf{H}$ is the Hessian matrix and $\mathbf{g}$ is the gradient vector. Unlike in a typical Newton iteration, in the above equation, the *Hessian* is always computed at the optimum $\hat{\mathbf{T}} = \hat{\mathbf{T}}^* = \mathbf{T}$ instead of the iteration point $\hat{\mathbf{T}}^k$. So, one of the key problems is, how to calculate the Hessian at the optimum prior to begining the iteration.

Let the vector $\mathbf{X}$ denote the coordinates in any image and $h : \mathbf{X} \rightarrow \mathbf{X}'$ a transformation from $\mathbf{X}$ to another set of coordinates $\mathbf{X}'$, characterized by a set of parameters collected into a vector $T$ i.e., $\mathbf{X}' = h(\mathbf{X}, \mathbf{T})$. The parameter vector $\mathbf{T}$ can represent any of rigid, affine, shearing, projective etc. transformations. Normally the Hessian at the optimum will explicitly depend on the optimum motion vector and hence can not be computed directly. However, a clever technique was introduced in [7], exploiting the facts that the *expectation is independent of coordinate systems and when motion is small, rotation and translation do commute.* Using these observations, as in [7], we introduce a moving coordinate system $\{\mathbf{X}^k\}$ and an intermediate motion vector $\tilde{\mathbf{T}}$ to develop the formulas for precomputing the Hessian. This intermediate motion vector gives the relationship between $\{\mathbf{X}^k\}$ of iteration step $k$ and $\{\mathbf{X}^{k+1}\}$ of iteration step $k+1$, given that

$\mathbf{X}^k = h(\mathbf{X}, \hat{\mathbf{T}}^k)$ , $\mathbf{X}^{k+1} = h(\mathbf{X}^k, \tilde{\mathbf{T}}^{k+1}) = h(h(\mathbf{X}, \hat{\mathbf{T}}^k), \tilde{\mathbf{T}}^{k+1}) = h(\mathbf{X}, \hat{\mathbf{T}}^{k+1})$. The Hessian at the optimum can be written as

$$\tilde{\mathbf{H}} = 2E\left\{ \left(\frac{\partial h(\mathbf{X},\mathbf{T})}{\partial \mathbf{T}}\right)^T \frac{\partial I_1(\mathbf{X})}{\partial \mathbf{X}} \left(\frac{\partial I_1(\mathbf{X})}{\partial \mathbf{X}}\right)^T \frac{\partial h(\mathbf{X},\mathbf{T})}{\partial \mathbf{T}} \right\}\Bigg|_{\mathbf{T}=0}. \quad (5)$$

Whereas, the gradient vector with respect to $\tilde{\mathbf{T}}$ is given by

$$\tilde{\mathbf{g}}(\hat{\mathbf{T}}^k) = 2E\left\{ e\left( \left(\frac{\partial I_2(\mathbf{X})}{\partial \mathbf{X}}\right)^T \left(\frac{\partial \mathbf{X}^k}{\partial \mathbf{X}}\right)^{-1} \left(\frac{\partial \mathbf{X}^{k+1}}{\partial \tilde{\mathbf{T}}^{k+1}}\right)\Bigg|_{\tilde{\mathbf{T}}^{k+1}=0}\right)^T \right\}. \quad (6)$$

Where $e = I_m(\mathbf{X}, \hat{\mathbf{T}}^k) - I_2(\mathbf{X})$. Thus the modified Newton algorithm consists of the following iteration: $\tilde{\mathbf{T}}^{k+1} = -\tilde{\mathbf{H}}^{-1}\tilde{\mathbf{g}}(\hat{\mathbf{T}}^k)$, and the estimate at step k+1 is given by: $\hat{\mathbf{T}}^{k+1} = f(\hat{\mathbf{T}}^k, \tilde{\mathbf{T}}^{k+1})$. Where, $f$ is a function that depends on the type of motion model used.

In the case of flow vector with 2D affine parameterization, $(\partial h(\mathbf{X},\mathbf{T})/\partial \mathbf{T})^T = block - diagonal(\mathbf{A}, \mathbf{A})$, where $\mathbf{A} = (\sum_j w_j \hat{x}_j, \sum_j w_j \hat{y}_j, \sum_j w_j)^T$. These formulas can be substituted into (5) to get $\tilde{\mathbf{H}}$. As for the gradient $\tilde{\mathbf{g}}$, we have

$$\frac{\partial \mathbf{X}^k}{\partial \mathbf{X}} = \begin{bmatrix} 1 + \sum_j (w_j)_x' \hat{u}_j^k & \sum_j (w_j)_y' \hat{u}_j^k \\ \sum_j (w_j)_x' \hat{v}_j^k & 1 + \sum_j (w_j)_y' \hat{v}_j^k \end{bmatrix} \quad (7)$$

and $\left(\frac{\partial \mathbf{X}^{k+1}}{\partial \tilde{\mathbf{T}}^{k+1}}\right)^T\Big|_{\tilde{\mathbf{T}}^{k+1}=0} = \begin{bmatrix} \mathbf{N} & \mathbf{0} \\ \mathbf{0} & \mathbf{N} \end{bmatrix}$, where $\mathbf{N} = (\sum_j w_j \hat{x}_j^k, \sum_j w_j \hat{y}_j^k, \sum_j w_j)^T$.

After computing $\tilde{\mathbf{H}}$ and $\tilde{\mathbf{g}}$ we compute $\tilde{\mathbf{T}}^{k+1}$ using equation $\tilde{\mathbf{T}}^{k+1} = -\tilde{\mathbf{H}}^{-1}\tilde{\mathbf{g}}(\hat{\mathbf{T}}^k)$ and update the motion parameter vector $\hat{\mathbf{T}}^{k+1}$.

The modified Newton scheme described here has a larger region of convergence [7] and is computationally more efficient – since Hessian is precomputed – in comparision to the traditional Newton scheme. In addition, the spline-based representation of flow field possesses the property of built-in smoothness. All of these features make our algorithm both robust and efficient.

## 4  Implementation Results

We tested our algorithm with the various types of motions and the error is reported as the relative error between optimum motion vector $\mathbf{T}_{opt}$ and the computed motion vector $\hat{\mathbf{T}}$: $error = \|\hat{\mathbf{T}} - \mathbf{T}_{opt}\|_2 / \|\mathbf{T}_{opt}\|_2$. We always use the zero vector as the initial guess to start the iterations.

First experiment involves 2d motion rests. We applied a known 2D affine motion to a slice of size $(256, 256)$ from the MR brain scan to generate a transformed data set. We then used these two data sets as input to the motion estimation algorithm. Table 1 summarizes the motion estimation results for different 2D affine motions. The computed motion results are shown for three different methods namely, the Lavenberg-Marquardt (LM) method used in [9] for minimization of the SSD error, the modified Newton method of Burkhardt [7] for minimizing the expectation of the measure error and our method. Note that our method outperforms the other two methods and is able handle large scaling fairly accurately. Our algorithm takes 19.54 seconds of CPU time on an Ultrasparc-1 to achieve the registration for the affine motion shown in the last row of the table 1. Table 2 summarizes results of comparison between the LM, Burkhard's method

| True Motion | Error from LM | Error from Burkhardt's | Error from ours |
|---|---|---|---|
| (1.5,0,0,0,1.5,0) | 3.114% | 19.54% | 1.16% |
| (2.5,0,0,0,2.5,0) | diverge | 1.45% | 1.34% |
| (0.8,0,0,0,0.8,0) | 26.32 % | 0.75% | 0.88% |
| (0.6,0,0,0,0.6,0) | diverge | diverge | 4.25% |
| (1.128,-0.410,2,0.410,1.128,4) | 0.69% | 0.25% | 0.27% |
| (1.449,-0.388,2,0.388,1.449,4) | 1.109% | 16.58% | 0.54% |

**Table 1.** Comparison of computed motion for the 2D affine motion model

and our method embeded in a Quasi-Newton scheme for the 3D affine motion applied to a volume data set namely, an MR brain scan of size $(128, 128, 35)$. The true motion column contains angle of rotation about a prespecified arbitrary axis(ten degrees to the Z-axis), with uniform scaling in (x,y,z) and a 3D translation. All the methods were initialized with zero intial guess and as seen from the table, our method outperforms the others. The LM method here refers to a 3D version of the scheme described in [9]. Figure 1 depicts results of applying our

| True Motion | Error from LM | Error from Burkhardt's | Error from our method |
|---|---|---|---|
| $(20°, 1.2, 2, 2, 2)$ | 4.12% | 12.3% | 0.56% |
| $(30°, 1.2, 2, 2, 2)$ | 2.87% | 13.3% | 0.51% |
| $(40°, 1.2, 2, 2, 2)$ | 91.5% | 21.5% | 2.47% |

**Table 2.** 3D affine motion: Accuracy comparasions

algorithm in 3D to register two MR brain scans of the same person. These two data sets were of size $(256, 256, 122)$ and $(256, 256, 124)$, respectively. We applied our algorithm to the raw 3D data, computed the motion using 8 control points in the $(u, v, w)$ representation,and then applied the inverse of the computed transformation to the second data set. For visualization purposes, heads from the two data sets were extracted and superimposed. The registration appears to be visually quite accurate. The evident misregistration could be attributed to the error in the head extraction process. The global registration results can be input to the local flow estimator to refine the registration as needed which however was not done in this example. Our algorithm takes and $16mins$. CPU time – on an Ultra-Sparc-1 – to register two $(256, 256, 122)$ MR brain scans.

## 5 Conclusion

In this paper, we presented a novel image/volume registration algorithm that can handle large motions and is computationally efficient. The algorithm proceeds

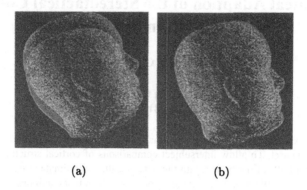

(a)          (b)

**Fig. 1.** Experiment on real 3D data,(a) before and (b) after registration.

to first globally register the data sets and then refines the registration locally if necessary. The effectiveness of the registration was measured quantitatively and the percentage error achieved by using our algorithm was compared with competing methods [9, 7]. it was shown that our algorithm outperforms the competing methods in robustness. Our future efforts will be focussed on further reducing the computational effort for the 3D registration.

## References

1. A. Black et al. "On the unification of line processes, outlier rejection and robust statistics with applications in early vision,". *Intern. J. Comput. Vision*, Vol.19:57–91, 1996.
2. C. A. Pellizari et. al. "Accurate three-dimensional registration of CT, PET and MR images of the brain". *J. Comput. Assist. Tomogr.*, 13(1):20–26, 1989.
3. G.E.Christensen et. al. "Individualizing neuroanatomical atlases using a massively parallel computer". *IEEE Computer*, 29(1):32–38, January 1996.
4. J.H.Duncan et. al. "On the detection of motion and the computation of optical flow". *IEEE Trans. Patt. Anal. Mach. Intell.*, PAMI-14(3):346–352, March. 1992.
5. L.Collins et. al. "Warping of computerized 3D atlas to match brain image volumes for quantitative neuroanatomical and functional analysis". In *Proc. SPIE Medical Imaging V*, volume (1445), pages 236–246, 1991.
6. W. M. Wells III et. al. "Multi-model volume registration by maximization of mutual information ". *Medical Image Analysis*, 1(1):35–51, March 1996.
7. H.Burkhardt and N.Diehl. "Simultaneous Estimation of Rotation and Translation in Image Sequences". *Proc. of the European Signal Processing Congerence*, pages 821–824, 1986.
8. J.Feldmar and N.Ayache. "Locally Affine Registration of Free-form Surfaces ". In *it Proc. of IEEE CVPR*, pages p496–501, 1994.
9. R. Szeliski and J. Coughlan. "Hierarchical spline-based image registration". In *IEEE Conf. Comput. Vision Patt. Recog.*, pages 194–201, Seattle, 1994.
10. J-P Thirion. "Extremal Points: definition and application to 3D registration". In *Proc. of IEEE CVPR*, pages 587–592, June 1994.

# Automatical Adaption of the Stereotactical Coordinate System in Brain MRI Datasets

F. Kruggel, G. Lohmann

Max-Planck-Institute of Cognitive Neuroscience
Inselstrasse 22-26, 04103 Leipzig, Germany

**Abstract:** Neuroanatomical and neurofunctional studies are often referenced to a high resolution MR brain dataset. To allow intersubject comparisons of cortical structures, one needs to remove the outer hulls of the brain, align the dataset with a coordinate system and introduce a spatial normalization. We describe an image processing chain that combines all these steps in a single, interaction-free procedure.

## 1 Introduction

The structural variability and complexity of the human brain has led to different attempts to define a common reference system in which an individual brain may be described. While today's most common approach was developed by Talairach 40 years ago [1], the high spatial resolution of recent neuroimaging techniques call for more precise methods of comparing individual brains. Most notably this has justified the foundation of a joint project to develop a computerized multimodal brain atlas, the "Human Brain Project" [2]. Common to all these approaches is the registration within a coordinate system and a method for the spatial normalization of the individual brain dataset. The "stereotactical coordinate system" has found the most widespread acceptance. It uses the anterior (AC) and posterior commissure (PC) as reference structures. Their midpoint defines the origin of a right-handed coordinate system. Much less agreement exists which method of spatial normalization will best serve the demands of the problem. First-order normalization methods like the system suggested by Talairach (the so-called Talairach space) have found widespread use [3,4]. Due to their limited accuracy, they will probably be superseded in the near future by second order methods like elastic or viscuous transformations [5] or symbolic atlases [6].

Today, high resolution MR brain datasets often serve as a reference system to which results of functional methods (like fMRI, PET, EEG or MEG) are mapped. They provide sufficient detail to allow the detection of AC and PC. In this article, we describe how a sequence of image processing steps and a few neuroanatomical heuristics work together to yield a stable procedure to detect these reference structures and adapt the stereotactical coordinate system automatically. In addition, this procedure can be comfortably combined with the removal of the non-brain parts ("brain peeling") in the dataset, which requires otherwise tedious manual work.

## 2 Details of the Procedure

For studying the individual brain anatomy as well as comparisions between brain structures of different subjects, it is advantageous to have a high resolution MR dataset, in which the non-brain parts are removed and which is aligned to a standard coordinate system. Such a dataset is stored in a "brain database" and available for further anatomical or functional studies. For the adaption, we need to (i) find and apply a binary mask to extract the brain, (ii) determine and apply an affine transform to align the brain with the coordinate system, and (iii) apply any method of spatial normalization. We cover only the analysis of single echo T1-weighted images, which commonly serve as a base for neuroanatomical analysis and are easily available on recent MR scanners within 15-30 minutes. In the context of this study, we also require that the MR scans of the head do not contain any pathologies. Most of the steps in this processing chain involve standard algorithms, so we simply refer to the literature for the algorithmic background. Only key processing steps and anatomical heuristics are discussed in more detail. Complete information is given in a technical report, which is available from the authors.

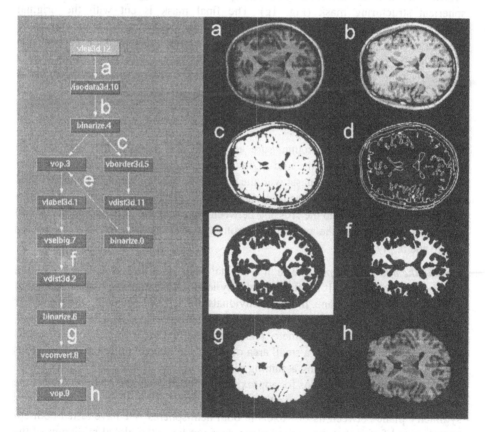

Fig. 1: Schematic overview over the peeling procedure and its intermediate results.

## 2.1 Brain Peeling

The first part of the processing chain will remove the non-brain parts in the MR tomogram, which is commonly referred to as "brain peeling". Our method is comparable to that of Brummer [7], who suggests a distance transform for the separation of the brain and its hulls. An overview of our chain and intermediate results are shown in Fig. 1. The dataset is preprocessed with a Lee filter to remove noise (Fig. 1a). A fast k-means algorithm segments the image into 5 classes, of which classes 2 and 3 typically contain grey matter, facial muscles, white matter, and connective tissue. Classes 2 and 3 are combined and binarized to form mask A (Fig. 1c). The set of border voxels is formed (Fig. 1d) and an Euclidean distance transform of this border image is computed (Fig. 1e). We threshold by a distance d1 to exclude all voxels too close to the border. We combine this image (binary 'and' operation) with mask A and select the largest connected component to form mask B (Fig. 1f). This mask is expanded by computing an Euclidean distance transform and thresholding with distance d2. We combine this image (binary 'and' operation) again with mask A. We fill the ventricles (which fall into class 1) by a morphological closing operation with a large spherical structuring mask (Fig. 1g). The final mask is cut with the original (unfiltered) image to extract the brain (Fig. 1h). This processing chain provides only two parameters, d1 and d2. The first distance specifies the separation between the brain and the outer hulls. Typical values range between 1.6mm and 3.0mm with a standard setting of 2.0mm. The distance d2 is used to enlarge the first mask and is usually set to 4.0mm.

## 2.2 Finding the Origin of the Coordinate System

The anterior and posterior commissure are small fiber bundles that connect both hemispheres and thus cross the mid-sagittal plane of the brain. To detect these fiber bundles and to register the dataset with the coordinate system, we need to perform the following steps: (i) determine the mid-sagittal plane, (ii) detect the anterior and posterior commissures, (iii) find the crossing between the plane and both commissures, (iv) compute the center and the axes, and (v) compute an affine transform for the peeled image and apply it.

*Finding the mid-sagittal plane.* The mid-sagittal plane is defined as a plane separating both brain hemispheres. It is often mistakenly identified as the interhemispheric cleft or the brain symmetry plane. In most individuals, the left hemisphere is slightly larger (especially in the posterior portions), so the interhemispheric cleft is bent to the right side. So the adoption of a "symmetry plane" is just a first order approximation. In this context, we are interested in a small area of this plane in the core brain and may thus introduce only a small error by assuming planarity.

One could think of two options for approximating the mid-sagittal plane: (i) detect the interhemispheric cleft by minimization of tissue voxels in a plane, (ii) determine a symmetry plane between tissue voxels in both hemispheres. We have tested both approaches and found that the desired plane does not lie in the global minimum of the parameter space. So we have to restrict the search space by introducing constraints.

An initial estimate for the mid-sagittal plane is determined most easily by segmenting the center of both eyes and defining a symmetry plane between them: For the detection of the vitrous body of the eyes, we select the class 1 voxels from the k-means classification in the brain peeling step. A morphological opening separates small bridges between the eyes and the skin. We label connected components and filter spherical objects of a certain size. If more than two components are found, we select the two most similar which are between 50 and 75 mm apart. The symmetry plane between both eyes is used as an estimate for the mid-sagittal plane. With this initialization we can restrict the rotation range to ± 5 degrees and the translation range to ± 10 mm. Then, we approximate the mid-sagittal plane by finding a symmetry plane between tissue voxels in both hemispheres. A Newtonian optimization scheme was found to be most stable here. This algorithm converges within 5-10 iterations and needs about 2 minutes computation time on a standard workstation.

*Detecting the anterior and posterior commissures.* The next and crucial step in the adaption of the stereotactical coordinate system is the detection of the two reference structures. Both commissures may be regarded as "shape bottlenecks". If we span a constant gradient field between both hemispheres, these bottlenecks are detectable in the steady state as regions of high flow [8]. Among other structures connecting both hemispheres, we find the anterior and posterior commissures as peak flow regions (Fig. 2). For a complete dataset this algorithm needs about 2h of computation time.

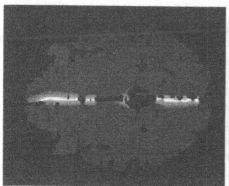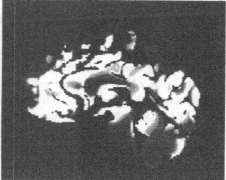

Fig. 2: Flow rate image computed from a binarized peeled dataset. Shown are an axial slice (left) in the AC-PC plane, and the mid-sagittal plane (right). One can easily detect AC and PC as flow maxima in this image.

To detect AC and PC only, it is advantageous to limit the search space to a small subvolume. We have tested several heuristics to define this subvolume. The center of mass in a peeled brain is found quite robustly in the area between the splenium of the corpus callosum, the habenula, and the adhesio interthalamica. On a line between the center of the eyes **CE** and the center of mass **CM**, the anterior commissure **AC** is found close to a point

(1) $\mathbf{a} = \mathbf{CE} + 0.7 * (\mathbf{CM\text{-}CE})$,

where an estimate for the posterior commissure **PC** is given by

(2) $\mathbf{p} = \mathbf{CM} - 0.1 * (\mathbf{CM\text{-}CE})_z$.

These heuristics were found to be valid in all available datasets with a deviation of less than 3mm. One can now limit the search space for **AC** and **PC** to a small subvolume of 50x50x30 voxels computed from **CM** and **CE**. The computation time of the flow algorithm on this grid is in the order of 2 minutes. We cut this flow rate image with the mid-sagittal plane and search for flow maxima using **a** and **p** as starting points. From these flow maxima, we adjust the coordinates to find the lower margin of AC and the upper margin of PC. We define the line passing through **AC** and **PC** as the x axis of the stereotactical coordinate system. The midpoint between **AC** and **PC** denotes the center. The y and z axis are found by introducing a right-handed system. We compute an affine transform to map the peeled brain image into this reference system which includes rescaling in 3D to form an isotropic resolution. We finally obtain a peeled brain dataset with isotropical resolution and registered to a standardized coordinate system. One should note that the steps to detect AC and PC are parameter-free and do not need any user interaction.

## 3 Implementation and Results

The image processing sequence outlined above was implemented and intregrated within the BRIAN environment [9]. The performance and robustness of this processing chain were tested with 26 high-resolution MR brain datasets, which were measured on 8 different MR scanners (Siemens Impact at 1.0 T, Siemens Vision at 1.5 T, Phillips Gyroscan at 1.5 T, GE Signa at 1.5 T, and Bruker at 3.0 T) at 5 different locations (see Acknowledgements). We used T1-weighted 3D sequences, including 3D GRE FLASH (16), SE FLASH (7), and MDEFT (3). Each dataset contained 128 sagittal (or axial) slices with an in-plane resolution between 0.86mm and 1.0mm and a plane-to-plane distance between 1.4mm and 1.5mm. All datasets were checked visually by an expert to exclude gross artifacts (motion, folding), developmental abnormalities, or the presence of pathologic structures.

In 17 of 23 cases (74%), this processing chain succeded on the first run. In the remaining 6 cases, the peeling was incomplete with parts of the neck still attached to brain structures. Raising the distance d1 from the default value of 2.0 mm to 2.5 mm resolved this problem in another 5 cases. A sufficient peeling was not achievable in one single case, where the left temporo-mesial cortex was attached to the meninges and thus was not separable. The higher the value of d1, the greater is the chance that portions of the cortical layer will be removed during peeling process. This will be noticable with values of d1 above 3.0 mm, so one should choose d1 to be small enough to warrant a successful peeling. In all successfully peeled cases (96%), the reference structures AC and PC were detected without problems and likewise a coordinate system adapted. To assess the quality of the procedure, we compared the position of the origin and orientation of the axes with reference alignments, which were manually generated. The deviation between the manually and automatically determined origin was 1.2mm (±0.4mm, range 0-2.5mm). The maximal rotational deviation before aligment were 4 degrees around x, 10 degrees around y and 8 degrees around z. After alignment, the deviation between the manually and automatically rotated axes were 0.8 degrees (±0.5 degrees, range 0-1.5 degrees).

## 4 Discussion

We have described an interaction-free procedure to remove the non-brain parts in an MR tomogram of the head and to adapt the stereotactical coordinate system. By adjusting only one parameter, we were able to segment 22 of 23 high resolution datasets measured on 8 different MR scanners within a few minutes. To our knowledge, no other algorithms to automatically detect the reference structures of the stereotactical coordinate system have been published so far. Minoshima et al. [10] have designed a two stage registration process that begins by identifying the interhemispheric cleft and then uses empirical rules to automatically locate four points along the AC-PC line. However, because this procedure was designed for PET experiments, these rules are dependent on the tracer distribution applied. Collins et al [4] use a multiscale cross-correlation for the registration of a sample dataset with an averaged MR brain volume that has been aligned with the Talairach space. They do not detect the reference structures directly and are thus dependent on a succesful registration with their model. The primary research focus of our institute is the study of cortical activity in the human brain. Our evaluations are based on a precise anatomical analysis of an *individual* brain. The first step in this analysis is the removal of the outer hulls of the brain and the alignment within a reference system. The procedure described in this paper performs this step automatically and with a high degree of accuracy.

# References

1. J. Talairach, M. David, P. Tournoux, H. Corredor, T. Ksasina: Atlas d'anatomie stereotactique des noyaux gris centraux. Masson Paris 1957.
2. J.C. Mazziotta, A.W. Toga, A. Evans, P. Fox, J. Lancaster: A probabilistic atlas of the human brain: theory and rationale for its development. Neuroimage 2, p. 89-101 (1995).
3. K. Friston: Statistical parametric mapping. in: Functional Neuroimaging: Technical Foundations, p. 79-91, Academic Press, Orlando 1995.
4. D.L. Collins, P. Neelin, T.M. Peters, A.C. Evans: Automatic 3D intersubject registration of MR volumetric data in standardized Talairach space. Journal of Computer Assisted Tomography 18 (2), p. 192-205 (1994).
5. P. Thompson, A.W. Toga: A surface-based technique for warping three-dimensional images of the brain. IEEE Transactions on Medical Imaging, 15 (4), p. 402-471 (1996).
6. F. Kruggel. Automatical adaption of anatomical masks to the neocortex. in: Computer Vision, Virtual Reality and Robotics in Medicine, Lecture Notes in Computer Science Vol. 905, p. 231-236, Springer 1995.
7. M.E. Brummer, R.M. Mersereau, R.L. Eisner, R.R.J Lewine: Automatic detection of brain contours in MRI data sets. IEEE Transactions on Medical Imaging 12 (2), p. 153-166 (1993).
8. J.F. Mangin, J. Regis, V. Frouin: Shape bottlenecks and conservative flow systems. in: Mathematical Methods in Biomedical Image Analysis, IEEE Press Washington, p. 319-328 (1996).
9. F. Kruggel, G. Lohmann: BRIAN (Brain Image Analysis) - A toolkit for the analysis of multimodal brain datasets. in: Computer Assisted Radiology, Elsevier Science BV p. 323-328, 1996.
10. S. Minoshima: Automated detection of the intercommisural (AC-PC) line for stereotactic localization of functional brain images. Journal of Nuclear Medicine 34, p. 322-329 (1993).

# Design of a Statistical Model of Brain Shape *

Lionel Le Briquer and James. C. Gee

GRASP Laboratory, University of Pennsylvania, Philadelphia, PA 19104, USA

**Abstract.** This paper describes a statistical shape model of the brain extending through the whole organ. The variability in a normal population is described by global deformation modes. The model is based on the analysis of homologous deformations mapping similar structures in brain images.

## 1 Introduction

Large variations exist across individuals in the morphology of the brain. Clinical diagnosis of diseases affecting the shape require the evaluation of the deviation from the normal anatomy. The large range of shape variations in a normal population (geometrical and topological) makes difficult the task of discriminating what is normal from what is pathological. To better address this problem, a shape model of normal variations must be identified. Although some shape variations can be explained by a mechanical model [1], a reliable model can only be inferred from a statistical study since the variations have morphogenic origins as well.

The morphometry is concerned with the study and classification of individuals based on a multivariate analysis of shape measurements. Its practical implementation for the brain is problematic: due to its geometrical complexity and its large variability among different individuals we need a number of shape measurements far too large to be collectable by a manual procedure. As an alternative, shape measurements can be derived from automatically computed homologous deformations, mapping similar structures in two individual studies. They provide a large amount of shape measurements making it possible to design a statistical model of brain shape. The deformation fields of a common reference to a set of individual studies are the shape measurements from which our statistical model is computed. The weak point about homologous mappings is that they only map corresponding structures and fail to capture the changes due to topological discrepancies (e.g. different sulcal patterns). Thus a morphometric analysis only partially describes the shape changes. This is illustrated in Figure 1: the deformation fields describe the variability of the deformed versions of the reference (second or third row) rather than the true variability (first row). An unresolved issue concerns the choice of the reference. As can be seen in Figure 1, different choices of the reference yield different interpretations of the individual images. What is not clear in Figure 1 is how much this choice affects

---

* This work was supported by the U.S.P.H.S. under grant 1-R01-NS-33662-01A1.

the measurement of shape variability: are the shape variations modeled by the first reference (second row) different from the ones modeled by the second reference (third row). This point is crucial, since the ability of any individual image to model the brain shape of other individuals is the basis not only of the work introduced here but also of all the applications in which the analysis is based on inter-subjects images comparison. Section 5 addresses this point and compares the shape models obtained using two different brain references.

## 2  Background

Thompson *et al* [9] developed an approach to quantify the variability of sulcal surfaces. Evans *et al* [3] constructed a probabilistic atlas by averaging 305 brain in a stereotactic space. The variability is illustrated by the sharpness of the grey level contours, but the method does not provide suitable information to derive a shape model. Both methods are local and disregards the global nature of the shape variations. Hill *et al* [6] performs a multivariate analysis on shape measurements derived from manually collected homologous points. Only objects having simple shapes and limited variations can be accounted. Therefore, the method is not applicable to modeling the whole brain. Martin *et al* [8] presents a variant where shapes are described as surfaces. Our shape model differs from previous global models in that it is volumetric and is intended to describe the whole brain (not only substructures). It differs from previous volumetric models in that the shape variations are described as whole organ (spatially correlated) deformations.

## 3  Matching of MR images

The matching problem consists in estimating the deformation $\delta$ defined on the continuous domain of the reference image ($\delta(x), \forall x \in \Omega$) maximizing the posterior distribution $p(\delta|d)$ where $d$ represents the data derived from the images. Using the Bayes rule, the matching process is ruled by the distribution $p(\delta)p(d|\delta)$. $p(d|\delta)$ is the likelihood and is derived from a normalized cross-correlation similarity function). $p(\delta)$ is the prior distribution. In these experiments it is a first order regularization, but as shown in [2], the prior can be inferred from the current statistical model of brain shape. The numerical approach for solving the matching problem is the finite element method (FEM) [5, 7] in which the deformation is sought in a space $\mathcal{H}_f$ of finite dimension. A set of basis polynomials (called shape functions) generate the space and any deformation $\delta$ of $\mathcal{H}_f$ can be expressed as

$$\delta = P_f \delta_f \in \mathcal{H}_f, \tag{1}$$

where $\delta_f$ is the FEM vector field of unknowns and $P_f$ interpolates these according to the shape functions. The full formulation of the method and its solution can be found in [4].

# 4    Method

We have a set of $k + 1$ MRI images of the brain, from which $k$ samples are used to measure the anatomical variability (Figure 1, first row). The $k$ datasets are globally aligned on the image that remains (reference). The homologous mappings from the reference to each of the individual studies are estimated. A statistical analysis of these provides is with a model of the brain shape. The mappings $(s(j), j = 1 \ldots k)$ are computed from the same FEM discretization, each has the FEM expression $s_f(j)$ (denoted in (1)). The FEM fields are too large to allow a direct computation of the variance matrix. They are therefore rewritten in basis of orthogonal FEM vectors:

$$s_f(j) = (v_{f,1} \ldots v_{f,n}) \begin{pmatrix} y_1(l) \\ \vdots \\ y_n(l) \end{pmatrix}, \qquad (2)$$

where $v_{f,j}$ is the $j^{th}$ FEM orthogonal basis vector and the coefficient vector $(y_1(l) \ldots y_n(l))$ is the expression of the deformation in this basis (see [2] for details). The mean deformation $\bar{y}_s(k)$ and its variance $w_s(k)$ are:

$$\bar{y}_s(k) = \frac{1}{k} \sum_{i=1}^{k} y(i), \qquad w_s(k) = \frac{1}{k} \sum_{i=1}^{k} y(i)y(i)^T - \bar{y}_s(k)\bar{y}_s(k)^T.$$

A principal components analysis (PCA) is performed on the variance. It determines the directions of maximum variation in the samples: the principal components (statistical deformation modes) which are the eigenvectors of the covariance matrix. The associated eigenvalues are the amount of variance in the direction of the corresponding eigenvectors. Let $\Lambda_m$ be the matrix of eigenvalues. The principal components $(e_{s,1} \ldots e_{s,n})$ are the columns of the matrix $E_{s,m}$ such that

$$w_s(k)E_{s,m} = \Lambda_m E_{s,m}.$$

The mean in the principal components space is $\bar{z}_m = E_{s,m}^T \bar{y}_s(k)$. The principal components are expressed in the cartesian space using equations (2) and (1)

$$E_m = (e_1 \ldots e_n) = P_f (v_{f,1} \ldots v_{f,n}) (e_{s,1} \ldots e_{s,n}).$$

Finally any deformation $\delta$ in the space of the deformations modes can be expressed as $\delta = E_m z_m$, where $z_m$ follows the Gaussian distribution

$$z_m \sim \mathcal{N}(\bar{z}_m, \Lambda_m). \qquad (3)$$

The statistical analysis of the homologous deformations provides us with the mean and the modes of principal variation along with their amplitude. When applied to the reference image, these yield the mean shape, the principal components of brain shape variation along with their amplitudes. Each of the deformation modes is separated from the others by the PCA and its effect on the brain shape can be visualized by applying it to the reference shape with a scaling coefficient in the range specified by the distribution (3). This emphasizes the spatial nature of the shape variations: we can see whether they are correlated or not, for different parts of the brain.

# 5 Experiments

Nine MRI exams ($0.937mm \times 0.9375mm$ pixel size; $5mm$ slice thickness) from normal subjects were used for this preliminary evaluation. The slices have been linearly interpolated to obtain datasets of size $224 \times 192 \times 160$ with square voxels. Two of them were picked to be the reference brains used to model the brain shape. The seven remaining individual studies were globally aligned to each reference so as to remove variations related to the head position during the data acquisition. The homologous mappings of the reference to each of them were then estimated. This yields for each reference seven individual measurements of brain shape (the deformed versions of the reference), from which we derive two statistical descriptions. The first and second principal components of brain shape are displayed in Figures 2 and 3. These indicate a globally smooth shape variation. It appears also that the next principal components have less smooth features, but since the covariance matrix was computed from only seven samples, these components are not reliably estimated so it is difficult to draw any additional conclusion about what is the morphological variability in this dataset.

Two models were trained using two different reference brains in order to assess the effect of a specific reference brain on modeling brain shape variability. A comparison of the first and second rows of Figure 2 shows that the model's first mode seems unaffected by the reference choice: the same variations in direction as well as magnitude are observed. A similar result can be seen in Figure 3 for the second deformation mode. To assess the resemblance of the shape models, a similarity measure for each pair of corresponding deformations modes is implemented: two deformation modes model the same shape variation if $i$) their variances are of the same order of magnitude and $ii$) their normalized cross-correlation is close to one (same direction). Table 1 summarizes the results for the six deformation modes of the two shape models. The results show that the two models broadly describe the same shape variations and thus are relatively alike. There is a limitation to this conclusion: the first deformation modes models the larger variations which correspond to the gross brain shape (i.e., the size and shape of the intra-cranial cavity). The homologous mappings can easily account for this kind of shape change and any individual brain can be used to model its effects. Therefore, it is not surprising that the two models are broadly identical. The choice of a specific reference could become more critical when it comes to the modeling of more localized structures. The current experiments cannot address this point not only because we do not have enough datasets, but also because the resolution of the MRI studies was low and it is likely that the fine cortical structures participated few to the homologous mappings estimation.

481

| Deformation Mode | 1 | 2 | 3 | 4 | 5 | 6 |
|---|---|---|---|---|---|---|
| Variance Reference 1 | 1887 | 948 | 624 | 348 | 177 | 153 |
| Variance Reference 2 | 2212 | 880 | 616 | 368 | 177 | 172 |
| Cross-correlation | | 0.88 | 0.70 | 0.73 | 0.69 | 0.70 | 0.58 |

Table 1. Comparison of deformation modes from two references.


# 6 Conclusion

The statistical shape model of the brain described here extends through the whole organ. It is constructed by principal components analysis of homologous mappings. The underlying assumption to its construction is that an individual anatomical image can model the morphometric variations observed in other individual images. It has been shown that to some extent (the gross brain shape) this assumption is valid. If performed from a larger set, the PCA would allow us to gain more insight into the nature of the shape deformations, as for instance, whether they are localized or imply whole brain variations, or whether some principal components affect the whole brain shape and some others only local structures. We need many more individual MRI studies with a highest resolution to validate the hypothesis that a specific brain can model the fine brain shape variations of a normal population. Future works will focus on the construction and validation of the model from more brain images.


# References

1. R. Bajcsy and S. Kovacic. Multiresolution elastic matching. In *Computer Vision, Graphics, Image Processing*, volume 46, pages 1–21, 1989.
2. L. Le Briquer. Statistical model of brain shape. Technical report, GRASP Laboratory, University of Pennsylvania, Philadelphia, 1997.
3. A. Evans, D. L. Collins, and C. J. Holmes. *Human Brain: the methods*, chapter Computational Approaches to Quantifying Human Neuroanatomical Variability, pages 343–361. Academic Press, 1996.
4. J. C. Gee. *Probabilistic matching of deformed images*. Ph.D. Thesis, Department of Computer and Information Science, University of Pennsylvania, Philadelphia, 1996.
5. W. Hackbusch. *Multi-Grid Methods and Applications*. Springer-Verlag, 1985.
6. A. Hill, A. Thornham, and C.J. Taylor. Model-based interpretation of 3d medical images. In 4th *British Machine Vision Conference*, pages 339–348, 1993.
7. T. J. R. Hugues. *The Finite Element Method*. Prentice-Hall INC, 1987.
8. J. Martin, A. Pentland, S. Sclaroff, and Ron Kikinis. Characterization of neuropathological shape deformations. Technical report, M.I.T. Media Laboratory Perceptual Computing, 1995.
9. P.M. Thompson, C. Schwartz, and A.W. Toga. High-resolution random mesh algorithms for creating a probabilistic 3d surface atlas of the human brain. *Neuroimage*, 1996.

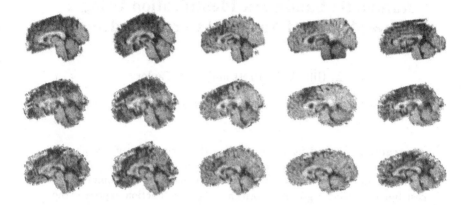

**Fig. 1.** Real and measured brain shape variability, sagittal view. First row, MRI brain volumes from different subjects. Second row, some reference brain volume deformed to match each of the individual brain volumes. Third row, second a different reference brain volume deformed to match the same individual images.

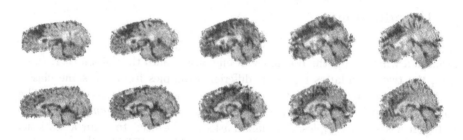

**Fig. 2.** First principal component of the brain shape, sagittal view (deformation mode corresponding to the largest variance in the samples). First row, Brain shape model derived from the first reference image. Second row, Brain shape model from the second reference image.

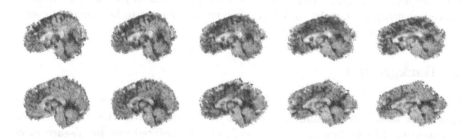

**Fig. 3.** Second principal component of the brain shape, sagittal view (deformation mode corresponding to the second largest variance in the samples). First row, Brain shape model derived from the first reference image. Second row, Brain shape model from the second reference image.

# Automatic Landmark Identification Using a New Method of Non-rigid Correspondence

A. Hill, A. D. Brett and C. J. Taylor

Department of Medical Biophysics, University of Manchester, Manchester, UK

**Abstract.** A method for corresponding the boundaries of two shapes is presented. The algorithm locates a matching pair of sparse polygonal approximations, one for each of a pair of boundaries, by minimising a cost function using a greedy algorithm. The cost function expresses the dissimilarity in both the shape and representation error (with respect to the defining boundary) of the sparse polygons. Results are presented for three classes of shape which exhibit various types of non-rigid deformation. The algorithm is also applied to an automatic landmark identification task for the construction of statistical shape models.

## 1 Introduction

A frequently encountered problem in computer vision is that of finding the transformation which maps the boundary of one object onto that of another. In our case, the two boundaries represent different examples from the same class of object (e.g. two hands) and the mapping is a non-rigid transformation. The application which motivates our work is that of generating *landmarks* automatically on a set of examples. The landmarks can be used to train a statistical flexible template known as a Point Distribution Model (PDM) [3].

In a previous publication [5] we described a framework for automatically generating landmarks for a training set of shapes. The algorithm generated a binary tree of merged pairs of shapes by pair-wise correspondence. The correspondence method we described was based on matching the curvature of the two boundaries using Dynamic Programming (DP). This DP approach to pair-wise correspondence has not proven to be sufficiently robust or accurate to be generally useful and does not extend easily to 3D.

## 2 Background

Kambhamettu and Goldgof [6] and Cohen *et al* [2] propose methods of correspondence based on the minimisation of a cost function involving the difference in curvature of two boundaries (or surfaces). As pointed out by Tagare *et al* [10], curvature is a rigid invariant of shape and its applicability to non-rigid correspondence is problematic.

The related methods of Shapiro and Brady [9] and Sclaroff and Pentland [8] describe methods of correspondence between two sets of points, the connectivity of which is not specified. The first of these methods is better suited to the determination of the correspondences arising from a *rigid* transformation of pointsets. Although the method of Sclaroff and Pentland [8] is proposed for non-rigid correspondence of pixellated boundaries, it has not proved sufficiently robust for our purposes.

## 3 Polygon-based Correspondence

In this section we describe a new correspondence algorithm which transforms a given pixellated boundary, $\mathbf{A} = \{A_i; 1 \leq i \leq n_A\}$, onto some other boundary, $\mathbf{B} = \{B_i; 1 \leq i \leq n_B\}$. The algorithm comprises three parts.

The first stage is the generation of sparse polygonal approximations to both $\mathbf{A}$ and $\mathbf{B}$, $\mathbf{A}''$ and $\mathbf{B}''$ respectively. No correspondences are established at this stage and the polygons will usually have a different number of sides i.e. $n_{\mathbf{A}''} \neq n_{\mathbf{B}''}$. To generate a sparse polygon, $\mathbf{A}''$, representing $\mathbf{A}$ we use the critical point detection (CPD) algorithm described by Zhu and Chirlian [11]. The result of applying this to various shapes is shown in Figure 1.

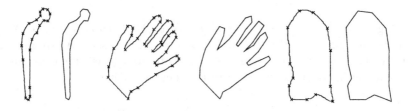

**Fig. 1.** Critical Points and Polygonal Approximations for Various Shapes

The second stage is to generate an initial estimate of the corresponding sparse polygons $\mathbf{A}'$ and $\mathbf{B}'$. The number of ordered pairs, $n_\Phi$, of corresponding points, $\Phi = \{\phi_i = (\alpha_i, \beta_i); 1 \leq i \leq n_\Phi\}$, is fixed at this stage, $n_\Phi = (n_{\mathbf{A}''} + n_{\mathbf{B}''})/2$. We use the assumption that $\mathbf{A}$ and $\mathbf{B}$ are similar shapes to predict that the spacing of the points $\mathbf{A}_{\alpha_i}$ with respect to the polygonal arc path-length of $\mathbf{A}$ will be similar to the spacing of the corresponding points $\mathbf{B}_{\beta_i}$ with respect to the polygonal arc path-length of $\mathbf{B}$. If two points on $\mathbf{A}'$, $\mathbf{A}_{\alpha_i}$ and $\mathbf{A}_{\alpha_{i+1}}$, are separated by 5% of the total path-length of $\mathbf{A}$, then we expect the corresponding points on $\mathbf{B}'$, $\mathbf{B}_{\beta_i}$ and $\mathbf{B}_{\beta_{i+1}}$, to be separated by 5% of the total path-length of $\mathbf{B}$. The polygonal arc path-length between two points $\mathbf{A}_i$, $\mathbf{A}_j$ is defined by $\sum_{k=i}^{j-1}\|\mathbf{A}_{k+1} - \mathbf{A}_k\|$. The path-matching correspondence algorithm exhaustively finds the pose transform which minimizes the sum of Euclidean distances between the sets of corresponding points, $\mathbf{A}_{\alpha_i}$ and $\mathbf{B}_{\beta_i}$.

In the third stage, the initial set of correspondences generated by the path-based correspondence algorithm is modified using an iterative local optimisation scheme in order to minimise a cost function of the form $E = \lambda E_S + (1-\lambda)E_R$. $E_S$ measures the difference in shape and $E_R$ the difference in *representation error* between the fixed polygon $\mathbf{A}'$ and its corresponding polygon $\mathbf{B}'$. The term $E_S$ is defined as:

$$E_S = \left( \frac{L(\mathbf{A'}) + L(\mathbf{B'})}{2n_\Phi} \right) \left( \frac{1}{n_\Phi} \sum_{i=1}^{n_\Phi} S(<\mathbf{A'}_{i-1}, \mathbf{A'}_i, \mathbf{A'}_{i+1}>, \\ <\mathbf{B'}_{i-1}, \mathbf{B'}_i, \mathbf{B'}_{i+1}>) \right) \tag{1}$$

where $L(\mathbf{A'}), L(\mathbf{B'})$ are the total polygonal arc path-lengths of the polygons $\mathbf{A'}$, $\mathbf{B'}$ respectively, the second term is illustrated in Figure 2.

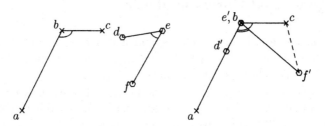

**Fig. 2.** Calculation of the local shape operator, $S(<\mathbf{a}, \mathbf{b}, \mathbf{c}>, <\mathbf{d}, \mathbf{e}, \mathbf{f}>)$. The triplet $<\mathbf{d}, \mathbf{e}, \mathbf{f}>$ is translated and rotated to $<\mathbf{d'}, \mathbf{e'}, \mathbf{f'}>$ so that $\mathbf{e'}$ and $\mathbf{b}$ are coincident and the directions $(\mathbf{b} - \mathbf{a})/\|\mathbf{b} - \mathbf{a}\|$ and $(\mathbf{e'} - \mathbf{d'})/\|\mathbf{e'} - \mathbf{d'}\|$ are equal. $S$ is then given by $2\|\mathbf{c} - \mathbf{f'}\|/(\|\mathbf{c} - \mathbf{b}\| + \|\mathbf{f} - \mathbf{e}\|)$.

It might well be possible to construct a $\mathbf{B'}$ on $\mathbf{B}$ which is similar to $\mathbf{A'}$ but which does not *represent* $\mathbf{B}$ in the same way that $\mathbf{A'}$ represents $\mathbf{A}$. We need also to ensure that the manner in which $\mathbf{A'}$ differs from $\mathbf{A}$ is as similar as possible to the manner in which $\mathbf{B'}$ differs from $\mathbf{B}$. Thus, we define:

$$E_R = \frac{2}{L(\mathbf{A'}) + L(\mathbf{B'})} \sum_{i=1}^{n_\Phi} R(\mathbf{A}, \alpha_i, \alpha_{i+1}, \mathbf{B}, \beta_i, \beta_{i+1}) \tag{2}$$

where $R$ is the local area difference operator for the corresponding polygonal segments $<\mathbf{A'}_i, \mathbf{A'}_{i+1}>$ and $<\mathbf{B'}_i, \mathbf{B'}_{i+1}>$. $R$ returns the absolute difference in the representation errors of $\mathbf{A}$ and $\mathbf{B}$ for the given segment $<i, i+1>$. The representation error is simply the area between the sparse polygon and its pixellated boundary.

The parameter $\lambda$ expresses the relative contribution of the two terms in the cost function. We have determined suitable values of $\lambda$ experimentally and found a range of 0.1–0.4 to be useful for real data. Note that both $E_S$ and $E_R$ are *local* operators, hence, we use a computationally efficient greedy descent algorithm for the optimisation of $E$.

## 4   Results

We present results for three classes of object – the right hand, the left ventricle of the heart and a hip prosthesis. Figure 3 shows the result of applying the polygon-based correspondence algorithm to pairs of shapes from each of these three classes. The value of $\lambda$ used to generate these and all the other results we present was 0.2.

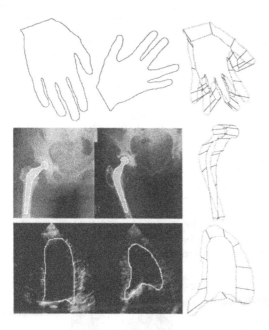

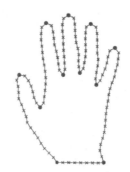

| | Landmark Error (Pixels) | |
|---|---|---|
| | $\sigma_{manual}$ | $\sigma_{auto}$ |
| Hand | 0.4 | 1.1 |
| Prosthesis | 0.5 | 1.3 |
| Heart | 0.9 | 2.7 |

**Fig. 4.** Manually Selected Major Landmarks, •, Equally-Spaced Minor Landmarks, ×, and Pixel Location Errors for Manual Landmark Identification, $\sigma_{manual}$, and Automatically Generated Landmarks, $\sigma_{auto}$.

**Fig. 3.** Polygon-based Correspondence Applied to Various Shapes. The first column represents shape **A**, the second **B** and the third shows the set of connections between the corresponding points of the sparse polygons.

Our goal is to identify a set of landmarks automatically on each of a set of examples in order to generate statistical shape models. Previously we have generated these landmarks manually by placing a small number of *major* landmarks on each example and generating *minor* landmarks equally-spaced between major landmarks. To investigate the accuracy of our correspondence algorithm for automatic landmarking, we have compared the position of landmarks placed manually (see Figure 4) with those generated using a binary tree of merged pairs of shapes, as described in [5], obtained using the polygon-based corresponder.

The values of $\sigma_{manual}$ and $\sigma_{auto}$ shown in Figure 4 represent the rms distance of manually-placed landmarks from their mean position (regarded as *ground truth*), and the rms distance of automatically generated landmarks from this ground truth, respectively. These results show that the errors (with respect to the ground truth landmarks) associated with generating the landmarks automatically are of the same order as the misplacement errors associated with identifying the landmarks manually.

In Figure 5 we present the results of building a PDM of the hand from both manually-placed and automatically generated landmarks. The figure shows the linearly independent modes of shape variation generated by a PCA of the landmark data [3]. Upon inspection, it is clear that these models are very similar.

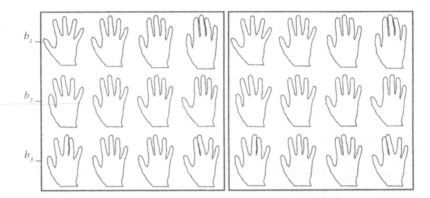

**Fig. 5.** Modes of Variation for the Hand Data. The modes are displayed by varying the shape parameters, $b_i$, of the PDM. The modes for the PDM built from the manual landmarks are shown on the left and from the automatic landmarks on the right.

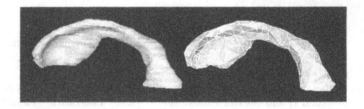

**Fig. 6.** Result of applying the decimation algorithm to the left lateral ventricle of the brain. On the left is the original dense triangulated surface with approximately 2000 points. On the right is the same surface decimated by 90%.

## 5 Extension to 3D

A major goal of our current research is to extend the correspondence algorithm presented in Section 3 for boundaries in 2D to surfaces in 3D. In our case a 3D surface is defined by a set of planar contours. A triangulated surface is generated from the contour data using the algorithm of Geiger [4].

For the initial decimation process in 3D we have used a modified version of the algorithm presented by Schroeder *et al* [7]. Rather than use a distance metric we have employed an estimate of the change in *volume* if the vertex were to be deleted. This is analogous to the CPD algorithm we have used in 2D in which the change in *area* is considered. A typical result for the decimation algorithm is shown in Figure 6. For the second phase of the algorithm we have used the iterative closest point (ICP) algorithm described by Besl and McKay [1]. The ICP algorithm is used to determine the Euclidean transformation required to map one pointset onto another without any initial correspondence information. The third stage of the algorithm shuffles the points defining the decimated surfaces over the original densely triangulated surfaces in order to bring the surfaces into better correspondence. This is an area of current research.

# 6   Conclusions

We have presented a novel method for the non-rigid correspondence of two closed, pixellated boundaries. No curvature estimation of either boundary is required and the algorithm requires only a single control parameter, $\lambda$, the value of which is not critical. We have presented results which demonstrate the ability of the algorithm to provide accurate, non-rigid correspondences.

We have also demonstrated that landmarks similar to those identified manually are produced when the polygon-based correspondence algorithm is employed as the method of pair-wise correspondence for automatic landmark generation. Extending the algorithm to multi-part objects and 3D surfaces are areas of current research.

# References

1. P. J. Besl and N. D. McKay. A method for registration of 3d shapes. *IEEE Transactions on Pattern Analysis and Machine Intelligence*, 14(2):239–256, 1992.
2. I. Cohen, N. Ayache, and P. Sulger. Tracking points on deformable objects using curvature information. In G. Sandini, editor, $2^{nd}$ *European Conference on Computer Vision, Santa Margherita Ligure, Italy*, pages 458–466. Springer-Verlag, May 1992.
3. T. F. Cootes, C. J. Taylor, D. H. Cooper, and J. Graham. Active shape models - their training and application. *Computer Vision and Image Understanding*, 61(1):38–59, Jan. 1995.
4. B. Geiger. Three-dimensional modeling of human organs and its application to diagnosis and surgical planning. Technical report no. 2105, Institut National de Recherche en Informatique et Automatique, Dec. 1993.
5. A. Hill and C. J. Taylor. Automatic landmark generation for point distribution models. In E. Hancock, editor, $5^{th}$ *British Machine Vison Conference, York, England*, pages 429–438. BMVA Press, Sept. 1994.
6. C. Kambhamettu and D. B. Goldgof. Point correspondence recovery in non-rigid motion. In *IEEE Conference on Computer Vision and Pattern Recognition*, pages 222–227, 1992.
7. W. J. Schroeder, J. A. Zarge, and W. E. Lorensen. Decimation of triangle meshes. *Computer Graphics*, 26(2):65–70, 1992.
8. S. Sclaroff and A. P. Pentland. Modal matching for correspondence and recognition. *IEEE Transactions on Pattern Analysis and Machine Intelligence*, 17(6):545–561, 1995.
9. L. S. Shapiro and J. M. Brady. A modal approach to feature-based correspondence. In P. Mowforth, editor, $2^{nd}$ *British Machine Vison Conference, Glasgow, Scotland*, pages 78–85. Springer-Verlag, Sept. 1991.
10. H. D. Tagare, D. O'Shea, and A. Rangarajan. A geometric criterion for shape-based non-rigid correspondence. In $5^{th}$ *International Conference on Computer Vision, MIT, Cambridge, Massachusetts*, pages 434–439, June 1995.
11. P. Zhu and P. M. Chirlian. On critical point detection of digital shapes. *IEEE Transactions on Pattern Analysis and Machine Intelligence*, 17(8):737–748, 1995.

# Non-rigid Curve Correspondence for Estimating Heart Motion

Hemant D. Tagare

Department of Diagnostic Radiology,
Department of Electrical Engineering,
Yale University, New Haven, CT 06520

**Abstract.** The boundaries of many biological objects are two-dimensional curves which evolve non-rigidly with time. This paper contains a theory and experiments for estimating motion of such curves using local shape. Beginning from first principles, a symmetric and explicitly non-rigid formulation is developed. The formulation uses the topology of correspondences and its associated geometry.

A numerical implementation of the resulting algorithm is also reported. The algorithm is used to estimate non-rigid motion of the endocardium in 21 MRI image sequences of normal and post-infarct dog hearts. Over 500 correspondences were computed. The measured average return error of the algorithm was less than 1 pixel.

## 1 Introduction

Accurate estimates of heart motion are believed to be a key factor in evaluating the health of the myocardium following a heart attack. One technique for estimating heart motion is to outline the endocardium in an image sequence and then track the outlined curves [1][2][4][6]. Motion is estimated by considering consecutive pairs of curves and establishing a non-rigid correspondence between their points such that "curved" and "flat" parts of the first curve are matched to corresponding "curved" and "flat" parts of subsequent curves. Figure 1 shows a typical example. Such non-rigid correspondences are said to be *shape-based*.

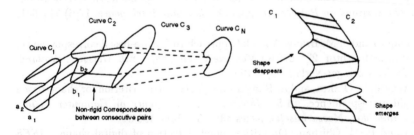

**Fig. 1.** Motion Estimation from Curves.  **Fig. 2.** A Symmetric Correspondence.

A new theory of shape-based non-rigid correspondence is proposed in this paper and a motion estimation algorithm is derived from the theory. The algorithm is used to track heart motion in MRI images of dog hearts.

Shape-based non-rigid correspondences are used in other applications as well [7] and it is useful to consider the problem more generally: Given a pair of curves, determine the set of all feasible correspondences (the search space). Then, select a criterion (the objective function) for evaluating how well any correspondence from the set aligns the shapes of the curves. Finally, design a numerical procedure to find the correspondence which best aligns the shapes according to the criterion.

For many problems, the search space and the objective functions are required to be symmetric. That is, they are required to remain the same if the labels of the two curves are switched. A further requirement is that the correspondence should model the emergence of new shape features and the disappearance of old shape features (fig. 2). Any such correspondence, when viewed in its entirety does not look like a function from one curve to another. However, locally the correspondence looks like a function from one curve to the other in some places and looks like a function from the second curve to the first in other places. A final requirement is that the differential geometry used in the shape comparison should be consistent with non-rigidity.

The author and his colleagues have recently formulated an approach to non-rigid correspondence that has all of these properties [7][9], and the aim of this paper is to present the theory and a new motion estimation algorithm based on it. Due to lack of space, proofs of various propositions and properties are omitted here.

## 2  Correspondences and Bi-morphisms

We begin from first principles, by defining a correspondence.

**Definition:** A *correspondence* between closed curves $C_1$ and $C_2$ is a subset of $C_1 \times C_2$ whose projections on $C_1$ and $C_2$ are onto. The *image* of a point $x$ under a correspondence is the set of points that $x$ is paired with.

Note that the product space $C_1 \times C_2$ comes equipped with natural projections. These are functions $p_1 : C_1 \times C_2 \to C_1$ and $p_2 : C_1 \times C_2 \to C_2$ which project an element of $C_1 \times C_2$ onto its first and second component, $p_1((x, y)) = x$ and $p_2((x, y)) = y$.

We can now proceed to define a particular type of correspondence, which we will call a *bi-morphism*. Recall from figure 2 that the sort of correspondence we want looks like a function from $C_1$ to $C_2$ in some places and like a function from $C_2$ to $C_1$ in other places. To make this intuition precise, we cover $C_1$ and $C_2$ with pairs of open sets $U_\alpha$ and $V_\alpha$ (fig. 3a) and require that the correspondence restricted to the subset $U_\alpha \times V_\alpha$ look like a function from one of the curves to the other.

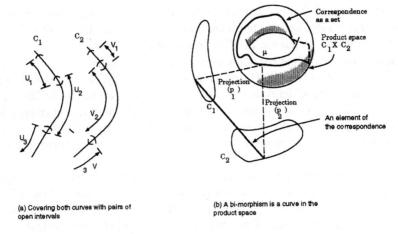

(a) Covering both curves with pairs of open intervals

(b) A bi-morphism is a curve in the product space

**Fig. 3.** Structure of a Bi-morphism.

**Definition:** Let $\alpha$ belong to some index set and let $U_\alpha$ and $V_\alpha$ be open sets covering $C_1$ and $C_2$ (fig. 3a ). Further, let $\Phi$ be a correspondence between $C_1$ and $C_2$. The correspondence is a *bi-morphism* if the following properties hold:

1. The image of every point in $U_\alpha$ is contained in $V_\alpha$ and vice versa (this simply means that the indexing convention for the $U$'s and $V$'s is consistent),
2. For each $\alpha$, the correspondence $\Phi$ restricted to $U_\alpha \times V_\alpha$ can be written either as

$$\{(x, \phi_\alpha(x))\} \text{ for some function } \phi_\alpha : U_\alpha \to V_\alpha, \text{ or as}$$
$$\{(\phi_\alpha(y), y)\} \qquad \text{for some function } \phi_\alpha : V_\alpha \to U_\alpha,$$

where, the function $\phi_\alpha$ is differentiable and non-decreasing with respect to arc-length (This implies that the image of every point under the correspondence is connected.).

Bi-morphisms have the desired symmetry property – any bi-morphism between $C_1$ and $C_2$ is also a bi-morphism between $C_2$ and $C_1$ and vice versa. Further, the set of all bi-morphisms is identical to a particular class of curves in $C_1 \times C_2$[1]:

**Theorem 1:** $\Phi$ is a bi-morphism between $C_1$ and $C_2$ if and only if $\Phi$ is a regular curve in $C_1 \times C_2$ such that its projections on $C_1$ and $C_2$ are onto and are non-decreasing with respect to arc-length.

By "its projections ..[are].. non-decreasing with respect to arc-length" we mean that as a point moves along the bi-morphism (which, according to theorem

---

[1] Reference [7] contains a slightly different, but equivalent theorem and proof.

1, is a curve in $C_1 \times C_2$), the arc-lengths of the projections of the point on $C_1$ and $C_2$ are non-decreasing.

Theorem 1 defines the topology of bi-morphisms and is illustrated in figure 3b. The product space of the two curves is a torus and is shown as one. Each element of a correspondence is an ordered pair $(x, y)$ and, hence, is a point on the torus. Theorem 1 guarantees us that the set of points corresponding to a bi-morphism is a regular curve on the torus. Figure 3b illustrates one such curve.

Since the bi-morphism is a regular curve we can parameterize it as $\mu(t)$, $\mu : [0, 1] \to C_1 \times C_2$. The arc-length $ds$ between the points $\mu(t)$ and $\mu(t + dt)$ can be defined as

$$ds = \sqrt{\mid p_1(\mu(t + dt) - \mu(t))) \mid^2 + \mid p_2(\mu(t + dt) - \mu(t))) \mid^2},$$

where, $\mid \mid$ is the Euclidean length of the projections.

The topological and metric structure of bi-morphisms give a simple geometry for non-rigid curve matching. Let $\mu(s)$ be an element of a bi-morphism $\Phi$ at arc length $s$ along $\Phi$ and let $p_1(\mu(s))$ and $p_2(\mu(s))$ be its projections on $C_1$ and $C_2$. Then, the angular orientations of the normals at these points are $\Theta_1(p_1(\mu(s)))$ and $\Theta_2(p_2(\mu(s)))$. The geometric criteria we propose is the following – since a bi-morphism is a curve, as $\mu$ moves along it, the derivatives of $\Theta_1(p_1(\mu(s)))$ and $\Theta_2(p_2(\mu(s)))$ with respect to the arc-length of $\Phi$ give the local shapes of $C_1$ and $C_2$ *as viewed from the bi-morphism*. The difference in the derivatives expresses the difference in local shapes. Integrating the square of this quantity gives an overall index $J(C_1, C_2; \Phi)$ of the dissimilarity of the shapes of $C_1$ and $C_2$ as viewed from $\Phi$. Thus,

$$J(C_1, C_2; \Phi) = \int_\Phi \left( \frac{d\Theta_1(p_1(\mu(s)))}{ds} - \frac{d\Theta_2(p_2(\mu(s)))}{ds} \right)^2 ds$$

$$+ \lambda \int_\Phi \left\{ \left( \frac{d^2 p_1(\mu(s))}{ds^2} \right)^2 + \left( \frac{d^2 p_2(\mu(s))}{ds^2} \right)^2 \right\}, \qquad (1)$$

where, we have added regularizing terms with $\lambda$ as the regularizing parameter.

The optimal bi-morphism between $C_1$ and $C_2$ is the one that minimizes $J()$ subject to the constraint that the projection of the bi-morphism on the curves has non-decreasing arc-length. It is easy to check that the above objective function is "symmetric" with respect to $C_1$ and $C_2$.

## 3    Numerical Algorithm and Experiments

For numerical implementation, the bi-morphism is approximated by piece-wise linear finite-elements. The optimization of $J()$ has two phases. The first phase obtains a discrete solution by minimizing $J()$ while restricting the knot points of the finite-element approximations to lie on a mesh on the torus. The minimum is obtained by dynamic programming. The second phase starts from this value and conducts a continuous descent minimizing $J()$.

During tracking, a sequence of curves $C_k$, $k = 1, N$ is available and the above algorithm is applied to each consecutive pairs of the curves $C_k, C_{k+1}$ in the sequence. The optimal bi-morphism between $C_k$ and $C_{k+1}$ shows how points of $C_k$ move onto points of $C_{k+1}$.

This algorithm was used to track the endocardium of dog hearts imaged in MRI. A total of 21 studies were available. The image plane just below the papillary muscle was chosen as the site to evaluate motion. This convention has been used by others [4]. In each study, starting from end-systole, four images (uniformly separated in time) were chosen from the sequence of 16 images. A B-spline active contour algorithm (snake) was used to interactively outline the endocardium. Figure 4 shows the images in one sequence with overlayed contours.

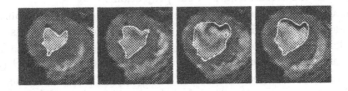

**Fig. 4.** MRI Images of a beating heart.

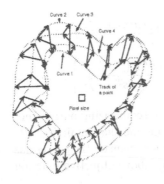

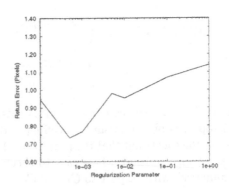

**Fig. 5.** Tracking the Endocardium.

**Fig. 6.** Return Error as a Function of Regularization.

Figure 5 shows the result of applying the algorithm to the contours of figure 4. The square in the center of the figure shows the size of single pixel. This is provided to visually evaluate the return error of the tracked points (the return error is discussed below).

With current technology, it is impossible to obtain ground truth about the motion of all points on the endocardium. In absence of ground truth, we use a performance measure called return error. Since heart motion is periodic, at the end of the period, each point should return to its initial location. Any error introduced by the algorithm would cause the point to return to a different location and the difference, which we call *return error*, measures how consistent the algorithm is under the presence of noise. The return is a function of the regularization parameter $\lambda$.

Figure 6 shows the average return error for all 21 image sequences as a function $\lambda$. There is a clear minimum at $\lambda = 0.005$ showing that it is the optimum value of $\lambda$. At the optimal value of $\lambda$, the return error is less than one pixel.

## 4 Conclusions

Starting from first principles, a non-rigid motion tracking algorithm was developed which tracks motion using local shape. By insisting on a completely symmetric formulation and by explicitly using a non-rigid formulation, the algorithm overcomes drawbacks of previous formulations.

Experimental evaluation of the algorithm over 21 sequences and over 500 bimorphisms shows that the algorithm performs well in tracking the endocardium.

## Acknowledgments

This research was supported by the grant 1WF181#94 from the Whitaker Foundation, and the grant 1-R01-LM05007 from the National Library of Medicine.

## References

1. Ayache N., Cohen I., Herlin I., "Medical Image Tracking," in *Active Vision*, ed. Blake A., Yuille A., M.I.T. Press, 1992.
2. Duncan J. S., Owen R. L., Staib L. II., Anandan P., "Measurement of Non-Rigid Motion Using Contour Shape Descriptors," Proc. CVPR, Maui, HI, 1991, 318-324.
3. Gold S., Lu C. P., Rangarajan A., et al., "New Algorithms for 2D and 3D Point Matching," Advances in Neural Inf. Proc. Sys., 7, 1995.
4. McEachen J. C., Duncan J. S., "A Constrained Analytic Solution for Tracking Non-rigid Motion of the Left Ventricle," IEEE 18th Annual Northeast Bioengineering Conf., Univ. of Rhode Island, March 1992, 137-138.
5. McEachen J. C., Duncan J. S., "Shape-based Tracking of Naturally Occurring Annuli in Image Sequences," CVPR, New York City, NY, 1993, 613-614.
6. Shi P., Robinson G., Duncan J. S., "Myocardial Motion and Function Assessment using 4D Images," Visualization in Biomedical Computing, 1994, 148-159.
7. Tagare H. D., O'Shea D., "The Topology and Geometry of Non-rigid Shape-based Correspondence," Technical Report, 95-3, Yale University, 1995.
8. Tagare H. D., O'Shea D., "Non-rigid Shape-based Correspondence: The Manifold Formulation," Technical Report (*Forthcoming*).
9. Tagare H. D., O'Shea D., Rangarajan A., "A Geometric Criterion for Shape-Based Non-Rigid Correspondence," *Intl. Conf. on Computer Vision*, Boston, 1995.

# Tracking of Tagged MR Images by
# Bayesian Analysis of a Network of Quads

Delman Lee, John T. Kent, and Kanti V. Mardia

Department of Statistics, University of Leeds, Leeds, LS2 9JT, U.K.

**Abstract.** Automatic tracking of tagged MR image sequences is done frame-by-frame. For each frame, a quadrilateral (quad) detector is run over the image to give a set of "potential quads". A likelihood function is specified for the detection of potential quads from an image. Quads are picked from the set of potential quads to form a "quilt". Quads are present where a grid structure is apparent in the image. A prior is specified to govern how the quads should be joined up to form the quilt. The prior for the quilt (i) encourages quads to be close to their positions predicted from the last frame, (ii) encourages neighbouring quads to be close to each other, (iii) discourages intersecting quads, (iv) avoids "tears" in the quilt, and (v) encourages connectedness of quads. With the likelihood and prior densities, a Bayesian analysis is carried out using the Markov Chain Monte Carlo method on the posterior density to give an estimate of the posterior mode.

## 1 Introduction

A non-invasive method for monitoring the deformation of the heart wall is by tagged Magnetic Resonance Imaging (MRI) [1]. A typical tagged MRI frame of the left ventricle (long-axis) is shown on the left of Fig. 1. The dark lines forming the grid are "tagged" to the material points (in planes perpendicular to the imaging plane), and as such follow the material points through time. In subsequent time frames, the contrast between the tagged and non-tagged materials decreases, and, furthermore, lines tagged to fluid material (e.g. blood) disappear. Tracking the grid through time provides deformation information that is useful for diagnosis of certain heart diseases. This paper addresses the issue of tracking the tagged grid through time.

Many past tracking techniques for tagged MRI images [2–5] follow the dark tagged lines through time with deformable splines. In this paper we investigate the dual problem of tracking the network of (approximate) quadrilaterals formed by the grid lines, rather than the lines themselves. *Quadrilateral* will hereafter be shortened to *quad*.

## 2 Principles of the Method

Tracking of tagged MR image sequences is done frame-by-frame. For each frame, a quad detector is run over the image to give a set of "potential quads". Quads are picked from the set of potential quads to form a "quilt". The quads in the quilt are connected by a square graph structure and can be either alive or dead. For a particular frame, live quads account for tagged materials, for example heart wall, that are visible, and dead quads

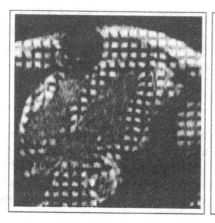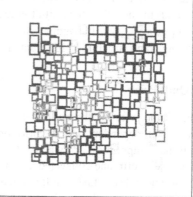

**Fig. 1.** The right picture shows the potential quads generated by the quad detector on the left image (the third frame of a sequence). The darker the potential quad, the higher the certainty.

account for tagged materials whose structure is no longer apparent, for example blood. A prior $f(x)$ is specified to govern how the quads should be joined up to form the quilt $x$ (§ 2.2). A likelihood function $f(y, \mu|x)$ is specified for the detection of potential quads $y$ (and some unobserved data $\mu$) from a quilt $x$ (§ 2.3).

A Bayesian strategy is used to infer about the quilt $x$ and the unobserved data $\mu$ from the observed data $y$. Information about the model and the unobserved data are contained in the posterior distribution given by $f(x, \mu|y) \propto f(y, \mu|x)f(x)$. Inference about the posterior density is done by sampling using the Markov Chain Monte Carlo (MCMC) method (§ 3) [6]. The MCMC method is chosen in favour of a deterministic method to avoid the solution being trapped in minor subsidiary modes of a "bumpy" posterior.

## 2.1 Notations

Let a quad be represented by $q_i = (c_i, v_i)$, where $c_i$ is the centre of the quad, and $v_i$ is the set of the four vertices of the quad. The centre of the quad $c_i$ is not strictly necessary, but it is kept in the representation for convenience. For each frame, the image is pre-processed by a quad detector to give a set of $P$ "potential quads" $\breve{q} = \{\breve{q}_p\}_{p=1}^P$, $\breve{q}_p = (\breve{c}_p, \breve{v}_p)$ and their "certainties" $e = \{e_p\}_{p=1}^P$. The certainty $0 < e_p < 1$ is a measure of how sure we are of the existence of the quad $\breve{q}_p$. Fig. 1 shows a sample output of the quad detector. The set of potential quads and their certainties $y = (\breve{q}, e)$ is our observed data.

Let $\mathcal{G}$ be an $n$-node undirected graph associated with a subset of a 2D square lattice. Nodes in the graph are indexed by $i = (i_1, i_2) \in \mathbb{Z}^2$, and are connected with 8-adjacency. The extent of the square lattice is specified by the user in the first frame. In subsequent frames, $\mathcal{G}$ is the output from processing of the previous frame.

Once $\mathcal{G}$ is specified at a time frame, the components of our model $x$ are (i) the maximum number of quads, $n$, that can make up a quilt, (ii) the positions and vertices of the quads, $q = \{q_i\}_{i \in \mathcal{G}}$, and (iii) the statuses, dead ($s_i = 0$) or alive ($s_i = 1$), of the quads, $s = \{s_i\}_{i \in \mathcal{G}}$. Two quads $q_i$ and $q_j$ are neighbours if the nodes $i$ and $j$ share an edge in the graph $\mathcal{G}$, and we write $i \sim j$ in such a case.

The set of live quads in $x$ forms the "fabric" of the quilt, while the set of dead quads corresponds to "holes" in the quilt. Let $\mathscr{L}$ denote the set of indices of the live quads in $x$, and $n_{\text{alive}}=\sum_{i\in\mathscr{G}} s_i$ the number of live quads. Thus the model $x=(q, s)$ (taking the underlying graph structure $\mathscr{G}$ for granted) defines a quilt in a certain region.

## 2.2 Quilt Prior

We model the prior for the quilt $x=(q, s)$ by $f(x)=f(q)f(s)$, where $q$ and $s$ are assumed to be independent. For the prior on the status, we assume an Ising model truncated to have support on $\mathscr{S}$, where $\mathscr{S}\subset\{0, 1\}^n$ is the set of configurations such that the live quads form one connected component. The truncated Ising model encourages neighbouring nodes to take similar values, discouraging a checkerboard pattern for $s$. We model the prior on the quads by

$$f(q) \propto \exp\left(-\frac{1}{2}\sum_{i\in\mathscr{G}}\Delta_i^T R_i\,\Delta_i\right) \times \exp\left(-\frac{1}{2}\sum_{i\sim j}\Delta_j^T S_{ij}\,\Delta_i\right) \times$$

$$\prod_{\substack{i\sim j,k \\ j\neq k}} \mathrm{I}\left[\cos(\psi_{jik} - \theta_{jik}) > \cos\phi\right] \times \exp\left(-\gamma \sum_{i,j\in\mathscr{G}} q_i \cap q_j\right) \tag{1}$$

with the following notations.

Based on information from previous frames, we have a set of $n$ predicted quad positions for the current frame $\hat{c}=\{\hat{c}_i\}_{i\in\mathscr{G}}$ and a set of $n$ $2\times2$ covariance matrices $\Sigma_i$ of the prediction error. Let $\Delta_i = c_i - \hat{c}_i$ be the deviation from the predicted position of the centre of the quad $i$. The first factor in (1) enforces our belief that the positions of the quads are not too far away from their predicted values, while the second factor in (1) encourages departures from predicted positions to be similar for neighbouring quads. The matrices $R_i$ and $S_{ij}$ are chosen such that the covariance matrix of the resultant quadratic form, when the first and second factors are combined, is positive definite.

Let $\psi_{jik}$ denote the angle formed by the three points $(c_j, c_i, c_k)$ with $c_i$ at the apex, and $\theta_{jik}$ be the predicted angle formed by the centres of the three quads $(q_j, q_i, q_k)$ with $q_i$ at the apex. Thus, with $\mathrm{I}\,[\cdot]$ denoting the indicator function, $\phi$ in the third factor of (1) is the allowed deviation from the expected angle $\theta_{jik}$. For an 8-adjacency graph, we chose $\phi=\pi/4$. The third factor in (1) aims to preserve the regularity of the quilt, avoiding tears.

Let $q_i\cap q_j$ denote the area of intersection of the interior of the two quads $q_i$ and $q_j$. With $\gamma>0$, the fourth factor in (1) penalizes against intersecting quads, and allows quads to be packed more closely in regions of small quads. This is the only factor in (1) which depends on the vertices of the quads.

## 2.3 Incomplete Data and Likelihood

Consider a hypothetical quad detector which takes a quilt $x$ as input and generates a list of $P$ potential quads $\check{q}$, their certainties $e$, and a mapping $\mu(\cdot)$. The function $\mu(\cdot)$, which maps $\mathscr{G}$ to $\{0, 1, \cdots, P\}$, describes which potential quad in $\check{q}$ corresponds to which model quad in $x$. Further $\mu(i)=0$ means that quad $i$ does not correspond to any potential quads in $\check{q}$. Let $z(\mu)$ be the number of zeros in $\{\mu(i)\}_{i \in \mathscr{G}}$. We assume that all live quads in $x$ are detected exactly once, i.e. the mapping from the set $\mathscr{L}=\{i : \mu(i) > 0\}$ to $\{1, \cdots, P\}$ is injective. The actual quad detector takes an image as input and generates the potential quads $\check{q}$ and their certainties $e$. The mapping $\mu$ is unobserved and represents missing data, while $y=(\check{q}, e)$ are the observed, incomplete data.

To specify the likelihood for $(y, \mu)$ given $x$, we need to answer the question: given a quilt $x$, what is the probability of the hypothetical quad detector generating potential quads $\check{q}$, certainties $e$, and mapping $\mu(\cdot)$? We model our likelihood function $f(y, \mu|x)$ as a product of three factors: $f(y, \mu|x) = f(\check{q}, e, \mu|x) = f(\check{q}|\mu, x)f(e|\mu, x)f(\mu|x)$, where $\check{q}$ and $e$ are assumed to be independent given $\mu$ and $x$.

Given the quilt $x$, we place a uniform weight on all permissible mappings $\mu$. Thus $f(\mu|x)$ is a discrete distribution with probability $(P - n_{\text{alive}})!/P!$ if $z(\mu) = P - n_{\text{alive}}$, and 0 otherwise. Given the quilt $x$ and the mapping $\mu$, the potential quad that corresponds to a live quad should have a certainty close to unity, and one that does not correspond to any live quads should have a certainty close to zero. We model these two cases with beta densities $e^2/3$ and $(1-e)^2/3$ for $0<e<1$, respectively. Assuming independence between the certainties of different potential quads, $f(e|\mu, x)$ is thus a product of $P$ independent beta densities.

Finally, given the quilt $x$ and the mapping $\mu$, the quad detector is assumed to detect all live quads in $x$ precisely, and gives out $P-n_{\text{alive}}$ artefactual potential quads. The artefactual potential quads are assumed to be uniformly distributed on the space of possible outputs of the quad detector. We denote the "volume" of such 8-dimensional space by $V$. We thus have $f(\check{q}|\mu, x) = V^{-z(\mu)} \prod_{i \in \mathscr{L}} I[\check{q}_{\mu(i)} = q_i]$ . Note that an artefactual potential quad $\check{q}_i$ has a probability density on $\mathbb{R}^8$ if $s_i=0$, and has a point mass if $s_i=1$.

## 3 Posterior Sampling

In order to gain information about the posterior, we used the MCMC method with a Metropolis-Hastings type algorithm that allows jumps between different dimensional spaces [7, 8]. The dimension changing aspect of our model comes from sites being alive or dead. Due to page limitations, only an outline of the algorithm is provided here.

At each MCMC iteration, the algorithm proposes one of four types of transitions: live-displacement, dead-displacement, birth and death. The live- and dead-displacement transitions displace the positions of a live and dead quad, respectively. The birth and death transitions toggle the statuses of a (feasible) dead and live quad, and propose a new position for them, respectively. The birth and death transitions are constrained so that the live quads in the quilt remain a single connected component.

The four types of transitions are proposed with equal probabilities. For each type of transition, a node $i$ is chosen randomly from the feasible nodes, and new values for the component $i$ of the quilt $(q_i, s_i)$ and for the component $i$ of the mapping $\mu(i)$ are proposed with a certain probability. The proposed values are then accepted with a certain acceptance probability. The proposal distributions and acceptance probabilities for the four types of transitions are carefully chosen to satisfy detailed balance so that the Markov chain has the desired stationary distribution.

Samples from the Markov chain are collected after a burn-in period. The posterior is summarized by its "restricted" marginal modes, arrived at by the following procedure. For a fixed node $i \in \mathcal{G}$, consider the histogram of the mapping $\mu$, $h_{\mu(i)}(p)$, whose entry is the frequency that the $p$th potential quad is picked by quad $i$ in the quilt during simulation. Picking a potential quad of 0 means that the quad is dead. For all the nodes that have been alive for more than a certain percentage of iterations of the chain (10% in our simulations), rescale the histogram $h_{\mu(i)}(p)$ to sum up to 1 for $p \neq 0$. We scan through the nodes according to the entropies of their rescaled histograms. Nodes with lower entropies are scanned first. For each scanned node $i$, the potential quad $\check{q}_p$ is picked, where $p$ is the mode of the rescaled histogram. Node $i$ is then born if $\check{q}_p$ is not already associated with a live node. After scanning through all the nodes, the set of live quads which forms the largest single connected component is our estimate of the quilt for the current frame.

## 4 Results & Discussion

The successful tracking in a region of interest of an image sequence is shown in Fig. 2, where the nodes of the graph correspond to the centres of the quads. Four selected frames of a long-axis sequence are shown. The results are for a MCMC simulation with 300 sweeps, of which 100 are for burn-in. The tracking for the nine frames took 20mins and 5mins on an i486-133MHz and UltraSPARC-167MHz, respectively. Note the successful tracking in Fig. 2 where a noticeable proportion of the live quads dies through time.

The number of burn-in sweeps of the MCMC is arrived at by inspection. Many convergence diagnostics have been proposed recently (see e.g. [9]) and will be incorporated into the algorithm. Related to the rate of convergence is the mixing property of the Markov chain. Our current algorithm proposes single-node transitions. Transition that updates a block of nodes at a time should improve the mixing property of the chain.

Since there is no substantial inter-frame motion, the following approximations work satisfactorily: (i) the estimated positions of quads from the previous frame is used as the initial estimate in the current frame, and (ii) a quad detector that handles only mild deformation from a square. If the inter-frame motion becomes severe, more sophisticated motion prediction and quad detection will be necessary. The paper has focussed on the problem of tracking the tagged grid. The next step is to deduce the full 3D motion of the left ventricle accounting for "through-plane motion" (see e.g. [10]).

## References

1. L. Axel and L. Dougherty, "Heart wall motion: Improved method of spatial modulation of magnetization for MR imaging," *Radiology*, **172**:349–350, 1989.

Acknowledgment: The work is supported under the EPSRC Stochastic Modelling in Science and Technology programme. We would like to thank Liz Berry, Bill Crum, John Ridgway and U. Sivananthan for useful discussions and for providing us with the data set.

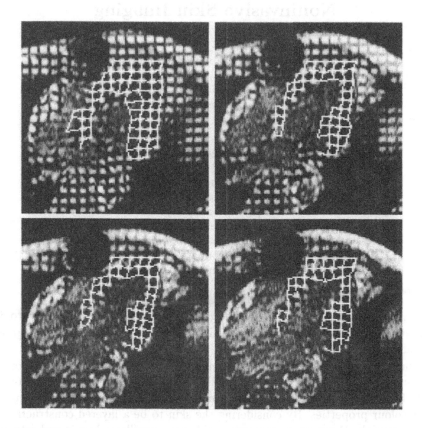

**Fig. 2.** The graph structure of the network of quads for four selected frames of a nine-frames long-axis sequence of the left ventricle. For clarity, only the 4-adjacent edges of the graph are drawn.

2. M. Guttman, J. Prince, and E. McVeigh, "Tag and contour detection in tagged MR images of the left ventricle," *IEEE Trans. Med. Imaging*, **13**:74–88, 1994.
3. S. Kumar and D. Goldgof, "Automatic tracking of SPAMM grid and the estimation of deformation parameters from cardiac MR images," *IEEE Trans. Med. Imaging*, **13**:122–132, 1994.
4. D. Kraitchman, A. Young, C. Chang, and L. Axel, "Semi-automatic tracking of myocardial motion in MR-tagged images," *IEEE Trans. Med. Imaging*, **14**:422–433, 1995.
5. P. Radeva, A. Amini, J. Huang, and E. Martí, "Deformable B-solids and implicit snakes for localization and tracking of SPAMM MRI-data," in *Proceedings of the IEEE Workshop on Mathematical Methods in Biomedical Image Analysis*, 192–201, June 1996.
6. J. Besag, P. Green, D. Higdon, and K. Mengersen, "Bayesian computation and stochastic systems," *Statistical Science*, **10**:3–66, 1995.
7. C. Geyer and J. Møller, "Simulation procedures and likelihood inference for spatial point processes," *Scandinavian J. of Statistics*, **21**:359–373, 1994.
8. P. Green, "Reversible jump Markov chain Monte-Carlo computation and Bayesian model determination," *Biometrika*, **82**:711–732, 1995.
9. M. Cowles and B. Carlin, "Markov chain Monte Carlo convergence diagnostics: A comparative review," *J. of the American Statistical Association*, **91**:883–904, 1996.
10. J. Park, D. Metaxas, and L. Axel, "Analysis of left ventricular wall motion based on volumetric deformable models and MRI-SPAMM," *Medical Image Analysis*, **1**:53–71, 1996.

# Noninvasive Skin Imaging

Symon Cotton[1], Ela Claridge[1], Per Hall[2]

[1] School of Computer Science, University Of Birmingham, B15 2TT, UK
[2] Consultant plastic surgeon, Addenbrooke's Hospital, Cambridge, UK

**Abstract.** An earlier model of colour formation within normal human skin was extended to include architectural distortions associated with various pigmented skin lesions, including malignant melanoma. The extended five-layer model makes it possible to derive parameters characterising the thickness and pigment composition of the skin layers from calibrated colour and infrared images of skin lesions. The extracted parameters can be used to reconstruct a full 3-dimensional model of the skin architecture which conveys information grossly comparable to that available through microscopical examination of biopsied skin tissue.

This work forms a part of research at the University of Birmingham into developing theories and techniques which aim to aid clinicians in the early diagnosis of malignant melanoma.

Our previous paper [2] presented a model of colour formation within normal human skin. The model is based on the Kubelka-Munk theory [5] of scattering and absorption within inhomogeneous materials and the physics pertaining to their colour properties. By considering the skin to be a layered construction of such materials, the stratum corneum, epidermis, papillary dermis and reticular dermis, and by exploiting the physics related to the optical interface between these layers, the model generates all possible colours occurring within normal human skin. In particular, the model predicts that all normal skin colours lie on a simple curved surface patch within a three-dimensional colour space bounded by two physiologically meaningful axes, one corresponding to the amount of melanin within the epidermis and the other to the amount of blood within the dermis.

The model postulated that abnormal skin conditions would cause the skin colours to deviate from the predicted surface in the colour space. This paper exploits this idea further. In particular, it demonstrates that it is possible to derive detailed information about the internal skin architecture and composition grossly comparable to information available through the microscopical examination of tumour tissue but without incurring the problems inherent in obtaining a biopsy. The central premise explored here is, therefore, that as abnormal skin often has a different internal architecture to normal skin it is a fair proposition that the coloration may not be bounded to this surface; if this is true, then the nature of the deviation may yield important information about the skin architecture.

To explore this the model presented in the previous paper was extended to predict the skin coloration associated with conditions where melanocytes penetrate into the dermis[3]. These are commonly seen in such conditions as the benign blue nevus and invasive skin cancer, such as melanomas, often leading to the blue hues characteristic with these conditions [1]. The "form" and depth of this invasion is an extremely important diagnostic factor in determining the nature of a skin lesion and, if abnormal, the relevant treatment and prognosis; currently the only reliable method of obtaining this information is by biopsy.

To account for the architectural distortion where dermal melanocytes occupy a region of the papillary dermis the model of normal skin needed to be extended to include additional layers. As can be seen from Figure 1, there are now five distinct layers which can be combined to construct an extended model: a layer within the upper papillary dermis containing no melanin; a layer within the upper papillary dermis containing melanin; a layer within the lower papillary dermis containing melanin; and a layer within the lower papillary dermis containing no melanin and finally the epidermis. The extended model [3] specifies how the magnitude of any colour primary depends on these model parameters thus allowing exploration of the coloration expected for various skin conditions.

A first such "computational experiment" modelled *in vitro* dermal tissue, that is bloodless skin with the epidermis removed. This analysis showed that the coloration "does indeed move off the surface corresponding to normal skin" in situations where melanocytes have penetrated the dermis. Further analysis led to the conclusion that "In principle, therefore, if presented with a section of *in vitro* dermis it should be possible to assess both the presence, concentration and position of melanocytes by an examination of the coloration" [3].

For such an approach to be useful when applied to living, *in vivo*, tissue it was necessary to include the effect of both melanin absorption within the epidermis and blood within the dermis. The result of this analysis showed that although the amount of blood could be quantified directly through an analysis of the remitted skin colour, when combined with dermal penetration of melanocytes, the amount of epidermal melanin could not. It was, however, possible to ascertain that "an amount" of dermal invasion had occurred, thus allowing areas of normal and abnormal skin to be segmented, but it was impossible to unravel the relative amounts of each.

To gain insight into the internal architecture therefore requires that either the amount of epidermal melanin, penetration of dermal melanocytes or the concentration of these melanocytes are known. If one of these parameters can be specified then it becomes possible to disentangle the other two from a measure of the coloration. Through further research it is hoped to be able to measure one of these parameters directly for every point within a lesion image. At present, however, the following approach has been adopted. First, the normal areas of skin are identified - that is areas with no dermal penetration of melanocytes - and within these areas the amount of epidermal melanin is ascertained; this is then followed by an interpolation of these surrounding melanin values into the abnormal areas. This approach assumes that the amount of epidermal melanin does not change by a significant amount within these areas or if it does it varies

---

[3] In normal skin melanocytes are restricted to the epidermis.

in a predictable manner thus allowing the variation to be modelled.

As described in [3] however it is necessary to ascertain one further parameter before such analysis can be undertaken. This parameter, the papillary dermal thickness, has a pronounced effect on the light remitted from a skin lesion. Indeed the change in coloration due to a variation in this parameter is almost identical to that due to melanocytic descent thus leading to lesions only varying in this parameter being wrongly classified. As an example it is possible to find malignant invasive melanomas with an identical coloration to that of simple warts.

This result casts doubt on the effectiveness of using purely colour information in the diagnosis of malignant melanoma and may offer itself as an explanation for the "moderate success achieved" by Umbaugh et al. [6] when they attempted to classify lesion types by an investigation of coloration. However, this is not to dismiss the usefulness of colour information when combined with other extracted lesion features such as that demonstrated by Dhawan and Sicsu [4] when they combined colour with a texture analysis; and Umbaugh et al. [7] when they applied artificial intelligence techniques to variations in lesion colour.

From the extended skin model the variation of remitted light with papillary dermal thickness can be ascertained. Therefore if this thickness were known for each image point it should be possible to calculate a transformation that adjusts the measured coloration to that of any specified papillary dermal thickness thus removing the metameric problems previously discussed.

The problem, therefore, is how can the papillary dermal thickness be measured noninvasively? In formulating a solution to this problem it is useful to recall that the amount of light remitted from the skin becomes highly dependent upon this factor as the wavelength increases [3]. When this is combined with the observation that both melanin and blood absorption drop significantly with increasing wavelength it seems it may be possible to find a wavelength range where the amount of remitted light depends largely on the papillary dermal thickness. This is never the case within the visible portion of the spectrum. However, it becomes plausible if the considered wavelength range is extended into the infrared. For instance, in the wavelength range 600–800 nm the absorption of melanin drops to around one tenth of its peak within the visible portion of the spectrum; the absorption of blood drops by around a factor of a hundred whilst the sensitivity of remitted light to variations in papillary dermal thickness increases. This difference becomes even more marked as longer wavelengths are considered; for example, the absorption of melanin drops by a further order of magnitude in the wavelength range 800–1000 nm. Indeed, within these wavelength ranges the thickness of the papillary dermis is the major parameter affecting skin coloration.

As these wavelength ranges are easily accessible with existing infrared film and infrared digital cameras it should be possible to use this information to provide the desired calibration. As an example of how this may be performed consider Figure 1 where the intensity of remitted light for *in vivo* skin between 600–800 nm is plotted against that measured between 800–1000 nm. As can be seen from this graph the amount of remitted light falls, with increasing melanin, faster for the 600–800 nm primary than for the 800–1000 nm primary. This is as one would expect; more interesting, however, is the significant variation in both primaries with papillary dermal thickness. This observation then allows construction of the lines of constant papillary dermal thickness as shown in the graph. A measurement of this thickness parameter can thus be recovered by obtaining images acquired within the given wavelength ranges and looking-up the corresponding papillary dermal thickness from the graph.

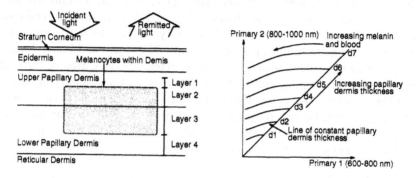

**Fig. 1.** Left: Extended skin model; Right: Variation of infrared primary intensities with epidermal melanin, blood, and papillary dermal thickness

The ideas outlined above give theoretical foundations for development of a noninvasive system capable of extracting information about the internal architecture of human skin. The complete process can be summarised as follows. Firstly, skin images are obtained using two infrared primaries and from these the thickness of the papillary dermal layer is computed across the image. This measurement is then used to "calibrate" the image so that the coloration for each image point is adjusted to that of a standard papillary dermal thickness[4]. Abnormal regions within the image can now be identified as they deviate, in a three dimensional colour space, from the surface of expected coloration for skin at this standard papillary dermal thickness. For those points identified as normal the amount of epidermal melanin can now be computed from the position, of their coloration, on this surface. By a process of interpolation, and possibly the use of a model, the amount of epidermal melanin within the abnormal regions is estimated. The points identified as abnormal can now be compared with those generated by the theoretical model for different concentrations and positions of melanocytes within the dermis as well as for differing amounts of dermal blood and these parameters quantified.

At the end of this process we now have information pertaining to the amount of epidermal melanin, dermal blood, thickness of the papillary dermis along with the concentration and position of dermal melanocytes for each point within the image. This can be presented using a number of methods ranging from simply reporting the maximum depth to which melanocytes have descended within the

---

[4] Even at this early stage, with the perturbing effect of variations in papillary dermal thickness removed, the calibrated images should prove useful to a clinician.

dermis to using the data to generate either a cross section, or a fully three dimensional representation, of the internal skin structure.

As a pre-cursor to a clinical trial the effectiveness of the system was assessed using computer generated phantoms of various skin lesions. Given knowledge of the internal structure of various skin conditions the appearance of the lesion was generated by the extended model producing both colour RGB images and infrared images. As examples of this consider the cross sectional representations, (b) and (f), of the two skin lesions shown in Figure 2. Within the left hand lesion, lesion A, there is no dermal invasion of melanocytes with the only architectural point of note being the thinned papillary dermis. The right hand lesion, lesion B, however represents a blue nevus with melanocytes, the dark area in the center of cross section (f), existing within the lower section of the papillary dermis. Although these lesions have markedly different internal architectures the observed coloration predicted by the extended model within the RGB colour space[5], (a) and (e), are very similar. It is this similarity which leads to problems when a diagnostic technique uses this coloration as its sole input.

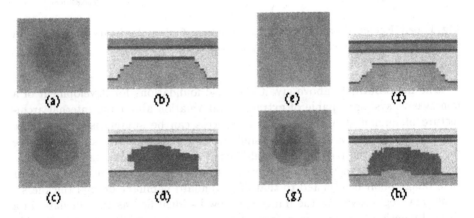

**Fig. 2.** Left: (a) RGB image of lesion A calculated from (b) internal structure input to system; (c) RGB image of lesion A calibrated to constant papillary thickness and (d) internal structure calculated by system; Right: (e) ... (h) the same for lesion B

After the infrared images are obtained the papillary dermis thickness can be ascertained for all points within the image. This then allows calibration of the lesion images to that of a standard papillary dermal thickness resulting in images (c) and (g) seen in Figure 2. As can be seen the appearance of lesion A has changed markedly which is as would be expected given that the major architectural feature within this lesion was a thinned papillary dermis. Given that the images are now calibrated to a standard papillary dermal thickness, processing can now proceed as described above resulting in measures for the parameters outlined earlier. These are shown within Figure 2 as cross sections

---

[5] These figures are black and white representations of the colour images.

(d) and (h) comparing favourably with the actual internal structure (b) and (f).

The work presented here outlines a noninvasive system allowing the investigation of internal skin architecture. It has been shown that provided with one standard colour and two infrared images, the developed system can recover a number of parameters characterising skin structure, including the amount of epidermal melanin, dermal blood, papillary dermal thickness along with the position and concentration of melanocytes within the dermis.

This work is of both theoretical and practical importance. The theoretical model of interaction of light with a multi-layer optical system, which is at the foundation of this work, can serve as a powerful simulation system for other medical applications. Moreover, the model can generate *explanations* and thus increase understanding of why skin diseases manifest themselves through particular appearances. Examples include malignant melanoma, port wine stains, naevi, wound healing etc. The practical importance of this work has two strands. Firstly, it gives clinical researchers a powerful and noninvasive tool with which to study skin diseases. At present dermatologists have a very limited choice of noninvasive tools with which to examine skin conditions and methods, such as biopsy, which are invasive and can sometimes adversely affect the outcome of the disease (as, for example, in malignant melanoma). Consequently, knowledge about the physical progress of the disease can be scant. Secondly, the system can be used as an aid in the diagnosis of skin diseases such as melanoma; the importance of this cannot be overstressed. A clinical trial is currently being undertaken at Addenbrooke's hospital in Cambridge where the predicted internal architecture generated by the system will be compared with the actual architecture found through biopsy.

# References

1. Anderson, R., Parrish, B. S., Parrish, J. A.: The Optics of Human Skin. The Journal of Investigative Dermatology **77(1)** (1081) 13–19
2. Cotton, S. D., Claridge, E.: Developing a Predictive Model of Human Skin Colouring. SPIE Proceedings Vol. 2708 Medical Imaging 1996: Physics of Medical Imaging (April 1996) 814–825
3. Cotton, S. D., Claridge, E.: A Noninvasive Skin Imaging System. Technical Report CSR-97-3. University of Birmingham School of Computer Science (1997)
4. Dhawan, A. P., Sicsu, A.: Segmentation of Images of Skin Lesions Using Color and Texture Information of Surface Pigmentation. Computerized Medical Imaging and Graphics **16(3)** (1992) 163–177
5. Egan, W. G., Hilgeman, T. W.: Optical Properties of Inhomogeneous Materials. Academic Press (1979)
6. Umbaugh, S. E., Moss, R. H., Stoecker, W. V.: Automatic Color Segmentation of Images with Application to Detection of Variegated Coloring in Skin Tumors. IEEE Engineering in Medicine and Biology Magazine (December 1989) 43–52
7. Umbaugh, S. E., Moss, R. H., Stoecker, W. V.: Applying Artificial Intelligence to the Identification of Variegated Coloring in Skin Tumors. IEEE Engineering in Medicine and Biology Magazine (December 1991) 57–62

# Modelling Interreflections in a System Based on the Differential Absorption of Light (DAL) for the Measurement of Range Images

Robert Wolfe and Denis Laurendeau

Computer Vision and Systems Laboratory, Université Laval, Québec (Québec)
CANADA, G1K 7P4 [wolfe, laurend]@gel.ulaval.ca

## 1 Introduction

Shape-from-shading methods have been developed for determining the shape of objects. However, interreflections between surface facets play an important role in the precision of the depth [4]. Most of the work concerning interreflections has concentrated on the direct problem: modeling interreflections for a given scene and source lighting. The solutions to this problem employ tools such as the hemi-cube [1]. Until recently, little work existed on the solution to the inverse problem in *computer vision*: the precise determination of shape in the presence of interreflected light. Nayar *et al* present a principle for separating surface light intensity into components due to direct source illumination and indirectly reflected light [4]. By applying the technique to photometric sampling with Lambertian surfaces, they succeeded in determining more precisely not only the shape of an unknown surface but the albedo of each surface facet or pixel.

In this work, interreflections are modelled by applying the Neumann series solution to the radiosity equation for Lambertian surfaces to the DAL technique [3]. Then, by applying Nayar's principle to the DAL technique, we develop an iterative refinement algorithm destined to improve the precision of depth images.

Working only with diffuse lighting and Lambertian surfaces of known constant albedo, the DAL technique does not need to know the location and luminance of source lighting [3].

This paper is divided as follows. Section 2 presents an introduction to the DAL system. In Section 3, we present system optical analysis and the interreflection kernel. In section 4, we develop a refinement algorithm destined to iteratively remove the component of interreflected light. Results and comparisons are presented. In section 5, conclusions are given.

## 2 The DAL system

The DAL method was originally developed for analyzing dental imprints in the framework of an expert orthodontics system [2]. The steps for the extraction of range are given in [3], only the final resuling equation is given here:

$$z = \frac{1}{a}ln\left(\frac{m\frac{dE_{\lambda_1}}{dE_{\lambda_2}} - c}{b}\right) = \frac{1}{a}ln\left(m\frac{dE_{\lambda_1}}{dE_{\lambda_2}} - c\right) + b' \tag{1}$$

The first indication that interreflected light plays a role in the interpretation of depth is indicated in the infrared image for which concave regions, especially at the bottom of individual tooth imprints, supercedes the maximum expected intensity of a flat surface oriented perpendicularly to the optic axis. Referring to (1), this leads to the theory, for a concave surface, that depth is systematically overestimated due to an exaggerated contribution of the infrared component.

## 3    System optical analysis

In Fig. 1 (A) we examine the absorption image (at $\lambda_1$) (the infrared image (at $\lambda_2$) is just

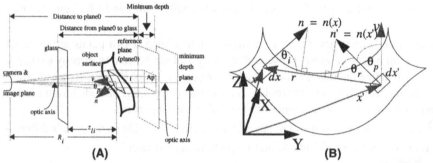

**Fig. 1 (A) Orthogonal projection of a facet i on the pixel i of the image plane in the DAL system (B) Concave surface in 3D Cartesian coordinates showing two surface elements.**

a special case of absorption (with $\alpha = 0$)). The area $A_p$ is the real surface area represented by a pixel of the image plane without accounting for the orientation of the represented facet. In the absorption case, the luminance $L_{(I,i)}$ of a pixel $i$ in the image plane due to the luminance $L_{(O,i)}$ of a surface facet $i$ projected orthogonally is given by:

$$L_{(I,i)} = L_{(O,i)} e^{-\alpha z_{li}} \tag{2}$$

where $z_{li}$ is the depth $z_l$ of the immersed facet $i$. The illuminance $dE_{(I,i)}$ received at pixel $i$ in the image plane is given by:

$$dE_{(I,i)} = \frac{L_{(I,i)} A \cos\theta_p}{R_i^2} = \frac{L_{(I,i)} A_p}{R_i^2} \tag{3}$$

where $A$ is the real facet area, $R_i$ is the distance from the image plane to the facet, $\theta_p$ is the angle between the facet normal $n$ and the camera direction $v$, and $A_p = A\cos\theta_p$. Combining (2) and (3), it is possible to express $dE_i$ in the following manner [5]:

$$dE_{(I,i)} = \frac{A_p e^{-\alpha z_{li}} L_{(O,i)}}{R_i^2} \tag{4}$$

In order to examine how the value of $L_{(O,i)}$ may be affected by interreflections, we borrow the concept of the interreflection kernel from Nayar [4]. To understand the role of the interreflection kernel, one considers two points on a concave surface as in Fig. 1 (B) where regions $dx$ and $dx'$ are infinitesimal surface elements. We would like to know the luminance $L(x)$ at point $x$ caused by the luminance $L(x')$ at point $x'$. This luminance is zero if the two points are not mutually visible. This is explicitly expressed in the following manner [4]:

$$Vue(x, x') = \frac{n \cdot (-r) + |n \cdot (-r)|}{2|n \cdot (-r)|} \cdot \frac{n' \cdot r + |n' \cdot r|}{2|n' \cdot r|} \tag{5}$$

Function $Vue$ is 0 for pairs of points that are not mutually visible and 1 for pairs that may be.

Surface orientation is not the only criterion in determining if two points are mutually visible. If an occlusion exists between them, they will not be able to directly exchange energy. We define the function $Occ$ which produces a value of 0 for each pair of points which are in occlusion and 1 otherwise. The fact that one point is occluded from another is, in general, a very complex function of global surface geometry.

For a Lambertian surface, the luminance $L(x)$ of point $x$ depends on the point's differential illumination $dE(x)$ and albedo $\rho(x)$ in the following manner:

$$L(x) = \frac{\rho(x)}{\pi} dE(x) \tag{6}$$

where $\frac{\rho(x)}{\pi}$ is the surface reflectivity coefficient and $\frac{1}{\pi}$ the bidirectional reflectance distribution function for a Lambertian surface. Applying the inverse square law and including exponential attenuation, the differential illuminance of the surface element $dx$ caused by the luminance $L(x')$ at $dx'$ is then expressed as:

$$dE(x) = \left[ \frac{[n \cdot (-r)] [n' \cdot r]}{[r \cdot r]^2} \right] e^{-\alpha r} Vue Occ L(x') dx' \tag{7}$$

Combining (6) with the visibility function $Occ$ we may write:

$$L(x) = \frac{\rho(x)}{\pi} \left[ \frac{[n \cdot (-r)] [n' \cdot r]}{[r \cdot r]^2} \right] e^{-\alpha r} Vue Occ L(x') dx' \tag{8}$$

The interreflection kernel is then defined as:

$$K(x, x') = \left[ \frac{[n \cdot (-r)] [n' \cdot r]}{[r \cdot r]^2} \right] e^{-\alpha r} Vue Occ \tag{9}$$

where $Vue$ and $Occ$ are still functions of $x$ and $x'$. For discrete elements (facets) resulting from surface sampling, the form of the interreflection kernel is given by:

$$K_{ij} = K(x_i, x_j) dx_j \tag{10}$$

where $x_i$ and $x_j$ are the centres of the facets associated with points $i$ and $j$ and $dx_j$ is the area of the facet associated with $x_j$. We denote $A_p$ as the area represented by the projection of the surface facet $dx_j$ onto a plane perpendicular to the optic axis. The real area represented by a pixel is then given by:

$$dx_j = \frac{A_p}{v \cdot n_j} = \frac{A_p}{\cos\theta_p} \tag{11}$$

where $v$ is the unit vector in the projection direction, $n_j$ is the associated unit surface normal at $x_j$ and $\theta_p$ the angle between these latter vectors. From (10) and (11), the discrete interreflection kernel may then be written as:

$$K_{ij} = \left[\frac{[n_i \cdot (-r_{ij})] \, [n_j \cdot r_{ij}]}{[r_{ij} \cdot r_{ij}]^2}\right]\left[\frac{A_p}{v \cdot n_j}\right]e^{-\alpha r_{ij}}VueOcc \tag{12}$$

where *Vue* and *Occ* both functions of $x_i$ and $x_j$ [4]. A sythentic image generator was designed to corroborate the presence of interreflections in DAL images. It is also used to furnish input images to confirm the validity of the depth refinement algorithm presented in Section 4. The description of this software package may be found in [5].

# 4 DAL depth refinement algorithm

Instead of considering the system of light-exchanging surface facets as tending towards an equilibrium (as in [4]), we consider that the system is already in a state of equilibrium and that an infinity of interreflections has already occurred. This is directly expressed in the radiosity equation for a Lambertian surface. All interreflections except the last are already *implicitly* treated while the last interreflection is *explicitly* treated. Applying a discrete version of the radiosity equation for a Lambertian surface to the case of a 3 facet surface with identical albedos, the luminance of the facets is given by:

$$L_1 = L_{1s} + \frac{\rho}{\pi}K_{12}L_2 + \frac{\rho}{\pi}K_{13}L_3$$

$$L_2 = L_{2s} + \frac{\rho}{\pi}K_{21}L_1 + \frac{\rho}{\pi}K_{23}L_3 \tag{13}$$

$$L_3 = L_{3s} + \frac{\rho}{\pi}K_{31}L_1 + \frac{\rho}{\pi}K_{32}L_2$$

This may be reorganized into the following form:

$$\begin{bmatrix} L_1 \\ L_2 \\ L_3 \end{bmatrix} = \begin{bmatrix} L_{1s} \\ L_{2s} \\ L_{3s} \end{bmatrix} + \left(\frac{\rho}{\pi}\right)\begin{bmatrix} 0 & K_{12} & K_{13} \\ K_{21} & 0 & K_{23} \\ K_{31} & K_{32} & 0 \end{bmatrix}\begin{bmatrix} L_1 \\ L_2 \\ L_3 \end{bmatrix} \tag{14}$$

or expressed in the compact form $L = L_s + \frac{\rho}{\pi}KL$ or $L_s = L - \frac{\rho}{\pi}KL$.

When a shape-from-intensity technique is applied, without considering interreflections, to extract the 3-D shape of the object surface, the total luminance of the facets, $L$, is considered to be due solely to direct source illumination ($L = L_s^1$). Obviously, the estimate of $L_s^1$ is too large as $L$ is a constant which includes both direct and indirect (inter-reflection) illumination. However, this estimate of the total luminance may be substituted into the above compact equations such that $L_s^{n+1} = L - \frac{\rho}{\pi} K^n L$ where $L_s^n$ and $K^n$ are values after $n$ iterations and $L_s^1 = L$. $L_s^{n+1}$ is iteratively calculated and expected to converge to a lower limit as the inital estimate of $K$, $K^0$, from the inital estimate of shape (computed with (1)), is successively refined by a shape-from-intensity algorithm that determines $K$ based on increasingly accurate estimates of $L_s$ with each iteration. For a single facet $i$ at the object surface, successive iterations may then be expressed as follows [4]:

$$L_{s(O,i)}^{n+1} = L_{(O,i)} - \frac{\rho}{\pi} \sum_{i \neq j} K_{ij}^n L_{(O,j)} \tag{15}$$

Applying (4) to both the direct and indirect illumination components in the case of DAL, the appropriate absorption intensity of pixel $i$ for successive iterations leading to correct interpretation of depth by the DAL technique is given by:

$$dE_{s(I,i)}^{n+1} = dE_{(I,i)} - \frac{\rho e^{-\alpha z_{ii}^n}}{\pi \left( R_i^n \right)^2} \sum_{i \neq j} K_{ij}^n \frac{\left( R_j^n \right)^2 dE_{(I,j)}}{e^{-\alpha z_{ij}^n}} \tag{16}$$

We set $\alpha = 0$ to obtain successive infrared intensities.

The algorithm for DAL refinement includes a filtering stage which begins with edge detection in the infrared image using the convolution of a LOG filter . The zero-crossings of this operation identify edges of the object which segment the image into distinct object surface areas. During filtering, masks centered on a given pixel respect the segmentation by including only the pixels of the mask which belong to the same object surface area as the central pixel. In median filtering, the median of all retained mask pixel values is applied to the central pixel. In average filtering, it is the average of all retained values which is applied to the central pixel. The algorithm was applied to the synthetic and real images of the V form in Fig. 2 (A,B). Fig. 2 (C) illustrates profiles, passing through the lengthwise symmetric axis, of the corrected depth images.

In addition, the profile of a canine tooth region in a corrected depth image of a dental imprint is shown.

Results indicate that the depth refinement algorithm consistently provides a significant correction of the depth image in the right direction, towards the camera. In processing the synthetic images, the correction ranges up to 2 mm or approximately 15% of the relative relief of the V form. The accuracy of the correction appears to be excellent everywhere except in the bottom of the V where interreflections have been shown to be strongest. In the case of the real V form, the correction appears to be slightly less significant but may lack the accuracy of the synthetic case due to image noise. Still, the correction partly compensates the overestimation of surface facet distance from the camera.

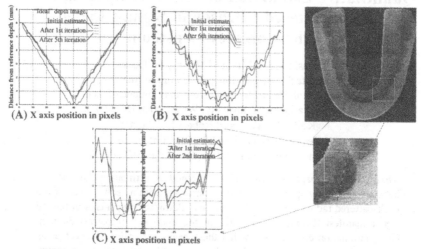

**Fig. 2 (A) Corrected depth image profile of the synthetic V form. (B) Corrected depth image profile of the real V form. (C) Corrected depth image profile of a tooth imprint.**

Much of the depth refinement algorithm was implemented on a MasPar MP-1 SIMD computer 5.

## 5   Conclusion and future work

This paper has presented a study of interreflected light in the context of a system designed to acquire 3-D images of dental imprints.

A discretized solution of the radiosity equation was applied to the DAL method in order to reproduce observed anomalies in the infrared and absorption images taken by the system. The location and intensity of the modelled interreflected light indicates that interreflected light is most likely responsible for the brightest image artifacts and any overestimation of depth in the 3-D images.

Following the work of Nayar et al [4], a discretized form of the radiosity equation was modified and adapted to the DAL method in order to develop a depth image refinement algorithm. The depth refinement algorithm succeeds in accurately correcting depth images everywhere except in the regions of greatest interreflection.

### References

1  Cohen, M.F.,Greenberg, D.P., "The hemi-cube: a radiosity solution for complex environments", *SIGGRAPH 85*, San Francisco, July 1985, pp. 31-40.

2  Coté, J, *Locating Interstices Between Teeth in Range Images of Dental Imprints: An Application in Orthodontics*, master's thesis, Laval Univ, Canada, 1991, 83 p.

3  Laurendeau, D., Guimond, L., Poussart, D., "A Computer-Vision Technique for the Acquisition and Processing of 3-D Profiles of Dental Imprints: An Application in Orthodontics", *IEEE Trans. on Med. Im.*, Vol. 10, No. 3, Sep. 1991, pp. 671-679.

4  Nayar, S. K., Ikeuchi, K., Kanade, T.,"Shape from Interreflections", *Proc. Third ICCV*, 1990, pp. 2-11.

5  Wolfe, R., *"Modelling Interreflections in a System Based on the Differential Absorption of Light"*, master's thesis, Laval Univ., Québec, P.Q., Canada, 1996.

# Quantitative Estimation of Scatterer Spacing from Backscattered Ultrasound Signals Using the Complex Cepstrum

Rashidus S. Mia and Murray H. Loew
Institute for Medical Imaging and Image Analysis
Department of Electrical Engineering and Computer Science
George Washington University, Washington, DC 20052
Keith A. Wear and Robert F. Wagner
Center for Devices and Radiological Health,
Food and Drug Administration, Rockville, MD 20850

**Abstract.** This paper presents a new method of estimating the distance between regularly-spaced coherent scatterers within soft tissue from backscattered radio-frequency (RF) signals. Periodic components in the RF signal manifest themselves as peaks in the quefrency (cepstral) domain. Using simulation data, we show that these peaks are easier to detect using the complex cepstrum rather than the commonly used power cepstrum. Similar improvements are seen using phantom and *in vivo* liver data.

## 1 Introduction

Quantitative analysis of backscattered ultrasound from biological tissue has been used successfully to characterize tissue types and to diagnose soft tissue diseases. The backscattered RF signal has been shown to have two principal components. The first component is a highly incoherent, diffuse scatter due to many randomly-distributed scatterers [1,2,3]. The second component is highly coherent and is caused by scatterers that are spaced periodically [4,5], such as the portal triads in the liver [6,7,8], the nephrons in the kidney [9], and trabeculae in the spleen [8].

Fellingham and Sommer [8] used the average scatterer spacing to diagnose cirrhosis and hepatitis in the liver and Hodgkin's disease in the spleen. Suzuki *et al.* [10] used the mode and kurtosis of the scatterer spacing to diagnose cirrhosis and hepatitis. Garra *et al.* [6,9] showed that the mean scatterer spacing was an important feature in diagnosing hepatitis, Gaucher's disease, and diffuse kidney disease.

A critical task that is integral to all of these approaches is the quantitative estimation of scatterer spacing from the backscattered RF signal. Fellingham and Sommer [8] estimated this spacing by computing the distance between peaks in the power spectrum of the RF signal. Varghese and Donohue [11] computed the autocorrelation matrix of the frequency spectrum and searched for ridges. Lizzi *et al.* [12] were the first to use the cepstrum to estimate features from the RF signal. They used it to measure the thickness of the wall of the hepatic vein. Suzuki *et al.* [10] used the cepstrum to estimate average scatterer spacing.

The power spectrum- and cepstrum-based approaches to computing the scatterer spacing discard useful information present in the phase component of the signal. In this work, we propose a new approach to computing scatterer spacing based on the use of the complex cepstrum. Since it uses the complex logarithm of the frequency spectrum rather than the logarithm of the power spectrum, the complex cepstrum retains the phase information of the original signal.

## 2 Theoretical Development

The power cepstrum of a signal is defined as the Inverse Fourier Transform of the logarithm of the power spectrum of the signal. This can be expressed as:

$$C_p(n) = IFT\{Log(|X(w)|^2)\}, \quad \text{and } X(w) = FT\{x(n)\}$$

Where $FT\{\}$ is the Fourier transform operator and $IFT\{\}$ is inverse Fourier transform operator. When the magnitude of $X(w)$ is found prior to computing the logarithm, the phase information in the original signal is discarded.

By contrast, the complex cepstrum is defined as the Inverse Fourier Transform of the logarithm of the frequency spectrum of the signal. This can be expressed as:

$$C_c(n) = IFT\{Log(X(w))\}, \quad \text{where } X(w) = FT\{x(n)\}$$

Here the logarithm is performed on the complex quantity $X(w)$. The logarithm of a complex number is defined as:

$$Log(X(w)) = Log(A) + j\theta, \quad \text{where } X(w) = Ae^{j\theta}$$

To compute the inverse Fourier transform after performing the complex logarithm, both the real and imaginary parts must be continuous signals. The real part is continuous. The phase angle, however, can be a discontinuous signal. It is necessary to first unwrap the phase signal to yield the continuous- phase signal.

## 3 Methods

The goal of this work is to provide an improved tool to extract a key feature (scatterer spacing) from backscattered ultrasound that can be used to diagnose various diseases. To verify the effectiveness of this technique, we use the normal-patient data collected by Garra *et al.* for their work on diffuse liver disease [6].

The patient data were not very useful, however, in quantifying the ability of the complex cepstrum to estimate scatterer spacing because the true spacings present in the patients were not known. As an intermediate step, the phantom data collected by Wear *et al.* [13] were used.

While this phantom provides a more controlled data set than the *in vivo* liver data and can be used to assess the effectiveness of the complex cepstrum using real ultrasound data, there are still important factors that cannot be controlled or even known. Specifically, the variation in the actual spacing is not known; the diffuse scatterer density cannot be controlled; and the relative strengths of the diffuse and periodic components cannot be varied.

Simulation data were used to quantify the performance of the complex-cepstrum approach to scatterer spacing estimation. The simulation consists of generating a scattering medium that consists of Poisson-distributed point scatterers. Wagner *et al.* [2] have shown that when the number of those scatterers per resolution cell of the transducer is sufficiently large, diffuse scattering having Rayleigh statistics results. The scattering medium also contains regularly-spaced scatterers whose spacing, variation in spacing, and relative strength can be controlled. The RF backscattered signal is simulated by convolving this scattering medium with an RF pulse. An exponential decay is then imposed on this RF signal to simulate the depth-dependent attenuation. Finally, measurement noise is added to the RF signal. The resulting simulated RF signal of a single A-line scan is shown in Figure 1.

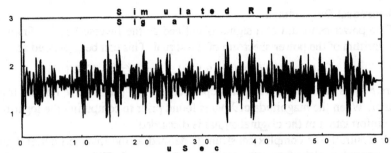

**Figure 1.** A simulated RF signal of a single A-line produced by the convolution of a transmitted pulse with a tissue scattering medium containing a high density of diffuse scatterers per resolution cell along with uniformly spaced scatterers 1.54 mm apart.

The periodic component of the scattering is not evident in the power (or complex) cepstrum of a single A-line. However, if N of these cepstra are summed, the signal due to the periodic scatterers increases by a factor of N while those due to the random scatterers increase by a factor of √N. This provides a gain of √N for the periodic component. The averaged (N=40) power and complex cepstrum are shown in Figures 2a and 2b, respectively. The effect of the periodic scatterers is clearly visible as a peak at the characteristic spacing. Peaks also occur at multiples of this spacing.

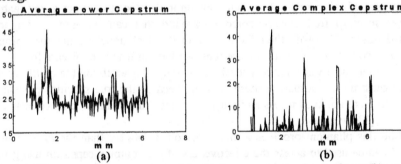

(a)  (b)

**Figure 2.** The average power cepstrum (a) and the average complex cepstrum (b) computed by summing the power and complex cepstra from 40 individual A-line scans.

The immediate task is to detect the main peak in the cepstra shown in Figure 2. The detectability of these peaks under various conditions will serve as a measure of effectiveness for each approach. One objective measure of the detectability of a peak in the presence of noise is the number of standard deviations separating the peak from the mean value [14]. Thus, our objective measure of performance will be the signal excess (SE), defined as SE = [peak-mean]/StdDev in units of standard deviations. The SE is computed for peaks in the cepstrum that satisfy all of the following conditions:

1) Its location is within a defined range (in the present case, 0.75-3.0mm).
2) It has the largest signal excess in that range.
3) It is a fundamental peak (i.e., it has no sub-harmonics).

The latter condition ensures identification of the fundamental period in the time domain. That period identifies the scatterer spacing in the material.

## 4 Results

We first consider simulated signals. Figure 3a displays the signal excess as a function of the relative strength of the regularly-spaced scatterers. Figure 3b shows the dependence on the variation in the scatterer spacing. The number of A-lines used in the average and the length of each A-line will also affect the detectabilities of the peaks in the quefrency domain. These dependencies are clearly evident in figures 3c and 3d, respectively. Each point represents the mean signal excess (with one standard deviation error bars) computed from 100 independent simulations.

It is clear from the plots that computing the complex cepstrum of each A-line and then averaging the resulting complex cepstra provides a larger signal excess as compared to averaging the power cepstra.

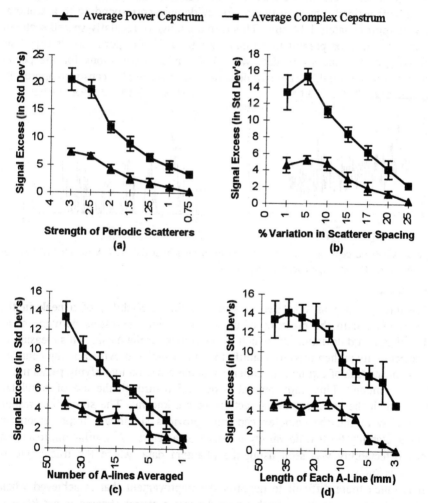

**Figure 3.** Signal excess, in units of standard deviations, as a function of: (a) the relative strength of regularly-spaced scatterers; (b) the variation in scatterer spacing; (c) the number of A-lines used in the average; and (d) the length of each A-line.

Using the phantom data, the signal excess for the power cepstra method was 5.1 Std Dev's. The complex cepstra approach yielded a signal excess of 7.0 Std Dev's. These values are consistent with the results from the simulations as presented above.

For the *in vivo* liver data, we started with data from 64 patients. For some patients the two techniques did not yield the same scatterer spacing estimate. Since the true scatterer spacing is not known, only the 48 cases where both of the approaches produced the same estimate are considered. For this data, the power cepstrum approach yielded a signal excess of $3.31 \pm 0.91$ Std Dev's compared to $4.18 \pm 0.56$ Std Dev's for the complex cepstrum approach. Again, we see that complex cepstrum approach yields a more detectable peak in the quefrency domain.

A typical set of cepstra derived from *in vivo* liver data is shown in Figure 4. Both methods yielded a peak in the quefrency domain corresponding to a scatterer spacing of approximately 1.14 mm. This is in the range of regularly-spaced scatterer spacing believed to be present in normal liver tissue due to portal triads [6]. The signal excesses for this set of data were 3.90 standard deviations for the power cepstrum approach and 4.32 standard deviations for the complex cepstrum approach.

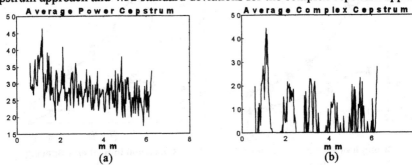

**Figure 4.** Averaged cepstra from a typical set of *in vivo* liver data (27 A-lines): (a) Average power cepstrum, (b) Average complex cepstrum.

## 5 Discussion

We have defined an objective measure for the detectability of a peak in the quefrency domain in the presence of noise. The signal excess is defined as the number of standard deviations by which the peak exceeds the mean. This measure of peak detectability is then used to quantify the improvement provided by the complex cepstrum at the task of estimating scatterer spacing based on identifying peaks in the quefrency domain. This improvement is quantified through the use of simulated data for which the exact signal characteristics are known. The simulation results show that averaging the complex cepstrum provides significant improvement in signal detectability for a wide variety of tissue parameters. A similar improvement in peak detectability was seen using the phantom data, where the true scatterer spacing was known.

It is much more difficult to quantify the improvement that is achieved when processing *in vivo* liver data. In this case the true scatterer spacing is not known. For this reason, only cases where there was agreement regarding the scatterer spacing estimate were considered. In this sub-set of the data, the complex cepstrum approach did provide some improvement in detection capability. An important question that needs to be addressed is the following: when the approaches yield different estimates, which one, if either, is correct?

The new method of estimating scatterer spacing proposed here is a tool to extract a feature for the diagnosis of diffuse diseases in soft tissue organs. Several researchers [6,8,9, and 10] have shown that scatterer spacing is an important feature in diagnosing various disease conditions. In the future, we hope to use the improved estimates of scatterer spacing described here, along with other features, to improve the diagnostic capability of quantitative ultrasound.

## 6 Acknowledgments

R. S. M. and M. H. L. gratefully acknowledge the support of this work under DHHS/FDA Order No. 363914.

## 7 References

1. C. Burckhardt, "Speckle in ultrasound B-mode scans," *IEEE Trans on Sonics and Ultrasonics,* vol. 25, no. 1, pp. 1-6, January 1978.
2. R. Wagner, S. Smith, J. Sandrik, and H. Lopez, "Statistics of speckle in ultrasound B-scans," *IEEE Trans on Sonics and Ultrasonics,* vol. 30, no. 3, pp. 156-163, May 1987.
3. R. Wagner, M. Insana, and D. Brown, "Statistical properties of radio-frequency and envelope-detected signals with applications to medical ultrasound," *Journal of the Optical Society of America A,* vol. 4, pp. 910-922, May 1987.
4. M. Insana, R. Wagner, B. Garra, D. Brown, and T. Shawker, "Analysis of ultrasound image texture via generalized Rician statistics," *Opt Eng,* vol. 25,pp.743-748, June 1986.
5. L. Landini and L. Verrazzani, "Spectral characterization of tissue microstructure by ultrasound: A stochastic approach," *IEEE Trans on Ultrasonics, Ferroelectrics, and Frequency Control,* vol. 37, no. 5, pp. 448-455, September 1990.
6. B. Garra, M. Insana, T. Shawker, R. Wagner, M. Bradford, and M. Russell, "Quantitative ultrasonic detection and classification of diffuse liver disease, comparison with human observer performance," *Invest Radiol,* vol. 24, pp. 196-203, March 1989.
7. M. Insana, R. Wagner, B. Garra, R. Momenan, and T. Shawker, "Pattern recognition methods for optimizing multivariate tissue signitures in diagnostic ultrasound," *Ultrasonic Imaging,* vol. 8, pp. 165-180, 1986.
8. L. Fellingham and F. Sommer, "Ultrasonic characterization of tissue structure in the *in vivo* human liver and spleen," *IEEE Trans on Sonics and Ultrasonics,* vol. 31, pp. 418-428, July 1984.
9. B. Garra, M. Insana, I. Sesterhenn, T. Hall, R. Wagner, C. Rotellar, J. Winchester, and R. Zeman, "Quantitative ultrasonic detection of parenchymal structural change in diffuse renal disease," *Invest Radiol,* vol. 29, no. 2, pp. 134-140, February 1994.
10. K. Suzuki, N. Hayashi, Y. Sasaki, M. Kono, Y. Imai, H. Fusamoto, and T. Kamada, "Ultrasonic tissue characterization of chronic liver disease using cepstral analysis," *Gastroenterology,* vol. 101, no. 5, pp. 1325-1331, November 1991.
11. T. Varghese and K. Donohue, "Mean-scatterer spacing estimates with spectral autocorrelation," *Journal Acoust. Soc. Am.,* vol. 96, pp. 3504-3515, December 1994.
12. F. Lizzi, E. Felepa, N. Jaremko, D. King, and P. Wai, "Liver-tissue characterization by digital spectrum and cepstrum analysis," *Proc 1981 IEEE Ultrason Symp,* pp. 575-578.
13. Wear, R. Wagner, M. Insana, and T. Hall, "Application of autoregressive spectral analysis to cepstral estimation of mean scatterer spacing," *IEEE Trans on Ultrasonics, Ferroelectrics, and Frequency Control,* vol. 40, no. 1, pp. 50-58, January 1993.
14. M. Skolnik, *Introduction to Radar Systems.* McGraw-Hill. New York, NY, 1980.

# Spatial Compounding of 3-D Ultrasound Images

Robert Rohling[1], Andrew Gee[1] and Laurence Berman[2]

[1] Department of Engineering, Cambridge University, Cambridge, UK, CB2 1PZ
[2] Department of Radiology, Addenbrooke's Hospital, Cambridge, UK, CB2 2QQ

**Abstract.** In this paper we investigate the use of spatial compounding to reduce speckle in 3-D ultrasound. 3-D voxel arrays are reconstructed by compounding a large number of overlapping B-scans. The reconstruction algorithm uses a novel landmark-based registration technique to accurately register each B-scan as it is inserted into the voxel array. In a series of *in-vitro* and *in-vivo* trials, we demonstrate that 3-D spatial compounding is very effective for improving the signal to noise ratio, but correction of registration errors is essential.

## 1 Introduction

Conventional diagnostic ultrasound imaging is performed with a hand-held probe which transmits ultrasound pulses into the body and receives the echoes. The magnitude and timing of the echoes are used to create a 2-D grey-level image (B-scan) of a cross-section of the body in the scan plane. 3-D free-hand ultrasound imaging is a technique used to create 3-D data sets from a series of 2-D B-scans. In this paradigm, a 3-D position sensor is attached to the probe, so that each B-scan is labelled with the position and orientation of the scan plane. Subsequent processing can build up a 3-D description of the imaged anatomy, analogous to stacking a deck of cards, except the B-scans may intersect each other.

Automatic interpretation of ultrasound data is often limited by noise, especially speckle. Speckle is common to all ultrasound images, a product of constructive-destructive interference of the ultrasound echoes. Spatial compounding has been previously suggested as an effective way to reduce speckle [6], but a thorough analysis of 3-D spatial compounding has never yet been performed.

The principle behind spatial compounding is to image the region of interest repeatedly, from different look directions, and then average the values from the intersecting B-scans when reconstructing the 3-D data set. The speckle signal, which de-correlates from different look directions, is suppressed by the averaging operation. Conversely, real anatomical features (tissue boundaries, for example) will be observed in the same location from all look directions. Provided the registration of the scan planes is accurate, the averaging operation will reduce the speckle without blurring real anatomical features.

The key to effective spatial compounding is to achieve very accurate registration [5]. Relying on the position sensor alone is usually not sufficient: there may be small errors in its calibration, and it does not take into account motion of the target or within-plane imaging artifacts. It is therefore necessary to improve the registration using image-based techniques.

In this paper we tackle three objectives. The first is to demonstrate a novel image-based registration technique using both *in-vitro* and *in-vivo* examinations. The second is to demonstrate how spatial compounding improves the signal to noise ratio (SNR) of the reconstructed data. Our final objective is to establish agreement between the observed and predicted improvements in SNR.

## 2 Acquisition system and test subjects

The acquisition system comprises a Toshiba ultrasound scanner, a standard 2-D probe, and a Polhemus FASTRAK position sensor. The phantom study used a 7 MHz probe while the *in-vivo* study used a 3.75 MHz probe. Images from the scanner and the related position data are recorded by a Sun workstation.

An investigation on SNR was first performed on a phantom comprising a latex balloon filled with a mixture of water, ultrasound coupling gel and talcum powder. An *in-vivo* examination was also performed on the gall bladder of a healthy human subject.

## 3 3-D Reconstruction *Without* Registration

Each B-scan is represented as a 2-D array $\mathbf{P}$ of intensity values. The reconstruction volume takes the form of a 3-D voxel array $\mathbf{C}$. The voxel size is typically chosen to be larger than the pixel dimensions in order to avoid large gaps in the reconstructions and reduce the memory requirements. The position sensor measurements are used to calculate the transformation $\mathbf{T}$ between the coordinate systems of the B-scan and the voxel array.

Before the start of the examination, the voxels in the reconstruction volume are all set to zero. As each B-scan is acquired, each voxel is adjusted according to the pixels which intersect it. A single voxel will envelop many pixels if the voxel size is larger than the B-scan pixel size. Each voxel may also be intersected again by future B-scans. The average value of all pixels that intersect the voxel is stored in $\mathbf{C}$. The array $\mathbf{C}$ can be then be displayed on a computer monitor, for example by the any-plane slicing method used in this paper.

## 4 3-D Reconstruction *With* Registration

As mentioned, small errors in B-scan position measurements and imaging artifacts need to be corrected for accurate registration. We attempt registration via *landmarks*: edge elements (edgels) automatically extracted by the Canny edge detection algorithm [3] at the resolution corresponding to the voxel size.

In this study, each examination commences with a quick pass over the region of interest, so that nearly all of the voxels are filled. No attempt is made to register these initial B-scans: they act as the baseline. Subsequent passes over the region of interest, from different look directions, are compounded into the voxel

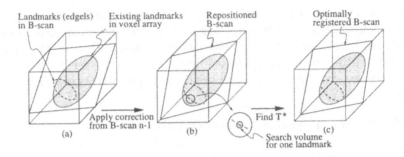

**Fig. 1. Landmark-based registration.** In (a), B-scan $n$ is inserted into the voxel array at the location indicated by the position sensor. Significant registration errors are evident. Since B-scans are acquired in rapid succession, any registration error varies slowly from one B-scan to the next: we use this observation to effectively *track* the registration error, which is more efficient than performing unconstrained registration for each B-scan. After applying the correction found from registering B-scan $n$-$1$, only small residual errors remain (b). These are corrected by landmark-based registration. A small ellipsoidal search volume is defined around each re-positioned landmark in **P**: any landmarks in **C** found within this volume are marked as candidate correspondences for the landmark in **P**. RANSAC regression [4] is used to find the optimal transformation **T*** which aligns as many of the corresponding landmarks as possible. Finally, the B-scan is compounded into the voxel array using **T*** (c).

array to reduce the noise. The inevitable registration errors are automatically corrected by landmark alignment as each new B-scan is acquired — see Figure 1.

In this study, the optimal transformation **T*** is constrained to a rigid 6 DOF transformation, consistent with the expected sources of registration error (rigid motion of the target and inaccurate B-scan position measurements). This assumption precludes use of the registration algorithm on organs which exhibit significant non-rigid motion, such as the heart. The registered image is added to **C** in the same manner as in the standard algorithm (Section 3).

## 5   Results

The purpose of the phantom study is to investigate the effect of compounding on the SNR. SNR is defined in this study as the ratio of the mean grey level to the standard deviation for an image with no resolvable structures. This applies to the interior (region 1) and exterior (region 2) of the latex balloon.

The phantom was scanned in a continuous series of sweeps from one end of the balloon to the other, producing many overlapping B-scans. Each sweep was carried out with the probe at a look direction slightly displaced from the previous sweep. Two reconstruction volumes were created, one with registration (using the novel reconstruction algorithm of Section 4), the other without (using the standard algorithm of Section 3). Figure 2 shows slices of the reconstructions.

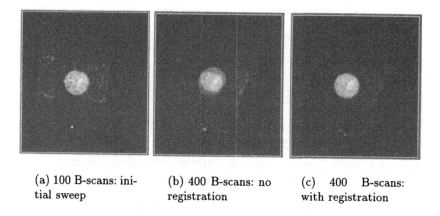

(a) 100 B-scans: initial sweep

(b) 400 B-scans: no registration

(c) 400 B-scans: with registration

**Fig. 2. Reconstructions** *with* **and** *without* **registration.** Slices (a–c) are taken at the same location in the reconstruction volume. In (b), speckle is reduced both inside and outside the object, but registration errors result in substantial blurring of the object boundary. Notice the speckle reduction yet minimal blurring in (c).

To investigate the improvement in SNR with spatial compounding, we analysed grey level statistics in the two reconstruction volumes at various stages of reconstruction: after 100 B-scans (initial sweep, no compounding), then 150, 200, 250, 300, 350 and finally 400 B-scans (heavy compounding). For each case we segmented volumetric regions 1 and 2 with a volumetric mask, then calculated the SNR of filled voxels in each region.

The improvement in SNR can be predicted by statistical theory. Previous research has demonstrated a $\sqrt{n}$ improvement in SNR for 2-D compounding of $n$ uncorrelated B-scans [2]. Since the voxels are not all compounded the same number of times, and there is a reduction in resolution from B-scan to voxel array, a more general theory has been derived [7]. Figure 3 shows that the measured increase in SNR closely matches the theoretical increase, demonstrating that the compounded scans are mostly uncorrelated. Only a modest improvement in SNR is achieved by compounding 400 scans since this represents only an approximate four-fold increase in the average number of intersections per voxel.

A measure is required to quantify the effect of registration errors on the reconstruction. In essence, we want a measure for the loss of spatial resolution, or blurring between regions 1 and 2. Instead of attempting to measure spatial resolution directly, we chose to focus on *volume* estimation of the phantom interior. Volume is estimated by "live-wire" segmentation [1] of slices through the reconstruction. Blurring of the object results in poorer segmentation and therefore worse estimates of volume — see Table 1. Organ volume is also a measure that is often sought after by physicians. Furthermore, it can be compared to the real phantom volume, measured with a graduated cylinder at 7.0 ml ± 0.2 ml.

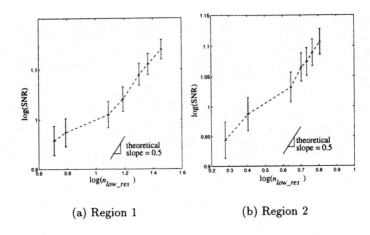

(a) Region 1                 (b) Region 2

**Fig. 3. Effect of compounding on SNR for registered reconstructions.** Each '+' data point represents a SNR calculated at 100, 150, 200, 250, 300, 350, and 400 B-scans. The x-axis variable $n_{low\_res}$ is the average number of intersections per voxel for low resolution reconstructions. A log-log plot is used because a slope of 0.5 indicates agreement with the theoretical increase of SNR as $(n_{low\_res})^{0.5}$ [7].

| Number of B-scans | | 100 | 150 | 200 | 250 | 300 | 350 | 400 |
|---|---|---|---|---|---|---|---|---|
| Volume | Unregistered | 7.20 | 7.17 | 7.19 | 7.27 | 7.31 | 7.43 | 7.56 |
| (ml) | Registered | 7.20 | 7.16 | 7.19 | 7.20 | 7.14 | 7.20 | 7.18 |

**Table 1. Volumes calculated by "live-wire" segmentation.**

Figure 4 shows the results of the *in-vivo* study. *In-vivo* registration errors are significant but can be minimised by landmark-based registration. A more subtle effect is that the high intensity cloud-like artifact is slightly reduced by compounding. Previous hardware limitations restricted this study to only 60 B-scans. With higher numbers of compounded B-scans, the artifacts should be further reduced, as in the phantom study.

## 6 Conclusions

We have shown how spatial compounding can improve the SNR of 3-D ultrasound images in agreement with theoretical predictions. The inevitable registration errors which come with higher levels of compounding can be corrected using an automatic, incremental landmark-based registration algorithm. The resulting high quality 3-D reconstructions are particularly well suited to automatic segmentation for visualisation and volume measurement.

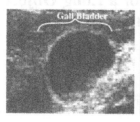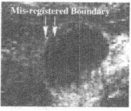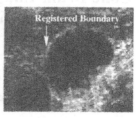

(a) Original B-scan    (b) Compounding: no registration    (c) Compounding: with registration

**Fig. 4. Registration of an *in-vivo* transverse and longitudinal gall bladder examination.** Figure (c) shows the elimination of a double boundary, evident (b), that is produced by mis-registered B-scans.

Future work will investigate higher levels of compounding in *in-vivo* scans, and improving the speed and robustness of the registration algorithm. We anticipate that the key to efficient registration will lie with more reliable landmark detection at larger scales, allowing registration of *contours* in the B-scans onto *surfaces* in the voxel array.

# References

1. W.A. Barrett and E.N. Mortensen. Fast, accurate, and reproducible live-wire boundary extraction. In K.H. Hohne and R. Kikinis, editors, *Lecture Notes in Computer Science: Visualization in Biomedical Computing, Proc. VBC '96*, volume 1131, pages 183–192. Springer-Verlag, Heidelberg, Germany, 1996.
2. C.B. Burckhardt. Speckle in ultrasound B-mode scans. *IEEE Trans. Sonics and Ultrasonics*, 25(1):1–6, 1978.
3. J. Canny. A computational approach to edge detection. *IEEE Trans. PAMI*, 8(6):679–698, 1986.
4. M. A. Fischler and R. C. Bolles. Random sample consensus: a paradigm for model fitting with applications to image analysis and automated cartography. *Communications of the ACM*, 24(6):381–395, June 1981.
5. A. Moskalik, P. L. Carson, C. R. Meyer, J. B. Fowlkes, J. M. Rubin, and M. A. Roubidoux. Registration of three-dimensional compound ultrasound scans of the breast for refraction and motion correction. *Ultrasound Med. Biol.*, 21(6):769–778, 1995.
6. T.R. Nelson and D.H. Pretorius. 3D ultrasound image quality improvement using spatial compounding and 3D filtering. *Med. Phys.*, 21(6):998, 1994.
7. R. N. Rohling, A.H. Gee, and L. Berman. Spatial compounding of 3-D ultrasound images. Technical Report CUED/F-INFENG/TR 270, Cambridge University Department of Engineering, October 1996. Also in press in *Medical Image Analysis*.

# Cone Beam Imaging of a Section of a Long Object with a Short Detector

K.C. Tam

Siemens Corporate Research, Inc.
755 College Road East
Princeton, NJ 08540

**Abstract.** Imaging a sectional region within an object with a detector just big enough to cover the sectional region-of-interest is analyzed. We show that with some suitable choice of scanning configuration and with an innovative method of data combination, all the Radon data can be obtained accurately. The algorithm is mathematically exact, and requires no iterations and no additional measurements. The method can be applied to inspect portions of large industrial objects in industrial imaging, as well as to image portions of human bodies in medical diagnosis.

## 1 Introduction

Cone beam x-ray computerized Tomography takes much shorter time than scanning the 3-dimensional object slice-by-slice with conventional fan beam x-ray, and promises to generate reconstructed images with sharper contrast, and better spatial resolution between slices. In the case of small objects that completely fit inside the FOV of the detector high quality images can be reconstructed using one of a number of exact algorithms [1,2].

Some objects which are of interest in medical as well as industrial inspections, however, are in the form of a relatively small sectional region in a long object. It is therefore desirable to employ a detector just big enough to cover the sectional region. However, such arrangement presents serious difficulties for the image reconstruction problem. From the perspective of reconstructing the entire object, some of the cone beam data penetrating portions of the object other than the region-of-interest are missing because of the insufficient size of the detector. From the perspective of reconstructing the region-of-interest, some of the x-ray paths penetrate other portions of the object as well as the region-of-interest, and thus the cone beam data collected no longer represent the region-of-interest exclusively but are corrupted by the overlaying materials. A technique of reconstructing a sectional region of an object has been previously addressed by Chen [3]. However, Chen's method assumes that the cone beam data for the entire object are available. Kudo and Saito [4] have investigated the use of the circle-plus-line scan path to handle truncated cone beam data. In this paper region-of-interest imaging with truncated cone beam data is analyzed, and a method to image the region without corrupted or missing data using a detector just big enough to cover half of the sectional region is presented. The results in this paper were first disclosed in [5,6].

## 2 Data Corruption

Because of the one-to-one correspondence between the points in Radon space and the planes of integration in the object space, the data corruption situation in the former can be analyzed by studying the corresponding situation in the latter. All the planes that intersect the region-of-interest can be classified into the following 3 types:

1. those that intersect the region-of-interest only;
2. those that intersect the region-of-interest and also either the region above or the region below, but not both;
3. those that intersect the region-of-interest and also both the region above and the region below.

These three types of planes are illustrated in Figure 1. Consider a region-of-interest with a cylindrical support with parallel top and bottom surfaces. The cylinder has height $2b$ and radius $a$. Take any vertical plane in Radon space containing the $z$ axis. Without loss of generality label the horizontal axis as the $y$ axis. The projection of the cylinder on the vertical plane is a rectangle of dimension $2a \times 2b$, as illustrated in Figure 2. It can be easily shown from geometry that the boundary of the support of the Radon transform of the region-of-interest on the vertical plane is the curve A shown in Figure 2. In polar coordinate a point $(r,\theta)$ in the first quadrant on curve A is given by the equation:

$$r = \sqrt{a^2 + b^2}\, \cos(\theta - \tan^{-1}\frac{b}{a}) \quad \theta \in \left[0, \frac{\pi}{2}\right] \tag{1}$$

The curve A in other quadrants are obtained by folding the curve in the first quadrant about the $y$ axis and $z$ axis respectively.

The three regions in Radon space which correspond to these three types of planes are illustrated in Figure 3 for the cylindrically shaped region-of-interest. With otherwise complete (for small objects) cone beam scanning configurations, only the Radon data (more precisely, the radial derivative of the Radon data) corresponding to the first type of planes of integration can be computed without corruption. The region in Radon space corresponding to this type of plane is indicated in the figure and is characterized by the equation:

$$r_1 = \sqrt{a^2 + b^2}\, \cos\left[\tan^{-1}\frac{a}{b} + \frac{\pi}{2} - \theta\right] \tag{2}$$

The line through any Radon point in this region perpendicular to the line connecting the point to the origin does not intersect the top and the bottom edges of the rectangle which is the projection of the cylindrical region-of-interest on the plane of the figure.

The support for the third type of planes is in the form of two pockets along the $y$ axis. The boundary is given by the following equation:

$$r_3 = \sqrt{a^2 + b^2}\, \cos\left[\theta + \tan^{-1}\frac{b}{a}\right] \tag{3}$$

The line through any Radon point in this region perpendicular to the line connecting the point to the origin intersects both the top and the bottom edges of the rectangle which is the projection of the cylindrical region-of-interest on the plane of the figure.

## 3 Elimination of Data Corruption

Usually, the cone beam data for the second and third types of planes are corrupted. However, by suitably manipulating x-ray beam coverage from various source positions, it would be possible to avoid data corruption by overlying material and at the same time achieve complete Radon space coverage. Consider the second type of planes. Take any scan path which includes a scan on the top level plane of the region-of-interest, viz. the $z = b$ level, or a scan on the bottom level plane of the region-of-interest, viz. the $z = -b$ level. The scan path on the top or bottom planes can take the form of any closed curve, not necessarily circular nor convex. For the ease of illustration, however, we assume these scan paths to be circular in the discussion below.

Consider the case of the top level, the $z = b$ level. In Figure 4 is illustrated a plane of integration intersecting the region-of-interest and its top surface, but not the bottom surface. When the x-ray source is located at this level, each x-ray path originating from the source intersects either only the region of the object above the $z = b$ level, or only the region below it, or only the $z = b$ level itself; but the path will not intersect more than one of these three regions. Which one of these three regions the path intersects can be identified from the position on the detector the x-ray path intersects. Thus the unwanted contribution of the portion of the object above the $z = b$ level to the computation of Radon derivatives can be eliminated by discarding all the x-ray data whose paths traverse the portion above the $z = b$ level. By considering a scan at the bottom level, i.e. the $z = -b$ level, and using a procedure similar to the one described above for the top ($z = b$) level scan with obvious modification, data corruption due to the portion of the object below the $z = -b$ level can also be eliminated.

With another innovative procedure, even data corruption due to the third type of planes can be eliminated. This is achieved by properly combining the cone beam data from the top scan and the bottom scan for each plane of integration intersecting both the top level and the bottom level of the region-of-interest. The method is illustrated in Figure 5, which features a plane of integration through the object intersecting portions of it above the $z = b$ level and below the $z = -b$ level, together with the two x-ray source positions T and B on the plane which are located on the top scan and the bottom scan respectively. We shall refer to the portion of the plane of integration covered by the cone beam rays emitted at source position T between the top level and the line TB as the partial plane A, and the portion of the plane covered by the cone beam rays emitted at source position B between the bottom level and the line TB shall be referred to as the partial plane B. Note that both partial planes do not intersect the portion of the object above the top level and that below the bottom level, and in combination they constitute the cross section of the region-of-interest intersected by the plane of integration.

If for the source position T only the portion of the cone beam data on the plane between the top level and the line TB is used in computing the Radon derivative datum, one can obtain the radial derivative of the planar integral of the object density on partial plane A. Similarly, for the source position B the computation of the Radon derivative datum using only the cone beam data on the plane generated between the bottom level and the line TB yields the radial derivative of the planar integral of the object density on partial plane B. Their sum yields the radial derivative of the planar integral of the density over the cross section of the region-of-interest. Since only about half of the cone beam data illuminating the entire cross section is needed at each source position, the detector size is only required to cover half of the sectional region (at the axis of rotation), as is evident in Figure 5. It should be noted that the method of obtaining the Radon transform of the object by combining cone beam data from the top and bottom level scans is possible if the operation which computes the function of the Radon transform from cone beam data is linear and local, such as Radon derivative computation [1,2].

## 4 Data Completion

Some planes which intersect the region-of-interest do not intersect the top and bottom scan paths. It can be readily shown that these planes only intersect the region-of-interest, and therefore there is no data corruption problem to deal with. The Radon derivative data for such planes can be filled in by adding any scan path connecting the top and the bottom level scan paths, as illustrated in Figure 6.

## 5 Discussion

We have analyzed the problem of imaging a section region-of-interest of an object using cone beam x-rays, and have developed a method to image the region without corrupted or missing data requiring only a detector big enough to cover half of the sectional region. The method is mathematically exact, and no iterations and no additional measurements are required. The region of the object is reconstructed without compromising the image quality. As a result the method can be applied to inspect portions of large industrial objects in industrial imaging, as well as to image portions of human bodies in medical diagnosis, with the same kind of image quality as in conventional x-ray CT. The size of objects to be inspected with cone beam CT are no longer limited by the detector dimension. In a sense the method presented in this paper extends CT from inspecting objects one slice at a time to one section at a time.

# References

[1]    R. Clack and M. Defrise, "Overview of reconstruction algorithms for exact cone-beam tomography", Proc. SPIE Vol. 2299, 1994, pp. 230-241.

[2]    K.C. Tam, "Exact image reconstruction in cone beam 3D CT", Review of Progress in Quantitative Non-Destructive Evaluation, Eds. D.O. Thompson and D.E. Chimenti (New York: Plenum Press) Vol. 4A, pp.657-664).

[3]    J. Chen, "A theoretical framework of regional cone-beam tomography", IEEE Trans.Med. Imag., MI-11 (1992) 342.

[4]    H. Kudo, T. Saito, "An extended completeness condition for exact cone-beam reconstruction and its application", IEEE Conf. Record 1994 Nuclear Science Symposium and Medical Imaging Conference, Norfolk, VA, 1710-14, 1995.

[5]    K.C. Tam, "Method and apparatus for acquiring complete Radon data for exactly reconstructing a three dimensional computerized tomography image of a portion of an object irradiated by a cone beam source", US. Patent 5,383,119, Jan 17, 1995.

[6]    K.C. Tam, "Helical and circle scan region of interest computerized tomography", US. Patent 5,463,666, Oct 31, 1995.

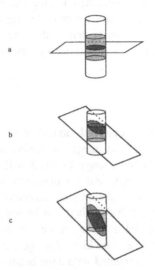

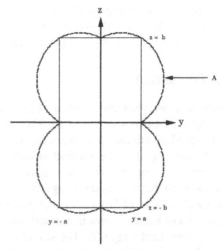

**Figure 1.** The three ways in which a plane intersects the region-of-interest: a. intersecting the region-of-interest only; b. intersecting the region-of-interest and also either the region above or the region below, but not both; c. intersecting the region-of-interest and also both the region above and the region below.

**Figure 2.** The vertical middle cross section of the Radon transform of the cylindrical region-of-interest.

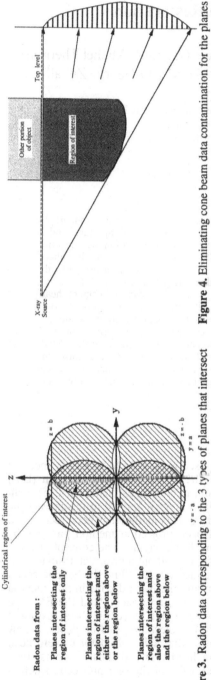

**Figure 3.** Radon data corresponding to the 3 types of planes that intersect the region-of-interest as depicted in Figure 1.

**Figure 4.** Eliminating cone beam data contamination for the planes that intersect the region-of-interest and also the region above.

**Figure 5.** Eliminating cone beam data contamination for the planes that intersect the region-of-interest and also both the region above and the region below.

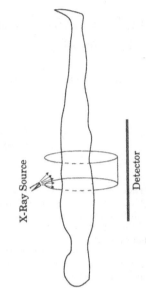

**Figure 6.** 2 circles + line scan path for ROI cone beam CT.

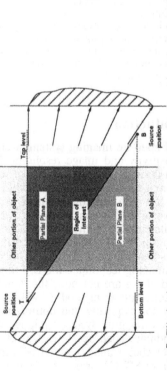

# New Methods for SPECT Imaging and Pre-reconstruction Restoration

Yi-Hwa Liu[+], Anand Rangarajan[†], Daniel Gagnon[*], Michel Therrien[*],
Albert J. Sinusas[+], Frans J.Th. Wackers[+] and George Zubal[†]

[+]Department of Medicine, [†]Department of Diagnostic Radiology
Yale University, School of Medicine
New Haven, CT 06520, USA

[*]Park Medical Systems Inc.
Lachine, Quebec H8T 1C4, Canada

**Abstract.** A novel dual single photon emission computerized tomography (SPECT) imaging system equipped with a modular coded aperture and a conventional parallel hole collimator is introduced. An expectation maximization type blind deconvolution algorithm (EMBD) based on maximum likelihood estimation is derived for restoration of SPECT planar projections acquired by the dual imaging system. The uniformly redundant array (URA) technique is used for decoding the shadowgram acquired by the coded aperture camera head. Results of real phantom data are presented. The new configuration of the dual SPECT imaging system considerably improves the count sensitivity while still maintaining (or slightly improving) the conventional resolutions of high resolution collimation. The results also demonstrate the feasibility of the EMBD algorithm in improving image resolution and reducing background noise and non-uniformity artifacts of the decoded images. Thus, the new imaging system associated with the image restoration algorithm may be an advance of low-count nuclear imaging.

## 1 Introduction

Coded aperture imaging systems were proposed previously by others to increase count sensitivity and image resolution [1-4]. The expectation maximization (EM) algorithm derived from the concept of maximum likelihood estimation (MLE) is an iterative image reconstruction method [5-7] which is often applied to reconstruct the source distribution from the acquired camera data. This method has been recognized to be superior to the commonly used filtered back projection method partially by virtue of its suitable mathematical model for nuclear imaging. The concept of blind deconvolution [8-12] is to restore a corrupted signal without a prior determination of the point spread function (PSF) of a linear imaging system. While the generic coded aperture imaging technique, the EM algorithm and the blind deconvolution method mentioned above are not new, the dual SPECT imaging systems and the EM-type blind deconvolution method (EMBD) presented herein have not been explored previously for acquiring and optimizing SPECT projections. In this paper, a new dual SPECT imaging system equipped with a parallel hole collimator camera head and a modular coded aperture (MCA) camera head (Park Medical Systems, Inc., Lachine, Quebec, Canada) are introduced. The EMBD method for pre-reconstruction restoration of SPECT projections is derived, and results of real brain phantom data are presented.

## 2 The Dual Imaging Configuration

A schematic of the dual image SPECT systems is shown in Fig. 1(a). The two camera heads are opposed in $180^0$ and are allowed to rotate in a $360^0$ orbit. The modular coded aperture configuration (see Fig. 1(b)) is constructed so as to have very little depth dependence (variability along the z-axis). This novel design minimizes the artifacts caused by the defocusing and overlapping of the photon detection [3-4]. For data acquisition, projections (planar images) are simultaneously acquired by the dual-headed SPECT camera systems. In this setup, the coded aperture head will acquire a count-rich image by virtue of the excellent count sensitivity of the coded aperture detector. On the other hand, the images acquired by the parallel hole collimator head will provide the uniformity and background information of the object.

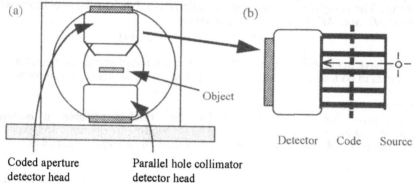

(a)  (b)

Object

Detector   Code   Source

Coded aperture  Parallel hole collimator
detector head  detector head

Fig. 1. A schematic of, (a) dual SPECT imaging system and, (b) the modular coded aperture camera head.

## 3 Derivation of the Dual Imaging EM Algorithm

### Table 1. Table of Symbols

| | |
|---|---|
| $i$ | pixel index in object space, (2D planar image) |
| $j$ | pixel index in parallel hole collimator space |
| $l$ | pixel index in coded aperture space |
| $\varepsilon$ | pixel index for the PSF of coded aperture |
| $\gamma$ | pixel index for the PSF of parallel hole collimator |
| $k$ | iteration number |
| $\mu 1, M1$ | projection data, associated random field for coded aperture space |
| $\mu 2, M2$ | projection data, associated random field for parallel hole collimator space |
| $\langle A \rangle_{x,y}$ | expected value of the random variable A conditioned on X = x and parameter y |
| $n, N$ | expected value of complete data, associated random variable |
| $\lambda$ | 2D source function |
| $\hat{\lambda}$ | maximum likelihood estimate of $\lambda$ |
| $\hat{\lambda}^{(k)}$ | maximum likelihood estimate of $\lambda$ at iteration k |
| $h_{li}$ | forward projection operator for coded aperture |
| $p_{ji}$ | forward projection operator for parallel hole collimator |

The incomplete data likelihood equation for the coded aperture system is expressed as,

$$\Pr(M1 = \mu 1 \mid \lambda) = \prod_i \frac{\left(\sum_i h_{li}\lambda_i\right)^{\mu l_i} \exp\left(-\sum_i h_{li}\lambda_i\right)}{\mu l_i !}, \quad (1)$$

and the incomplete data likelihood equation for the parallel hole collimator system is expressed as,

$$\Pr(M2 = \mu 2 \mid \lambda) = \prod_j \frac{\left(\sum_i p_{ji}\lambda_i\right)^{\mu 2_j} \exp\left(-\sum_i p_{ji}\lambda_i\right)}{\mu 2_j !}. \quad (2)$$

To relate the two incomplete data likelihoods, we begin with a complete data description which encompasses both systems - coded aperture and parallel hole collimator. The complete data random variable $N$ is related to the two incomplete data sets, $M1$ and $M2$ in the following manner:

$$\sum_{ij} N_{ijl} = M1_l, \quad (3), \quad \sum_{il} N_{ijl} = M2_j, \quad (4)$$

where we have made the usual assumption that the forward projection operators are probabilities in both detector spaces (coded aperture and parallel hole collimator):

$$\sum_l h_{li} = \sum_j p_{ji} = 1. \quad (5)$$

Given this definition for the complete data random variable, it is fairly straightforward to construct the complete data probability distributions and expected values. The expected value of the complete data random variable is defined as

$$\langle N_{ijl} \rangle \overset{def}{=} n_{ijl} = h_{li}p_{ji}\lambda_i. \quad (6)$$

with the <·> notation indicating expected values. Given the expected value of $N$ defined above, we may write the complete data likelihood equation as

$$\Pr(N = n \mid \lambda) = \prod_{ijl} \frac{(h_{li}p_{ji}\lambda_i)^{N_{ijl}} \exp(-h_{li}p_{ji}\lambda_i)}{N_{ijl}!}. \quad (7)$$

Possessed with the complete data likelihood equation, we may start the entire expectation-maximization (EM) steps in order to produce an algorithm for the estimation of the two dimensional (2D) source intensities given the dual-imaging counts - coded aperture and parallel hole collimator. We also assume that the coded aperture and the parallel hole collimator counts are conditionally independent of each other given the 2D source. This is a reasonable assumption since it is equivalent to assuming that the counts obtained from the coded aperture system are independent of the counts obtained by the parallel hole collimator system when the same object is imaged in both. Thus, based on the Bayes theorem and the two constraints shown in (3) and (4), we have

$$\Pr(N = n \mid M1 = \mu 1, M2 = \mu 2, \lambda) = \frac{\prod_{ijl} \frac{(h_{li}p_{ji}\lambda_i)^{N_{ijl}}}{N_{ijl}!}}{\sum_{\left[\substack{\{N_{ijl} = \{0,1,\ldots\} \forall i,j,l\} \\ \sum_{il} N_{ijl} = \mu 2_j, \\ \sum_{ij} N_{ijl} = \mu 1_l\}}\right]} \prod_{ijl} \frac{(h_{li}p_{ji}\lambda_i)^{N_{ijl}}}{N_{ijl}!}}. \quad (8)$$

The constrained summation over all configurations in (8) above is not trivial as in the more familiar single set of counts situation. When only one set of counts, say $M = \mu$ is available, we get instead of (8)

$$\Pr(N = n | M = \mu, \lambda) = \frac{\prod_{il} \frac{(h_{il}\lambda_i)^{N_{il}}}{N_{il}!}}{\sum_{\substack{\{N_{il}=\{0,1,...\} \forall i,l\} \\ \sum_i N_{il}=\mu_{1l}\}}} \prod_{il} \frac{(h_{il}\lambda_i)^{N_{il}}}{N_{il}!}} = \prod_i \frac{\mu_l!}{\prod_i N_{il}!} \prod_i \left(\frac{h_{il}\lambda_i}{\sum_i h_{il}\lambda_i}\right)^{N_{il}}. \quad (9)$$

This is a multinomial distribution. Since the $(N=n \mid M=\mu, \lambda)$ has such a simple and well known closed distribution form, calculation of the E-step is simple. Recall from (7) that the E-step requires the expected value of only those terms that depend on $\lambda$. Any terms in the E-step that are additively independent of $\lambda$ need not be evaluated since they are not needed in the M-step:

$$\langle \log \Pr(N = n | \lambda) \rangle_{\mu 1, \mu 2, \hat{\lambda}^{(k)}} = \sum_{ijl} \langle N_{ijl} \rangle_{\mu 1, \mu 2, \hat{\lambda}^{(k)}} \log(h_{il} p_{ji} \lambda_i) - \sum_{ijl} h_{il} p_{ji} \lambda_i. \quad (10)$$

Once the E-step has been evaluated, the M-step can be carried out by

$$\hat{\lambda}_i^{(k+1)} = \frac{\sum_{jl} \langle N_{ijl} \rangle_{\mu 1, \mu 2, \hat{\lambda}^{(k)}}}{\sum_{jl} h_{il} p_{ji}}. \quad (11)$$

We now present our heuristic for the E-step. Since satisfaction of the two incomplete data constraints is central to the E-step and separates it in complexity terms from the more simple single projection data case, our heuristic involves iterating so as to satisfy the two constraints:

$$\langle N_{ijl} \rangle_{\mu 1, \mu 2, \hat{\lambda}}^{(2k+1)} = \mu_{1l} \frac{h_{il} p_{ji} \hat{\lambda}_i^{(2k)}}{\sum_{ij} h_{il} p_{ji} \hat{\lambda}_i^{(2k)}} \quad (12), \quad \langle N_{ijl} \rangle_{\mu 1, \mu 2, \hat{\lambda}}^{(2k+2)} = \mu_{2j} \frac{h_{il} p_{ji} \hat{\lambda}_i^{(2k+1)}}{\sum_{il} h_{il} p_{ji} \hat{\lambda}_i^{(2k+1)}}. \quad (13)$$

This iterative algorithm completes our E-step. From (5) and (11), Eq.'s (12) and (13) above can be written as:

$$\hat{\lambda}_i^{(2k+1)} = \hat{\lambda}_i^{(2k)} \sum_l \frac{h_{il}}{\sum_i h_{il} \hat{\lambda}_i^{(2k)}} \mu_{1l} \quad (14), \quad \hat{\lambda}_i^{(2k+2)} = \hat{\lambda}_i^{(2k+1)} \sum_j \frac{p_{ji}}{\sum_i p_{ji} \hat{\lambda}_i^{(2k+1)}} \mu_{2j}, \quad (15)$$

respectively.

## 4 The EM-type Blind Deconvolution

The EM-based blind deconvolution was first derived by Holmes for fluorescence microscopy [11] in which only one incomplete data was considered. Because the linear model of the dual imaging system is analogous to that of fluorescence microscopy, we adapt this method to SPECT pre-reconstruction restoration of the dual projections, while *two* incomplete data sets are taken into account. Using the modified EMBD method, we estimate the tracer activity of the projected object as expressed in (14) and (15), and estimate the PSFs of the dual imaging systems by

$$\hat{h}_\varepsilon^{(k+1)} = \hat{h}_\varepsilon^{(k)} \sum_l \frac{\hat{\lambda}_{l-\varepsilon}^{(2k+2)}}{\sum_z \hat{\lambda}_{l-z}^{(2k+2)} \hat{h}_z^{(k)}} \mu_{1l} \quad (16), \quad \hat{p}_\gamma^{(k+1)} = \hat{p}_\gamma^{(k)} \sum_j \frac{\hat{\lambda}_{j-\gamma}^{(2k+2)}}{\sum_z \hat{\lambda}_{j-z}^{(2k+2)} \hat{p}_z^{(k)}} \mu_{2j}. \quad (17)$$

Notice that a spatially invariant linear system is assumed here.

## 5 Results

An elliptically cylindrical brain phantom was used in our experiments. The bottom of the phantom was filled with approximately 15 mm thick of a diluted solution of Tc-99m radio-active isotope. The phantom was placed at the midpoint between coded aperture and parallel hole collimators. The distances of the phantom from the coded aperture and from the parallel hole collimators were 8.5 and 8.0 inches, respectively. The coded aperture image (shadowgram) and parallel hole image of the phantom were acquired simultaneously using the SPECT systems illustrated in Fig. 1. The total counts acquired for the shadowgram and parallel hole collimator image were 13,577K (Fig. 2(a)) and 805K (Fig. 2(b)), respectively. The decoded image is shown in Fig. 2(c) which was obtained from decoding the shadowgram using the URA technique [3]. The matrix size for the images was 256×256 with a pixel size of 0.67 mm/pixel. As seen in Fig. 2(b), the parallel hole image is very noisy and contains almost no information about the rod structures of the phantom. The decoded image shown in Fig. 2(c) appears to be sharper than the parallel hole image. However, it suffers from severe non-uniformity and background noise artifacts caused by the coding and decoding processes.

In the EMBD restoration processes, we used the decoded image as a first guess for the object, a flat sheet image (constant pixel values) for the coded aperture PSF and a 2D Gaussian function image with a standard deviation of 5 pixels (3.35 mm) both in the x and y directions for the parallel hole collimator PSF. The selection of the width of 5 pixels for the PSF was arbitrary. Fig. 2(d) shows the image restored from Fig.'s 2(b,c) after 50 iterations of the EMBD method. As shown in Fig. 2(d), the image resolution, background noise and non-uniformity are significantly improved as compared to Fig.'s 2(b,c). Fig.'s 2(e) and (f) show the restored PSFs of the coded aperture and parallel hole collimator imaging system, respectively. Apparently, the restored PSF of the coded aperture has a better contrast than that of parallel hole collimator, since the coded aperture collimator has a higher count sensitivity than the conventional parallel hole collimator. Fig. 2(g) is the plot of log-likelihood for the restored images, and Fig. 2(h) is the plot of mean-squared-error (MSE) between the estimated and observed images, from 1 to 50 iterations. As seen, the log-likelihood increases and MSE decreases as a function of iterations, which implies the improvement of the restored images as iterations proceed.

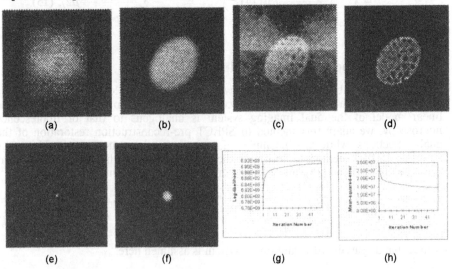

Fig. 2. (a) Shadowgram of the phantom, (b) parallel hole collimator image, (c) decoded image from the shadowgram using the URA technique; (d) restored image, (e) restored coded aperture PSF, (f) restored parallel hole collimator PSF, at 50 iterations of the EMBD; (g) log-likelihood plot and (h) MSE plot, for the restored images at 1-50 iterations of the EMBD.

# 6 Discussions and Conclusions

We have introduced a novel dual SPECT imaging system and derived a new EM-type blind deconvolution algorithm for pre-reconstruction restoration of SPECT projections. The method have been tested previously on computer simulated data (not shown in this paper). The results were quite encouraging. The results of real phantom data presented herein further demonstrated the feasibility of this method in improving the resolution and eliminating the background noise and non-uniformity artifacts of the decoded images. The background and uniformity information provided by the parallel hole collimator image was quite helpful for the dual restoration processes.

Pre-reconstruction restoration has an advantage over post-reconstruction restoration for SPECT images if a suitable model can be chosen for the planar projections [13]. The results presented herein demonstrates that our methods work quite well for the dual planar projections. By rotating the camera gantry and obtaining such projection data around $360^0$, we envision that the improved projections may result in a significant improvement on SPECT volume reconstructions.

*Acknowledgments*: The authors thank Dr. Gabriele Zacek for her helpful discussions.

# References

[1] M.M. Rogulski, H.B. Barber, H.H. Barrett, R.L. Shoemaker and J.M. Woolfenden, "Ultra-high-resolution brain SPECT imaging: simulation results," *IEEE TNS*, vol. 40, no. 4, pp. 1123-1129, 1993.

[2] T.A. Gooley and H.H. Barret, "Evaluation of statistical methods of image reconstruction through ROI analysis," *IEEE TMI*, vol. 11, no. 2, pp.276-283, 1992.

[3] E.E. Fenimore and T.M. Cannon, "Uniformly redundant arrays: digital reconstruction methods," *Applied Optics*, vol. 20, no. 10, pp. 1858-1864, 1981.

[4] G.R. Gindi, "Use of a priori information for improved tomography imaging in coded-aperture systems," *U. of Arizona, Ph.D. Thesis*, 1982.

[5] A.P. Dempster, N.M. Laird and D.B. Rubin, "Maximum likelihood from incomplete data via the EM algorithm," *J. Royal Statist. Soc. (London) Series B*, vol. 39, pp. 1-38, 1977.

[6] L.A. Shepp and Y. Vardi, "Maximum likelihood reconstruction for emission tomography," *IEEE TMI*, vol. 1, pp. 113-121, 1982.

[7] R.E. Carson and K. Lange, "The EM parametric image reconstruction algorithm," *J. Amer. Statis. Ass.*, vol. 80, pp. 20-22, 1985.

[8] B.C. McCallum, "Blind deconvolution by simulated annealing," *Optics Comm.*, vol. 75, no. 2, pp. 101-105, 1990.

[9] J.H. Seldin and J.R. Fienup, "Iterative blind deconvolution algorithm applied to phase retrieval," *J. Opt. Soc. A*, vol. 7, no. 3, pp. 428-433, 1990.

[10] G.R. Ayers and J.G. Dainty, "Iterative blind deconvolution method and its applications," *Optics Let.*, vol. 13, no. 7, pp. 547-549, 1988.

[11] T.J. Holmes, "Blind deconvolution of quantum-limited incoherent imagery: maximum-likelihood approach," *J. Opt. Soc. Am. A*, vol. 9, no. 7, pp. 1052-1061, 1992.

[12] V. Krishnamurthi, Y.H. Liu, S. Bhattacharyya, J.N. Turner and T.J. Holmes, "Blind deconvolution of fluorescence micrographs by maximum-likelihood estimation," *Applied Optics*, vol. 34, no. 29, pp. 6633-6647, 1995.

[13] D. Boulfelfel, R.M. Rangayyan, L.J. Hahn and R. Koliber, "Prereconstruction restoration of myocardial single photon emission computed tomography images," *IEEE TMI*, vol. 11, pp. 336-341, 1992.

# Reconstruction of the Intracerebral Vasculature from MRA and a Pair of Projection Views

Elizabeth Bullitt, Alan Liu, Stephen Aylward, Stephen M. Pizer

Medical Image Display and Analysis Group,
University of North Carolina, Chapel Hill, NC

**Abstract.** Clinicians cannot easily visualize 3D intracerebral vascular anatomy in adequate detail. We present methods of creating a detailed, 3D vascular map from an MRA and a pair of x-ray angiograms. The MRA provides a 3D reconstruction base. Core-based methods segment the datasets and provide 3D-2D registration. Angiographic data not included in the MRA are automatically reconstructed into 3D, using methods capable of dealing with viewplane error. We provide algorithms for automatically associating 2D curves and test our methods in phantom data.

## 1. Introduction

For the neurosurgeon, it is often critical to visualize intracranial vessels in 3 dimensions (3D). Unfortunately, 3D datasets such as magnetic resonance angiograms (MRA) often contain insufficient detail. Projection angiograms (angiograms) provide high detail from a fixed point of view. Reconstruction of angiograms into 3D would therefore be helpful.

Reconstruction of the intracerebral vasculature from projection views is difficult for several reasons. First, the intracranial vasculature is so overlapped on projection that the human eye cannot identify associated points or structures on separated views. Second, the number of available views is small. Third, reconstruction that does not depend upon user identification of points requires the computer to make associations under conditions of error. Although many groups have attempted 3D intracerebral vascular reconstruction from small numbers of views, a clinically useful solution has proven elusive.

This report describes a new approach to intracerebral vascular reconstruction. We use "core" methods of segmentation and registration and employ reconstruction algorithms capable of dealing with viewplane error. A preliminary description has been published [3]. We have also performed limited but clinically useful reconstructions from true angiograms [4,5]. This paper describes methods of large volume reconstruction in the presence of error, provides algorithms for automatic 2D curve pairing, and tests the curve-pairing methods in phantom data in the presence of error.

## 2. Method of 3D Angiographic Reconstruction

The approach uses a pair of angiograms and an MRA obtained from the same patient. Vessels extracted from the MRA are used as a 3D base. The finer network of vessels seen only by angiography are then reconstructed into 3D, building upon the MRA base. This process requires 5 steps, listed below and described in more detail later. We use the terms 2- and *3D curve* to refer to skeletons of 2- and 3D tubular objects. All objects also have widths.

1) *3D segmentation of MRA*: The MRA is segmented into individual, unbranched 3D curves, used both for registration and as the initial 3D base.

2) *2D segmentation of angiograms:* Each angiogram is segmented into a set of 2D curves. 2D curves associated with projections of the MRA are used for registration. 2D curves not associated with MRA vessels are reconstructed into 3D.

3) *Registration of each angiogram with the MRA*: The pose of the MRA relative to each angiogram is computed, using 3D curves and their projections as fiducial markers.

4) *Reconstruction of a 3D curve from 2D curves in the presence of error*: For tubular objects, the projection of a 3D object's skeleton generally coincides with the skeleton of the object's projection. One can create 3D curves by pairing selected points along 2D curve pairs. Our methods estimate the capacity of two 2D curves to combine to create a 3D object. This *match value* is used to help pair 2D curves.

5) *Pairing of 2D curves:* For any given 2D curve on view A, the program must select among tens or hundreds of choices the correct 2D curve on view B. If 2D curves are paired incorrectly, a spurious 3D curve will be created. Our approach to automated 2D curve pairing involves both an assessment of 2D connectivity and match values.

## 2.1 3D Segmentation of MRA Data

Our 3D segmentation methods are based upon core and medialness methodology [11, 12, 13], as adapted by Aylward [1]. For tubular figures, each core represents a 3D curve running longitudinally down the center of the figure in spatial coordinates, with an associated scale σ giving the approximate width at each point.

MRA vessels are close to circular in cross-section and have central intensity extrema. The spatial locus of such objects can be located as an image intensity ridge [1]. This ridge is calculated beginning from an interactively provided seed point. A calculation of the local maximum in medialness is automatically performed at each ridge point via gradient ascent from the previous ridge point's maximum, thus assuring continuity of width. This method has the advantage of speed [1].

For extraction of vessels from an MRA dataset, the user is presented a set of MRA slices and provides seed points by clicking upon a point within a vessel, simultaneously supplying an estimate of width. Given this seed point, vessel extraction is automatic.

## 2.2 2D Segmentation of Angiographic Data

2D angiographic segmentation is performed by core-based methods, as described by Fritsch [8]. The 2D curves and widths extracted are ridges of medialness in x, y, σ. As with the 3D segmentation method, the user supplies seed points and a simultaneous estimate of expected width. The program then automatically extracts an individual vessel projection represented continuously across crossings of smaller vessel projections.

## 2.3 Registration of Each Angiogram with the MRA

The 3D-2D registration process uses as primitives the 2D curves extracted from an angiogram at sub-pixel resolution and the 3D curves extracted from an MRA at sub-voxel resolution. The registration program is given these skeletons with about 8 vessels paired interactively, and a rough approximation of the 3D dataset pose. No point-to-point mapping is provided by the user. Given the initial pose approximation, the program optimizes, on the projection plane, an objective function based on the iterative closest point measure [2] between the angiogram skeletons and the projections of the MRA skeletons. Newton's method on the pose parameters in 3D is used to iteratively refine the solution until the optimum of the objective function is reached. This process is repeated for a preset number of iterations or until convergence criteria are met [9].

## 2.4 Reconstruction of a 3D Curve from a Pair of 2D curves

We can automatically reconstruct a pair of directed 2D curves into a 3D curve in the presence of error. The last point mapped into 3D space, together with the two viewplane points used to create this point, define an epipolar plane. It is impossible to determine the course of a 3D curve within an epipolar plane. However, one can identify the next point lying outside of the current epipolar plane along each directed 2D curve, thus providing a new seed point that permits reconstruction to continue [6].

We define a *viewplane error* as any error in the set of 2D points describing a 2D curve. When reconstruction is performed by the rules of epipolar geometry, viewplane error may prevent appropriate ray intersections from occurring. It is possible to accomodate for small viewplane errors by increasing the area upon which a 3D point is allowed to project, such as by defining 2D curves in pixel units. The cost of such accomodation is a fuzzy reconstruction. Bullitt [7] analyzes these costs, which are dependent upon several factors including the relative angle of the reconstruction views.

Missing 2D points or errors producing point projections outside of the correct pixel must be handled differently. If a sequence of points is missing at the start of one 2D curve or if registration error precludes ray intersections at a loop apex, reconstruction will stop. In such cases, we search for a new seed point along each of the two 2D curves, looking for the shortest possible distance along both curves for a pixel pair that produces a ray-ray intersection. The search length is limited both in 2- and 3D, contributing both to program speed and curve-pairing specificity. Width of the reconstructed vessel is determined by the viewing geometry, the location of the 3D skeleton points, and the widths of the 2D curves. Specific algorithms [6] and error analysis [7] exist.

This method produces an ordered set of 3D points separated by explicitly delineated regions of uncertainty that, if needed, can be filled in by a third view. When viewplane errors interrupt reconstruction, the program automatically approximates the error's location and quantifies lost information by the search length for the next seed point. The number of 3D points, decremented by a penalty proportional to search lengths, approximates the ability of a 2D curve pair to combine to create a 3D object. This *match value* can be used to help associate 2D curve pairs.

## 2.5 Algorithms for Automatic 2D curve Pairing

Our methods use 2D connectivity, the match values provided by our curve creation methods, and the presence of a 3D base to automatically associate 2D curve pairs.

The algorithm repeatedly calls a function that maps a single, new branch if

1) A 2D curve on view A (curveA) identifies a 2D curve on view B (curveB) as providing a match value clearly greater than any other choice on view B,

2) CurveB identifies curveA as its clearly superior numerical match,

3) The proposed match is numerically superior to any other match involving curveA or curveB, and

4) CurveA and curveB each have at their bases the projections of a vessel already mapped in space. A line between the projections of the parental connection point and the child's start point fails to cross empty space on either projection (2D connectivity).

Since a long 2D curve on one view may map to a sequence of short 2D curves on the second view, match calculations often must evaluate competing 2D curve chains. Views containing short 2D curves and heavy projection overlap may produce many hundreds of possible curve combinations.

Once a new vessel is selected it is added to the 3D base to serve as a potential parent for future generations. The 2D curves or curve portion used to create a new vessel are removed from further consideration. Match calculations are updated before the next choice is made. Since projection overlap and a variety of errors produce gaps in the 2D representation of 3D vessels, the program is allowed to bridge limited 3D gaps.

Ideally, the above function will be called repeatedly until all 2D curves are mapped. In practice, the program may be unable to make a decision because short 2D curves have similar match values, because viewplane error decrements the value of an appropriate match, or because a 2D curve is missing.

If ambiguity or error blocks reconstruction, a number of recovery functions are available. If a recovery function is successful in mapping a new branch, the program updates the match calculations and reenters its primary reconstruction loop. Recovery functions take several approaches. The stringency of a "clearly superior" match is first reduced. Match value ties and less desirable match choices are then examined. If the program is still unable to make a decision, a recovery function identifies the 2D curve pair whose match value is the greatest relative to any competing match involving that pair of 2D curves. A new root is thus created, allowing reconstruction to continue past a 3D gap unbridgeable by other means.

## 3. Tests of Reconstruction Methods

We tested this approach by reconstructing simulated angiograms in the presence of viewplane error. Vessels were segmented from MRA datasets and connected into trees. Vascular trees likely to be seen on an angiographic projection (e.g. a middle cerebral complex plus the anterior cerebral group) were projected onto viewplanes of 1024 x 1024 pixels using clinically used oblique and lateral views. For this test, 2D curves were defined mathematically, but several 2D curves were broken into multiple pieces to simulate the situation in which a long 2D curve on one view maps to a sequence of curves on the second view. Each view contained 45-65 2D curves. Pairs of 2D images were then reconstructed into 3D. A single vessel was used as the 3D reconstruction base.

Viewplane error was introduced by mistranslating the entire 3D dataset relative to one view at a time. We have previously tested our registration methods [10]. Following registration of clinically used views, the MAXIMUM 3D point placement error is less than 0.01cm in x, 0.01 cm in y, and 0.1 cm in z of the viewplane coordinate system, in which z represents the depth of the 3D point [9]. In order to relate the error tolerance of the reconstruction program to the likely errors produced by our registration method, mistranslations of the 3D dataset were introduced by multiples of 1-4 of the "error unit" (0.01, 0.01, 0.1). A total of 9 reconstructions were performed for each dataset: one reconstruction in the absence of registration error and, for each of the 2 views, 4 reconstructions in the presence of progressively severe registration error.

Results were evaluated by comparing the reconstructed vessels with the vessels used to create the projection images. For surgical planning purposes, results were judged acceptable if the reconstruction appeared correct from 3 mutually orthogonal angles of view and if mean point placement errors were less than 0.2 cm. For stereotactic surgery, an additional requirement was a limit of 0.5 cm on gap length and point placement errors. Three different datasets were reconstructed, for a total of 27 tests.

All 27 reconstructions met the requirements of utility for surgical planning. Mean point placement errors remained less than 0.2 cm for all 27 tests. No 3D point was misplaced by 0.5 cm or more. In the absence of registration error, mean point placement errors were $0.01 \pm 0.02$ cm or better. In the presence of registration error some 2D curves became incapable of pairing with their proper mates, thus producing missing and spurious 2D curves on each projection view. Although 2D curve pairing errors did occur, they were confined to closely adjacent, short, 2D curve segments.

Five reconstructions at high levels of registration error failed the additional criterion for stereotactic surgery because of a missing peripheral branch. Although our algorithms appear capable of preventing a cascade of 2D curve pairing errors produced by an initial error or by a missing 2D curve, and although we can bridge short internal gaps, we cannot reconstruct a peripheral branch if one of its 2D curves is undefined on one view or if viewplane error prevents the appropriate 2D curves from matching with each other.

## 4. Discussion

Reconstruction of the intracerebral vasculature is difficult largely because the human eye cannot associate paired points on separated views. This paper describes a method of reconstructing the intracerebral vasculature from a pair of widely separated projection views and an MRA, under conditions in which viewplane error is present and 2D curve pairings are performed automatically.

Reconstruction detail is directly related to pixel size. This report employs viewplanes subdivided into 1024x1024 pixels of 0.03x0.03 cm. Such reconstructions can provide much higher detail than is possible by traditional 3D imaging modalities.

The reconstruction algorithms are reasonably fast. Reconstruction of a pair of views each containing 50 2D curves takes 15-20 minutes on a DEC 5000/200. The time required to segment an MRA and 2 angiographic images is approximately an hour. Higher speed and efficiency are achievable in all modules. Methods to decrease user intervention during segmentation and registration are under development.

We have, at present, confined our efforts in true angiographic data to local reconstructions [4,5], since only local registration is required. Before performing large volume reconstructions, we need to correct both viewplane distortions and MRA magnetic distortion error, as described by others [e.g., 10].

In summary, this report describes a method of reconstructing projection angiograms of the intracerebral vasculature into 3D in the presence of viewplane error and at clinically useful levels of detail. In addition, the approach is applicable to segmentation and reconstruction of connected tubular objects in any part of the body. Examples include other vascular trees, nerves, long bones, and the bronchi. The 3D-2D registration algorithm is applicable to any situation in which tubular objects are present.

## References

1. S. Aylward, S.M. Pizer, E. Bullitt, D. Eberly: Intensity ridge and widths for 3D object segmentation and description. IEEE WMMBIA 96TB100056, 131-138 (1996).
2. P. Besl, N. McKay: A method for registration of 3D shapes. IEEE-PAMI 14, 239-256, (1992).
3. E. Bullitt, M. Soltys, J. Chen, J.R. Rosenman, S.M. Pizer: Three-dimensional reconstruction of intracranial vessels from biplane projection views. J Neurosci Meth 66,13-22 (1996).
4. E. Bullitt, A. Liu, S. Aylward, M. Soltys, J. Rosenman, S.M. Pizer: Methods of displaying intracerebral vascular anatomy. Amer J Neuroradiol (to appear 3/97).
5. E. Bullitt, A. Liu, S. Aylward, S.M. Pizer: Three-dimensional reconstruction of aneurysms from projection views. J Neurol Neurosurg Psychiatr (in press).
6. E. Bullitt, A. Liu, S.M. Pizer: Three-dimensional reconstruction of curves from pairs of projection views in the presence of error. I. Algorithms. TR# 96-047 (submitted Med Phys).
7. E. Bullitt, A. Liu, S.M. Pizer: Three-dimensional reconstruction of curves from pairs of projection views in the presence of error. II. Analysis of error. TR# 96-048 (submitted Med Phys).
8. D.S Fritsch, D. Eberly, S.M. Pizer, M.J. McAuliffe MJ: Stimulated cores and their applications in medical imaging. In: Y. Bizais, C. Barillot, R. DiPaola(eds): IPMI '95. Dordrecht: Kluwer Series Computational Imaging and Vision 1995, pp.365-368.
9. A. Liu, E. Bullitt, S.M. Pizer: 3D/2D registration using tubular anatomical structures as a basis. TR # 96-053 (submitted IEEE-TMI).
10. J. Michiels, P. Pelgrims, H. Bosmans, D. Vandermeulen, J. Gybels, G. Marchal, P. Suetens: On the problem of geometric distortion in magnetic resonance images for stereotactic neurosurgery. Mag Res Imag 12, 749-765 (1994).
11. B.S. Morse, S.M. Pizer, D.K. Puff, C. Gu: Zoom-invariant vision of figural shape: effects on cores of image disturbances. CVIU (in press).
12. S.M. Pizer, C.A. Burbeck, J.M. Coggins, D.S. Fritsch, B.S. Morse: Object shape before boundary shape: Scale-space medial axes. J Math Imag Vis 4, 303-312 (1994).
13. S.M. Pizer, D. Eberly, B.S. Morse, D.S. Fritsch: Zoom-invariant vision of figural shape: the mathematics of cores. CVIU (in press).

Supported by P01CA47982, R01CA67812 NCI-NIH.

# Two Alternative Forced Choice Evaluation of Vessel Visibility Increases Due to Zero-filled Interpolation in MR Angiography

Brian E. Chapman[1], K. Craig Goodrich[3], Andrew L. Alexander[2], Duane D. Blatter[3], Dennis L. Parker[1,2]

[1] Department of Medical Informatics, University of Utah, Salt Lake City, UT
Department of Radiology, University of Utah, Salt Lake City, UT
[2] Department of Radiology, LDS Hospital, Salt Lake City, UT

**Abstract.** The effects of reconstructing low resolution 3D time-of-flight MR images using zero-filled interpolation were examined using observer performance measures. Two alternative forced choice experiments using digital subtraction angiography images as a truth standard were performed. MR angiography data were acquired from six patient volunteers and were reconstructed with and without zero-filled interpolation. The MR angiography images were evaluated by generating divergent maximum intensity projection images with the same view as digital subtraction angiography images obtained on the patients as part of their clinical workup. The projection images were evaluated by three observers. Zero-filled interpolation significantly increased the detectibility of very small vessels (diameters less than 0.7 mm) but had no significant effect on larger vessels.

## 1 Introduction

Cerebral magnetic resonance angiography (MRA) is an important technology as it can visualize the vasculature in a less invasive and less expensive method than conventional x-ray angiography (XRA). However, standard MRA techniques fail to produce the small cerebral vessel detail which can be seen in XRA and which is important for the diagnosis of a variety of pathologies. Thus improving the visualization of small cerebral vessels is an important research topic.

Clinically viable MRA techniques need to be performed at a moderate resolution for which many vessels of interest are of sub-voxel diameter. Unfortunately the MRA imaging techniques are not uniformly sensitive to signals from these sub-voxel vessels. Depending on the actual position within the reconstruction voxel, a sub-voxel vessel may be well visualized or not visualized at all. A simple but effective method for improving the visualization of sub-voxel vessels is zero filled interpolation (ZFI) [1] which reconstructs the image on a finer grid than the acquisition. We hypothesize that applying ZFI will significantly increase the visualization of vessels of the size of a voxel or smaller but will have little effect on the visualization of larger structures.

An important question which arises in assessing the technical efficacy of MRA, is what measure should be used to quantify vessel visibility. Blatter *et al.*, examined vessel visibility in MRA based on expected anatomy [2]. This method suffered, however, from not having a truth standard since anatomy varies widely between patients. Contrast-to-noise ratio (CNR) is a convenient and quantitative measure of vessel visibility. But it is not precisely known how changes in CNR relate to changes in observer detection of vessels in a correlated background (*e.g.*, image artifacts, background tissue structures, *etc.*) although Eckstein and Whiting found that signal contrast energy was quite accurate in predicting detection of simulated arteries in a coronary angiogram background [3].

In this paper we present an observer performance evaluation of vessel visualization in cerebral MRA using a two alternative forced choice experiment (2AFC) [3, 4, 5] which directly measures an observers ability to differentiate vessel structures from correlated background.

## 2 Theory

### 2.1 Image Resolution in MRA

The intensity in the reconstructed image of a point located in the object being imaged in an MR scanner is determined by the voxel sensitivity function (VSF), which is nonuniform across the voxel [6]. Points in the imaged object which are smaller than a voxel may or may not appear in the reconstructed image, depending on where they lie within the voxel region. Sub-voxel vessel structures which lie near the edge of the voxel will be poorly visualized in the reconstructed image.

It has been demonstrated by many groups that increasing the image acquisition matrix improves the visualization of small vessels in MRA. However, increasing the acquisition matrix increases the acquisition time and decreases the signal-to-noise ratio for objects larger than a voxel.

ZFI is a post-processing means of increasing the visualization of sub-voxel structures without increasing the image acquisition matrix. Instead, the image reconstruction matrix is increased. ZFI data is acquired on an acquisition matrix of size N but is reconstructed on an image matrix of size LN, where L is the interpolation factor. The ZFI can be accomplished by zero-padding the MR spectral data to a larger size, as we did for the data examined in this paper, or equivalently using a voxel-shifted interpolation (VSI) technique [1].

ZFI does not increase the image resolution, since no estimates of the higher frequency components are made as they are in various superresolution techniques. However, by reconstructing on a finer grid, each point along sub-voxel structures will be found to lie closer to a voxel center and the maximum of the VSF and thus are better visualized in the image. Du *et al.* applied VSI to 3D MRA data and found a significant increase in vessel CNR and qualitative increases in vessel continuity and vessel edge definition [1].

### 2.2 2AFC Evaluation

2AFC is a signal detection measure which directly measures an observer's ability to differentiate a noise-only stimulus from a signal-plus-noise stimulus where the class of the stimulus is determined by some reference truth standard. In the context of our evaluations, a noise-only stimulus is a region-of-interest (ROI) containing background tissue, artifacts, and electronic noise. The signal-plus-noise stimulus is similar to the noise-only ROI except with the addition of a vessel imbedded in the background tissue. The 2AFC experiment simultaneously presents an observer with a randomly selected signal-plus-noise stimulus and a noise-only stimulus and forces the observer to choose which of the stimuli is signal-plus-noise. The proportion of correctly identified signal-plus-noise stimuli ($P_c$) can be shown to be equivalent to the area under the ROC curve [5].

The details of our 2AFC experiments are presented elsewhere [7, 8]. Here we provide just a brief summary. We use digital subtraction angiography (DSA) images acquired on patient volunteers as a truth standard for assessing the location, orientation, and size of the patients vasculature. We project a subregion of the 3D MRA data as a 2D image with the same view and magnification as the DSA image using a divergent maximum intensity projection (MIP) algorithm. The registration of the MRA MIP images to the DSA images is limited by geometric distortions present in both imaging modalities and the comparative quality of the MIP images is compromised both by the image misregistration and by imperfections in the volume subregioning. The divergent MIP images are evaluated by multiple observers. Observer responses to the ROIs in the MRA MIP images are compared to the DSA truth standard to calculate $P_c$ which is used as the figure of merit for image quality.

## 3 Methods

Six patients from two institutions undergoing intra-arterial cerebral angiography were invited to participate in an MR angiography study. The studies were performed in accordance with an Institutional Review Board approved protocol. All patients provided informed consent.

DSA images were acquired on GE Advantx digital angiography systems (General Electric Medical Systems, Waukasha, Wis.). Contrast injection was subselective into either the right or left internal carotid artery. The DSA images were acquired on a 1024x1024 grid and were corrected for pincushion and sigmoidal distortions.

MRA images were obtained on Signa 1.5 Tesla scanners operating with the 5.4 operating system (GE Medical, Waukasha, Wisconsin). The images we obtained were acquired in a single slab 3D time-of-flight (TOF) acquisition with a 256x256 acquisition matrix and 32 axial slices. Voxel dimensions were 0.86 mm x 0.86 mm x 0.80 mm. A fractional echo of 0.6 was collected. Magnetization transfer was used to suppress signal from the background tissue. The top two and bottom two slices of the slab were discarded.

Images were reconstructed using a homodyne reconstruction method as described by Noll, *et al.* to correct for the partial echo acquisition [9]. In one set of images the image was reconstructed on the same resolution grid as the image acquisition. The other set of images were obtained from the same raw data and reconstructed using the same homodyne algorithm, but the spectral data was zero-padded to a 512x512x56 grid before reconstructing.

ROIs for observer evaluation were defined by three closely spaced points connected by linear line segments. The ROIs were selected from the lateral DSA images without reference to the MRA images other than to confirm that the ROIs lie in the MRA imaged regions. Signal-plus-noise ROIs were selected along vessel centerlines. Noise-only ROIs were defined on the DSA by tracing out lines which mimic vessels in regions void of visible vessels. Between 100 to 150 ROIs, roughly equally split between signal-plus-noise and noise-only, were selected from each DSA image.

The signal-plus-noise ROIs were categorized according to estimated signal strength (vessel size). Vessel size was estimated from the DSA images by reference to the major cerebral vessels imaged. Vessels were categorized as "very small" (diameter less than 0.7 mm), "small" (between 0.7 mm and 1.2 mm) or "medium" (between 1.2 mm and 2.0 mm).

For a given image the signal-plus-noise ROIs were placed in a randomized list and the noise-only ROIs were placed in another randomized list. A signal-plus-noise ROI was randomly placed in either the right or left canvas of an observer panel which contained two image regions. The noise-only ROI was then placed in the remaining canvas. The observer was forced to choose whether the right or left ROI was the signal-plus-noise ROI. The process continued until all the ROI pairs for that image were evaluated. Then the next image was brought up and the process was repeated until all twelve images were evaluated.

Images were evaluated in either a ZFI then non-ZFI order or a non-ZFI then ZFI order. The ZFI and non-ZFI images from the same patient were separated by an average of five images.

The data from the three observers were pooled into one large data set of $N$ forced choices. $P_c$ was calculated for both the total forced choices and for the vessel size specific data. $P_c$ is a binomial random variable with standard deviation $s(P_c) = \sqrt{P_c(1 - P_c)/N}$. The statistical significance of differences between two $P_c$ values was determined by forming a $z$ statistic $z = (P_{c1} - P_{c2})/\sqrt{s^2(P_{c1}) + s^2(P_{c2})}$ which was tested as a two-tailed normal variable. Our estimate of the standard deviation neglects two factors: first, we do not account for the correlation between images which would serve to increase the significance of our results [10]; second, we do not account for the correlation between forced choices that results from pooling the data, which would tend to decrease our significance. We tried to reduce this correlation by randomly assigning each signal-plus-noise/noise-only pairing for each observation; that is, each observer is comparing a given signal-plus-noise ROI with a different noise-only ROI.

## 4 Results

Examples of both the non-ZFI and ZFI divergent MIP images are shown in Fig. 1. A total of 948 signal-plus-noise/noise-only ROI pairs were evaluated for both ZFI and non-ZFI images. For the ZFI images 827 ($P_c = 0.8724$) of the signal-plus-noise ROIs were correctly chosen while for the non-ZFI images 803 were correctly chosen ($P_c = 0.8470$). Overall the difference between the two techniques was not significant ($z = 1.59$, $p = 0.11$). However, when the data was analyzed by estimated vessel size (see Fig. 2), the very small vessels (estimated vessel diameter less than 0.7 mm) had a 0.17 increase in $P_c$ ($P_c = 0.6548$ vs. $P_c = 0.8235$) with the use of the ZFI which was the only statistically significant ($z = 2.5430$, $p = 0.01$) effect observed, as hypothesized.

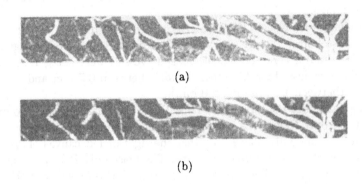

(a)

(b)

**Fig. 1.** Examples of the projective MIP images. (a) is the ZFI image from patient five while (b) is the non-ZFI image from the same patient. Note the improved continuity of vessels in the ZFI images as well as the increased visualization of small vessels.

## 5   Discussion

We have demonstrated the usefulness of ZFI for increasing the visualization of subvoxel sized vessels in 3D TOF MRA. The increase was achieved with moderate computational expense by reconstructing on a matrix twice the size of the acquisition matrix. Three observers used the 2AFC to evaluate both ZFI images and the non-ZFI images from six patients. The proportion correct for vessels with diameters less than 0.7 mm increased from 0.6548 to 0.8235 when ZFI was used. The detectibility of larger vessels was not statistically significantly different between the two reconstruction techniques. These results demonstrate the usefulness of ZFI for small vessel visualization in MRA. Future work will focus on evaluating MRA using the full 3D data.

## References

1. Y. P. Du, D. L. Parker, W. L. Davis, and G. Gao. Reduction of partial-volume artifacts with zero-filled interpolation in three-dimensional MR angiography. *Journal of Magnetic Resonance Imaging*, 4:733–741, 1994.

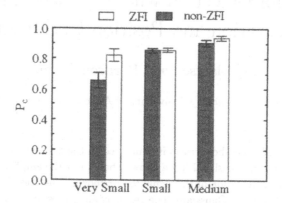

**Fig. 2.** Comparison of 2AFC $P_c$ for ZFI (white) and non-ZFI (gray) reconstruction. Vessel size categories are very small (diameter less than 0.7 mm), small (diameter between 0.7 and 1.2 mm), and medium (diameter between 1.2 and 2.0 mm). The effect on the very small vessels is the only significant effect, as hypothesized.

2. D. D. Blatter, D. L. Parker, and R. O. Robison. Cerebral MR angiography with multiple overlapping thin slab acquisition: part I. quantitative analysis of vessel visibility. *Radiology*, 179:805–811, 1991.

3. M. P. Eckstein and J. S. Whiting. Visual signal detection in structured background I. effect of number of possible spatial locations and signal contrast. *Journal of the Optical Society of America A*, 13:1777–1787, 1996.

4. A. E. Burgess. Comparison of receiver operating characteristic and forced choice observer performance measurement methods. *Medical Physics*, 22:643–655, 1995.

5. J. A. Hanley and B. J. McNeil. The meaning and the use of the area under a receiver operating characteristic (ROC) curve. *Diagnostic Radiology*, 143:29–36, 1982.

6. D. L. Parker, Y. P. Du, and W. L. Davis. The voxel sensitivity function in Fourier transform imaging: applications to magnetic resonance angiography. *Magnetic Resonance in Medicine*, 33:156–162, 1995.

7. B. E. Chapman, A. R. Sanderson, K. C. Goodrich, A. Alexander, D. D. Blatter, and D. L. Parker. A two alternative forced choice evaluation of blood vessel visibility in MR angiograms. In *Proceedings of the ISMRM 4th Scientific Meeting*, 1996.

8. B. E. Chapman, A. R. Sanderson, K. C. Goodrich, A. Alexander, D. D. Blatter, and D. L. Parker. Observer performance methodologies for evaluating blood vessel visibility in MR angiograms using accurate geometric registration to high resolution x-ray angiograms. to appear, *Magnetic Resonance in Medicine*.

9. D. C. Noll, D. G. Nishimura, and A. Macovski. Homodyne detection in magnetic resonance imaging. *IEEE Transactions on Medical Imaging*, 10:154–163, 1991.

10. J. A. Swets and R. M. Pickett. *Evaluation of Diagnostic Systems*. Academic Press, New York, 1982.

# Bayesian Detection with Amplitude, Scale, Orientation and Position Uncertainty

Eric Clarkson and Harrison Barrett

Department of Radiology, University of Arizona, Tucson, AZ 85724

**Abstract.** The likelihood ratio is computed in the case where the background is known, the signal has a known shape, but the amplitude, scale, orientation and location of the signal are unknown. The noise is assumed to be additive i.i.d. Gaussian. The result is an expression involving the mutidimensional wavelet transform of the data with respect to the signal. The linear and quadratic approximations to the full likelihood statistic are examined in detail and are seen to involve operations commonly used in this context. Finally the full nonlinear ratio is formulated in terms of an amplification and modulation mechanism from the data to the prior probabilty distribution on the unknown parameters.

## 1  Introduction

The detection of signals with parameter uncertainty has been studied extensively for decades [8,9]. Various combinations of amplitude, scale, orientation and/or position uncertainty have been examined with both linear and non-linear discriminants [2,3]. These are particularly useful in optical pattern recognition, for example [1,4]. In this article we examine the likelihood ratio for a signal with additive i.i.d. Gaussian noise in the presence of all of these uncertainties. Therefore the signal to be detected has a known shape but unknown amplitude, scale, orientation and position. After formulating the general problem in terms of the average likelihood ratio, we first examine the linear and quadratic approximations. Many of the commonly used procedures - averaging over parameters, Fourier transforming or Mellin transforming the data and signal - show up at this stage. Finally, we show that the full likelihood ratio has a relatively straightforward interpretation involving modulating the prior parameter probability distribution with a nonlinear function of the wavelet transform of the data with respect to the signal. Since the parameters in this problem form a group, left invariant integration on this group is used for averaging. This is useful for displaying the symmetries of the likelihood ratio and also allows the wavelet transform to be introduced, which simplifies some calculations. However, the group structure of the parameter set is not crucial for many of the arguments.

## 2 The likelihood ratio

We consider the likelihood ratio in the case where the background $\mathbf{b}$ is known exactly and the signal $\mathbf{s}$ has parameters that are unknown. If $\mathbf{d}$ is the data, then we have $\Lambda(\mathbf{d}) = \frac{Pr(\mathbf{d}|H_1)}{Pr(\mathbf{d}|H_0)}$, with hypotheses $H_0 : \mathbf{d} = \mathbf{b} + \mathbf{n}$ and $H_1 : \mathbf{d} = \mathbf{b} + \mathbf{n} + \mathbf{s}(A, g)$, for some $A$ and $g$. In these equations $A$ is the signal amplitude, $g$ contains the other parameters of the signal and is an element of some group $G$, which will be specified later, and $\mathbf{f}, \mathbf{b}, \mathbf{n}, \mathbf{s}(A, g) \in \mathbb{R}^M$. We take the $n_m, m = 1, \ldots, M$ to be i.i.d. Gaussian with variance $\sigma^2$. Let $pr_n(\mathbf{n})$ be the probability density function for $\mathbf{n}$ and $\mathbf{f} = \mathbf{d} - \mathbf{b}$. Then $Pr(\mathbf{d}|H_0) = pr_n(\mathbf{f})$ and $Pr(\mathbf{d}|H_1) = \int_G \int_{\mathbb{R}^+} pr_n(\mathbf{f} - \mathbf{s}(A, g)) \, pr(A, g) dA dg$. The function $pr(A, g)$ is a prior distribution on the parameters $A$ and $g$, and $dg$ is the left invariant measure on the group $G$. All that we need to know about this measure is $\int_G w(g_0 g) dg = \int_G w(g) dg$ for any $g_0 \in G$. The likelihood ratio is now

$$\Lambda(\mathbf{f}) = \int_G \int_{\mathbb{R}^+} exp\left[\frac{\mathbf{f}^\top \mathbf{s}(A, g)}{\sigma^2}\right] exp\left[-\frac{\mathbf{s}(A, g)^\top \mathbf{s}(A, g)}{\sigma^2}\right] pr(A, g) dA dg. \quad (1)$$

Assume that the components of $\mathbf{f}, \mathbf{s}(A, g)$ are samples of corresponding functions $f, s(A, g)$ on a grid of points in $\mathbb{R}^N$. Also assume that $s(A, g)(\mathbf{x}) = A\pi_g h(\mathbf{x})$, where the map $g \to \pi_g$ is a representation of $G$ as unitary linear operators on $L^2(\mathbb{R}^N)$, and $h$ is a fixed function in this space. This representation is made explicit below. For a very large grid, the sums in the inner products may be approximated by integrals. Let $(f, f')$ be the usual Hilbert space inner product of $f, f' \in L^2(\mathbb{R}^N)$ and $\|f\| = (f, f)^{\frac{1}{2}}$. Then

$$\Lambda(f) = \int_{\mathbb{R}^+} exp\left[-\frac{A^2}{2\sigma^2}\|h\|^2\right] \left\{\int_G exp\left[\frac{A}{\sigma^2}(f, \pi_g h)\right] pr(A, g) dg\right\} dA. \quad (2)$$

Now let $G$ be the group of scale, rotation and translation operations in $\mathbb{R}^N$. An element $g$ of $G$ is a triplet $(a, \sigma, \mathbf{t})$ where $a$ is a positive real number, $\sigma$ is an $N \times N$ real matrix satisfying $\sigma^\top \sigma = I$ and $det(\sigma) = 1$, and $\mathbf{t} \in \mathbb{R}^N$. The group multiplication rule for $G$ is $(a, \sigma, \mathbf{t})(a', \sigma', \mathbf{t}') = (aa', \sigma\sigma', \mathbf{t} + a\sigma\mathbf{t}')$. The representation $\pi$ of $G$ on $L^2(\mathbb{R}^N)$ is given by $\pi_g h(\mathbf{x}) = a^{-\frac{N}{2}} h\left(\frac{1}{a}\sigma^{-1}(\mathbf{x} - \mathbf{t})\right)$. This corresponds to scaling the function $h$ by a factor of $a$, rotating it with the rotation matrix $\sigma$, and translating it by the vector $\mathbf{t}$. The group multiplication law is precisely the one needed so that $\pi_g \pi_{g'} = \pi_{gg'}$, i.e. that $\pi$ gives a representation of the group $G$. The $a^{-\frac{N}{2}}$ factor in front makes $\pi$ a unitary representation, so that $\|\pi_g h\| = \|h\|$ for any $h$ and $g$. Now we have

$$\Lambda(f) = \int_{\mathbb{R}^+} exp\left(-\frac{A^2}{2\sigma^2}\|h\|^2\right) \left\{\int_G exp\left[\frac{A}{\sigma^2} w(g)\right] pr(A, g) dg\right\} dA \quad (3)$$

where $w(g) = (f, \pi_g h)$ is the $N$-dimensional wavelet transform on the group $G$ of $f$ with respect to the signal $h$ [1,6,7]. We write $w = W\{f, h\}$.

One reason for using the left invariant measure on $G$ can now be shown. If we include the prior probability in the argument of $\Lambda$ and let $L_{g_0} pr(A, g) = pr(A, g_0^{-1} g)$, then $L$ is a representation of $G$ as operators on the space of prior probabilities and $\Lambda(pr, f) = \Lambda(L_g pr, \pi_g f)$ for all $g \in G$. In other words, applying the same scale, rotation and translation to the data and to the prior leaves the statistic $\Lambda$ invariant. If, for example, $pr(A, g_0^{-1} g) = pr(A, g)$ for elements $g_0$ of the rotation subgroup of $G$, then $\Lambda(f)$ is invariant under rotations of the data. Whatever symmetries the prior probability has will be reflected in the statistic $\Lambda$.

# 3   The linear and quadratic terms

If we expand the inner exponential we have $\Lambda(f) = \Lambda_0(f) + \Lambda_1(f) + \Lambda_2(f) + \ldots$, where $f$ appears to order $n$ in $\Lambda_n$. Each $\Lambda_j(pr, f)$ has the same symmetry property as described above for $\Lambda(pr, f)$. The zero-order term is independent of $f$ and has no effect on statistical inference as long as $h$ is fixed. For the first order term let

$$q_1(g) = \frac{1}{\sigma^2} \int_{\mathbb{R}^+} pr(A, g) exp\left(-\frac{A^2}{2\sigma^2} \|h\|^2\right) A dA. \tag{4}$$

(For non-random $A$, $q_1(g)$ is a multiple of $pr(g)$.) Then $\Lambda_1(f) = \int_G w(g) q_1(g) dg$, an inner product in the Hilbert space $L^2(G)$. This can also be written as $\Lambda_1(f) = \int_{\mathbb{R}^N} f(\mathbf{x}) s_1(\mathbf{x}) d^N x$, where $s_1(\mathbf{x}) = \int_G q_1(g) \pi_g h(\mathbf{x}) dg$ is a weighted average of the signal $h$ over all scales, orientations and positions with weight function $q_1(g)$. This is the standard type of result for linear discriminants with parameter uncertainty.

It is interesting to examine $\Lambda_2$ in the case where $pr(A, g) = pr(A, a, \sigma, \mathbf{t})$ is independent of $\sigma$ and $\mathbf{t}$. A real probability density, of course, could not be independent of $\mathbf{t}$ since this would violate the normalization condition. Nevertheless, we may treat this as an approximation to the case where the prior probability is constant over a large range of $\mathbf{t}$ and drops to zero outside of that range.

$$\Lambda_2(f) = \int_{\mathbb{R}^+} q_2(a) \left[ \int_{SO(N)} \int_{\mathbb{R}^N} w^2(a, \sigma, \mathbf{t}) d^N t d\sigma \right] a^{-N-1} da, \tag{5}$$

where $d\sigma$ is the left invariant measure on $SO(N)$, the group of $N$-dimensional rotation matrices, and

$$q_2(a) = \frac{1}{2\sigma^4} \int_{\mathbb{R}^+} pr(A, a) exp\left(-\frac{A^2}{2\sigma^2} \|h\|^2\right) A^2 dA. \tag{6}$$

(For non-random amplitude, $q_2(g)$ is a multiple of $pr(a)$.)

If $F$ and $H$ are the Fourier transforms of $f$ and $h$ respectively, then let $S_H(k) = \int_{S(k)} |H(\mathbf{k})|^2 d^{N-1}\Omega$ and $S_F(k) = \int_{S(k)} |F(\mathbf{k})|^2 d^{N-1}\Omega$, be angular averages over $S(k)$, the sphere of radius $k$. Then

$$\Lambda_2(f) = \int_{\mathbb{R}^+} S_H(r) \left[ \int_{\mathbb{R}^+} q_2\left(\frac{r}{k}\right) S_F(k) k^N \frac{dk}{k} \right] \frac{dr}{r}. \tag{7}$$

The inner integral is the Mellin convolution of $q_2(k)$ with $S_F(k)k^N$. This is also the group convolution on the scale group $\mathbb{R}^+$. The outer integral is then the inner product in $L^2(\mathbb{R}^+)$ of this convolution with $S_H$. We might call this the Mellin inner product. To summarize, we arrive at $\Lambda_2(f)$ by following these steps, starting with $f$ and the signal $h$:
1) Fourier transform and compute $|F(\mathbf{k})|^2$ and $|H(\mathbf{k})|^2$.
2) Perform angular averaging on these functions to get $S_F(k)$ and $S_H(k)$.
3) Multiply $S_F(k)$ by $k^N$ and Mellin convolve with $q_2(k)$.
4) Compute the Mellin inner product of the result with $S_H(k)$.
   If we have a power series expansion for $q_2(a)$ we can get a different form for $\Lambda_2(f)$. Suppose that $q_2(a) = \sum_{j=1}^{\infty} q_{2j} a^j$. Then

$$\Lambda_2(f) = \sum_{j=1}^{\infty} q_{2j} \left[ \int_{\mathbb{R}^+} r^j S_H(r) \frac{dr}{r} \right] \left[ \int_{\mathbb{R}^+} k^{N-j} S_F(k) \frac{dk}{k} \right] \tag{8}$$

If $\mathcal{M}$ indicates the Mellin transform operator, then let $M_H = \mathcal{M}\{S_H\}$ and $M_F = \mathcal{M}\{S_F\}$. If we define $q_{2j} = 0$ for $j < 0$, then this is

$$\Lambda_2(f) = \sum_{j=-\infty}^{\infty} q_{2j} M_H(j) M_F(N-j), \tag{9}$$

which is the convolution, on the additive group of integers, of the function given by $Q_H(j) = q_{2j} M_H(j)$ with $M_F(j)$. This is often called discrete convolution. In this case the steps leading to $\Lambda_2(f)$ are
1) Fourier transform and compute $|F(\mathbf{k})|^2$ and $|H(\mathbf{k})|^2$.
2) Perform angular averaging on these functions to get $S_F(k)$ and $S_H(k)$.
3) Mellin transform to get $M_H(j)$ and $M_F(j)$.
4) Multiply $M_H(j)$ by $q_{2j}$ to get $Q_H(j)$.
5) Compute the discrete convolution of $Q_H(j)$ with $M_F(j)$.
The effect of the prior is to weight the transformed signal $M_H(j)$ before convolving it with the transformed data $M_F(j)$. the operations involved in both of these procedures have been used by others in deriving scale, rotation and translation invariant statistics. Here we see how they arise from the quadratic term of the likelihhod ratio for Gaussian noise.

# 4  The full nonlinear likelihood ratio

We return to $\Lambda(f)$ now. Let $b(w) = \frac{1}{w}(e^w - 1)$. Then $b$ is a monotonic increasing function with $0 < b(w) \le 1$ for $w \le 0$ and $1 < b(w)$ for $w > 0$. Now we have

$$\Lambda(f) = \Lambda_0 + \int_{\mathbb{R}+} exp\left(-\frac{A^2}{2\sigma^2}\|h\|^2\right)\left\{\int_G b\left(\frac{A}{\sigma^2}w(g)\right)pr(A,g)w(g)dg\right\}dA. \tag{10}$$

Let $pr_f(A,g) = b\left(\frac{A}{\sigma^2}w(g)\right)pr(A,g)$. This depends on the data $f$ through $w = \mathcal{W}\{f,h\}$. If $s_f(A,\mathbf{x}) = \int_G pr_f(A,g)\pi_g h(\mathbf{x})dg$ and $\lambda_A(f) = \int_{\mathbb{R}^N} s_f(A,\mathbf{x})f(\mathbf{x})d^N x$, then

$$\Lambda(f) = \Lambda_0 + \int_{\mathbb{R}+} exp\left(-\frac{A^2}{2\sigma^2}\|h\|^2\right)\lambda_A(f)dA. \tag{11}$$

We can now see a way to describe how the $\Lambda$ statistic works. Suppose that the signal is present in the data at some scale, orientation and location described by $g_0$. Then $w(g)$ has a maximum at $g = g_0$. The function $b\left(\frac{Aw(g)}{\sigma^2}\right)$ has a maximum at $g_0$ also and, due to the nonlinearity of this function, it is a sharper maximum than $w(g)$ has. This sharply peaked positive function is used to modulate $pr(A,g)$ to produce a weighting function $pr_f(A,g)$. This function therefore tends to be more peaked at $g = g_0$ than the original prior. Then the signal $h(\mathbf{x})$ is averaged over scale, orientation and position with this weighting function to produce $s_f(A,\mathbf{x})$. The inner product in $L^2(\mathbb{R}^N)$ of $s_f(A,\mathbf{x})$ and $f(\mathbf{x})$ produces $\lambda_A(f)$. Finally, a gaussian weighted average, with variance $\frac{\sigma^2}{\|h\|^2}$, of this quantity gives $\Lambda(f) - \Lambda_0$.

In summary we can produce $\Lambda(f) - \Lambda_0$ by following these steps:
1) Compute the wavelet transform $w = \mathcal{W}\{f,h\}$.
2) Amplify any maxima by forming $b\left(\frac{Aw(g)}{\sigma^2}\right)$.
3) Modulate the prior with this function to get the weighting function $pr_f(A,g)$.
4) Find $s_f(A,\mathbf{x})$ by averaging the signal $h$ over $g$ with this weighting function.
5) Take the inner product of this average with the data $f$ to get $\lambda_A(f)$.
6) Integrate this with a Gaussian over $A$.
If we replaced $b(w)$ with 1, then this procedure would result in $\Lambda_1(f)$. The difference between $\Lambda - \Lambda_0$ and $\Lambda_1$ is contained in the amplification and modulation steps 2) and 3). If we replaced $b(w)$ with $w$ we would get a multiple of $\Lambda_2$. Thus $\Lambda_2$ contains the modulation mechanism without the amplification step.

# 5  Conclusion

We constructed the likelihood ratio in the case of amplitude, scale, orientation and position uncertainty for i.i.d. Gaussian noise and background known exactly. The linear term is pretty much what we would expect - average the signal over the parameters and compare to the data. The quadratic term turned out to involve many of the operators commonly used in this situatation - the Fourier transform, angular averaging, and the Mellin transform. Finally, the total likelihood ratio can be described in terms of an inner product of the data with a weighted average of the signal, if we account for the fact that the data itself affects the weighting via an amplification and modulation procedure.

This publication was made possible by grant number R01 CA52643 from the National Cancer Institute. Its contents are solely the responsibility of the authors and do not necessarily represent the official views of the National Cancer Institute.

# References

[1] J.-P. Antoine et. al.: Image analysis with two-dimensional continuous wavelet transform. Signal Processing 31, 241-272 (1993)

[2] H. H. Barrett and C. Abbey: Bayesian Detection of Random Signals on Random Backgrounds. (In this volume)

[3] H. H. Barrett et. al.: Linear discriminants and image quality. Image and Vision Computing 10, 451-460 (1992)

[4] D. Casasent and D. Psaltis: Position, rotation and scale invariant optical correlation. Applied Optics 15, 1795-1799 (1976)

[5] J.-M. Combes, A. Grossmann and P. Tchamitchian (eds.): Wavelets, Time-Frequency Methods and Phase Space. Berlin: Springer 1989

[6] A. Grossmann, J. Morlet and T. Paul: Transforms associated to square integrable group representations I. Journal of Mathematical Physics 26, 2473-2479 (1985)

[7] R. Murenzi: Wavelet transforms associated to the n-dimensional euclidean group with dilations: signal in more than one dimension. In: [4], pp. 239-246

[8] L. W. Nolte,: Theory of signal detectability: adaptive optimum receiver design. Journal of the Acoustical Society of America 42, 773-777 (1967)

[9] L. W. Nolte and D. Jaarsma: More on the detection of one of M orthogonal signals. Journal of the Acoustical Society of America 41, 497-505 (1967)

# Author Index

# Lecture Notes in Computer Science

For information about Vols. 1–1156

please contact your bookseller or Springer-Verlag

Vol. 1195: R. Trappl, P. Petta (Eds.), Creating Personalities for Synthetic Actors. VII, 251 pages. 1997. (Subseries LNAI).

Vol. 1196: L. Vulkov, J. Waśniewski, P. Yalamov (Eds.), Numerical Analysis and Its Applications. Proceedings, 1996. XIII, 608 pages. 1997.

Vol. 1197: F. d'Amore, P.G. Franciosa, A. Marchetti-Spaccamela (Eds.), Graph-Theoretic Concepts in Computer Science. Proceedings, 1996. XI, 410 pages. 1997.

Vol. 1198: H.S. Nwana, N. Azarmi (Eds.), Software Agents and Soft Computing: Towards Enhancing Machine Intelligence. XIV, 298 pages. 1997. (Subseries LNAI).

Vol. 1199: D.K. Panda, C.B. Stunkel (Eds.), Communication and Architectural Support for Network-Based Parallel Computing. Proceedings, 1997. X, 269 pages. 1997.

Vol. 1200: R. Reischuk, M. Morvan (Eds.), STACS 97. Proceedings, 1997. XIII, 614 pages. 1997.

Vol. 1201: O. Maler (Ed.), Hybrid and Real-Time Systems. Proceedings, 1997. IX, 417 pages. 1997.

Vol. 1202: P. Kandzia, M. Klusch (Eds.), Cooperative Information Agents. Proceedings, 1997. IX, 287 pages. 1997. (Subseries LNAI).

Vol. 1203: G. Bongiovanni, D.P. Bovet, G. Di Battista (Eds.), Algorithms and Complexity. Proceedings, 1997. VIII, 311 pages. 1997.

Vol. 1204: H. Mössenböck (Ed.), Modular Programming Languages. Proceedings, 1997. X, 379 pages. 1997.

Vol. 1205: J. Troccaz, E. Grimson, R. Mösges (Eds.), CVRMed-MRCAS'97. Proceedings, 1997. XIX, 834 pages. 1997.

Vol. 1206: J. Bigün, G. Chollet, G. Borgefors (Eds.), Audio- and Video-based Biometric Person Authentication. Proceedings, 1997. XII, 450 pages. 1997.

Vol. 1207: J. Gallagher (Ed.), Logic Program Synthesis and Transformation. Proceedings, 1996. VII, 325 pages. 1997.

Vol. 1208: S. Ben-David (Ed.), Computational Learning Theory. Proceedings, 1997. VIII, 331 pages. 1997. (Subseries LNAI).

Vol. 1209: L. Cavedon, A. Rao, W. Wobcke (Eds.), Intelligent Agent Systems. Proceedings, 1996. IX, 188 pages. 1997. (Subseries LNAI).

Vol. 1210: P. de Groote, J.R. Hindley (Eds.), Typed Lambda Calculi and Applications. Proceedings, 1997. VIII, 405 pages. 1997.

Vol. 1211: E. Keravnou, C. Garbay, R. Baud, J. Wyatt (Eds.), Artificial Intelligence in Medicine. Proceedings, 1997. XIII, 526 pages. 1997. (Subseries LNAI).

Vol. 1212: J. P. Bowen, M.G. Hinchey, D. Till (Eds.), ZUM '97: The Z Formal Specification Notation. Proceedings, 1997. X, 435 pages. 1997.

Vol. 1213: P. J. Angeline, R. G. Reynolds, J. R. McDonnell, R. Eberhart (Eds.), Evolutionary Programming VI. Proceedings, 1997. X, 457 pages. 1997.

Vol. 1214: M. Bidoit, M. Dauchet (Eds.), TAPSOFT '97: Theory and Practice of Software Development. Proceedings, 1997. XV, 884 pages. 1997.

Vol. 1215: J. M. L. M. Palma, J. Dongarra (Eds.), Vector and Parallel Processing – VECPAR'96. Proceedings, 1996. XI, 471 pages. 1997.

Vol. 1216: J. Dix, L. Moniz Pereira, T.C. Przymusinski (Eds.), Non-Monotonic Extensions of Logic Programming. Proceedings, 1996. XI, 224 pages. 1997. (Subseries LNAI).

Vol. 1217: E. Brinksma (Ed.), Tools and Algorithms for the Construction and Analysis of Systems. Proceedings, 1997. X, 433 pages. 1997.

Vol. 1218: G. Păun, A. Salomaa (Eds.), New Trends in Formal Languages. IX, 465 pages. 1997.

Vol. 1219: K. Rothermel, R. Popescu-Zeletin (Eds.), Mobile Agents. Proceedings, 1997. VIII, 223 pages. 1997.

Vol. 1220: P. Brezany, Input/Output Intensive Massively Parallel Computing. XIV, 288 pages. 1997.

Vol. 1221: G. Weiß (Ed.), Distributed Artificial Intelligence Meets Machine Learning. Proceedings, 1996. X, 294 pages. 1997. (Subseries LNAI).

Vol. 1222: J. Vitek, C. Tschudin (Eds.), Mobile Object Systems. Proceedings, 1996. X, 319 pages. 1997.

Vol. 1223: M. Pelillo, E.R. Hancock (Eds.), Energy Minimization Methods in Computer Vision and Pattern Recognition. Proceedings, 1997. XII, 549 pages. 1997.

Vol. 1224: M. van Someren, G. Widmer (Eds.), Machine Learning: ECML-97. Proceedings, 1997. XI, 361 pages. 1997. (Subseries LNAI).

Vol. 1225: B. Hertzberger, P. Sloot (Eds.), High-Performance Computing and Networking. Proceedings, 1997. XXI, 1066 pages. 1997.

Vol. 1226: B. Reusch (Ed.), Computational Intelligence. Proceedings, 1997. XIII, 609 pages. 1997.

Vol. 1227: D. Galmiche (Ed.), Automated Reasoning with Analytic Tableaux and Related Methods. Proceedings, 1997. XI, 373 pages. 1997. (Subseries LNAI).

Vol. 1228: S.-H. Nienhuys-Cheng, R. de Wolf, Foundations of Inductive Logic Programming. XVII, 404 pages. 1997. (Subseries LNAI).

Vol. 1230: J. Duncan, G. Gindi (Eds.), Information Processing in Medical Imaging. Proceedings, 1997. XVI, 557 pages. 1997.

Vol. 1231: M. Bertran, T. Rus (Eds.), Transformation-Based Reactive Systems Development. Proceedings, 1997. XI, 431 pages. 1997.

Vol. 1232: H. Comon (Ed.), Rewriting Techniques and Applications. Proceedings, 1997. XI, 339 pages. 1997.

Vol. 1233: W. Fumy (Ed.), Advances in Cryptology — EUROCRYPT '97. Proceedings, 1997. XI, 509 pages. 1997.

Vol 1234: S. Adian, A. Nerode (Eds.), Logical Foundations of Computer Science. Proceedings, 1997. IX, 431 pages. 1997.

Vol. 1235: R. Conradi (Ed.), Software Configuration Management. Proceedings, 1997. VIII, 234 pages. 1997.

Vol. 1240: J. Mira, R. Moreno-Díaz, J. Cabestany (Eds.), Biological and Artificial Computation: From Neuroscience to Technology. Proceedings, 1997. XXI, 1401 pages. 1997.